Giulio Preti ■ Prosthetic Rehabilitation Part II: Technical Procedures

Giulio Preti ■ Prosthetic Rehabilitation Part II: Technical Procedures

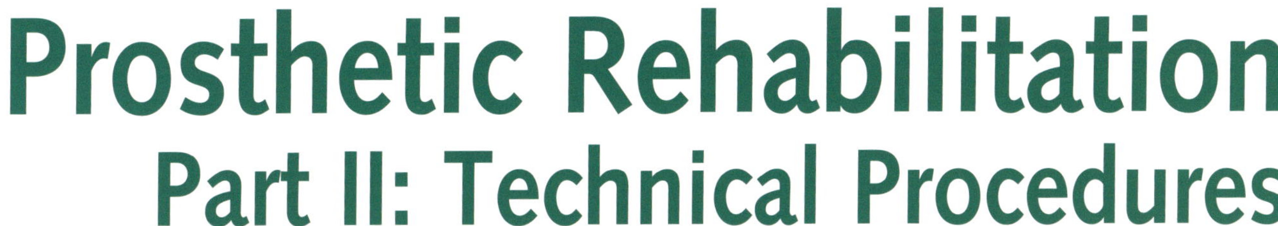

Prosthetic Rehabilitation
Part II: Technical Procedures

Edited by

Giulio Preti, MD, DDS

Professor Emeritus
Section of Oral and Maxillofacial Rehabilitation
School of Dentistry
University of Turin
Turin, Italy

Translated by

Jennifer Sardo Infirri

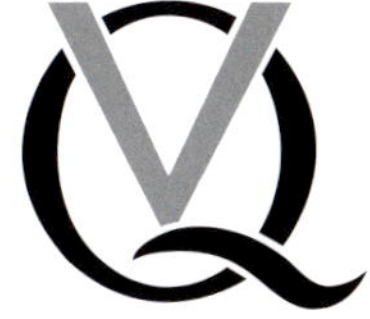

Quintessence Publishing Ltd.
London, Berlin, Chicago, Tokyo, Barcelona, Istanbul, Milan, Moscow, New Delhi, Paris, Beijing, Prague, São Paulo, Seoul, and Warsaw

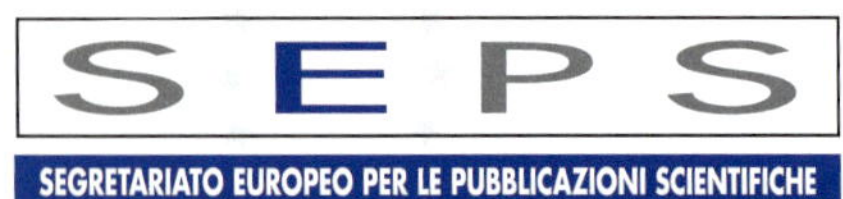 SEGRETARIATO EUROPEO PER LE PUBBLICAZIONI SCIENTIFICHE

The translation of this work has been funded by SEPS
SEGRETARIO EUROPEO PER LE PUBBLICAZIONI SCIENTIFICHE
Via Val d'Aposa 7 - 40123 Bologna - Italy
seps@seps.it - www.seps.it

Title of the original Italian edition: Riabilitazione protesica
Copyright © 2004 UTET – Unione Tipografico-Editrice Torinese S. p. A.

Dedication

To the professors of the University of Turin—Dino Roccia, Giuseppe Ceria, and Remo Modica—who, more than anyone else, contributed to the development of the School of Dentistry in the late 1950s with their hard work, their passion for dentistry, their professionalism, and their dynamic teaching. The Section of Oral and Maxillofacial Rehabilitation was established in the mid 1970s in the culturally favorable environment created by these professors.

© 2011 Quintessence Publishing Co, Ltd

Quintessence Publishing Co, Ltd
Grafton Road
New Malden
Surrey KT3 3AB
United Kingdom
www.quintpub.co.uk

ISBN: 978-1-85097-198-6
Printed in Germany

Contents

Foreword

The past two decades of the 20th century were extraordinary ones for my discipline of predilection—prosthodontics. They ushered in a strong biologic focus, which gradually matched and perhaps even eclipsed traditional exclusive concerns with dental materials and techniques. The change was an inevitable and welcome one, and it belatedly paralleled the shift toward emphasis in basic and clinical sciences that had influenced development in the discipline. Neurophysiology, bioengineering, and health economics emerged as profound concerns in the effort to provide predictable treatment outcomes that recognized both patient as well as dentist-mediated concerns.

It is perhaps impossible to identify a specific text or event that catalyzed the much-needed changes. Most seminal events in history or breakthroughs in science tend to have similar origins—often unrelated, but ultimately convergent occurrences. Small streams of thought and experiment gradually converge to create a river full of force and momentum, which will in turn irrigate new sources of creativity.

My own academic development was influenced by particular Scandinavian works. The first was the 1977 article by Brill et al, "Ecologic changes in the oral cavity caused by removable partial dentures."[1] The second was the 1977 monograph by Brånemark et al on osseointegrated implants.[2] Both sets of authors indirectly framed the prosthodontist's twin concerns that must dominate evidence-based clinical decisions. These concerns can be posed as two questions: *(1)* What is the biologic price paid as a result of the diverse sequelae and consequences of loss of teeth? and *(2)* What is the biologic price inherent in the prosthodontic intervention? The very perceptive, if understandably limited, ecologic focus of Brill et al[1] gradually expanded from the notion of adverse ecologic shifts to far beyond those of plaque-induced and mechanical trauma. Brånemark et al,[2] on the other hand, proposed an entirely new model in pursuit of understanding the therapeutic benefits resulting in a scientific transition from an uncontrolled to a controlled induced interface. The impact of both ideas cannot be underestimated, particularly in the context of the subtle, yet profound, differences in dental, as opposed to medical, biotechnology.

Prosthodontics has been in the "spare parts" business for a long time, although we have done it with only a small degree of the anguish found in the medical field. As a result, we have not been unduly burdened with the sort of tricky ethical questions associated with genetics and organ transplantation.

However, our commitment to enriching our patients' lives, rather than prolonging them, demands the same degree of scientific rigor in the way we make clinical decisions and carry out prosthodontic therapy.

The need for outstanding texts that articulate this new vision for prosthodontic rehabilitation has therefore become a serious and major priority. Professor Giulio Preti and his colleagues have provided us with such a text, and all of us in the discipline have been enriched by this masterful effort. I have been studying the Turin team's contribution to dental scholarship—research, education, service—for several years, and theirs has been an exemplary record of commitment and leadership. They have distilled an enormous body of knowledge and wisdom in writing this book and presented their convictions in a lucid and highly organized manner. I have little doubt that this contribution stands out among those distinguished texts in the all-too-small canon of significant works in prosthodontics. Above all, the publication of this book is a compelling testimony to the purpose and meaning of clinical academics' lives. Giulio Preti and his Turin colleagues deserve our gratitude for their outstanding contribution.

George A. Zarb, BChD, DDS, MS, FRCD
Professor Emeritus, Department of Prosthodontics, Faculty of Dentistry, University of Toronto, Toronto, Canada

1. Brill N, Tryde G, Stoltze K, El Ghamrawy EA. Ecologic changes in the oral cavity caused by removable partial dentures. J Prosthet Dent 1977;38:138–148.
2. Brånemark PI, Hansson BO, Adell R, et al. Osseointegrated implants in the treatment of the edentulous jaw. Experience from a 10-year period. Scand J Plast Reconstr Surg 1977;16(suppl):1–132.

Preface

There can be no doubt that scientific advancement is today articulated by papers published in specialized journals. Such articles measure the progress made by research, even when the truths they state are subsequently denied or enriched by the onward march of research. The sum of articles published by a research group or a school is a chronicle of what they have contributed to a field of research. But a book . . . a book is not part of a chronicle. Rather, it expresses the history of the steps through which a school was born, matured, and changed—in short, its evolution.

Over the years, two philosophies have had a strong positive influence on our thinking: the Zurich School, with Professor Albert Gerber and Professor Sandro Palla, which remains a constant reference point for continuing and new students alike; and the UCLA School of Dentistry, first with Professor Jim Krachtovil and now Professor John Beumer, in a collaboration of more than 20 years that has contributed to the education of several of our collaborators in the difficult art of maxillofacial prosthetics. In addition, Professor Remo Modica has become our maestro in life as well as in our profession. These individuals, with their enthusiasm and their commitment to the psychosocial aspects of prosthetic rehabilitation, have strongly influenced the direction our school has taken.

During the past 25 years of teaching, treatment, and research, our biennial congress has provided us with an opportunity to compare our progress against the world's most prestigious schools. Since then thousands of patients have been treated and hundreds of students trained in our department. Some of our alumni are now professors in various Italian universities including Bari, Bologna, Brescia, Ferrara, and Genoa. Each of these institutions is committed to giving continuity to the tradition of our school. Today, both our alumni and I believe we have achieved sufficient maturity to communicate our philosophy through this book. This publication represents 25 years of collective knowledge and experience. Each book tells a story, and we would like to think that this is our story.

Although this book is the product of many authors' work, it has a uniformity of thought, thanks to our common approach

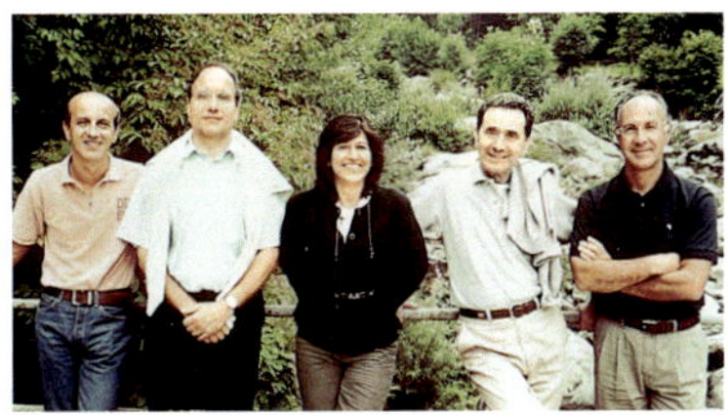

Boves, Italy, July 2001, from the left: Professors Bassi, Carossa, Bucca, Preti, Pera.

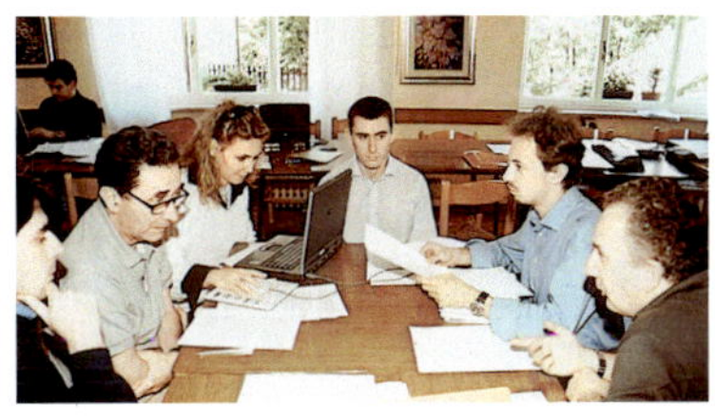

Boves, Italy, July 2001, a working group.

and the professional contacts we have maintained over the years. In compiling this book, two fundamental concepts have been dominant: our teaching methodologies and the importance of providing supporting documentation from the literature. Today, when critically analyzing the effectiveness of new therapies, the predictability of posttherapeutic success has become crucial. Following in the wake of evidence-based medicine, evidence-based dentistry has now arisen, and within this, evidence-based prosthodontics. This approach can only help our discipline make better progress, where in the past, randomized controlled trials were rare.

Scientific progress in prosthetic dentistry has, nevertheless, not yet led to the large-scale adoption of new, improved therapies. For example, implant dentistry offers enormous therapeutic possibilities, but only a tiny fraction of the population has been able to benefit from this treatment. When treatment costs are high and patients' economic situations must be taken into consideration, traditional therapies maintain their value in comparison to new methods of prosthetic rehabilitation.

This text was split into two distinct parts. The first volume in this series discussed diagnosis and the components of prepro-

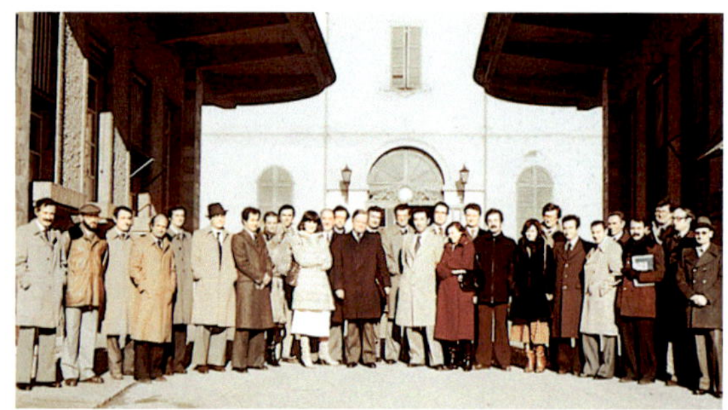

Cinzano, Italy, October 1978, on a seminar with Prof Gerber.

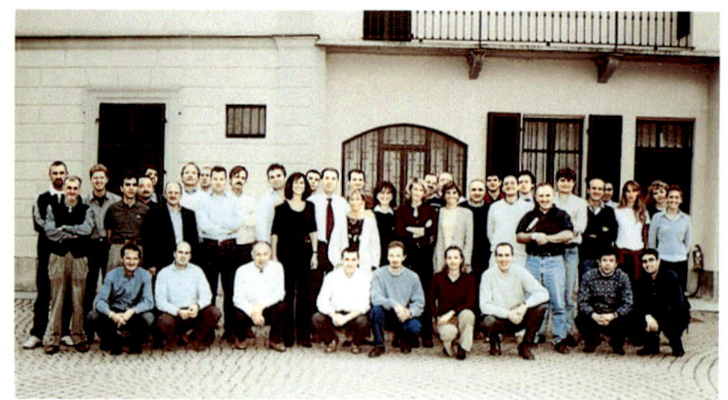

Pecetto, Italy, October 2001, a seminar for writing the book.

sthetic care, whereas this book discusses the clinical and technical aspects of fabricating functional prostheses for patients with different stages of edentulism. Taken together, these two books offer a more biologic and patient-centered approach to prosthetic treatment.

Some of these chapters have been written by our alumni who, while having worked as independent practitioners over the years, have maintained their professional ties with our department of prosthodontics, within which they have played or still play an active consultant role. These chapters, far from being exhaustive for those who are experts in the subject, discuss prosthetic aspects with two goals in mind: *(1)* to emphasize our department's philosophy of "comprehensive care"; and *(2)* to make the reader aware of his or her limits so that, on a case-by-case basis, he or she will refer to or consult with a specialist as required.

The multidisciplinary approach to prosthetic rehabilitation of the oral cavity is a complex process that proceeds through diagnosis and application of the necessary technical knowledge to design and construct a prosthesis to ensure long-term success.

Prosthetic treatment that modifies the oral cavity inevitably must consider the patient's physical as well as emotional needs. It is thus important to ensure correct communication so that we may understand our patients from psychologic, social, and cultural points of view.

Clinical evaluation continues with morphostructural and functional evaluation of the stomatognathic system. Whereas the former has long been considered indispensable and is routinely carried out, the same cannot be said for functional evaluation. Failure to appreciate disorders of the stomatognathic system before beginning treatment is frequently the cause of treatment failure.

The ecosystem of the oral cavity is modified by the presence of the prostheses, which may have a highly destructive effect if the mechanisms involved are not properly understood. Knowledge of these mechanisms is based on the awareness that long-term success of the rehabilitation is the product of patient compliance and consistent follow-up by the dentist.

In this book, the various modalities of prosthetic rehabilitation of a stomatognathic system compromised by loss of some or all teeth are next taken into consideration. The first subject addressed is total edentulism because rehabilitation of the edentulous patient presupposes knowledge that is often indispensable in rehabilitating the partially edentulous patient. The discussion of rehabilitation of different degrees of edentulism is developed by considering different therapeutic options, ranging from the simplest to the most sophisticated. One of our goals was to provide the independent dental practitioner or the dental student with all those elements necessary to select the most suitable treatment for each patient, always bearing in mind that the patient is at the center of our interest.

No dentist can neglect a careful evaluation of his or her patient as a whole, from medical history to social and psychologic status, before formulating a personalized treatment plan. For this purpose we propose a guide to diagnosis and to the prosthodontic treatment plan in which, among other factors, every treatment considered ideal must then be adapted to the requirements of the individual patient.

In the final analysis, the treatment plan must address the articulated or perceived concerns of each patient. These important determinants of any successful treatment outcome include a symptom-free, esthetic, and functional result that does not incur risks of morbidity or unnecessary expense.

Giulio Preti, MD, DDS
Professor Emeritus, Section of Oral and Maxillofacial Rehabilitation, School of Dentistry, University of Turin, Turin, Italy

Acknowledgments

Many people contributed to the writing of this book, and, at the risk of forgetting someone, we wish to thank:

Our students for the continuing contact we have had with them over the years, which has enriched us professionally as well as personally.

Prof Pietro Bracco, for the Department of Orthodontics' contribution to chapter 7.

Our colleagues Gaetano Calesini, Carlo Marinello, Giorgio Pedretti, Massimo Simion, and Carlo Tinti for the clinical cases that they generously made available to us.

Dental technicians Valerio Burello, Adolfo Camisotti, Enrico Hans Carlucci, Biagio Ciancio, Luigi Colleoni, Paolo Del Bianco, Daniele Fiengo, Cristiano Gaggio, Giovanni Giachero, Giorgio Perna, Paolo Riccio, and Alberto Sannazzaro.

Administrative assistants Antonella Baldin and Roberto Calcagnile, and a particular heartfelt acknowledgment to Rosalia Genchi for her unseen but essential secretarial work.

Carlo ed Alessandro Piacquadio for his invaluable collaboration on the illustrations.

Thank you to you all!

Contributors

Guido Audenino, DDS, Lecturer, Department of Prosthodontics, School of Dentistry, University of Turin, Turin, Italy

Eva Barabino, DDS, Private Practice, Turin, Italy

Sandro Barone Monfrin, DDS, Lecturer, Section of Oral and Maxillofacial Rehabilitation, School of Dentistry, University of Turin, Turin, Italy

Francesco Bassi, MD, DDS, Professor, Department of Prosthodontics, School of Dentistry, University of Turin, Turin, Italy

Matteo Bonifacino, DDS, Private Practice, Turin, Italy

Mario Bresciano, DDS, Lecturer, Section of Oral and Maxillofacial Rehabilitation, School of Dentistry, University of Turin, Turin, Italy

Vincenzo Bruno, DDS, Private Practice, Naples, Italy

Dario Caire, DDS, Private Practice, Turin, Italy

Stefano Carossa, MD, DDS, Lecturer, Center for Cancer Epidemiology, San Giovanni Battista Hospital, Turin, Italy

Marco Carrozzo, MD, DDS, Professor of Oral Medicine, School of Dental Sciences, University of Newcastle upon Tyne, Newcastle upon Tyne, England

Santo Catapano, MD, Professor, Istituto di Clinica Odontoiatrica, University of Ferrara, Ferrara, Italy

Paola Ceruti, DDS, Assistant Professor, Faculty of Medicine and Surgery, School of Dentistry, University of Turin, Turin, Italy

Massimo Corsalini, MD, DDS, Assistant Professor, School of Dentistry, University of Bari, Italy

Francesco Erovigni, DDS, Tutor, Department of Prosthodontics, School of Dentistry, University of Turin, Turin, Italy

Sergio Gandolfo, MD, Professor, Section of Oral Pathology, School of Dentistry, University of Turin, Turin, Italy

Gianfranco Gassino, MD, DDS, Assistant Professor, Department of Prosthodontics, School of Dentistry, University of Turin, Turin, Italy

Giorgio Gastaldi, MD, DDS, Professor, Department of Removable Prosthodontics, School of Dentistry, University Of Brescia, Brescia, Italy

Gianni Giannella, DDS, Tutor, Department of Prosthodontics, School of Dentistry, University of Turin, Turin, Italy

Bartolomeo Griffa, DDA, Private Practice, Turin, Italy

Stefano Lombardo, DDS, Lecturer, Department of Prosthodontics, School of Dentistry, University of Turin, Turin, Italy

Carlo Manzella, DDS, Private Practice, Turin, Italy

Marco Mozzati, MD, DDS, Director SSCVD, Oral Surgery, Department of Dentistry, San Giovanni Battista Hospital, Turin, Italy

Giovannino Muci, DDS, Private Practice, Nardo, Italy

Paola Pera, MD, DDS, PhD, Professor and Chair, Department of Health Sciences, Section of Biostatistics, Genoa University, Genoa, Italy

Denis Pettenò, DDS, Private Practice, Turin, Italy

Enrico Poglio, DDS, Private Practice, Turin, Italy

Giulio Preti, MD, DDS, Professor Emeritus, Section of Oral and Maxillofacial Rehabilitation, School of Dentistry, University of Turin, Turin, Italy

Riccardo Preti, DDS, Private Practice, Turin, Italy

Valter Previgliano, MD, DDS, Lecturer, Department of Prosthodontics, School of Dentistry, University of Turin, Turin, Italy

Alessio Rizzatti, DDS, Assistant Professor, Department of Oral and Maxillofacial Rehabilitation and Dental Implants, University of Turin, Turin, Italy

Gianluca Santià, DDS Private Practice, Turin, Italy

Gianmario Schierano, MD, DDS, Professor, Department of Prosthodontics, University of Turin, Turin, Italy

Roberto Scotti, DDS, Professor and Chair, Department of Prosthodontics, School of Dentistry, Alma Mater Studiorum, University of Bologna, Bologna, Italy

Vassili Valentini

Patrizia Zoccola

An Explanation of the Criteria Used for Evaluating the Dental Literature

Mario Bresciano, DDS, University of Turin, Turin, Italy
Giovannino Ciccone, San Giovanni Battista Hospital, Turin, Italy

> Man prefers to believe what he prefers to be true.
> Francis Bacon, *Novum Organum*, 1620

> Experiments are the only means of knowledge
> at our disposal; the rest is poetry, imagination.
> Max Planck

A new scientific publication is the product of authors elaborating on the present knowledge of a specific subject through the mediation and integration of their personal experiences. A scientific text is, therefore, the product of detailed research from many sources that is presented in a natural and logical order. The success of this process is based on the ability of the authors to explain their arguments and the validity of what they have written. Even if the reader can easily judge the quality of the authors' ideas, this is not the case for the scientific accuracy of the ideas cited from other sources. How many readers take the trouble to check the bibliographic sources cited in a text? In order to provide readers with an additional means to substantiate their learning, every reference cited in this volume has been ranked by scientific weight, following the evaluation criteria and methodology published by Jacob and Carr.[1] In particular, every reference has been categorized according to the type of article (Table 1).

Scientific Validity

Technologic innovations of the last 20 years have forced dentists to acquire new knowledge and techniques to stay in step with the advances in the profession. Remaining up-to-date and assessing the efficacy and safety of new products, procedures, and techniques are becoming increasingly difficult, if not impossible, given the constant flow of information (not always of high quality) presented in scientific journals, textbooks, and continuing education courses.

Making sense of these often contradictory sources requires a new skill—that of being able to select information that is valid and useful in clinical practice. The questions that dentists must pose to themselves are: *(1)* Is the information scientifically correct, and if this is the case, is it new and valid? and *(2)* Is it clinically important? We propose a hierarchical scale of assessment (see Table 1), based on the quality of the experimental evidence, to assist clinicians to select therapies for their patients that are supported by reliable verified data and to set aside those based only on personal opinion or equivocal data. Differences in scientific weight are determined by the type of source and the type of experimental study from which the data are obtained. The clinical relevance and practical utility depend instead on external evaluation of the research.

Sources

Scientific information that is the product of valid and repeatable experiments is published almost exclusively in professional journals that use a review system for selecting articles for publication. Such information is rarely obtained from books, courses, or continuing education conferences. Textbooks logically present the results of research that has already been published, and so is not new, as well as the opinions, usually implicit, of the authors. Often new results of experimental research are presented for the first time at conferences. However, given the limitations of the lecture format, it is not possible to present all of the information needed to evaluate or replicate the results of the studies and therefore determine their veracity. In addition, much research presented at conferences is not subsequently published.

All dental journals do not have the same scientific importance. The most prestigious journals ensure that all articles are evaluated by a group of experts (peer review) before being accepted for publication. Other less rigorous journals accept articles at the discretion of the editor alone.

One system of valuing scientific journals, called *impact factor* (IF), is based on the number of citations of the journal or its articles found in other journals. The IF index thus permits a valuation of the scientific weight of a publication. Articles published in a journal with a high IF have greater probability of being considered valid by the scientific community.

It is timely to recognize that nearly all dental journals that have a high IF are published in English. As in the 17th century the language of music was Italian, so in the 21st century the language of science is English.

Types of Scientific Articles

The Council of Science Editors has defined a *scientific article* as "the first publication containing sufficient information to allow colleagues to understand the observations, repeat the experiment, and evaluate the intellectual process."[2] Clearly this definition is based on scientific methods enunciated by Bacon and Galileo in the 17th century. Essentially, to determine the validity of information, it is necessary above all to verify the methodology by which the study was made. For this reason, we have classified the various types of articles based on the hierarchy proposed by Jacob and Carr[1] (see Table 1).

Personal communications

Not everything printed in scientific journals is scientific. Personal opinions expressed as editorials, letters, or contributions to roundtable discussions are usually cited as *personal communications*. They are judged as hypotheses, ideas, opinions, and comments that are not to be confounded with data of scientific relevance, especially if the primary argument concerns questions that can be tested in experimentation. More rigorous critical evaluation must be applied to informative leaflets provided by manufacturers to publicize and promote the sale of their products.

Case reports

These articles introduce a new technique or results of a new product used in a limited number of cases. Their scientific importance is exclusively chronological, only establishing the author as the first person to propose the innovation. It is clearly impossible to draw extensively applicable conclusions based on the results of one or two cases that were followed for a very limited time period and, above all, derived from observations that have no analytical design.

Reviews of the literature

Traditional review articles are narratives, often the work of only one author, that comment on publications on a specific topic, in a uniform fashion, from the author's point of view and experience. The scientific data reported in such articles are drawn from various types of studies, often not selected in a systematic manner, and not evaluated in a standard mode. Reviews with these characteristics, though useful as a synthesis of a particular argument, risk presenting conclusions that are not reproducible and that reflect, in some measure, the opinion of the author as well as those expressed in the reviewed literature.

In vitro experiments

In vitro experiments are carried out in laboratories using models to, more or less, reproduce clinical reality. They are the overwhelming majority of studies published in dentistry and prosthodontics because of the ease of execution and limited expense. Numerous types of models are used, including mechanical, computerized, and those using extracted teeth. The conclusions that can be drawn from such experiments are often difficult to accept as conclusive scientific proof, due to their evident limitation as only partially reproducing the clinical reality, which is decidedly more complex and practically impossible to represent using such defined models.

Animal studies

Animal studies provide a first approximation of what happens in the human oral cavity; the higher the animal subjects are in the evolutionary scale, the better the experiment will approximate results found in humans. Because animals can be sacrificed in experiments, important data can be obtained, particularly in the area of histology. Obvious differences between the oral cavity of animals and that of humans, however, limit the validity of this type of study.

Clinical studies

Studies with consenting humans are without doubt the principal sources from which we can draw reliable information for daily clinical practice. For the numerous types of clinical studies, the scientific weight increases as study variables that may influence the results are strictly controlled. Schematically, clinical studies can be divided into two primary categories: *(1) analytical studies*, in which there are two groups of subjects, one that receives the experimental treatment and the other that serves as a control; and *(2) descriptive studies*, in which there is no control group. These categories, in turn, can be subdivided into two types: *experimental*, in which treatment is assigned to randomly defined groups of subjects according to a research protocol; and *epidemiologic* or observational, in which the treatment is assigned to subjects without the control of the researcher.

Experimental studies

Prospective controlled, randomized studies, in which the experimental treatment is assigned to two homogenous groups, represent the "gold standard" on the methodologic plane for evaluation of efficacy. In a randomized controlled trial the inclusion of a group of subjects that is identical to the group under treatment serves as a control to verify the real efficacy of the therapy or the experimental diagnosis. For example, in pharmacologic investigations, the control group is given either a pharmaceutical placebo or a drug that is considered the present standard treatment. In these studies, it is important that the distribution of the subjects between the two groups is completely randomized and double blind, in which neither the participating patients nor the researchers know which type of treatment is being followed. This allows a probable uniform distribution of the various prognostic factors and of possible unpredictable variables.

Studies in which subjects are assigned to a group in a manner that is not completely random are known as *quasirandomized controlled trials*. When the control group is made up of the same subjects who receive the various treatments (experimental and comparative) in two different periods, this is called a *randomized crossover trial*.

Observational studies

Nonexperimental epidemiologic studies can be of two types: *(1) case controlled studies*, in which a group of subjects with a certain problem are confronted with a homologous control group that does not have the problem to identify the relevant factors that might be responsible; and *(2) cohort studies*, in which subjects who have received different treatments are followed over time to evaluate the incidence of relevant clinical events.

Systematic review of the literature (meta-analysis)

Systematic literature reviews are conducted according to a rigorous and explicit protocol that prescribes criteria for the search, selection, and evaluation of the literature on a defined topic. Meta-analysis studies gather together and statistically analyze similar clinical studies, often with limited samples, providing reliable scientific data because of the overall higher num-

bers of subjects involved. Fundamental to this kind of analysis is the comparability of the various clinical studies taken together. The scientific relevance of these analyses is given by the affiliation of the studies that are compared.

Descriptive studies

Clinical studies are defined as *descriptive* if an analytical control of the experiment is not possible because of the lack of subjects that can act as a control group. If the therapy or the diagnostic procedure for analysis was already accomplished before the patients were selected for the study, it is called a *retrospective study*. If, instead, the individuals were selected prior to the experiment proceeding, it is a *prospective study*. Because of the possibility of controlling patient participation and the execution of the study, prospective studies are more relevant from the scientific point of view than retrospective studies.

Conclusion

The majority of studies presented in the prosthodontic literature fall into the categories described here. Undertaking experimental or observational studies is very difficult because of practical concerns (eg, the difficulties of always having a control group), economic funding (ie, scarce economic resources available for dental research), and the high degree of individualization in prosthodontic therapy.

Most articles in the prosthodontic literature are derived from in vitro studies, which are easier and more economical to carry out but of inferior scientific weight. The few clinical experiments of long duration concern, above all, retrospective epidemiologic analyses without control groups. Despite the infrequent publication of prospective clinical studies, such articles (eg, work on implant osseointegration) have been essential to advancements in dentistry in recent years.

Table 1 Evaluation categories for cited references

Category 1	Experimental clinical analytical studies
Category 2	Observational clinical analytical studies
Category 3	Prospective descriptive clinical studies
Category 4	Descriptive clinical studies
Category 5	Animal studies
Category 6	In vitro studies
Category 7	Books and narrative reviews of the literature
Category 8	Case reports
Category 9	Personal communications

References

1. Jacob RF, Carr AB. Hierarchy of research design used to categorize the "strength of evidence" in answering clinical dental questions. J Prosthet Dent 2000;83:137–152.
2. Day RA. How to Write and Publish a Scientific Paper. Philadelphia: ISI Press, 1979:2.

Total Edentulism

In the past several decades, the Western world has witnessed a general improvement in living conditions. Important progress in the field of medicine has contributed to an increase in the average age of the population. Dentistry has also progressed to serve this older and healthier population with advances in prophylactic and operative techniques that have raised the age at which people become edentulous.[1]

At the same time, in terms of general and oral health, new problems have arisen, which the edentulous patient and clinician must together resolve in order to arrive at and maintain a functionally and esthetically adequate denture. It is important to bear in mind that a patient's dissatisfaction with a complete denture may be linked to problems of a psychologic nature whose solutions lie outside the field of dental prosthetics. However, osseointegration has supplied new ways in which edentulism, especially mandibular edentulism, can be treated, with good functional and esthetic results.

The following chapters discuss traditional prosthetic rehabilitation as well as the use of implants, such as in the implant-retained overdenture. The choice has been dictated by the desire to promote a rehabilitation technique that is geared toward a prevalently older population while taking into account the often economically limited possibilities for such patients.

Physiopathology of the Edentulous Mouth

Edentulism can profoundly alter oral and extraoral tissues and functions. The most evident sign of these alterations is the resorption of the alveolar bone, which demonstrates the disease-like process of edentulism, with its chronic, progressive, and mutilating course.

The alveolar bone is maintained by the support of the teeth and periodontium, the health of which depends on local and systemic factors. The correlation between maintaining the alveolar bone and oral function is, on the other hand, less clear. Oral function and the presence of teeth are so intimately correlated that the effects of these two factors are difficult to distinguish.[2]

The adult maxillary bones comprise two components: a structural support that is tendentially stable, represented by the periosteal cortical bone and the lamina dura, and a metabolic component whereby the trabecular bone provides a calcium reserve.

The skeletal support of the oral structures is a clear example of form linked to function. According to the loads to which it is subjected, the trabecular bone may appear to be relatively thin, and the cortical bone may be relatively compact.

The distinction between the effects on osseous resorption caused by systemic pathologies and those caused by an altered masticatory function is further complicated by the fact that most edentulous patients are elderly people and usually women, who are more frequently affected by hormonal and metabolic alterations. Many studies[3–5] have investigated the effects that systemic illnesses have on resorption of the alveolar bone, but there is a lack of inherent information regarding oral function.

A study[6] of more than 1,000 edentulous subjects divided into three age groups and either wearing or not wearing complete dentures concluded that the use of a complete denture accelerates osseous resorption. Information on the systemic conditions of the subjects was not provided, however.

In light of current knowledge, resorption of the alveolar bone in the edentulous patient is considered the result of a complex interaction among genetic, hormonal, metabolic, and biomechanical factors. The maxillary bones are under stress by forces of compression, traction, and cutting, and as well as flexion and torsion. The variations in direction, intensity, frequency, and distribution of these stresses with respect to the physiologic situation caused, for example, by a prosthetic rehabilitation, can in turn cause relatively severe osseous rearrangements.

Normal mechanical physiologic stress on connective tissues evokes a tissue response that guarantees maintenance; on the contrary, excessive and abnormal stress causes pathologic changes and tissue damage.[7]

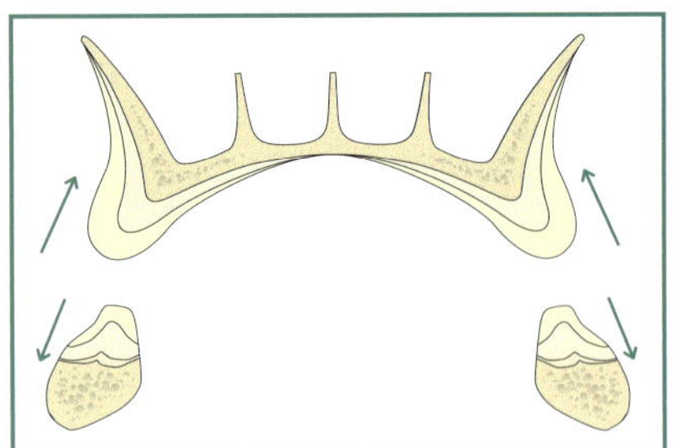

Fig 1-1 Centripetal resorption of the maxilla and centrifugal resorption of the mandible.

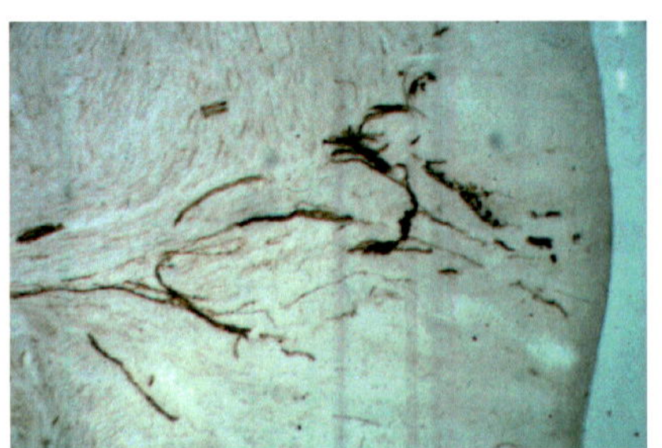

Fig 1-2 Histology of the mucosa of a dentate subject with clear receptors (in brown) and an immunochemical reaction.

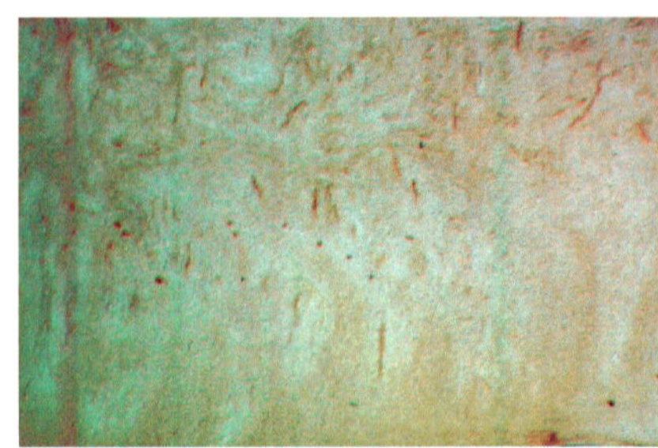

Fig 1-3 Mucosal histology of an edentulous patient. The number of receptors is greatly reduced.

The osseous response to mechanical stress is managed at a biomolecular level by cytokines, proteins produced by cells to modify the behavior of other cells. Some cytokines encourage bone resorption; others inhibit it.

Mechanical stresses to tissues in the edentulous patient differ notably from the normal mechanical stresses subjected by the tissues of an integral oral structure. In the latter case, the functional loads are transmitted with the same intensity but in opposite directions to the maxilla and mandible, and the periodontal ligament transforms the stress (compression, traction, cutting, flexion, and torsion) transmitted to the alveolar bones into forces of traction and compression. Through the maxilla, a great deal of the masticatory load is transferred to the cranial bones, usually in the form of compression forces. The mandible, being a suspended bone, absorbs the functional loads, with heightened stresses generated by traction and torsion. As a consequence, the osseous morphology of the two jaws differs substantially.[8]

The maxilla is made up of a palatine cortex of moderate thickness connected to the vestibular cortex, which is thinner, through the internal trabeculae which, in turn, transfer the masticatory loads to the cranium.[9]

In the mandible, on the other hand, the thick cortical bones are connected by trabeculae oriented toward the mandibular anatomic structures, such as the alveolar canals and dental alveoli.[9]

In the edentulous patient, the functional forces are prevalently compressive and are transmitted to the residual alveolar bone through the mucosa that covers the edentulous ridge. As a result, the protective action of the periodontal ligament and the inductive stimulus on the alveolar bone caused by the transmission of the loads through the dental roots is lacking.

Longitudinal studies have shown that osseous resorption is much more rapid in the first year of edentulism[10,11] and that resorption of the anterior portion of the mandible is four times that of the maxilla[12,13], thus provoking a forward and upward rotation of the mandible.[11]

The anterior rotation of the mandible and the loss of support of the perioral tissues are the cause of profound esthetic alterations of the face[14] that result in an older appearance. The maxilla is resorbed in a centripetal direction. After loss of teeth, the oblique position of the incisors leads to considerable narrowing and shortening of the maxilla in this area, while at the level of the molars the narrowing of the arch is decidedly less.

The mandible resorbs in a centrifugal direction. The lingual inclination of the teeth, especially the molars, causes an increase in the curvature of the residual arch.[10] In the anterior region of the mandible, the morphologic modifications vary in relation to the inclination of the incisors.[9]

Over time, most people with edentulism develop a spatial incongruity between the mandible and the maxilla that becomes more and more marked as osseous resorption progresses (Fig 1-1). However, the resorption of the alveolar ridges and the changes in the maxillomandibular relationships have significant individual variations.[15]

The oral mucosa, like the alveolar ridges, also undergoes structural modifications. The viscoelasticity of the mucosa does not allow an immediate recovery of the original dimensions when it is deformed by masticatory stresses. The collagen fibers of the oral mucosa diminish with age. For this reason, viscoelastic deformation lasts longer in the older patient than in the younger patient.[16,17]

Both mechanical and toxic insults, provoked primarily by poor hygiene, tend to accelerate inflammation of the mucosa. It has been shown that mucosal inflammation accelerates osseous resorption.[18]

Structural modifications of the mucosa also result in a significant decrease in the number of receptors[19] (Figs 1-2 and 1-3), which influence both sensitivity and oral motor functions. Subjects with their natural teeth have the capacity to detect interposed thicknesses between the dental arches of 10 to 20 µm, whereas edentulous subjects can only detect a thickness of 100 µm.[20] The clinical significance of good oral proprioception has not altogether been clarified. It is thought that it can

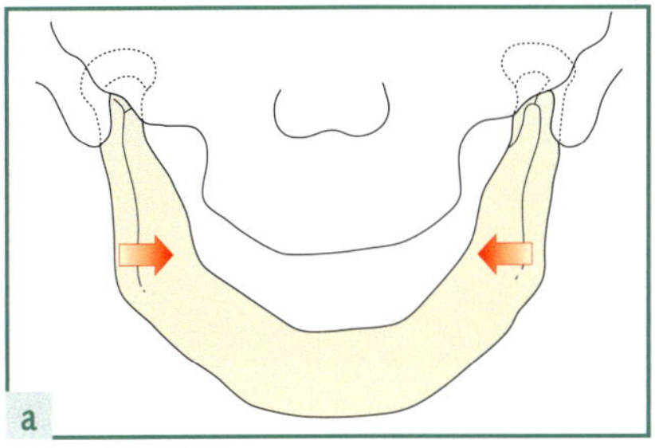 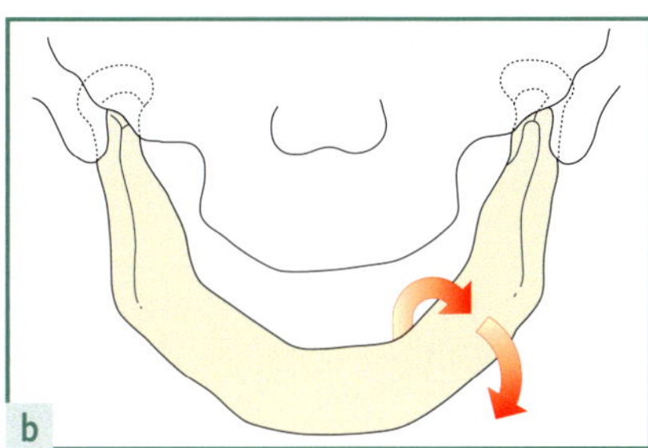 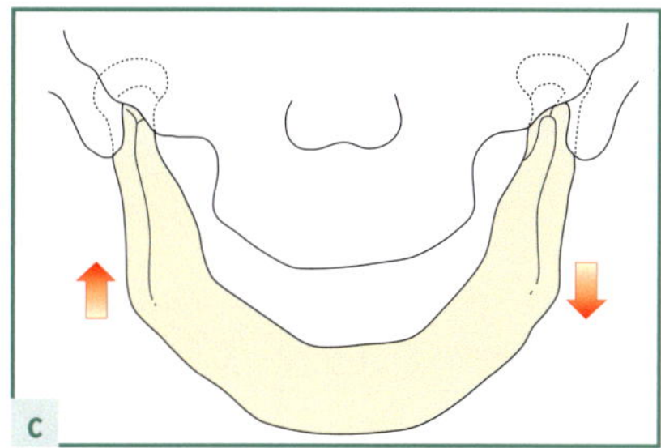

Fig 1-4 Deformation of the mandible during function: *(a)* medial convergence; *(b)* corporal rotation; *(c)* dorsoventral deformation.

favor the incorporation of the denture, allow the patient to more easily identify occlusal interferences, and influence the direction and intensity of loads.[21]

The extension of the masticatory cycle and masticatory efficiency are also reduced.[22–24] The masticatory cycle covers an area that is clearly inferior and more irregular in these patients, and the masticatory force is reduced to about a sixth. These two factors together contribute to reducing the extent of deformation of the mandible during the function. It has been shown[24] that, during functioning, the mandible is deformed because of a medial convergence, a corporal rotation, and deformation in the dorsoventral direction (Fig 1-4). This deformation results in a bilateral transmission of forces, part of which result in traction. The deformation of the mandible in the three spatial planes is correlated to the extent of the lateral movement and the intensity of the applied force. The more the lateral movement of the mandible is reduced, the more the applied forced on the alveolar ridge is likely to be of a compressive type, resulting in osseous resorption.

The masticatory loads and the force and muscle tone diminish with age and with the duration of edentulism. The reduction in muscular density can lead to muscular atrophy and a consequent increase in adipose tissue.[25] The decrease in masticatory forces and oral function means that masticatory efficiency (capacity to break a food sample into small fragments in a determined time) is reduced compared with that in a person with natural teeth.[26]

Masticatory efficiency is likewise correlated to the quality of the denture. A denture with good stability and retention increases the ability to break up food into small fragments and is subjectively perceived by the patient to do so. Edentulous patients who complain of difficulty in breaking up food into small fragments are not necessarily choosing foods that are easier to chew.[27,28] In the period of adaptation to a new denture, a more consistent bolus provokes a greater number of lesions. For this reason, at least at the beginning, the patient should be advised to eat softer foods.[29]

Edentulous patients follow a less rich and varied diet compared with subjects with natural teeth, who tend to consume foods that are higher in protein and vitamins and lower in fat and cholesterol.[28]

In the older patient, the correlation between oral condition and nutritional state is not so clear. A poor nutritional state in these patients can be due to many other factors, such as alterations in sense of taste, socioeconomic conditions, dietary habits, and a generally compromised state of health. Inadequate dentures could be a further obstacle to bettering the dietary habits of older persons.[30] Studies have shown a lack of influence of oral rehabilitation on nutrition in edentulous elderly subjects.[31,32]

The diets of such patients are often lacking in fiber, calcium, vitamins A, E, D, B_6, and magnesium,[32] which certainly has a negative influence on the general state of health. Dietary guidance should be provided for patients in need.

Conclusive Considerations and Therapeutic Approach

In the edentulous patient, the resorption of alveolar bone is progressive, continuous, and more accentuated in the first year. Inflammation of the mucosa accelerates osseous resorption through the effect of paracrine signaling. It is necessary to:

- Prepare a denture that guarantees optimal distribution of loads.
- Schedule follow-up to maintain optimal denture quality. Follow-up is particularly important during the first year.
- Bear in mind that a denture that is not liked will not function well.
- Provide psychologic support if needed.
- Provide dietary guidance, because edentulous patients usually choose less nutritionally rich and varied foods, even when fitted with a proper denture.

References

1. Douglass CW. Prosthodontics. Clinical practice-delivery of services. Review of the literature. J Prosthet Dent 1990;64:275–283. Cat. 7
2. Roberts WE, Holt WF, Arbuckle GR. The supporting structures and dental adaptation. In: McNeill C (ed). Science and Practice of Occlusion. Chicago: Quintessence, 1997:79–92. Cat. 7
3. Jaul DH, McNamara JA, Carlson DS, Upton LG. A cephalometric evaluation of edentulous rhesus monkeys (Macaca mulatta): A long term study. J Prosthet Dent 1980;44:453–460. Cat. 5
4. Klemetti E, Vainio P, Lasilla V, Alhava E. Trabecular bone mineral density of mandible and alveolar height postmenopausal women. Scand J Dent Res 1993;101:166–170. Cat. 4
5. Klemetti E, Vainio P. Effect of maxillary edentulousness on mandibular residual ridges. Scand J Dent Res 1994;102:309–312. Cat. 4
6. Jozefowicz W. The Influence of wearing dentures on residual ridges: A comparative study. J Prosthet Dent 1970;24:137–144. Cat. 4
7. Carvalho RS, Scott JE, Bumann A, Edwin HKY. Connective tissue response to mechanical stimulation. In: McNeill C (ed). Science and Practice of Occlusion. Chicago: Quintessence, 1997:205–219. Cat. 7
8. Atkinson SR. Normal jaws in action. Am J Orthod 1965;51:510–528. Cat. 9
9. Roberts WE. Fundamental principles of bone physiology, metabolism and loading. In: Naert I, Van Steenberghe D, Worthington P (eds). Osseointegration in Oral Rehabilitation. London: Quintessence, 1993:157–169. Cat. 7
10. Sicker H, Dubrul EL. Oral Anatomy. St. Louis: Mosby, 1975:Ch 4. Cat. 7
11. Tallgren A. Positional changes of complete dentures. A 7-year longitudinal study. Acta Odontol Scand 1969;27:539–561. Cat. 3
12. Tallgren A. The continuing reduction of the residual alveolar ridges in complete denture wearer: A mixed-longitudinal study covering 25 years. J Prosthet Dent 1972;27:120–127. Cat. 2
13. Lestrel PE, Kapur KK, Chauncey HH. A cephalometric study of mandibular cortical bone thickness in edentulous persons and denture wearers. J Prosthet Dent 1980;43:89–94. Cat. 2
14. Tallgren A. The effect of dental wearing on facial morphology. A 7-year longitudinal study. Acta Odontol Scand 1967;25:563–592. Cat. 4
15. Tallgren A, Tryde G, Mizutani H. Changes in jaw relations and activity of masticatory muscles in patients with immediate complete upper dentures. J Oral Rehabil 1986;13:311–324. Cat. 3
16. Picton DCA, Wills DJ. Changes in the mobility and resting position of incisor teeth in Macaque monkeys. Arch Oral Biol 1978;23:225–229. Cat. 5
17. Kydd Wl, Daly CH. The biologic and mechanical effects of stress on oral mucosa. J Prosthet Dent 1982;47:317–329. Cat. 4
18. Pendleton EC. Changes in the denture supporting tissues. J Am Dent Assoc 1951;42:1–15. Cat. 7
19. Desjardins RP, Winkelmann RK, Gonzales JB. Comparison of nerve endings in normal gingiva with those in mucosa covering edentulous alveolar ridge. J Dent Res 1971;50:867–879. Cat. 2
20. Lundquist S, Haraldson T. Occlusal perception of thickness in patients with bridges on osseointegrated oral implants. Scand J Dent Res 1984;92:88–92. Cat. 2
21. Jacobs R, Van Steemberghe D. Comparative evaluation of the oral tactile function by means of teeth or implant-supported prostheses. Clin Oral Implants Res 1991;2:75–80. Cat. 2
22. Benzing U, Weber H. Changes in chewing patterns after implantation in the edentulous mandible. Int J Oral Maxillofac Implants 1994;9:207–213. Cat. 2
23. Fontijn-Tekamp FA, Slagter AP. Biting and chewing in overdentures, full dentures, and natural dentitions. J Dent Res 2000;79:1519–1524. Cat. 2
24. Abdel-Latif HH, Hobkirk JA, Kelleway JP. Functional mandibular deformation in edentulous subjects treated with dental implants. Int J Prosthodont 2000;13:513–519. Cat. 4
25. Termote JL, Baert A, Crolla D, Palmers Y, Bulcke JA. Computed tomography of the normal and pathologic muscular system. Radiology 1980;137:439–444. Cat 3
26. Helkimo E, Carlsson GE, Helkimo M. Chewing efficiency and state of dentition. A methodologic study. Acta Odontol Scand 1978;36:33–41. Cat. 2
27. Gunne HJ. The effect of new complete dentures on mastication and dietary intake. Acta Odontol Scand 1985;43:257–268. Cat. 3
28. Greksa LP, Parraga IM, Clark CA. The dietary adequacy of edentulous older adults. J Prosthet Dent 1995;73:142–145. Cat. 2
29. Cleary T, Hutter L, Blunt-Emerson M, Hutton JE. The effect of diet on the bearing mucosa during adjustment to new complete dentures: A pilot study. J Prosthet Dent 1997;78:479–485. Cat. 1
30. David D, Watson RM. Significance of tooth loss in the elderly patient in aging osteoporosis and dental implants. Chicago: Quintessence, 2002:135–146. Cat. 7
31. Elmstahl S, Birkhed D, Christiansson U, Steen B. Intake of energy and nutrients before and after dental treatment in geriatric long-stay patients. Gerondontics 1988;4:6–12. Cat. 2
32. Sebring NG, Guckes AD, Li SH, McCarthy GR. Nutritional adequacy of reported intake of edentulous subjects treated with new conventional or implant-supported mandibular dentures. J Prosthet Dent 1995;74:358–363. Cat. 2

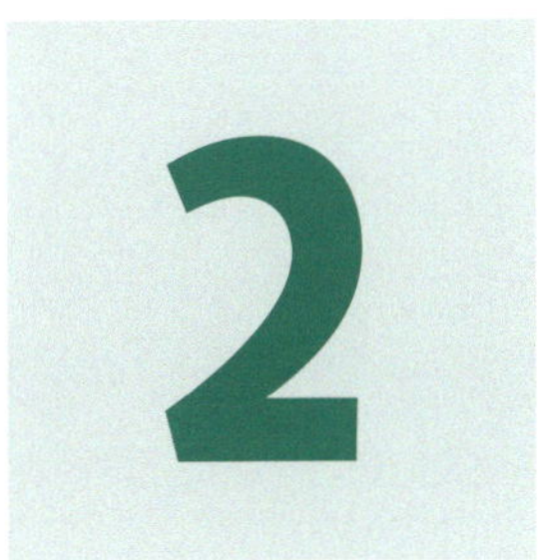

Constructive Principles of the Complete Denture: Retention, Stability, Support

The complete denture has three surfaces: (*1*) the inner edentulous ridge-bearing surface; (*2*) the external surface in contact with the cheeks, lips, and tongue; and (*3*) the occlusal surface. The interaction of these surfaces with anatomic structures and the biologic and functional characteristics of the edentulous oral apparatus is responsible for retention, stability, and support during rest and in function. For didactic purposes, retention, stability, and support will be treated separately even though they are closely interdependent.

Retention

Retention is the resistance to the forces that would otherwise distance the denture from the edentulous ridge in a vertical direction.[1] Retention is related to the interposition of a subtle layer of saliva between the mucosa and the inner surfaces of the prosthetic body. The intervening factors in retention are cohesion, surface tension, adhesion (Fig 2-1), and atmospheric pressure (Fig 2-2).

Cohesion is the physical force that acts between molecules of the same material. Adjacent molecules inside a material exercise an attractive force of the same intensity on each other but with opposite direction. Cohesion is responsible for the continuance of a droplet of water when it is put on the surface of a solid.

Surface tension is the cohesive force that acts between molecules of a liquid. At the surface, the force of cohesion is exercised exclusively between adjacent and underlying molecules, with the consequence that the resulting force on such molecules is directed toward the interior of the liquid, causing a tension tangential to the surface.

Adhesion is the physical force involved in the attraction between molecules of different bodies. The greater the force needed to distance a drop of water from the surface of a solid, the greater the force of adhesion exercised between the molecules of the water and the surface of the solid.

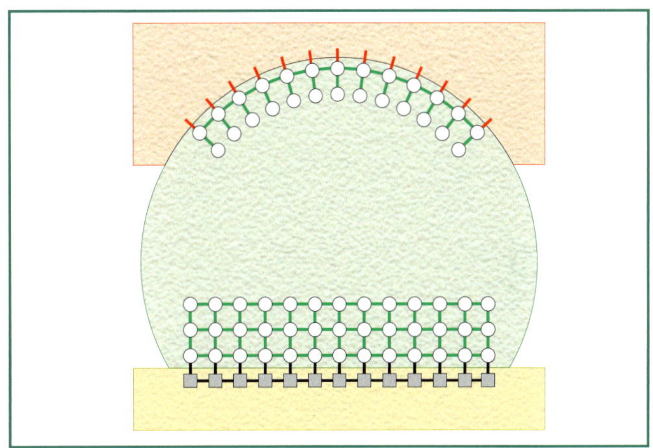

Fig 2-1 A schematic diagram of a drop of liquid on a plane surface of a solid material. The diagram shows adhesive forces *(yellow)*, cohesive forces *(green)*, and the surface tension *(red)*.

Atmospheric pressure is the hydrostatic pressure caused by the weight of the atmosphere on the earth's surface and on every surface in contact with the atmosphere.

The interaction of the factors involved in retention has been explained in the laboratory by interposing a fluid between two sheets of glass[2] (Fig 2-2a). The pressure on the interior of the fluid is of the same value as the atmospheric pressure, which acts on the exterior. When a force is applied, the fluid forms a concave surface, or meniscus. The surface tension at the meniscus maintains the difference in pressure between the interior of the fluid, which becomes negative, and the surrounding atmospheric pressure. When the applied force (F) is greater than the force of adhesion, cohesion, and surface tension, the two sheets separate (Fig 2-2b). The force necessary to separate the two sheets is inversely proportional to the thickness of the interposed liquid film[2] (Fig 2-3).

The saliva film interposed between the mucosa and the prosthetic body is subject to the same physical phenomenon that acts on the layer of liquid interposed between the two sheets of glass. The mucosa-saliva-denture interface has a variable

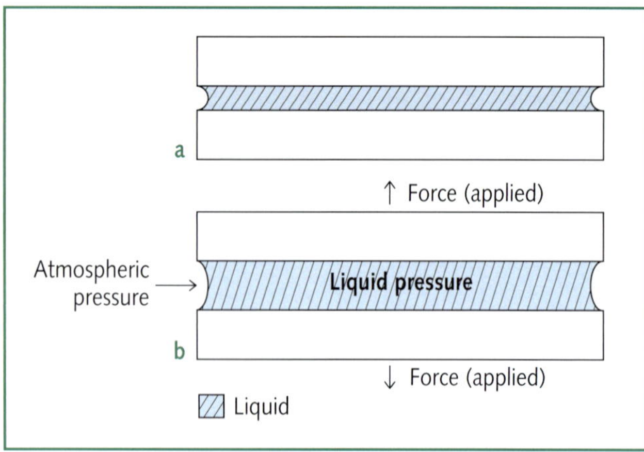

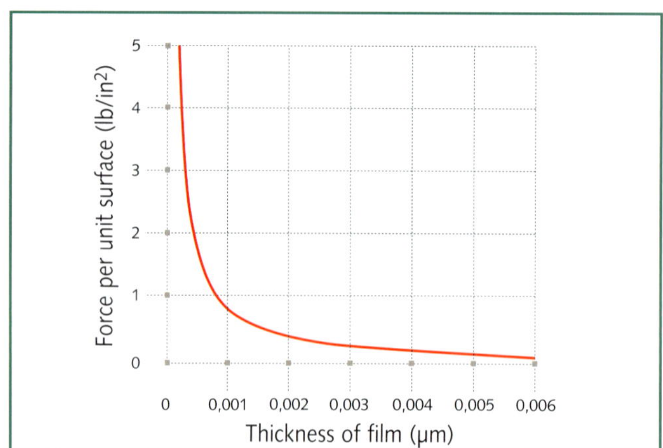

Fig 2-2 *(a)* Sheets of glass with interposed liquid; *(b)* forces that tend to separate the two sheets of glass. (Reprinted from Stanitz and Lakewood[2] with permission.)

Fig 2-3 Graph showing the forces per unit of surface needed to interrupt the liquid layer. The smaller the salivary layer the greater the force needed. (Reprinted from Stanitz and Lakewood[2] with permission.)

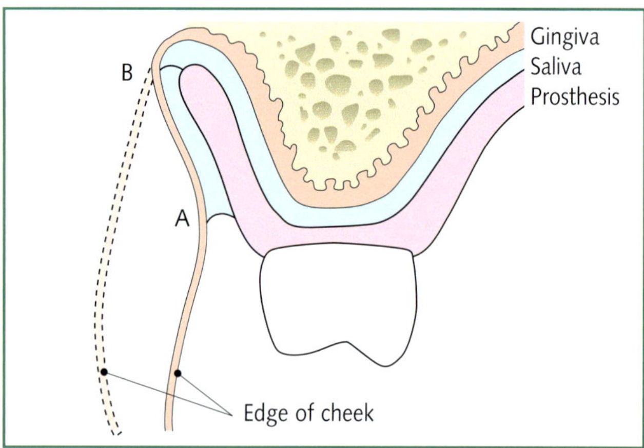

Fig 2-4 When the cheek is in contact with the denture, the meniscus is in position A. When the cheek is raised, it is in position B. (Reprinted from Jacobson and Krol[3] with permission.)

extension related to the position of the seal and therefore of the meniscus. When the cheek is moved away, the meniscus moves from position A to position B and, consequently, the surface of the saliva film is reduced (Fig 2-4).

Stability

Stability is the resistance to dislocating horizontal and rotational forces. The factors that participate in stability are the height and morphology of the alveolar ridges, the relationships between the alveolar ridges, neuromuscular control, and occlusal harmony.[4]

Height and morphology of the alveolar ridges

Ridges that are well adapted (tall and squared) contribute to the stability of the denture. At times, owing to the effect of resorption, the edentulous ridge can assume unfavorable morphologic characteristics. Insufficient height and width and the resultant superficial insertion of the muscles compromise the stability of the denture.

The edentulous ridge can present, in section, different profiles (Fig 2-5): round, serrated, and squared. A denture whose buccal and lingual flanges rest on steep walls, as in the case of a squared ridge, is more stable because it opposes the dislocating action of the lateral and perpendicular forces of the walls themselves. For the same physical reasons, the shape of the arch of the edentulous ridge is more favorable when it is more square.

Spatial relationships between the alveolar ridges

The more the ridges are congruent, the easier it is to position the diatoric teeth on the peak of the ridges and in the sphere of the neutral zone (Fig 2-6). The neutral zone is that in which the forces directed toward the interior, originating from the contractions of the buccinator muscle, are balanced by the externally directed forces exerted by the action of the tongue muscles.

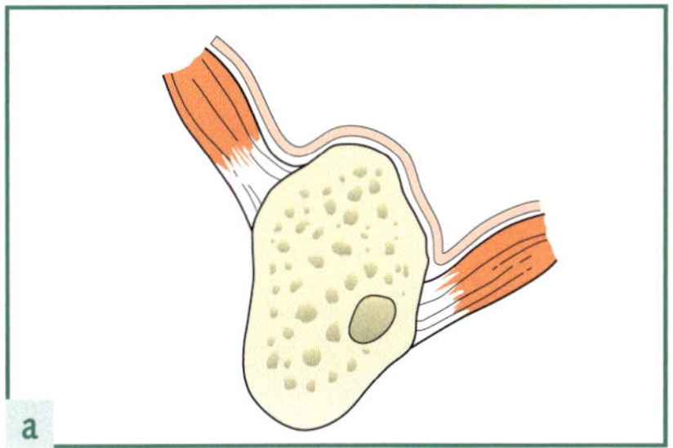 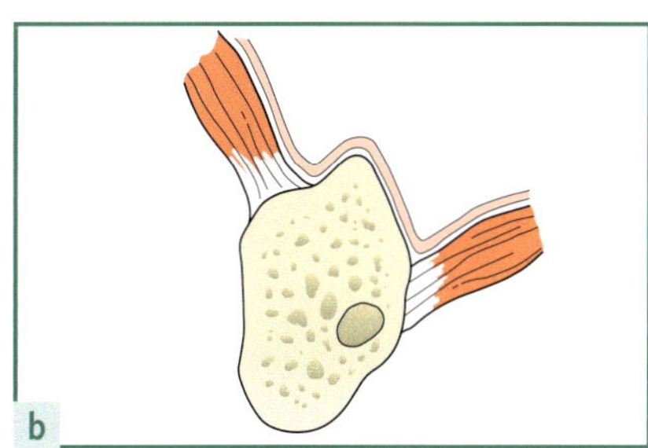 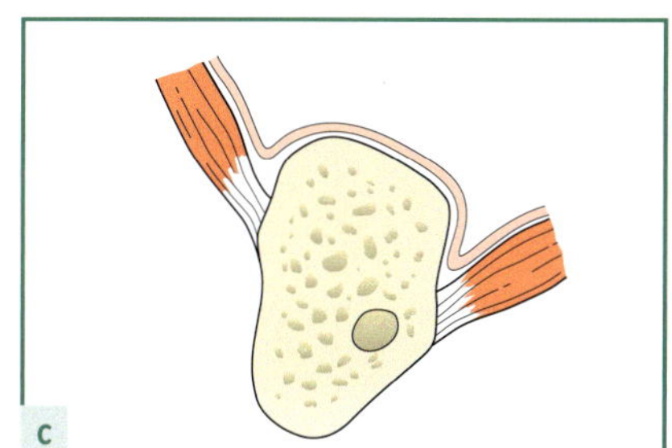

Fig 2-5 Different morphologies of the alveolar crest in section: *(a)* rounded, *(b)* serrated, or *(c)* squared.

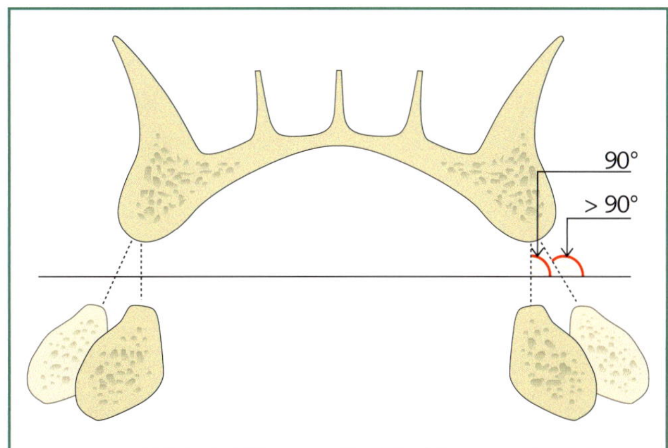

Fig 2-6 Depending on the different patterns of resorption, incongruities between the jaws can occur.

Neuromuscular control

In the 1930s, Fish[5] wrote that in a complete denture, "every part of every surface of the denture must be so modeled to adapt itself to the respective portion of the patient's tissue" and that one of the main stabilizing factors of the denture is the design of "that portion of the surface which comes into contact with the muscles of the cheek, of the tongue and of the lips."

The modeling of the external surfaces of the denture must take into consideration the variations of form and position that the inserted muscles and tendons are subjected to during function. The process of stabilization of the denture comes about through physiologic support of the muscles on the denture surfaces during rest and an equally physiologic seating during function.

The muscles responsible for the neuromuscular control of the denture are the buccinator, the mimic muscles (which are inserted in the modiolus), the orbicularis oris, and the tongue muscles (Fig 2-7).

The buccinator muscle (Fig 2-8) is made up of three segments. According to Fish,[5] the three segments have different functions during mastication in a patient who has a complete denture. The superior fibers contribute to maintaining the maxillary denture in situ, the intermediate fibers control the alimentary bolus and its positioning between the arches, and the inferior fibers contribute to the stability of the mandibular denture. This observation has been confirmed by an electromyographic study by Lundquist.[6] In the area where the buccinator fibers converge and cross, the fibers of other muscles are inserted, all of which have a single muscular insert at the angles of the mouth, or the modiolus (Fig 2-9). At the modiolus, the fibers of the quadratus labii superioris meet with those of the canine muscle, zygomaticus, risorious, triangularis, quadratus labii inferioris, and orbicularis oris. The contraction of the triangularis, the canine, and the zygomaticus muscles fixes the modiolus, thus allowing the buccinator to contract isometrically to maintain the bolus between the dental arches. If the modiolus is mobile, the contractions of the buccinator

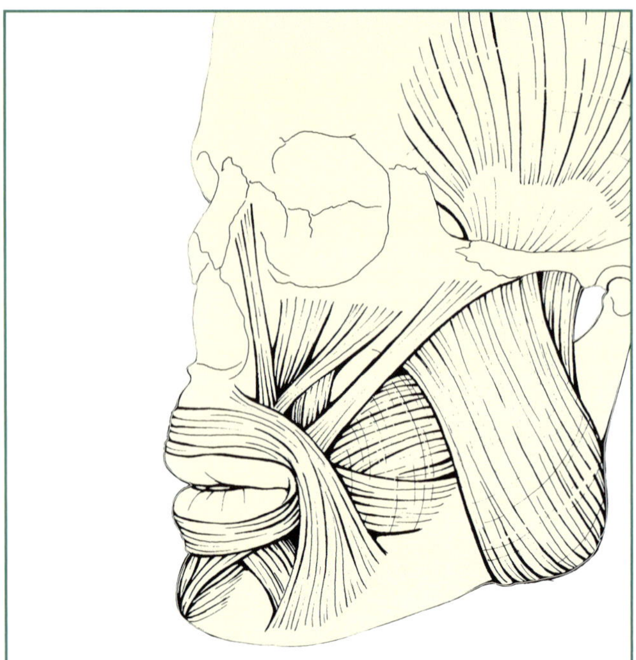

Fig 2-7 Mimic muscles.

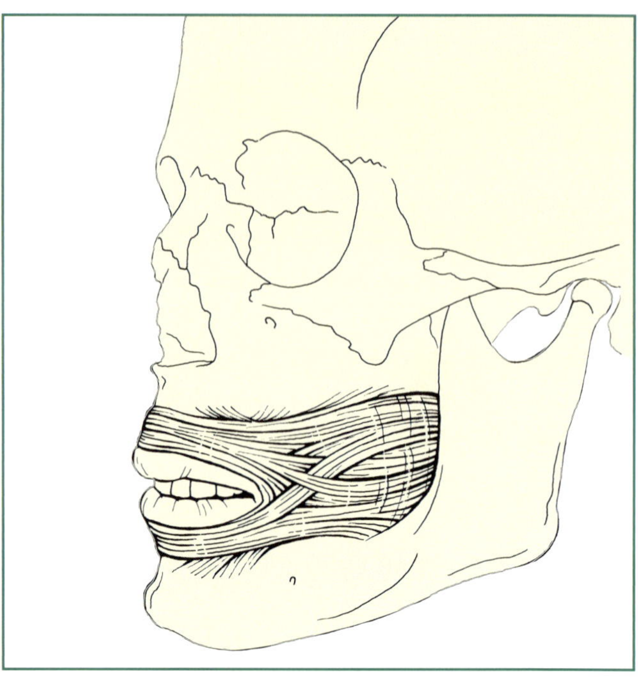

Fig 2-8 Buccinator muscles: superior, intermediate, and inferior fibers.

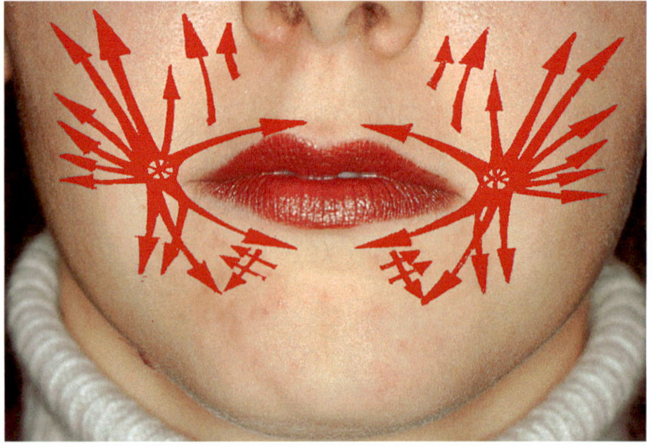

Fig 2-9 The modiolus: muscle tendon nodes at the angles of the mouth.

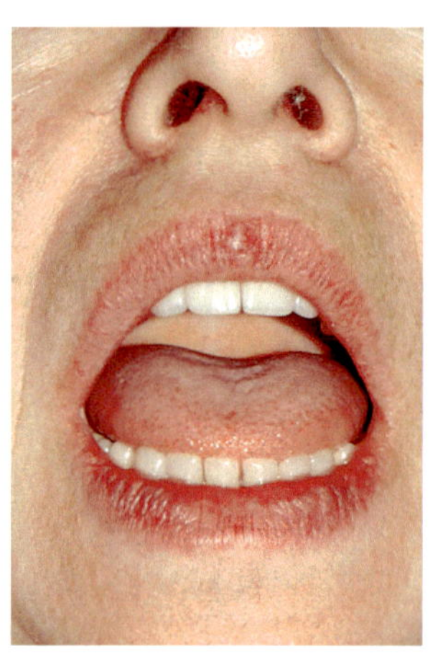

Fig 2-10 In cases of macroglossia, the occlusal plane of the mandible arc is positioned below the equator of the tongue.

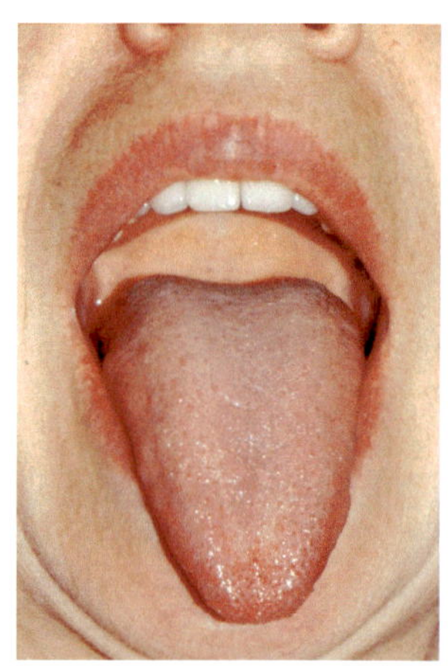

Fig 2-11 Patients with macroglossia can touch the chin with the point of the tongue, and exhibit hypertrophia of the muscles of the floor of the mouth. Note the typical indentation on the lingual border.

pull behind the angle of the mouth, bringing the bolus beneath the dental arches.

The tongue has a wide spectrum of movements, both during mastication and phonation. These functional movements must not interfere with the prosthetic body for stability of the denture. It is a good idea to remember that the lower occlusal plane must be situated at the level of the equator of the tongue.

In a patient with macroglossia, it is necessary to keep the teeth lower than the lingual equator (see chapter 3) (Figs 2-10 and 2-11).

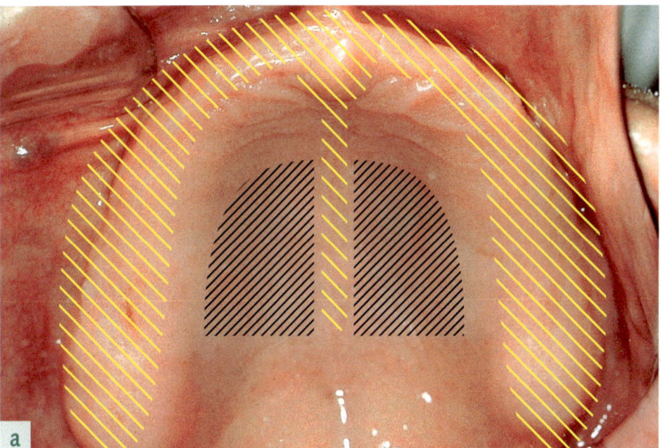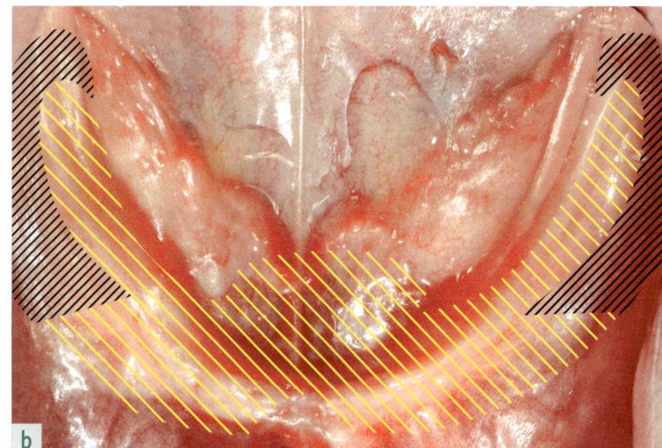

Fig 2-12 Areas of primary and secondary support in the maxilla (*a*) and mandible (*b*).

Occlusal harmony

Interdental contacts must be possible without interference in eccentric positions and in maximum intercuspidation.

Support

The support of the denture is subdivided into areas of primary and secondary support based on the characteristics of the mucosa and bone[7] (Fig 2-12). Primary support is characterized by keratinized masticatory mucosa, with the submucosa solidly anchored to the underlying osseous cortical tissue. They are found near muscular insertions, which impede resorption. The muscular fibers exercise a continuous traction on the bone, stimulating the remodeling process (eg, mylohyoid ridge, apophysis geni).

Secondary support is provided by alveolar ridges made up of bone that is susceptible to resorption, regions with thin mucosa lying directly on the cortical tissue without the interposition of a submucosa, and regions in which the mucosa covers vascular-nervous bundles.

In the maxilla, the hard palate is the area of primary support, and the alveolar ridge is the area of secondary support.

In the palate, laterally to the midline raphe, the masticatory keratinized mucosa covers a submucosa that contains adipose tissue anteriorly and glandular tissue posteriorly. This resilient layer of submucosa acts as a cushion for the functional stresses transmitted by the denture.

Primary support in the mandible is achieved by the retromolar pads and distal buccal osseous surfaces, and secondary support is achieved by the anterior buccal inclined plane.

The retromolar pads represent the distal limit of the masticatory keratinized mucosa of the mandibular alveolar ridge; they are formed by healed scar tissue from extraction of the third molar and its distal papilla. The retromolar pads constitute the primary support, as the superficial and deep tendons of the temporal muscles are inserted distally to them and impede resorption by exercising a continual traction on the underlying bone.

The posterior buccal osseous surfaces between the alveolar ridge and the external oblique line provide primary support because they are covered by thin mucosa, with submucosa containing connective glands and fibers of the buccinator muscle. The fibers of the buccinator run parallel to the buccal posterior surfaces, are oriented in an anteroposterior direction and include the retromolar pads posteriorly. Such orientation of the fibers impedes the dislocation of the denture during contraction. The anterior buccal inclined plane can be considered a secondary area of support because of the quality of mucosa.

The region of the apophysis geni is not subject to resorption because of the insertion of the genioglossal and geniohyoid muscles. However, the mucosa in this region is not keratinized and therefore is unsuited to bear high functional stresses.

In the mandible, the alveolar ridges provide primary support in some patients. If the alveolar ridge is not greatly resorbed and it is covered by masticatory mucosa, it can tolerate functional loading. But if it is very resorbed and covered by thin and friable mucosa, the alveolar ridge is considered an area of secondary support.

References

1. Jacobson TE, Krol AJ. A contemporary review of the factors involved in complete denture retention, stability, and support. Part I: Retention. J Prosthet Dent 1983;49:5–15. Cat. 7

2. Stanitz JD, Lakewood MS, An analysis of the part played by the fluid film in denture retention. J Am Dent Assoc 1948;37:168–172. Cat. 6

3. Jacobson TE, Krol AJ. A contemporary review of the factors involved in complete denture retention, stability, and support. Part II: Stability. J Prosthet Dent 1983;49:165–172. Cat. 7

4. Cox AM. A consideration of the fundamental physical principles involved in the retention of artificial dentures. Br Dent J 1926;47:1058–1070. Cat. 7

5. Fish EW. Using the muscles to stabilize the full lower denture. J Am Dent Assoc 1933;20:2163–2169. Cat. 9

6. Lundquist DO. An electromyographic analysis of the function of the buccinator muscle as an aid to denture retention and stabilization. J Prosthet Dent 1959;9:44–52. Cat. 2

7. Jacobson TE, Krol AJ. A contemporary review of the factors involved in complete denture retention, stability, and support. Part III: Support. J Prosthet Dent 1983;49:306–313. Cat. 7

Construction Principles for Complete Dentures

The construction of a complete denture entails detailed clinical and laboratory procedures. In this chapter the principles of the procedure are discussed and the following elements are considered:

- Requirements of the impression and the limits of the prosthesis body
- Maxillomandibular relationships
- Esthetic considerations and mounting the anterior teeth

Requirements of the Impression and Limits of the Prosthetic Body

A master cast that allows the preparation of a denture must be prepared with:

- The greatest possible extension, without the margins interfering with the perimaxillary musculature during function.
- Close contact with the mucosa, which must cover the osseous plateau without being compressed or stretched.
- A perfect peripheral seal, which is indispensable for obtaining retention and stability. These characteristics allow:
  - An increase in retention (R) that is directly proportional to the extension of the support surface (S) and inversely proportional to the thickness of the salival film (SF) interposed between the edentulous ridge and the internal surface of the prosthesis: $R = S/SF$
  - The reduction of the masticatory loads (C) per surface unit. Masticatory loads are directly proportional to the muscular force (MF) and inversely proportional to the extension of the surface (S): $C = MF/S$

The master cast is obtained using a customized impression tray constructed on an initial cast, which in turn is obtained by means of a prefabricated stock tray. The impressions are mucostatic[1] with light manual activation of the frena and the floor of the mouth by the operator.[2] Excessive voluntary movements of the cheeks, tongue, and lips may cause abnormal widening

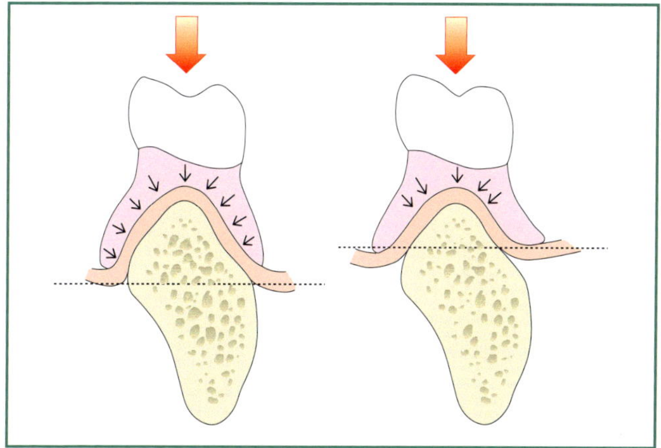

Fig 3-1 *(left)* The mucosa is correctly molded to the bone profile. *(right)* The mucosa is only adhering to the summit of the profile.

of the impression so that the margins remain unattached from the osseous plateau (Fig 3-1). The peripheral seal is obtained by border molding of the customized impression tray with a thermoplastic material.

Defining the limits of the individual impression tray and the prosthetic body requires knowledge of the clinical anatomy of the edentulous oral cavity.

Anatomy of the Edentulous Jaws
Maxilla

The maxillary anatomic regions and structures that must be taken into consideration are the following (Fig 3-2):

- Orbicularis oris muscle
- Buccal mucosa
- Posterior palatal region
- Region of the pterygomaxillary ligaments

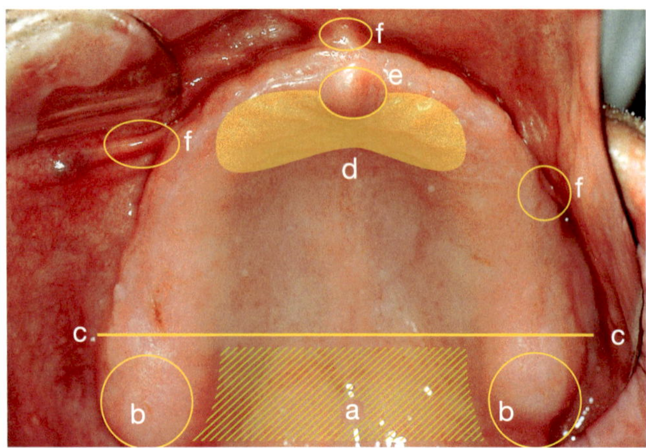

Fig 3-2 Anatomic areas of the maxilla: posterior palatal region *(a)*; tuberosity *(b)*; region of Schroeder *(c)* (see Fig 3-6); palatal line *(d)*; palatal rugae *(e)*; and anterior and lateral frena *(f)*.

- Tuberosities
- Paratuberosity regions
- Schroeder region
- Anterior and lateral buccolingual

The orbicularis oris muscle consists of a superior segment and an inferior segment, derived from the fibers of the buccinator muscle.

The customized impression tray must have a shield-shaped handle, which accommodates the orbicularis muscle and is positioned in line with the incisors.

The buccal mucosa comprises an area between the alveolar ridges and the posterior cheeks and the lips. The mobile buccal mucosa contacts the underlying bone in various relationships during function. It is possible to distinguish three fundamental positions of interest for the prosthodontist[2] (Fig 3-3). The first position is assumed in forced movements, for example, when the lips are strongly protruded forward. In such a situation, the floor of the vestibule runs in the direction of the alveolar margins, and the depth of the fornix is considerably reduced. This position represents the limit of movement of the mobile mucosa in the coronal direction. The second position (functional limit) is reached during the unforced movements carried out during mastication and phonation. The third position (stretching limit) is obtained with the stretching of the mucosa, upward in the maxilla and downward in the mandible.

The margin of the customized impression tray and the prosthetic body must maintain the mucosa in place over the osseous plateau in the second position. Clinically, this position can be adjusted individually by discretely moving the lips and the cheeks away from the alveolar ridges.

The soft palate and the sulci of the pterygomaxillary notches make up the posterior palatal region.[3] The pterygomaxillary

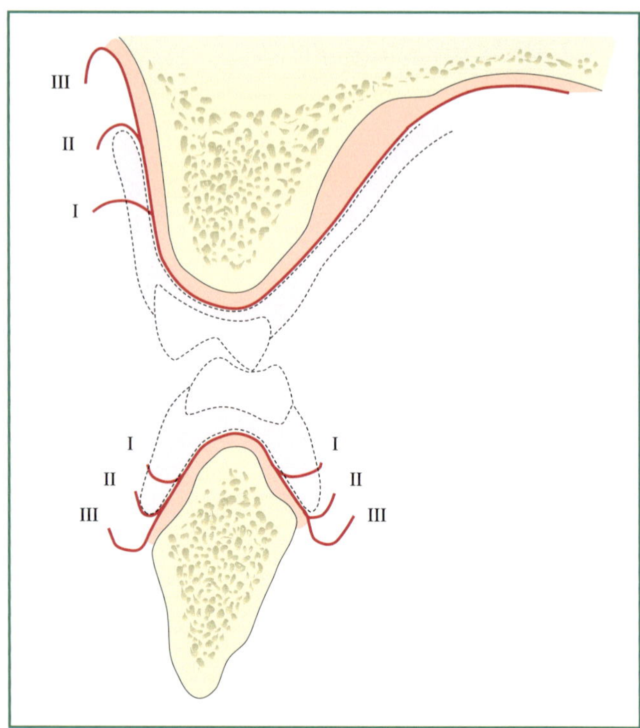

Fig 3-3 Schematic of possible positions of the mobile mucosa over the osseous plateau.

notches are formed by soft compressable tissues and are limited mesially by the distal portions of the maxillary tuberosities and distally by the pterygoid processes of the sphenoid. These notches consist of loose connective tissue and are covered by the pterygomandibular plica, which extends backward and downward from the posterior part of the tuberosity into the retromolar pad. Clinically, the position of the notches can be modified individually with the use of a burnisher. In patients with heightened resorption of the maxillary tuberosities, it is particularly difficult to observe this anatomic structure.

The soft palate is made up of a mesial membranous part (or aponeurosis), which constitutes the tendon of the tensor veli palatini muscle and is not very compressible, and a vibratile part, which is compressible. The soft palate is part of the velopharyngeal complex; its movement allows the closure of the nasopharynx during swallowing.

The vibratile line runs along the connection of the aponeurosis of the tensor veli palatini and the muscular portion of the soft palate. It can be viewed by making the patient pronounce the letter "A" with a normal voice and represents the limit of the posterior margin of the denture. The portion of the palate situated distal to this line is the portion subjected to the greatest movement during function.

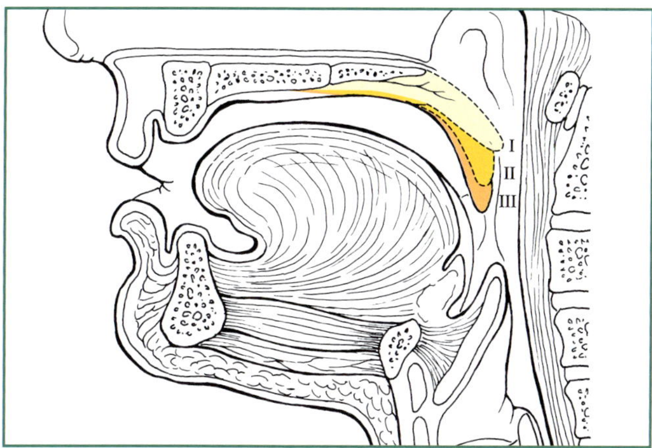

Fig 3-4 Typology of the soft palate.

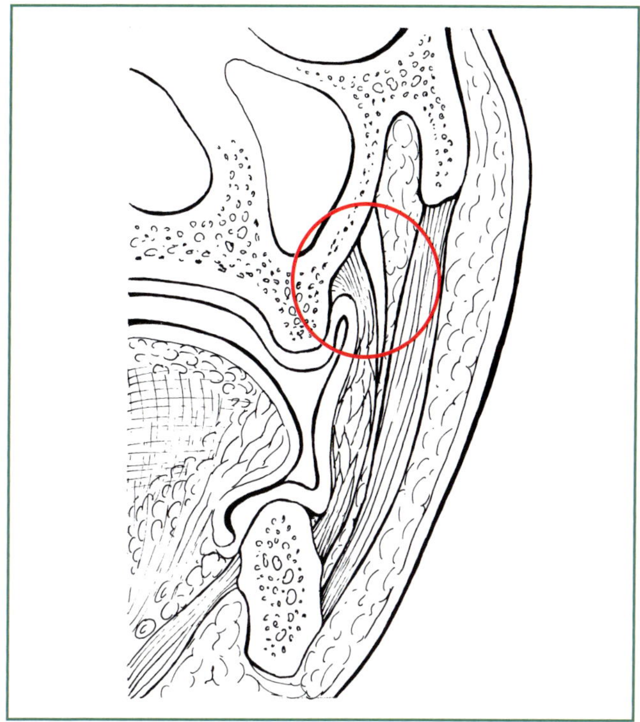

Fig 3-5 Paratuberosity regions.

The morphology of the soft palate can be characterized in three classes[4,5] (Fig 3-4):

- Class I: The straight soft palate follows the horizontal direction of the hard palate and has reduced mobility.
- Class II: The intermediate soft palate has a configuration between classes I and III.
- Class III: The long, flexible soft palate has marked mobility and may form a high arch. The inclination with respect to the hard palate is accentuated.

The palatine foveae constitute the ducts of mucous glands and are usually situated on either side of the midline in the posterior portion of the hard palate. They are situated about 1.31 mm anteriorly to the vibratile line.[6]

The customized impression tray must extend over the soft palate while compressing it, 4 to 6 mm beyond the palatine foveae. The limits of the prosthetic body are clinically determined and transferred to the master cast and positioned on the compressible tissues, which can guarantee the hermetical seal. The palatine foveae should not be used as a limit for the posterior margin of the denture; the area of the posterior palatal seal would be limited, with consequent reduction of retention of the prosthetic body.

The *Journal of Prosthetic Dentistry*'s "Glossary of Prosthodontic Terms" defines the area of the palatal seal as that which is made up of "soft tissues along the junction between soft palate and hard palate on which the denture applies a pressure within the physiologic limits of the tissues to enable the retention of the denture itself." A correct palatal seal gives the prosthetic body greater retention, maintaining continuous contact between mucosa and denture, impedes the accumulation

of food under the denture, and increases comfort by reducing nausea and the irritation caused by contact between the dorsum of the tongue and the prosthetic border.

The pterygomaxillary ligaments are inserted into the superior pharyngeal constrictor (on the posterior border) and into the intermediate edge of the buccinator (on the anterior border). The extension of the prosthetic body must respect these ligaments, which could interfere with the maxillary and the mandibulary dentures.

In the distal portion of the maxillary alveolar ridge are the tuberosities, which are covered by a fibrous mucosa of varying thickness. Pockets around the tuberosity region are created by the centripetal resorption of the maxilla and laterally delimited by the horizontal fibers of the buccinators.

The vertical fibers of the masseters do not interfere with the horizontal fibers of the buccinators, contrary to what happens in the mandibular vestibule, in which the contraction of the masseters affects the buccinators (Fig 3-5).

The customized impression tray must cover all of the tuberosities. The extension of the prosthetic body is clinically determined to avoid interference with the coronoid process during the opening of the mouth. The correct inclusion of the tuberosities and the filling of any paratuberosity pockets oppose the forces of diagonal dislocation.

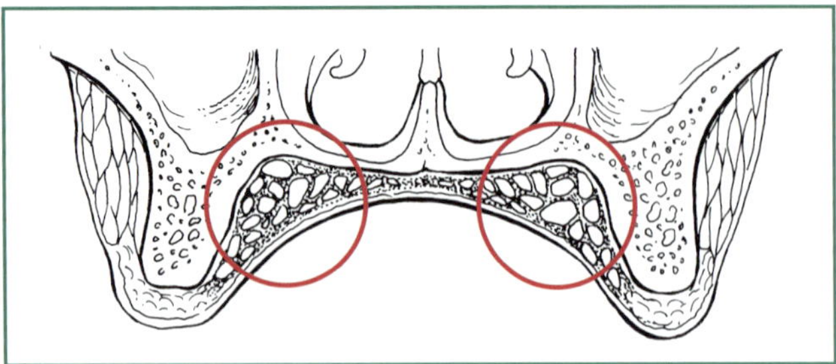

Fig 3-6 Regions of Schroeder (*red circles*); coronal section of the palate.

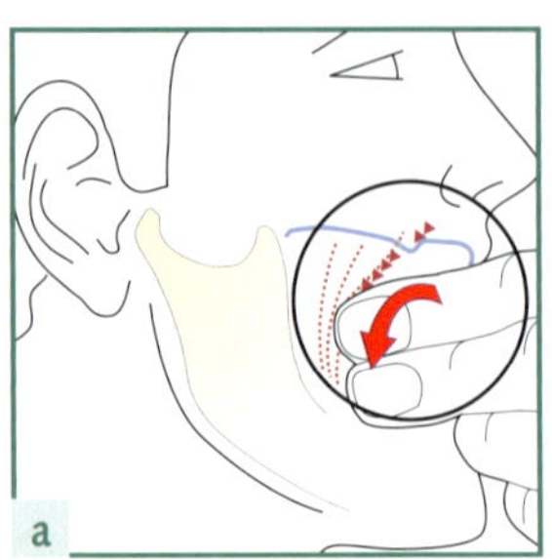

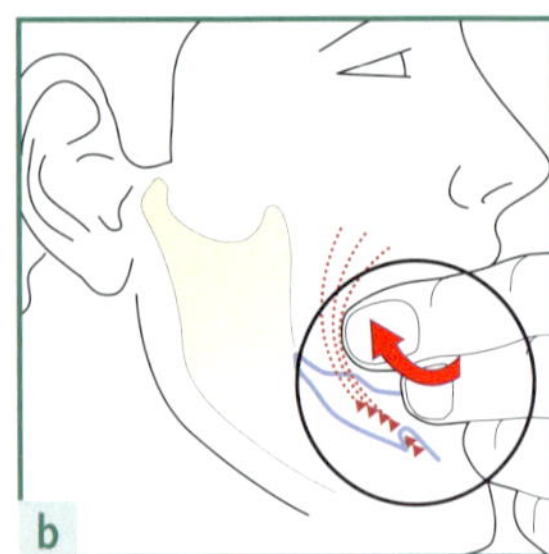

Fig 3-7 *(a)* Functioning of the maxilla frena acording to Gerber: Grasp the cheek with a thumb and index finger and pull it gently out and downward; *(b)* functioning of the mandibular frena: Grasp the cheek with the thumb and index finger and pull it gently out and upward.

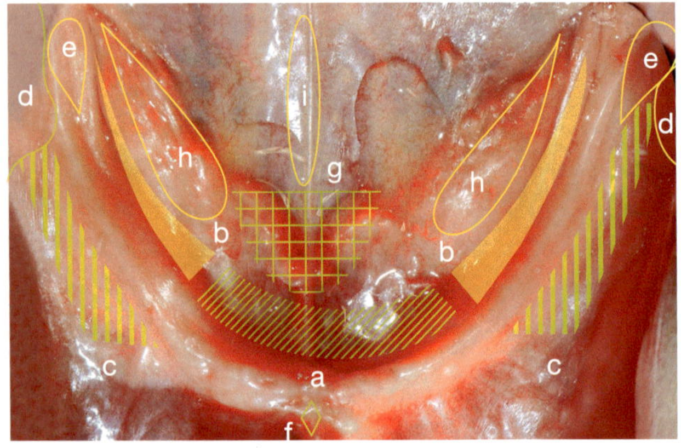

Fig 3-8 Anatomic regions of the mandible: anterior sublingual region (a); lateral sublingual region (b); region of Fish (c); masseter region (d); retromolar pads (e); inferior labial frenum (f); carungle (g); sublingual glands (h); and lingual frenum (i).

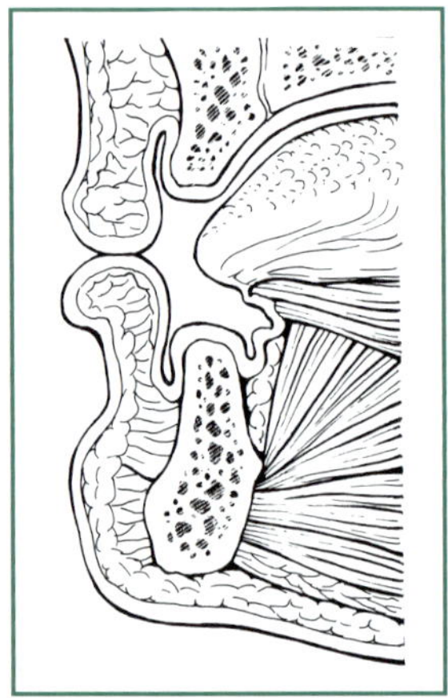

Fig 3-9 Sagittal section of the sublingual anterior region.

The Schroeder regions (Fig 3-6) are situated in the posterior portion of the palate, laterally to the median raphe. They are made up of adipose tissue in the anterior portion and adipose and glandular tissue in the posterior portion. When taking the definitive impression, the tray that corresponds to these areas must be perforated to allow the impression material to flow out without compressing them.

The frena are fibrous muscular formations covered by mucosa, and extend from the alveolar mucosa to the genial and labial mucosa. The anterior frenum and the lateral frena are found in the maxilla. The frena become tense during contraction of the perioral muscles.

In the tray, free spaces for the frena must be planned. During impression taking, the frena should be positioned by the clinician (Fig 3-7) in order to be correctly situated in the prosthetic body. To obtain a good seal and prevent dislocation, it is necessary to compress the less mobile portion at its base.

Mandible

The structures and anatomic regions that are important in mandibular denture construction[5] (Fig 3-8) are:

- Anterior sublingual region
- Mylohyoid ridges
- Posterior sublingual (retromylohyoid) regions
- Anterior buccal regions
- Region of Fish
- Masseter regions
- Retromolar pads
- Anterior and lateral buccal frena

The limits of the anterior sublingual region (Fig 3-9) are marked anteriorly by the lingual surface of the mandible, inferiorly by the mylohyoid and the genioglossus muscles, and posteriorly by the sublingual gland and the body of the tongue. The anterior sublingual region plays a fundamental role in the retention of

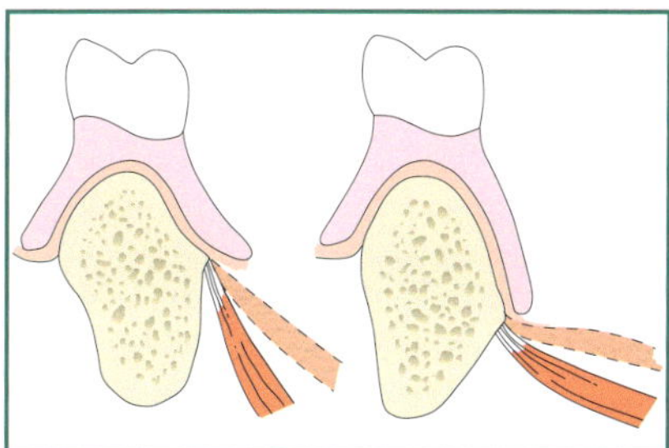

Fig 3-10 Inclination of the fibers of the relaxed mylohyoid muscle (*dotted lines*) in the anterior and posterior areas.

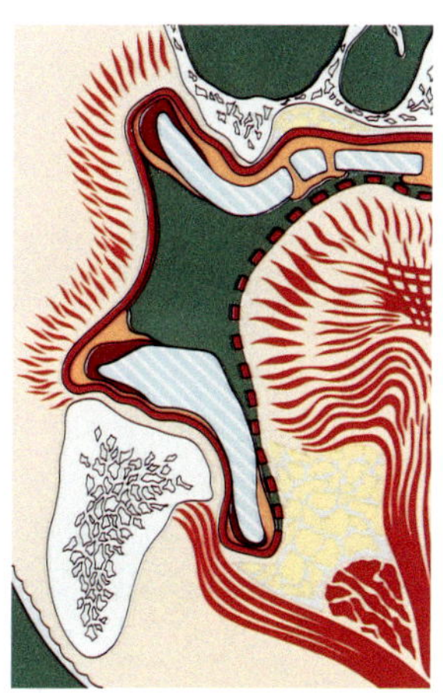

Fig 3-11 Individual impression tray above the mylohyoid ridge by 3 to 4 mm. (From Gerber[2].)

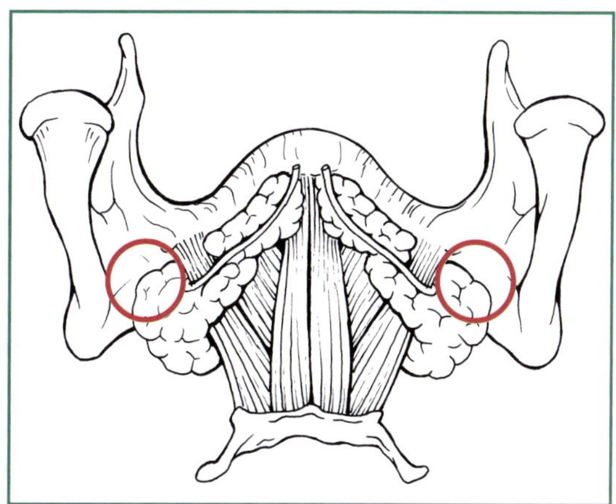

Fig 3-12 Sublingual posterior area (*red circles*).

the denture. The space between the lingual surfaces of the alveolar ridge and the sublingual caruncles must be completely occupied by the prosthetic body. The secretion ducts must be free.

The mylohyoid ridge on the sublingual lateral region is the site for the insertion of the mylohyoid muscle. In the anterior portion the muscular fibers follow an almost perpendicular direction with respect to the osseous plane; in the posterior portion these gradually assume a more vertical direction (Fig 3-10). The margin of the individual tray must extend beyond the mylohyoid ridge by at least 3 to 4 mm by molding the borders with thermoplastic paste to push the alveolar mucosa down on the osseous plateau. The prosthetic margin can extend beyond the ridge by about 1 mm. If the ridge is serrated and painful at palpation, it is necessary to intervene surgically with bone remodeling (Fig 3-11) or to resort to a technical defect (see chapter 9). The limits of the posterior sublingual region are defined posteriorly by the lingual head of the superior pharyngeal constrictor and anteriorly by the palatoglossus and the posterior margin of the mylohyoid muscle (Fig 3-12).

During swallowing and forward movement of the tongue, this region changes in form and dimension. The degree of change is individual, and three classes can be distinguished based on the characteristics that the region assumes during the movements of the tongue:

- Class I: The depth of the region is maintained.
- Class II: The depth of the region is appreciably reduced.
- Class III: The depth of the region is in between the previous classes.

If the changes in form in the sublingual region are not respected during preparation, the muscles will dislocate the prosthetic body during function. If the anatomic limits are respected, the region can represent an important area of retention, as in a class II.

The anterior buccal regions are between the anterior labial frenum and the lateral frena. The morphology of the buccolabial regions is not constant during the functional movement of the lower lip. The margins of both the customized impression tray and of the denture must be positioned in the second position of the mobile buccal mucosa (Fig 3-3).

The lateral buccal area (region of Fish) is between the anterior margin of the masseter muscle and the lateral buccal frena, and the limits are defined laterally by the external oblique ridge—the site of insertion of the buccinator muscle. The prosthetic body must reach the external oblique ridge without covering it. The masseter regions are found distal to the region of Fish. Here the fibers of the masseter muscle run perpendicular to the buccinator muscle. Both the customized impression tray and the denture must have a shape that avoids muscular interference during function.

The retromolar pads represent the most distal portion of the osteomucosal ridge (Fig 3-13). They consist of an anterior portion coated by attached mucosa and a more mobile posterior portion in which the pterygomaxillary ligaments are inserted. The tray must cover the retromolar pads and extend to the pterygomaxillary ligament. The prosthetic body only covers the part of the retromolar pads covered by the attached mucosa.

The anterior and lateral buccolabial frena vary in number and extention from subject to subject. The margin of the denture must extend to the base of the frena. The prosthetic body must seat the portion of the frena that is subjected to tension during muscular contraction (Fig 3-14).

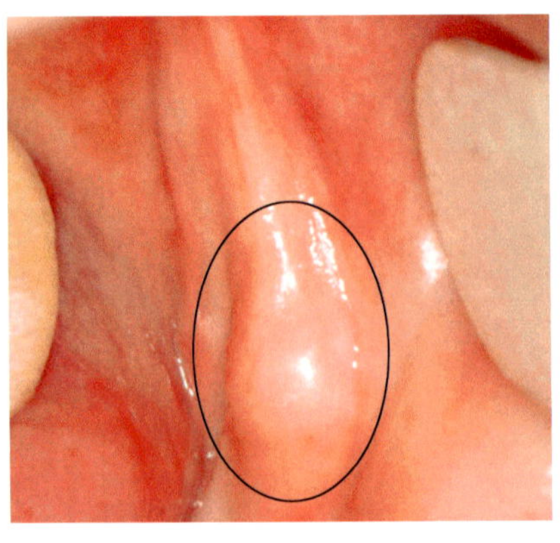

Fig 3-13 Retromolar pads.

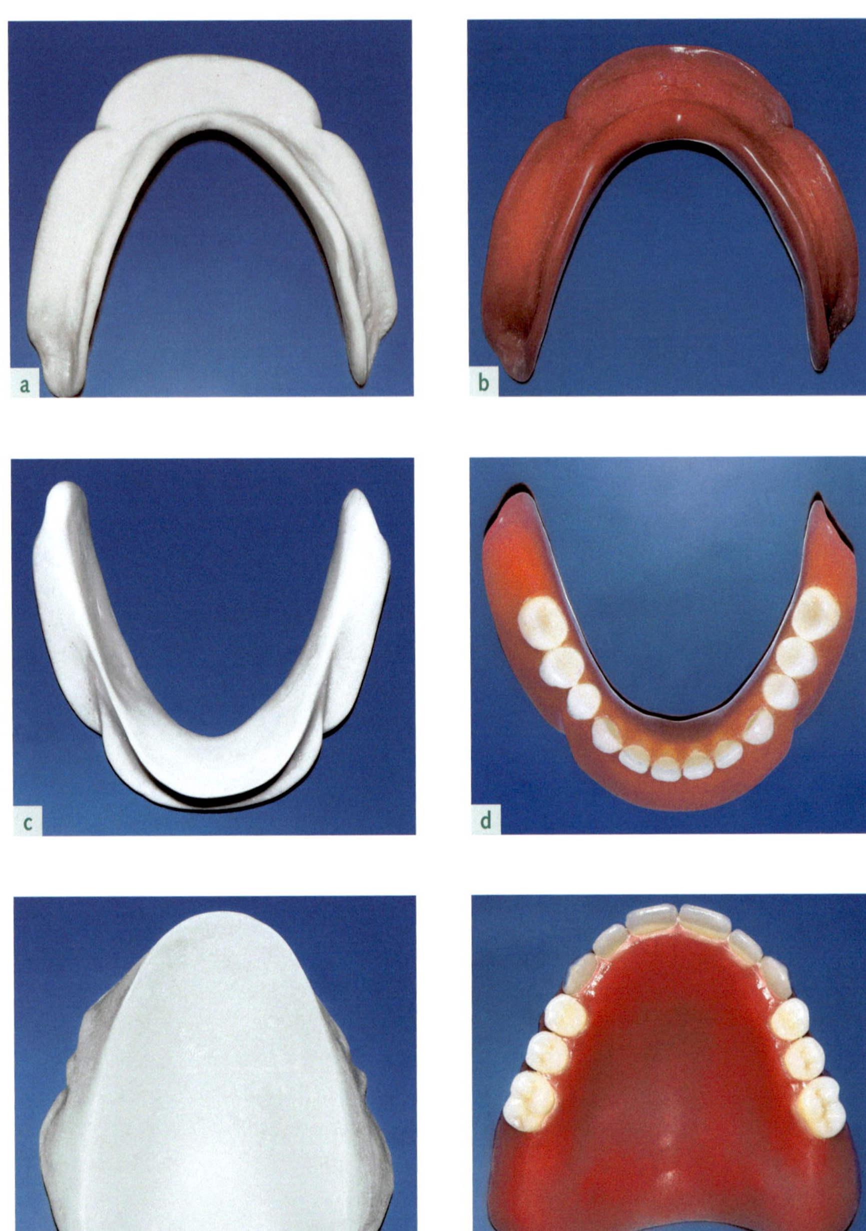

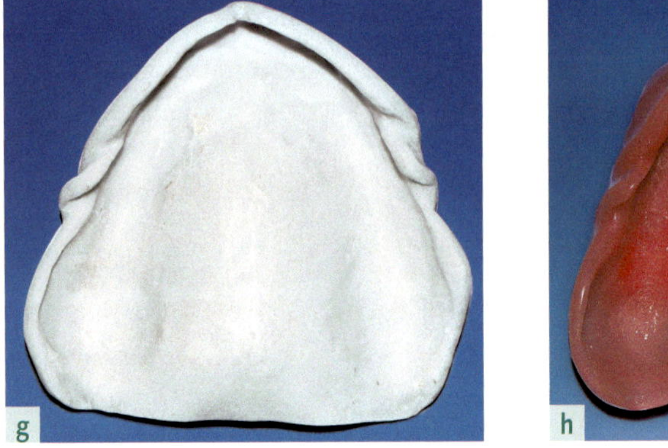

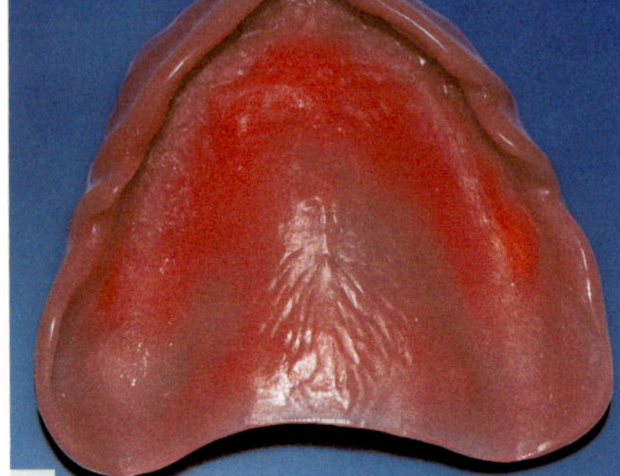

Fig 3-14 Individual mandibular impression tray and the respective prosthesis. The morphology of the individual impression tray is similar to the prosthetic body.

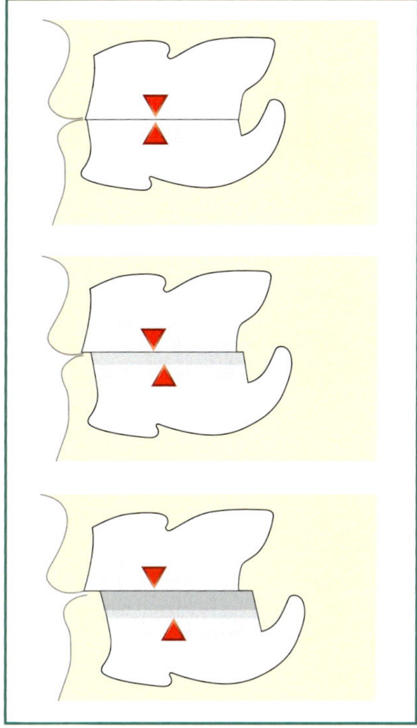

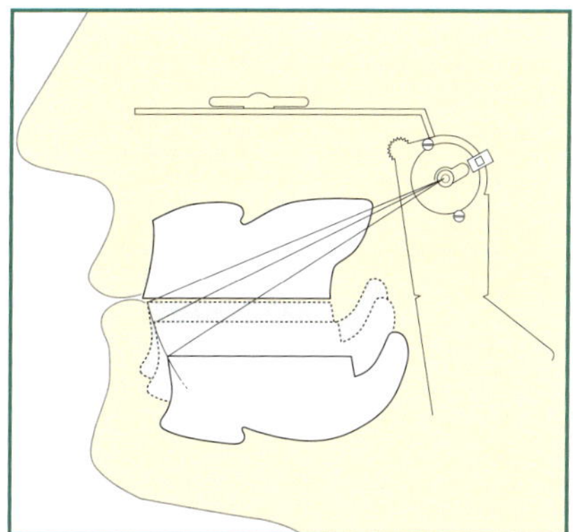

Fig 3-16 With the use of the facial arch, the terminal rotation axis of the patient and that of the simulator of movement coincide; it is therefore possible within certain limits to vary the vertical dimension without having to redetermine the relationship on the horizontal plane.

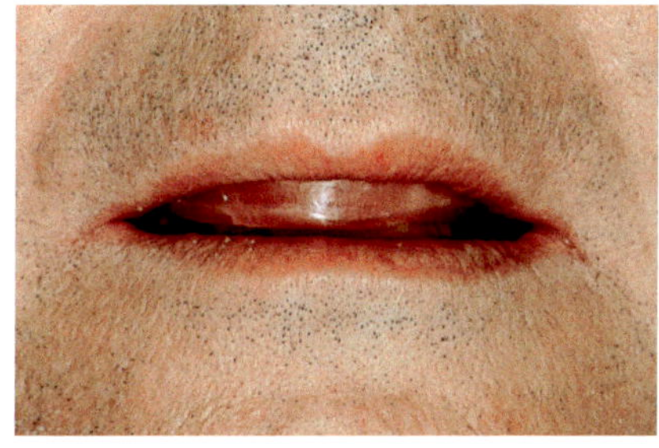

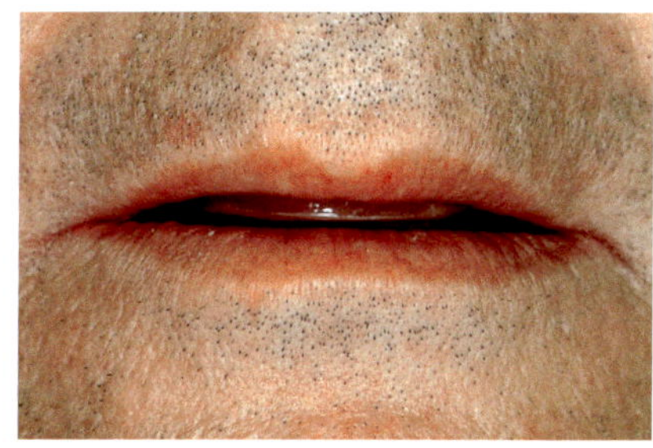

Fig 3-15 Changing the vertical dimension also changes the horizontal relationships.

Fig 3-17 ORP: The occlusal rim is too long.

Fig 3-18 ORP: The occlusal rim is correct.

Maxillomandibular Relationships

In the edentulous patient, the maxillomandibular relationships, once maintained by a natural complement of teeth, must be restored with a complete denture. The three-dimensional space between the edentulous jaws is occupied by the prosthetic body and the artificial dental arches, which determine the vertical dimension of occlusion (VDO) of the face.

During swallowing, the opposing dental arches often come into contact and determine maxillomandibular relationships on vertical and horizontal planes in the maximal intercuspal position (ICP). The ICP is only valid for the VDO for which it has been determined (Fig 3-15) unless the terminal rotational axis of the mandible and its spatial relationships with the cranium are transferred on an articulator by means of a facebow (Fig 3-16).

In determining the maxillomandibular relationships it is necessary to subdivide the space between the edentulous ridges to correctly orient the occlusal plane and to determine the VDO and the maxillomandibular relationships on the horizontal plane.

Subdivisions of the maxillomandibular space and orientation of the occlusal plane

The space between the edentulous ridges is subdivided by the adaptation of two occlusal wax rims stabilized on the respective resin baseplates. To determine the height of the maxillary occlusal rim, the upper lip is used as a landmark during the open rest position (ORP) of the mouth. This position is obtained by inviting the patient to relax the masticatory muscles and then delicately and repeatedly tapping with the tip of the index finger against the area of the lip philtrum and the chin on the labiomental crease.[7] The position of the upper lip also depends on the extension and thickness of the resin baseplate, on the position, form, and length of the occlusal rim, and on the correct lodging of the frena. The position of the upper lip is considered correct when the nasolabial crease has a normal depth, the philtrum appears natural, and there is not excessive reduction of the lip vermilion, particularly in the lip commissure region. In these conditions, the margin of the occlusal rim usually goes beyond the inferior margin of the lip by 0.5 to 1.0 mm in its median position, whereas at the commissure level it is about 3 mm[8,9] (Figs 3-17 and 3-18).

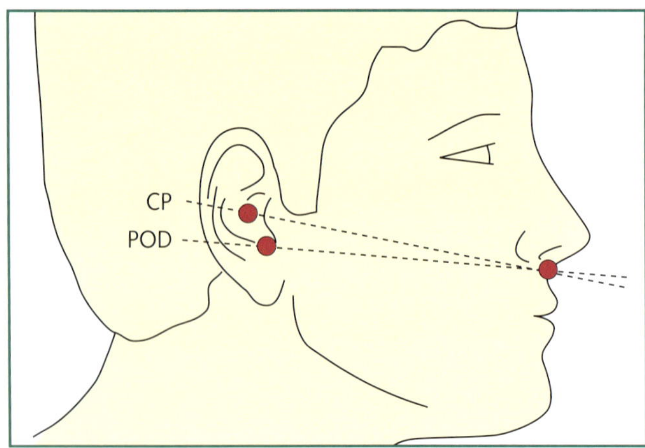

Fig 3-19 CP = Camper plane; POD = prosthetic occlusal plane. (From Koller et al.[11]).

The posterior part of the occlusal rim must be parallel to the bipupillar line on the frontal plane and to the Camper plane on the sagittal plane. The Camper plane can be identified by the lower part of the tragion posteriorly and by the lower margin of the nasal ala anteriorly. It is the reference plane that, even if not exactly superimposed, comes closest to the occlusal plane.[10] In determining the occlusal plane in the edentulous patient, the level of resorption of the alveolar ridges and the maxillomandibular relationships must be evaluated. When the mandibular alveolar ridge is greatly resorbed, the occlusal plane tends to diminish in height in the distal portion.

Some studies[11,12] have shown that, in edentulous patients with correctly made dentures, the occlusal plane is posteriorly inclined from 7 to 11 degrees with respect to the Camper plane. It is possible to affirm that the occlusal plane in the edentulous patient does not correspond to the proper Camper plane but to a cutaneous plane (ala-tragal plane) that runs from the lower margin of the alare to the inferior portion of the tragion[11] (Fig 3-19).

The occlusal surface of the inferior occlusal rim must be adapted in a uniform and continuous way to the superior rim, so that their contact does not dislocate one or both baseplates from the respective osteomucosal supports. The height of the anterior portion of the mandibular rim must correspond to the top of the lower lip.[13] It must run at the level of the equator of the tongue and finish posteriorly at two-thirds the height of the retromolar pad.[14] The height of the inferior occlusal rim is established only after the determination of the VDO.

Determination of the VDO

In the literature, many methods of determination of the VDO have been described based on statistical data, preextractive

data, and individual evaluations, none of which can guarantee, on their own, a correct result.

The clinical method described in this text refers to *(1)* the ORP of the mandible or postural position, *(2)* phonetic monitoring, and *(3)* esthetic monitoring. Each of these three parameters has some limits but yields useful information when correlated between each other.

ORP of the mandible

The distance between two landmarks, one above and one below the lip line, when the masticatory muscles are relaxed, defines the ORP of the mandible, sometimes called the *postural position*. The importance of the ORP as a landmark in the prosthetic rehabilitation of the edentulous patient has been based for a long time on the principle of its reliability independent of the age of the patient and the loss of teeth.[15–18] This principle later was proved to be wrong. Some authors[19,20] have observed variations in the ORP caused by a hypotonic or hypertonic state of the musculature. More in-depth studies have shown that other factors influence the ORP, such as posture of the body, posture of the head, psychic factors, age, proprioceptive stimuli, pain, articular and muscular pathologies, and medications. Furthermore, a variation of the ORP has been shown in edentulism[21,22] (Fig 3-20). It is therefore clear that the ORP, which is used to reestablish the VDO, cannot be considered a sufficient parameter itself. Nevertheless, owing to the lack of other objective criteria, the ORP can be a useful benchmark to achieve an acceptable VDO in the edentulous patient,[22] both functionally and esthetically.

Correct clinical determination of the ORP requires some useful expedients and skill:

- The patient must maintain the head and trunk erect[23–25] while looking at the horizon. The best results are obtained when the patient is standing.[26]
- The environment in which the examination takes place must be relaxed. In order to reduce the influence of cortical stimuli, the Jendrassick maneuver is useful. This maneuver is obtained by asking the patient to hold one hand in the other and pull hard, outward, for about 10 seconds.[27]
- The muscles, often hypotonic, can be briefly massaged in the areas in which they are more easily accessible, such as on the anterior temporal lobe, the temples, the posterior area above and behind the ear, the masseter, the cheek, the suprahyoid muscles with a combined intraoral and extraoral maneuver, and the floor of the mouth. Activation of the muscle tone is completed with a forced opening of the lips, which is obtained with bilateral traction on the commissure with protrusion of the tongue and maximum opening of the mouth.[27]

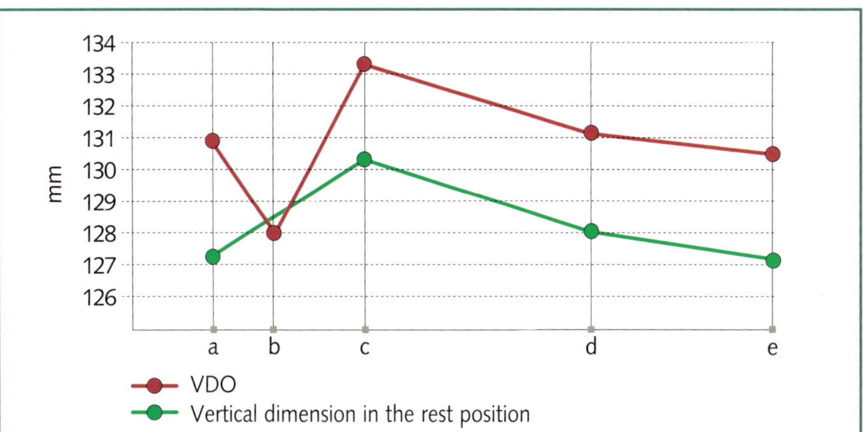

Fig 3-20 Changes of the VDO of the physiologic rest position from the time of extraction and 12 months after insertion of the prosthesis. The progressive diminution of the VDO is accompanied by a similar progressive vertical loss of the rest position (from Ismail et al[21]). a, before extraction; b, after extraction; c, before insertion of the prosthesis; d, after 6 months; e, after 12 months.

- The patient is asked to completely relax the mandible. In order to obtain such a position, swallowing and pronouncing words containing "m" can be useful.
- The lips are separated, and the degree of space between the two occlusal rims at the level of the premolars should be around 2 to 4 mm. This distance is defined as the interocclusal distance (ID).

The most common mistakes made in determining the ORP are:

1. Referring to cutaneous marks, one above and one below the lip line. It has been shown that no linear relationship exists between the true movement of the mandible in the passage from ORP and VDO and the measurement between the marked points.[28–30]
2. Determining the ORP when the baseplates with the respective occlusal rims are not in place. It has been observed that the ORP varies according to the presence or absence of the prosthetic plates in the mouth.[31] This variable is probably due to variations in the morphology of the tongue.

Phonetic monitoring

This measure consists of evaluating the ID while the patient pronounces words containing "s" associated with the sounds "ee" or "eh."[32] This ID is referred to as the *closed speaking space* (CSS) and is dynamically evaluated while the mandible and the relative muscles are functioning. The CSS can be correctly determined by reading a paragraph of text, a short phrase, or a single word containing sibilant sounds.[33] In clinical practice it is necessary to create a CSS of about 2 mm between the opposing incisors during the construction of the denture. It should be noted that this parameter is highly variable, between 0 and 10 mm, from patient to patient.[34–36]

Clémençon[36,37] found that it is possible to increase the dimensions of the CSS and thus increase the palatal thickness of the prosthetic body. This hypothesis has been confirmed by recent research.[38] The phenomenon could be due to oral sensory feedback evoked by the contact of the tongue with the back of the palate.[39] Such contact could cause a posterior positioning of the tongue as is found in macroglossia, and tightening of the pharyngeal-tracheal lumen diameter, which causes the patient to open the mouth wider.[40,41] Thickening the resin palatal plate could, as hypothesized by Clémençon, increase the VDO in cases in which it is too low from an esthetic point of view and its increase would cause contact between opposing teeth during speech. In this case the ID should be reevaluated. The common assumption that the CSS is less than the ID is not always true.[42]

Esthetic monitoring

This measure consists of evaluating the harmony of the relationship between the various parts of the face, in profile, in a position of maximum intercuspidation (MI). Esthetic monitoring is the more important type of monitoring.[43] The VDO and ORP in the edentulous patient gradually reduce because of osseous resorption and tooth wear,[21] with adverse esthetic consequences. To restore the esthetic harmony, an increase in the VDO of several millimeters is often necessary. Usually, the variation in the postural tone of the masticatory muscles helps maintain the ID.[21,22]

Maxillomandibular Relationships on the Horizontal Plane

After determining the VDO, the maxillomandibular position of reference on the horizontal plane must be recorded in order to place the artificial teeth and determine the occlusion. The occlusal relationship in complete dentures is important not only for the balance of the stomatognathic system but also

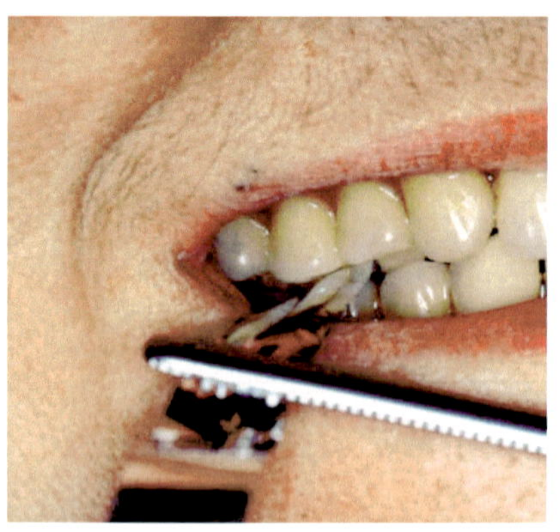

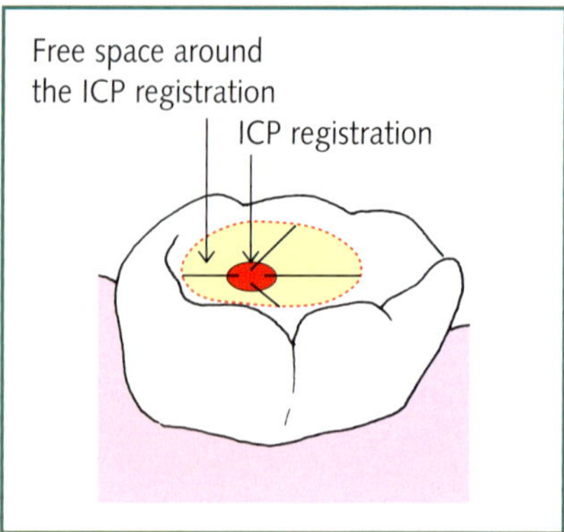

Fig 3-21 Shim stock metal foil. Examination by interpostion of a strip of shimstock foil with a thickness of 8 μm between the jaws. The strip can be folded and refolded until the patient can feel the thickness of the strip.

Fig 3-22 Freedom in ICP. Central length and width.

for retention of the denture itself.[43] When an MI is obtained without interferences, the retention of the denture increases. By inviting the patient to repeatedly close in ICP, the wide occlusal contact will cause the denture to be pushed against the respective osteomucosal supports: the saliva between the internal tissue-bearing surfaces of the prosthetic body, the mucosal flow,[44] and the thin residual salival film that enhances retention (see chapter 2). The same phenomenon should occur when the patient reaches the ICP while swallowing. If in ICP a premature contact comes about, the less retentive denture, usually in the mandible, will dislocate.[45] The level of retention of the denture is important in making the adaptation easier.

Extensive occlusal contact transfers and distributes the masticatory load onto support tissues homogeneously, avoiding overloads, which could cause pain.[46] Also, the absence of pain clearly eases the patient's adaptation. It has been demonstrated that a homogenous load distribution on the support tissues has a beneficial effect on patients' health. The tropism of the mucosa that covers the edentulous ridges increases in quality,[47] its receptors increase in number,[48] and the fibroblasts of the mucosa release osteogenic cytokines. By paracrine signaling these cytokines can oppose osseous resorption,[49] which is unavoidable with complete dentures. The wear of artificial teeth and the variations in muscle tone are responsible for the occlusal changes in the edentulous patient. The best occlusal contacts can be maintained only by using the remounting technique.[43] This technique must not be used in the first 2 weeks after delivery of the denture, because it is in this period that the greatest adjustments occur.[50]

A method to determine the need for a relining or remounting of the denture is to evaluate the capacity of the patient to discriminate thicknesses interposed between the arches (shimstock foil [Fig 3-21]). If the patient does not perceive a thickness less than 100 μm, the denture must be reevaluated.[51,52]

Problems in determining maxillomandibular relationship on the horizontal plane

In reestablishing the occlusion of the edentulous patient, the reference position should correspond not only to a physiologic relationship between the condyle, the articular disc, and the glenoid fossa, but also to the habitual muscular paths during closure of the mandible.

It is necessary to bear in mind that:

- There are patients with neuromuscular disorders in which the paths of mandibular closure do not correspond to an ideal condyle–articular disc–glenoid fossa relationship. Often they are patients who have difficulties in carrying out protrusion, retrusion, and lateral movements, and have a mandible that can only be manipulated with difficulty.[43] Furthermore, remember that after the extraction of teeth, the mandible tends to rotate anteriorly, moving forward and upward.[53] Therefore, in edentulous patients, the correct reference position can often only be acquired by degrees through a series of therapeutic positions.
- The muscular paths of closure depend on peripheral afferent signals and the position of the head and body. When the head assumes a dorsal position, the paths of muscular closure move dorsally and vice versa.[54] These variations cannot be foreseen when determining occlusal relationships. Therefore, a certain level of freedom in ICP[43] should be allowed in occlusion (Fig 3-22).

Determining maxillomandibular relationships on the horizontal plane

Different methods have been proposed, such as manual maneuvers, deglutition, use of the Myomonitor (Myotronics-Noromed), and intraoral and extraoral graphic registration. The intraoral and extraoral graphic registration offers the following advantages:

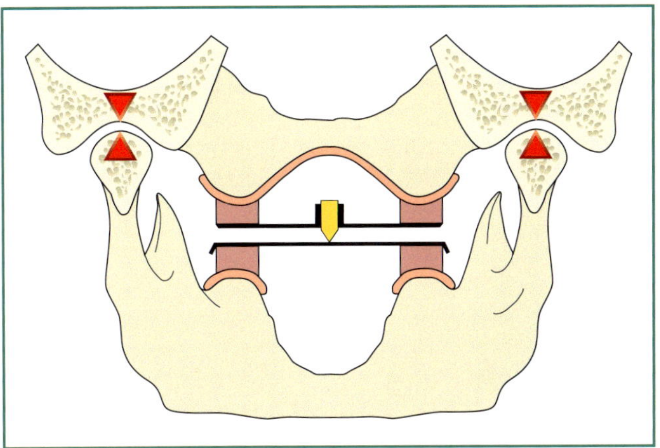

Fig 3-23 Dynamic support of the mandible on three points. Absence of contact between the wax occlusal rim during the registration reduces risk of slippage.

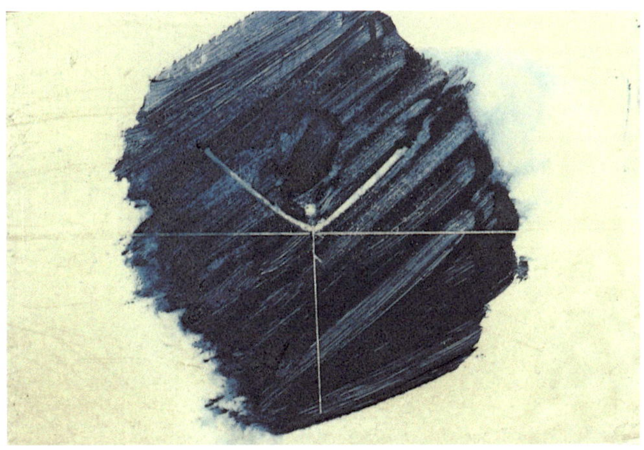

Fig 3-24 Apex of the gothic arch and the neuromuscular center *(white spot)*.

- Graphic intraoral registration (or *gothic arch technique*) makes use of three support points from the mandible to the cranium. The action of the muscles between the pivot and the temporomandibular joints could favor a correct repositioning of the condyles in the region of the glenoid fossa.
- Support of the baseplates on the respective alveolar ridges and the absence of contact between the maxillary and mandibular occlusal rims reduces the risk that during the recording the bases will abandon their osteomucosal support (Fig 3-23).
- Graphic intraoral recording helps visualize both the top of the gothic arch (articular centric or centric relation [CR]) and the neuromuscular center (the arrival point of the path of elevation of the mandible and its topographic relationships) (Fig 3-24).
- Extraoral graphic recording through the dynamic facebow allows graphic visualization of the sagittal condylar path to calculate the inclination of the occlusal plane and to transfer the spatial relationships of the mandible with respect to the cranium correctly onto the articulator.

These abilities allow the modification of the VDO within certain limits.

Esthetics in Complete Dentures

In a society in which the standard of education and well-being are continually on the rise, expectations for self-improvement have increased, especially in terms of esthetics. A certain level of narcissism exists in every person, and therefore the consequences of physical deformity are not only physical but also

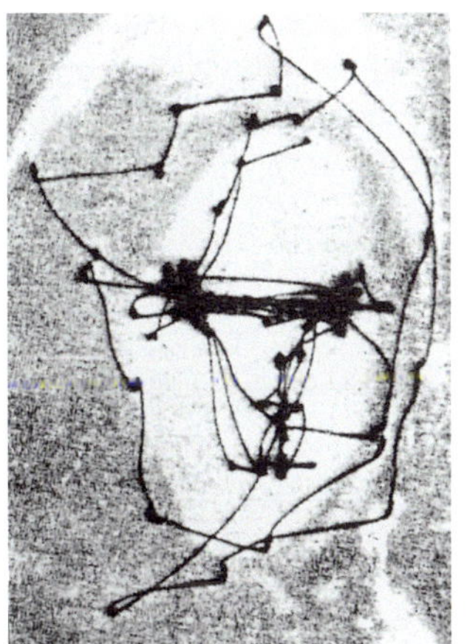

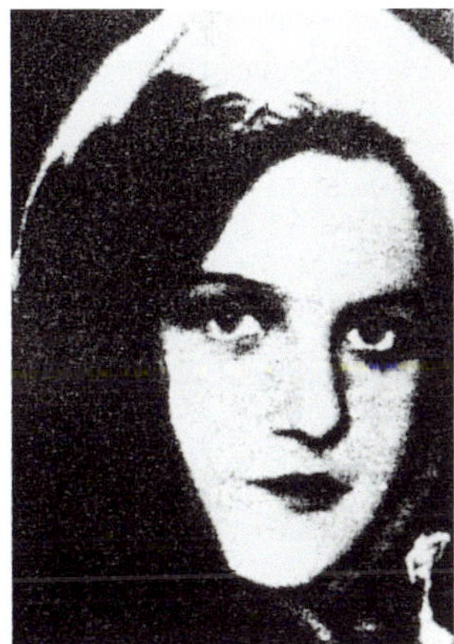

Fig 3-25 Monitoring eye movement for 3 minutes.

psychologic. The face is the body part most significant to body image. It has been written that, "We say hello to the world with the face."[55] The mouth and teeth play a primary role in manifesting our emotions and expressing language. Through changes of facial expression we are able to manifest joy, pain, fear, surprise, etc. Our interlocuters instinctively know this; they concentrate on mouths and eyes. This behavior has been documented scientifically by Yarbus[56] (Fig 3-25).

Edentulism has an enormous impact on the morphology of the face, because the lips and cheeks no longer have any physiologic support. The genial creases and the labiomental crease become deeper, and the vermilion of the lips tends to disappear. The lower third of the face diminishes in height and appears aged (Fig 3-26). The goal of morphologic repair of a face disfigured by the loss of teeth is to restore the harmony

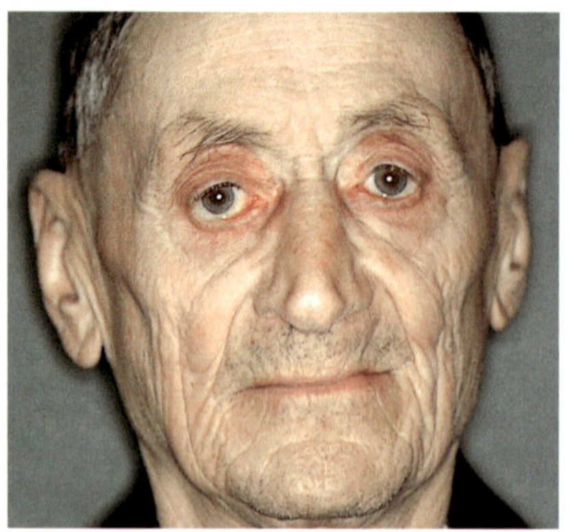

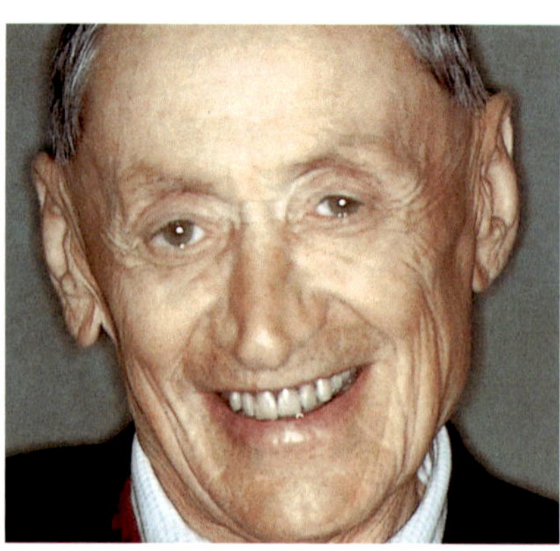

Fig 3-26 Patient before prosthetic rehabilitation.

Fig 3-27 Patient after prosthetic rehabilitation.

per il dott. PRETI
una "suggestione" che le vuole
indicare - attraverso questa
illustrazione - le mie preferenze
per la parte superiore (denti
leggermente distanti uno dall'altro)
la parte inferiore credo meriti
meno attenzione perchè meno
visibile. Molti cordiali saluti

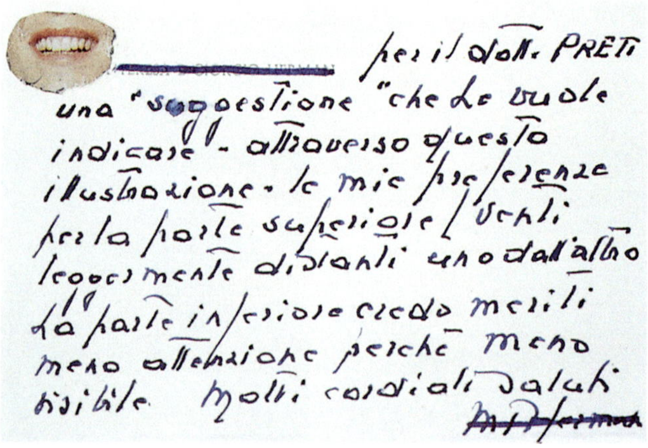

Fig 3-28 A letter from an elderly patient requesting a prothesis that imitates perfect dentition.

of relationships among the orofacial components through prosthetic rehabilitation (Fig 3-27).

Understanding and educating the patient

The planning of esthetics in a complete denture must involve psychologic in addition to geometric and biologic consideration.[57] It is important to get to know patients' tastes and preferences and to perceive their physiognomic characteristics and personality. A multicenter study[58] involving 203 clinicians, 197 dental technicians, and 604 volunteers belonging to different cultures concluded that esthetic evaluations for prosthetic rehabilitation should be individualized. Patients who participate in the choice and arrangement of teeth complain less, demand fewer corrections, and are more satisfied with their dentures according to one study.[59]

The crucial variable seems to be the involvement of the patient more than the result itself.[60] However, sometimes even if the patient has been involved throughout the process of planning and treatment, the esthetic result does not satisfy him or her.[61] The opinions of patients and clinicians regarding dental esthetics often diverge.[61,62] Elderly patients usually prefer white teeth[58] and teeth that are well aligned, maybe because the mass media proposes these characteristics as ideal (Fig 3-28). Clinicians tend to prefer a more realistic, age-appropriate appearance.

Clinicians must involve patients in decision-making and also educate them on realistic goals and realistic expectations in order to obtain acceptable results. For the older patient who prefers younger-looking teeth rather than teeth more appropriate for his or her age, the clinician can show photographs of older famous people who have natural-looking teeth.[63] This process of patient education requires the ability to sensitively transmit information to ensure that the patient is well informed and satisfied with the treatment plan.

In a natural-looking denture, there are spaces between the central incisors, the central and lateral incisors, and the lateral incisors and canines, the morphology of which has been described by Belser[64] (Fig 3-29). Nature itself offers us examples that we can imitate (Fig 3-30) when we want to place the teeth in a more irregular way to make the smile natural. A *natural* complement of teeth produces a space between the arches that Lombardi[65] defines as *dynamic* in contrast with the *static* space produced by unnaturally aligned arches (Figs 3-31 to 3-34). In some arches between the cheek and the premolars there is a space called a *dark corridor*.

Sometimes there is a diastema between the central incisors, which is accepted by European patients, probably because there are famous European actors and athletes who have this feature.[58] The central incisors are the biggest and most important teeth for the characterization of the face.[66] Portalier[67] wrote that "the mouth is like a theatre in which the lips are the curtains, the teeth the actors and amongst them the central incisors are the protagonists, whilst the other teeth make up the

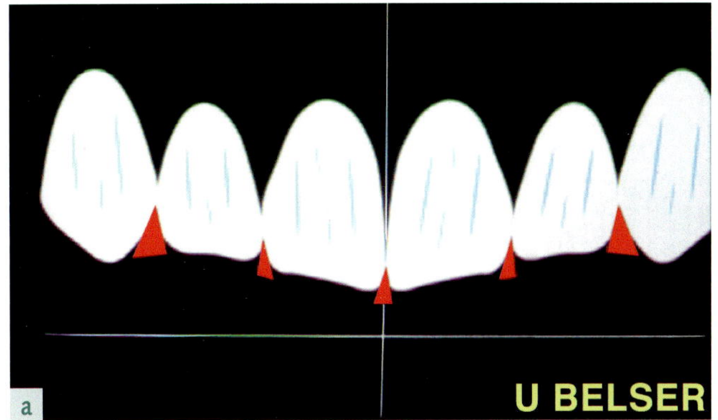

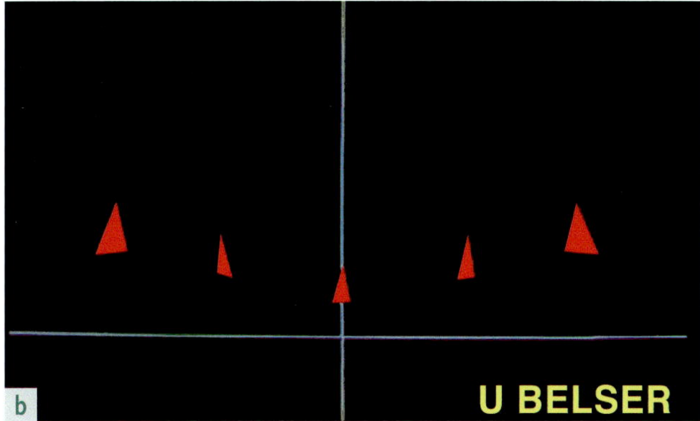

Fig 3-29 *(a)* Interdental spaces according to Belser[64]; *(b)* morphology of the interdental spaces of the same case.

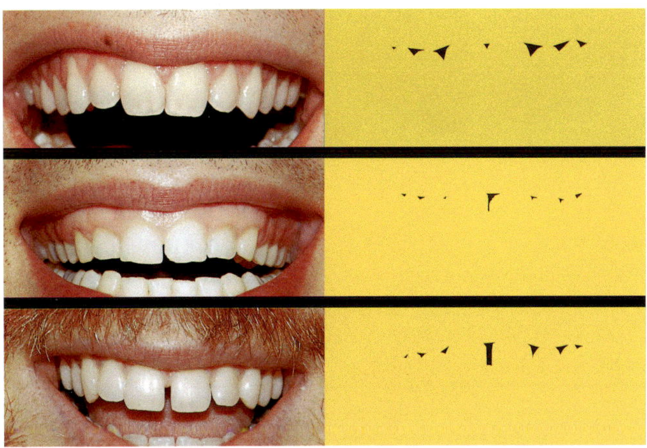

Fig 3-30 Different morphologies of black spaces in three young subjects.

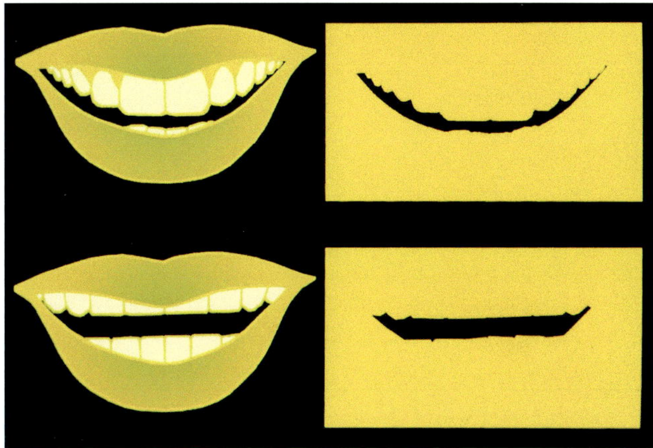

Fig 3-31 Dynamic spaces give vitality and realism. *(a)* Dynamic space; *(b)* static space. (From Lombardi[65].)

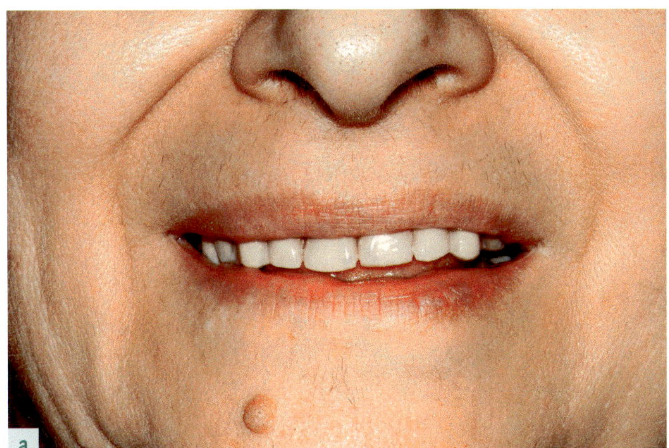

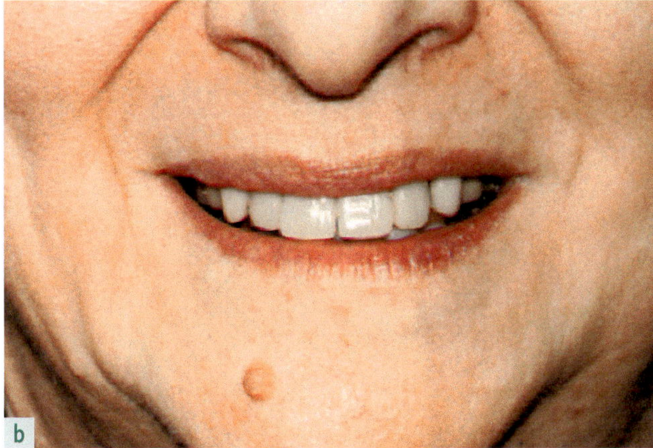

Fig 3-32 *(a)* Patient with an incongruent prosthesis; *(b)* the same patient with a correct esthetic prosthesis.

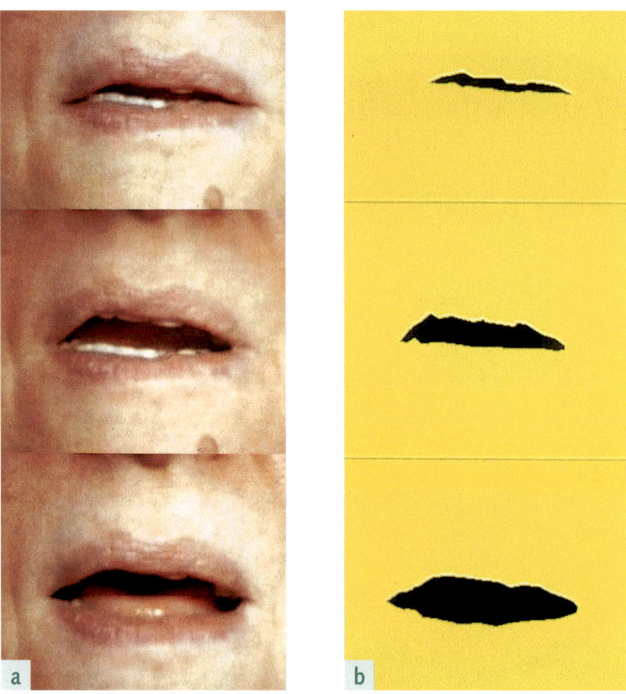

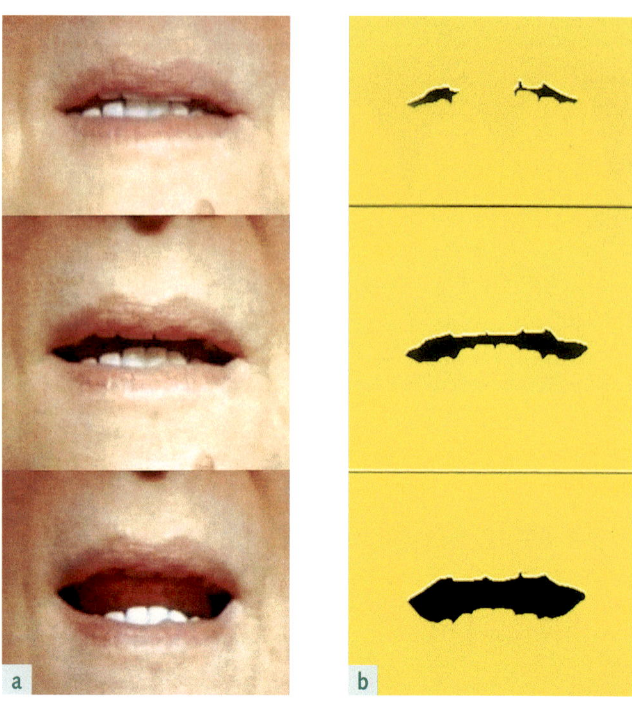

Fig 3-33 *(a)* Patient with an incongruent prosthesis. The patient was filmed while she pronounced certain phonemes; *(b)* the black space between the arches maintains an asymmetric morphology.

Fig 3-34 *(a)* Congruent prosthesis. *(b)* The black space between the arches is more realistic.

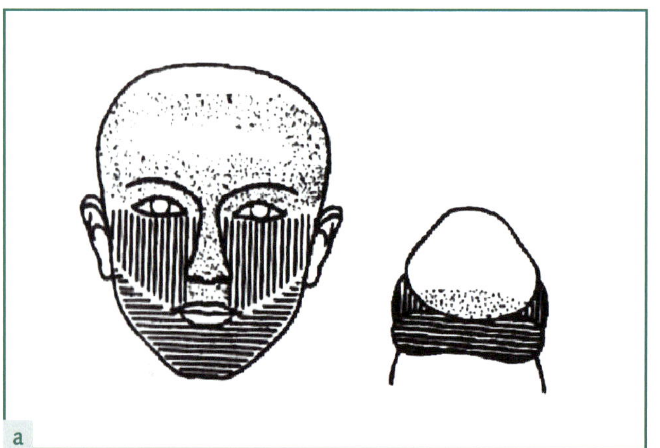

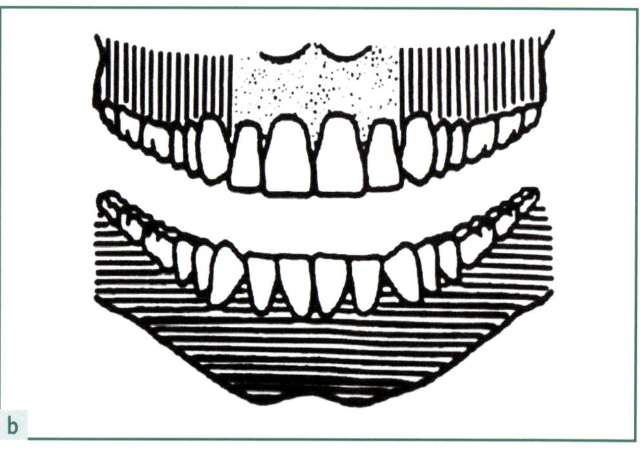

Fig 3-35 Embryogenic theory of Gerber[68].

chorus." Unfortunately, commercial teeth are generally smaller than natural ones.[66] In order to obtain a good result they often have to to be enlarged.

The embryogenic theory of Gerber[68] is very interesting even if it has not been validated by studies[69] carried out on an adequate number of people with a natural complement of teeth. Embryogenic formation of the face involves the frontonasal prominence; the right and left maxillary prominences; and the right and left mandibular prominences.

The four maxillary incisors, the nose, and the forehead derive from the frontonasal processes; the canines and the zygomatic bones from the maxillary processes; and the teeth of the mandibular arch from the mandibular processes (Fig 3-35).

According to Gerber[68], among the structures that have the same embryonic origins, there are morphologic relationships, which he defines as *harmonizations*. The central incisors would be dimensionally correlated with the base of the nose (distance between the alar), whereas the lateral incisors are correlat-

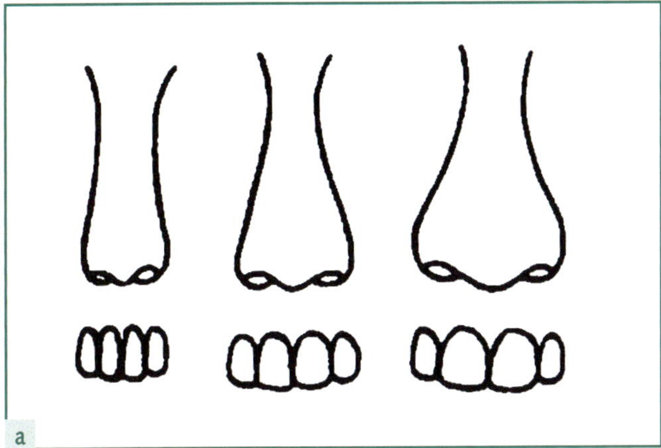

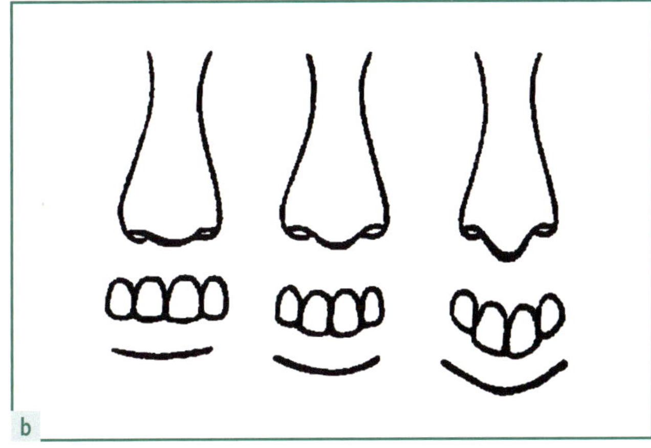

Fig 3-36 *(a)* Dimensional proportions bewteen central and lateral anterior teeth correspond to the proportions between the base and the root of the nose; *(b)* correspondence of the nasal and marginal incisal rim.

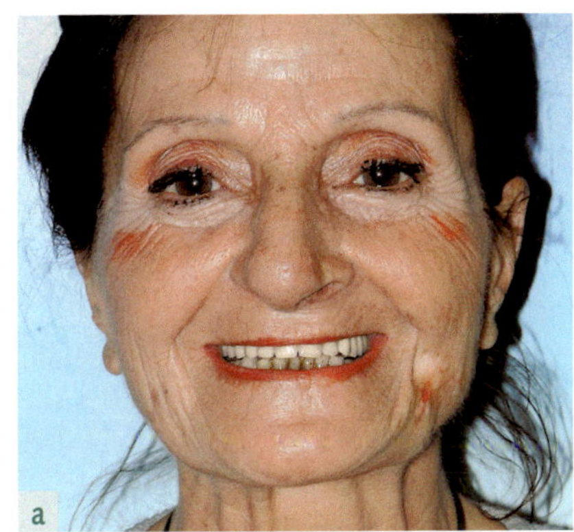

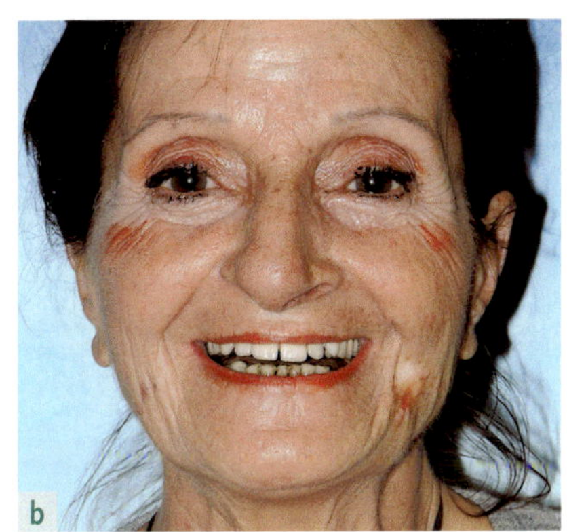

Fig 3-37 *(a)* Prosthesis without the centrolateral proportions; *(b)* the centrolateral proportions have been re-established, making the facial aspect more natural.

edwith the root of the nose (distance between one eye and another) (Figs 3-36 a, 3-37, and 3-38). Furthermore, in the presence of transient zygomatic bone, the canines are prominent and the arch is flat, and in the presence of protruding zygomatic bone, the four incisors align themselves in the shape of an arc and the canines are more retruded. The line of the incisal margin corresponds to that of the nostrils (Fig 3-36b).

The interview with the patient should be an opportunity for the clinician to evaluate the patient's physiognomic characteristics and personality and to get to know the patient's expectations. Both are important factors for an esthetic result that will "heal the spirit of the person who has lost his/her own teeth"[70].

Physiognomy is a school of thought that studies the facial characteristics of a person as they relate to his orher moral qualities. Ninth century and Renaissance writers suggested the possibility of deducing the nature of a person based on the structure of his other body. Although these writings do not seem to have a scientific basis, we cannot say that Eco[71] is wrong when he writes, "How is it not possible to consider that a person with black eyes, injected with blood, a prominent chin, a tubby nose, with two sharp canines is not the most adept person to trust our savings or the surveillance of our car with our children on board?"

A person who has lost his or her teeth has lost a great part of his or her physiognomic characteristics. The complete denture can either restore these characteristics or interfere with them in a negative manner, causing esthetic and physiognomic damage (Fig 3-39).

Personality is the result of the interrelationship of a number of character factors. The most appropriate esthetic solution should be guided in part by the patient's personality. For some people the Hollywood smile (technically perfect but artificial) is desirable; for others it is preferable to create imperfections that make the smile more natural and adapted to age (Figs 3-40 and 3-41) as proposed by Frush and Fisher.[72] The correct interpretation of the characteristics of the edentulous patient leads to the creation of a denture described as *dentogenic*.[73] Dentogenesis is an esthetic philosophy that considers a patient's sex, age, and personality to arrive at a denture that is complementary to the patient.

25

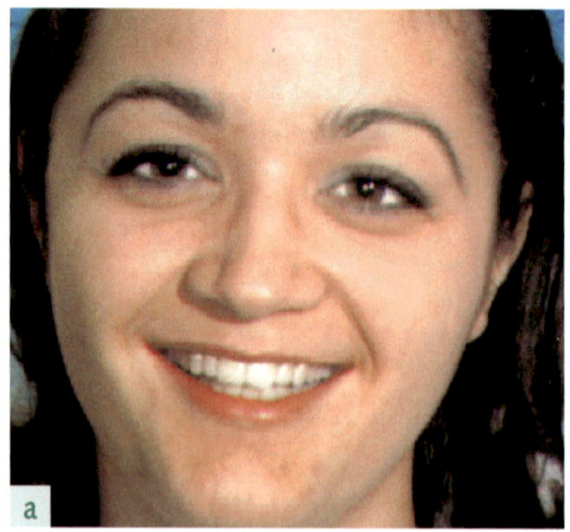
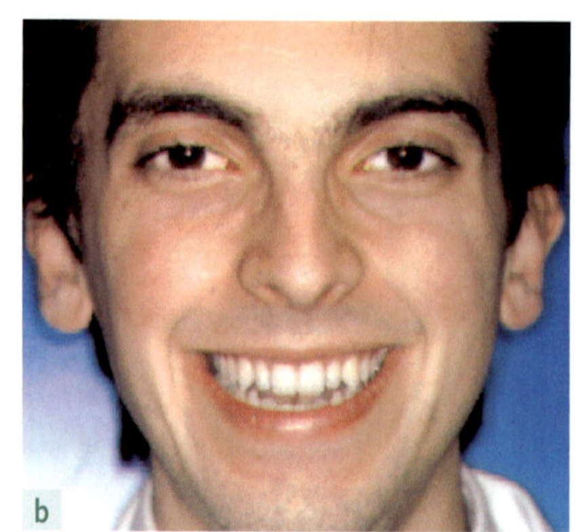

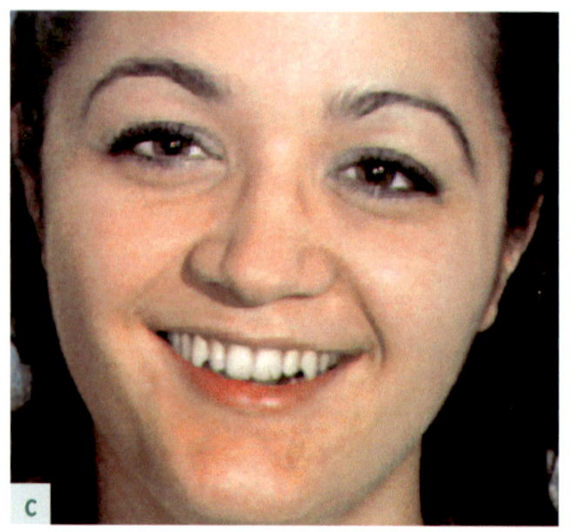
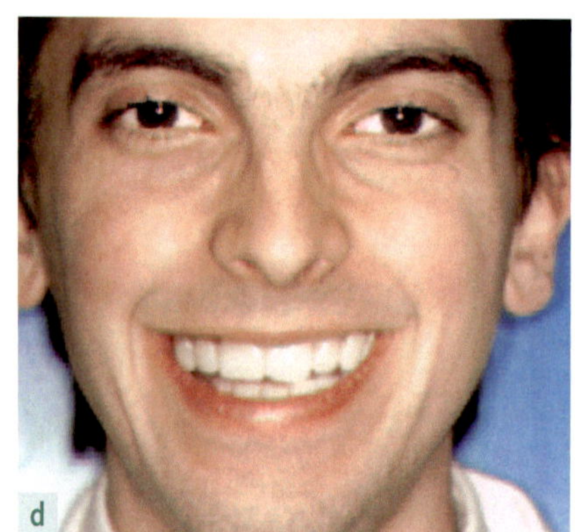

Fig 3-38 *(a and b)* Two patients with correct centrolateral proportions and a harmonious dentofacial aspect. *(c and d)* Computer-enhanced image of the same patients with the anterior groups interchanged. The images do not have the correct centrolateral proportions and so lack dentofacial harmony.

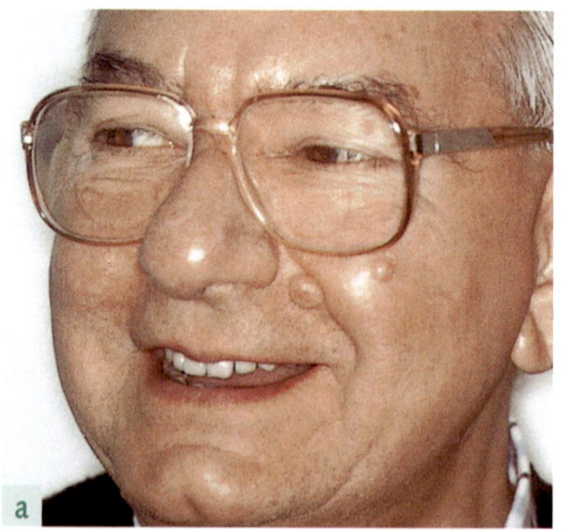
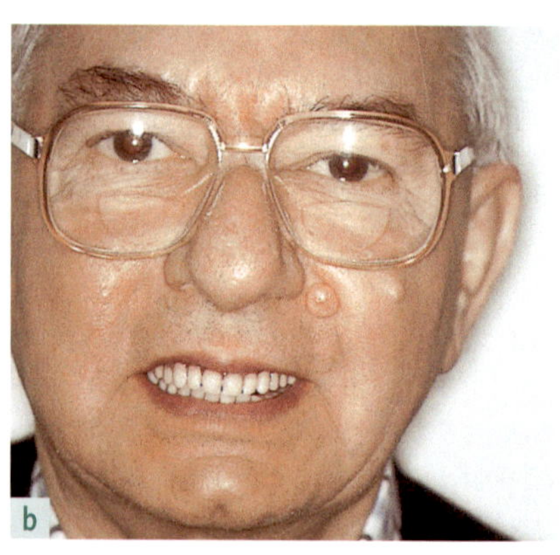

Fig 3-39 *(a)* A patient with an appropriate physiognomic rehabilitation. He looks like a gentle, accomodating person. *(b)* The same patient with an incorrect physiognomic rehabiltation looks more aggressive.

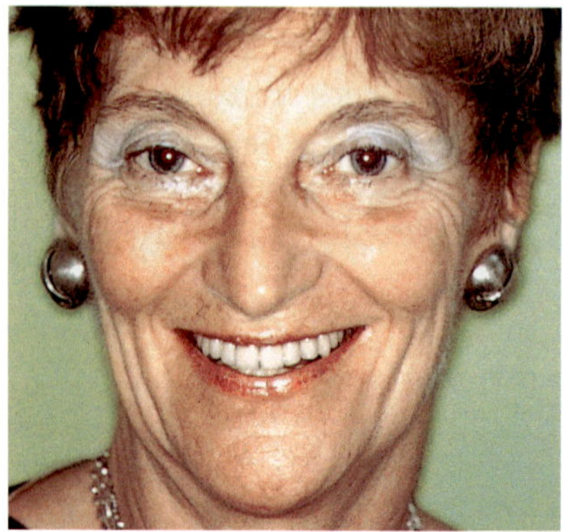
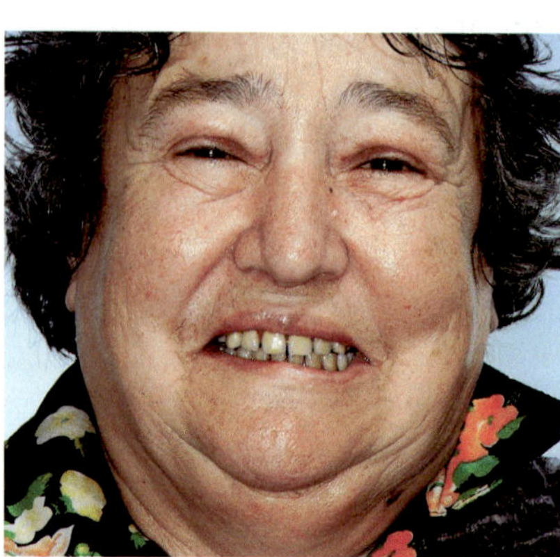

Fig 3-40 For a patient who appears to care a good deal about her appearance, it is appropriate to provide the same level of esthetic care when constructing her denture.

Fig 3-41 A patient who accepts the imperfections (of color and form) that reflect a natural dentition of her age.

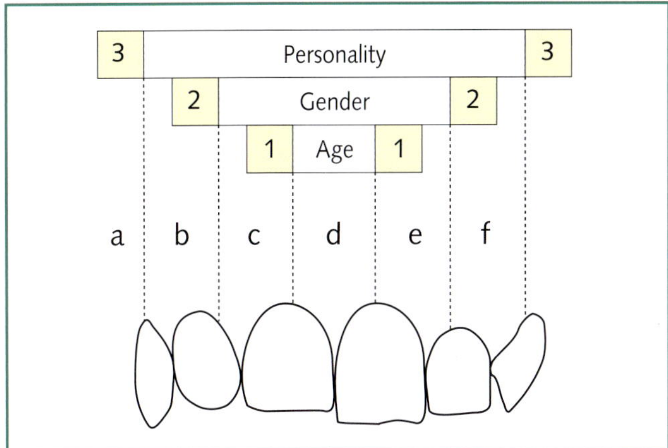

Fig 3-42 Lombardi's modified scheme: a Delicate; b Feminine; c Elderly; d Young; f Masculine; g Strong.

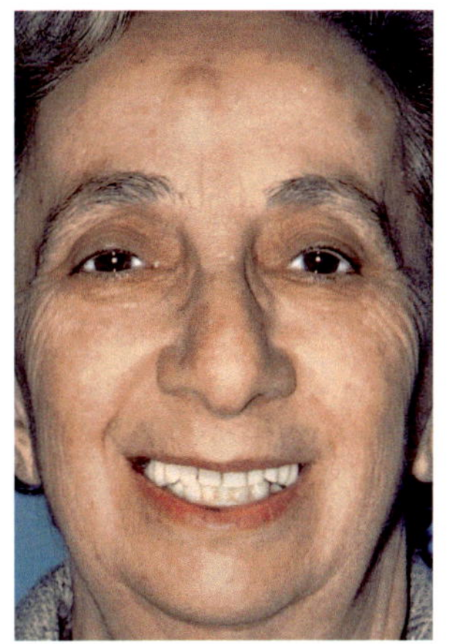

Fig 3-43 Frontal view of an incongruent occlusal plane for this face.

Lombardi[65] proposed, for didactic purposes, the rule of one, two, three. The rule is easy to remember and to apply: one is the central incisors and the expression of age, two is the lateral incisors and the expression of sex, and three is the canines and the expression of vigor or strength (Fig 3-42).

During the mounting of the teeth, the clinician has another opportunity to educate patients[73] on small modifications of placement that can have a great influence on general appearance. Also, patients who have worn incongruous dentures for many years can be guided to choose characteristics they had not considered previously.[63]

Impression taking

The thickness of the impression tray border must be adequate to obtain a denture that provides proper support for the facial musculature and a natural aspect. In long-term edentulous patients, in whom there is often notable resorption of the residual alveolar ridges, the space between the lips and the cheeks must be filled to allow the muscles to assume their natural positions. Adding resin to a completed prosthetic body at a second stage will not achieve the same results.[74]

In patients with minimal resorption of the alveolar ridges, the borders of the tray must not be too thick so as not to stretch the lip and make the philtrum and the labiomental crease disappear.

Orientation of the occlusal plane

The occlusal plane is important in relation to esthetics and to the frontal and horizontal planes. The best esthetic results are obtained by positioning the artificial teeth in the same position as the natural teeth. For this reason, the anterior occlusal plane must correspond to the top of the lower lip, run along the equator of the tongue, and end posteriorly at twothirds of the height of the retromolar pad. An incongruous occlusal plane confers an unnatural aspect (Fig 3-43).

Vertical dimension of occlusion

A correct VDO is determined by the position of the orbicular oris and other facial muscles. If the VDO is low, the patient looks aged. The genial and mental creases become deeper, the vermilion of the lip is reduced or disappears, and the labial rim appears wider (Figs 3-44 and 3-45). The clinician is sometimes persuaded by a patient to greatly increase the VDO to eliminate age-related wrinkles. This drastic procedure yields disastrous results, however. Besides an unnatural appearance, the contact of the lips is difficult, and during speech the arches come into contact with each other, producing a noise that is annoying for the patient and anyone nearby.

Maxillomandibular relationships on the horizontal plane

The resorption of the residual edentulous ridge in the anterior zone of the mandible is four times higher than in the anterior zone of the maxilla.[75–78] This different resorption rate provokes a forward and upward movement of the mandible,[78] and the denture tends to be pushed upward and backward. The negative esthetic consequences are easy to understand. If this dysfunctional position of the mandible is maintained for a long time, correcting maxillomandibular relationships on the horizontal plane and the consequent esthetic restoration can only be obtained gradually.

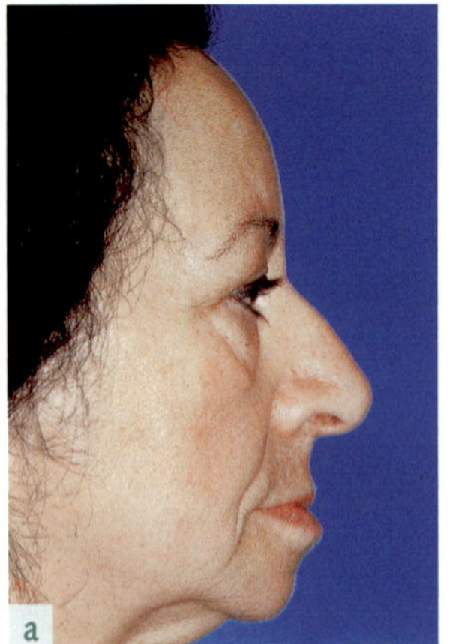
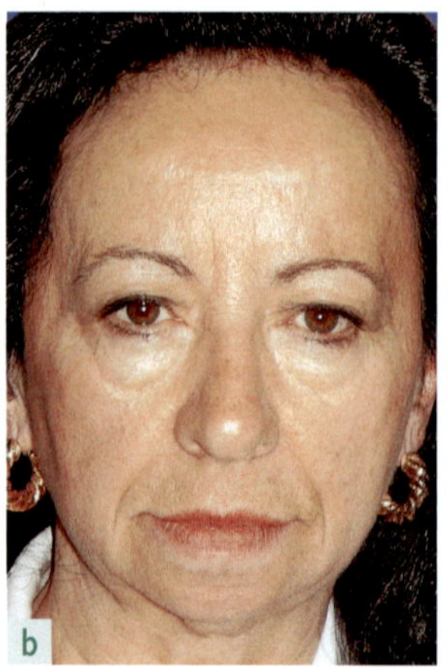

Fig 3-44 Patient with VDO that is too low.

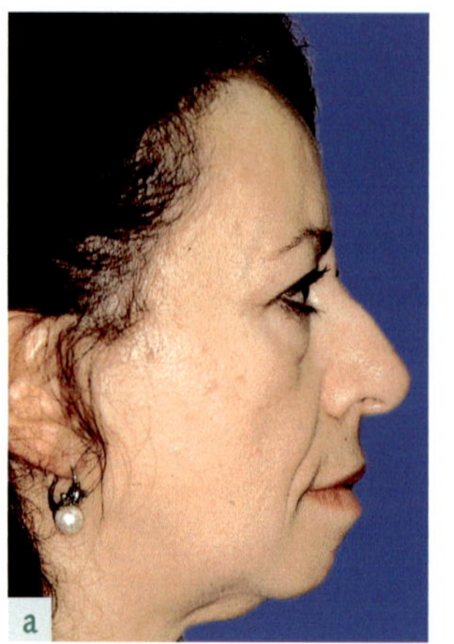
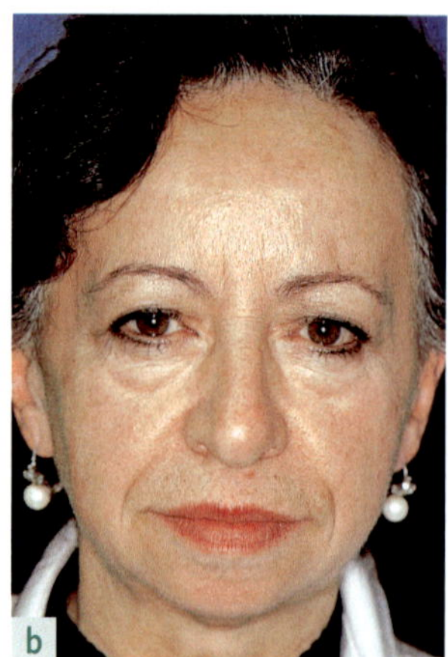

Fig 3-45 Patient correctly rehabilitated.

The prosthetic body

Among its other functions, the prosthetic body serves to substitute the resorbed alveolar bone, contributing with the teeth to provide the lips and cheeks physiologic support and therefore esthetic restoration. The prosthetic body must be modeled in a way that allows natural repositioning of the muscles.

Positioning of the maxillary incisors

The maxillary incisors should be mounted in the same position as the natural teeth.[79] One of the most common errors in the setting of the anterior teeth is the attempt to position them on top of the residual alveolar ridge independently of its level of resorption. This mistake often occurs when placement is assigned to a dental technician. For didactic purposes, it is necessary to distinguish the positioning of the teeth on the horizontal plane versus the vertical plane.

Positioning maxillary incisors and canines on the horizontal plane

Numerous studies carried out on plaster casts of jaws with natural teeth have examined the position of the maxillary incisors and canines. The anatomic references to be considered are the incisive papilla and the palatine rugae. The incisive papilla is a reliable benchmark, because it maintains its stable position despite osseous resorption.[80]

According to some studies,[81,82] the line between the cusps of the two canines passes through the center of the incisive papilla. Furthermore, the distance between the center of the papilla and the labial surface of the central maxillary incisors is ± 8 mm (Figs 3-46 and 3-47) in 75% of cases, and the distance between the labial surface of the canine and the external point of the first palatine ruga is 10.5 ± 1 mm in 87% of cases.

The possibility of determining the form and dimension of the anterior zone of the maxillary arch through the morphometric and angular relationships of the incisors and the incisive papilla has been the object of another study,[83] which sought to define a clinical method that was useful in setting up the anterior teeth. One thousand casts of maxillae with natural teeth were examined and the following measurements determined:

- The center of the papilla and most labial surface of every anterior tooth
- A line perpendicular to the midline passing through the center of the papilla
- A line through the center of the papilla and the labial surface of every tooth

These guidelines have made it possible to identify a parabola for every model (Fig 3-48).

In a second part of the study, three parabolic curves were identified: large, medium, and small. Each of the three curves was traced on a transparent baseplate modeled so that it could be applied intraorally (Fig 3-49). In subjects with natural teeth, the parabola corresponding to the arch was chosen, and at the same time the distance between the lateral frena was measured (Fig 3-50). A statistical study[83] has shown a very significant correlation between the distance between the frena and the different dimensions of the curve. The parabola can be applied for every edentulous patient, correlating it with the dimensions of his or her maxillary arch.

From a practical point of view, the three curves can be inserted into a single baseplate by making the hole on the baseplate correspond to the center of the papilla, automatically referenced to the large, medium, and small curves. This method

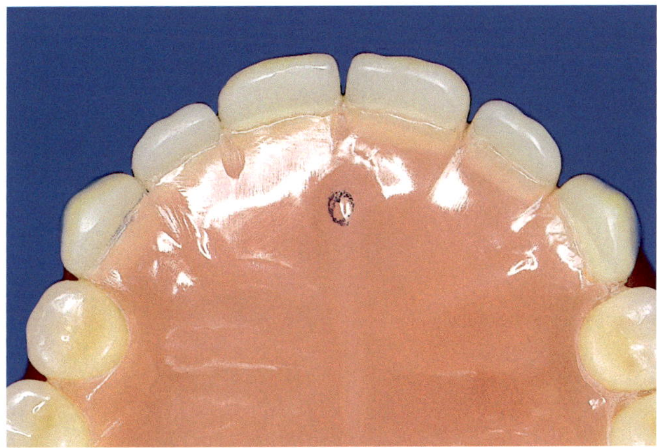

Fig 3-46 Distance between the center of the papilla and the labial surface of the incisors and between the palatine rugae and the labial surface of the canines.

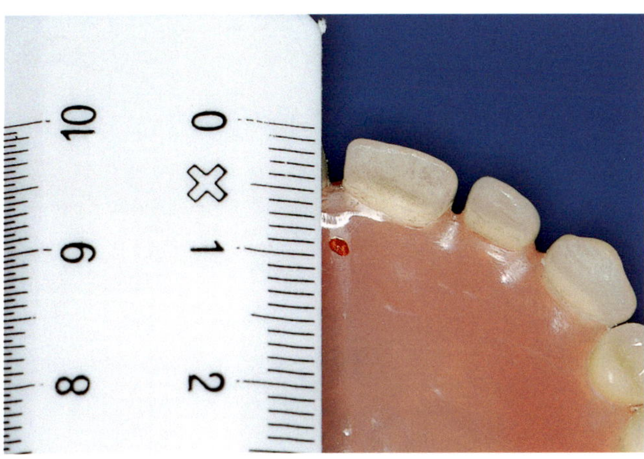

Fig 3-47 Distance between the center of the papilla and the labial surface of the incisors is correct.

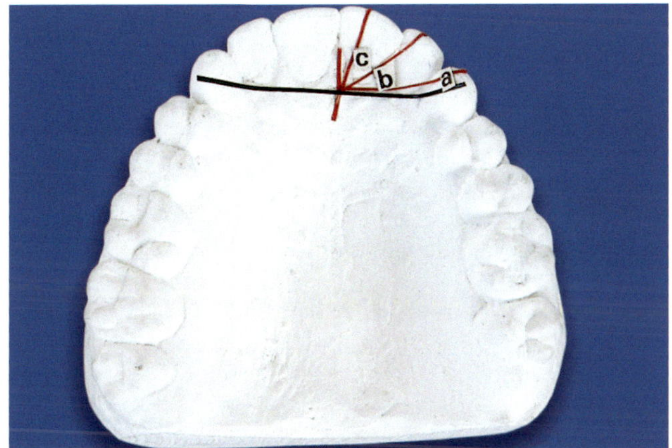

Fig 3-48 Distance from the center of the papilla and the most buccal surface of every tooth, and the angle between the perpendicular to the midline and the line that unites the center of the papilla and the most buccal surface of every tooth, have been measured.

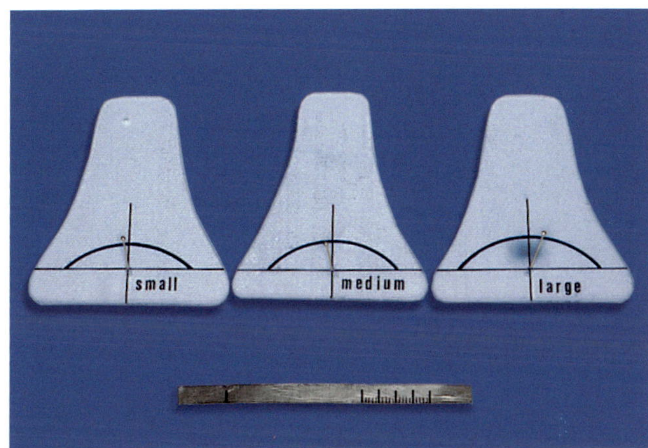

Fig 3-49 Parabolic curves: large, medium, and small.

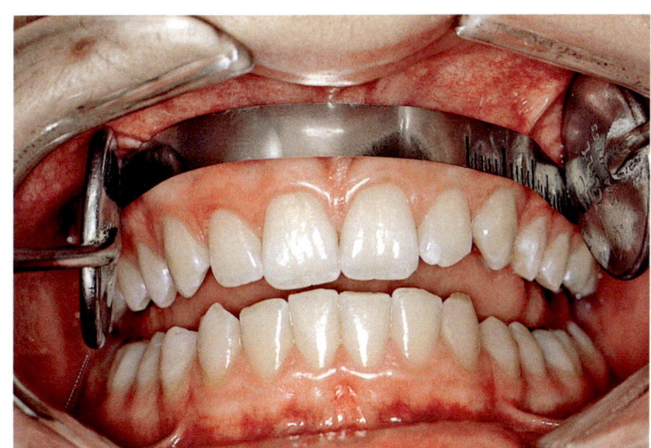

Fig 3-50 Distance between the lateral frena was measured in correlation with the corresponding parabolic curve.

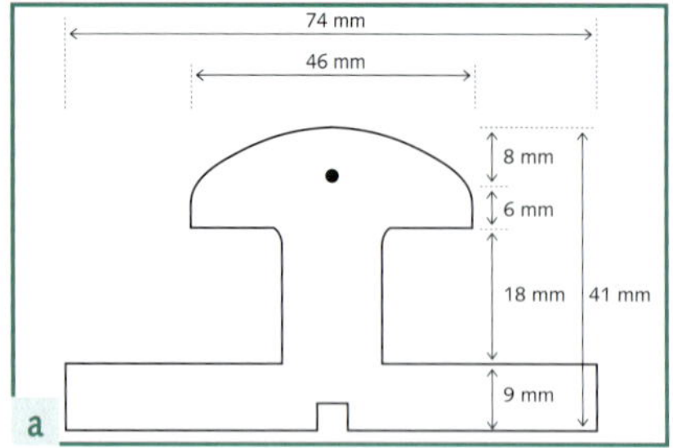
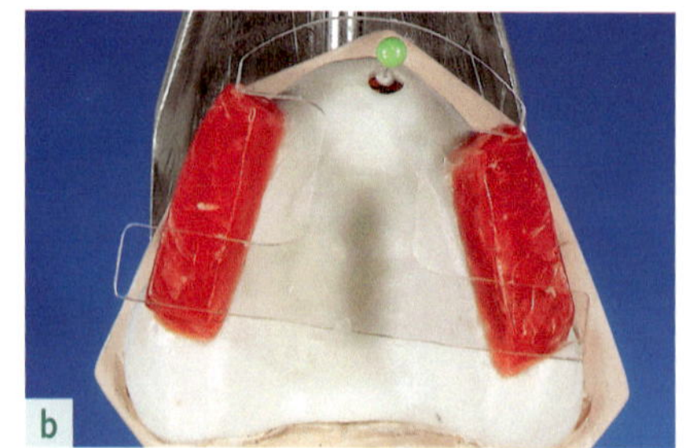
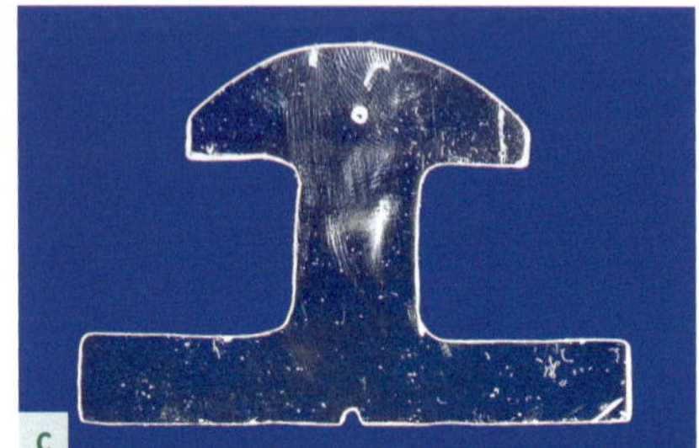
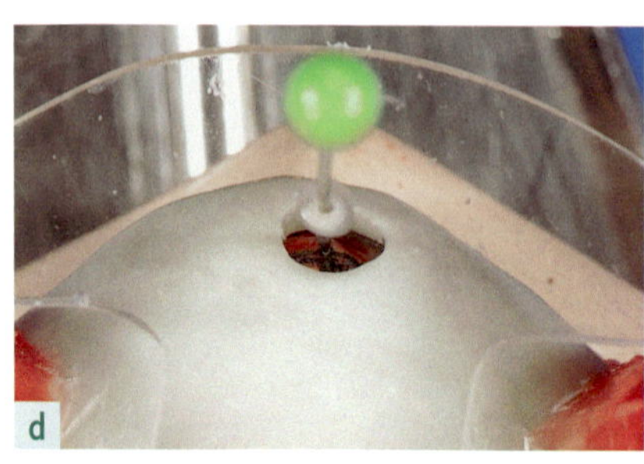

Fig 3-51 *(a)* Diagram to scale (at 8 mm from the highest protrusion and presenting a foro corresponding to the center of the papilla); *(b)* reproduction in transparent plexiglass of the diagram prepared by the lecturer, to be used by the dental technician to prepare the wax rim; *(c)* locating the center of the papilla; *(d)* wax is removed from the anterior part of the base, where a foro is then made corresponding to the center of the papilla; *(e)* the curve in Plexiglas is positioned by matching the hole in the center of the papilla; *(f)* the details; *(g)* the wax rim is constructed following the indication of the curve of the plexiglass model; *(h and i)* a patient smiling with the rim and then with the teeth positioned following the curvature of the wax rim, respectively.

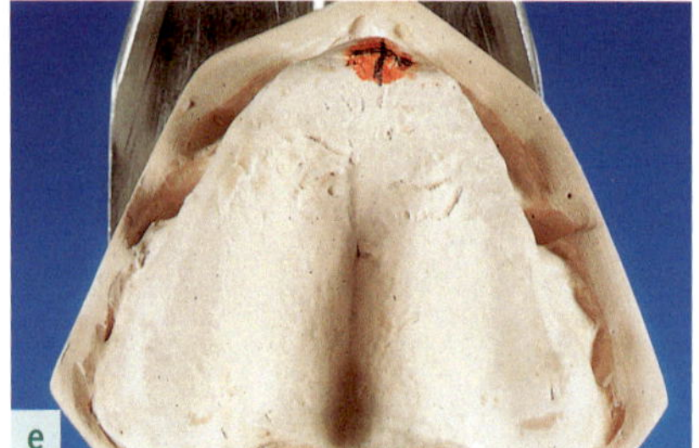
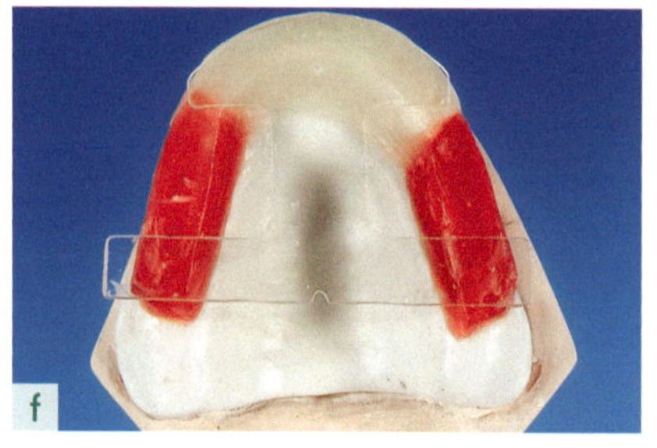
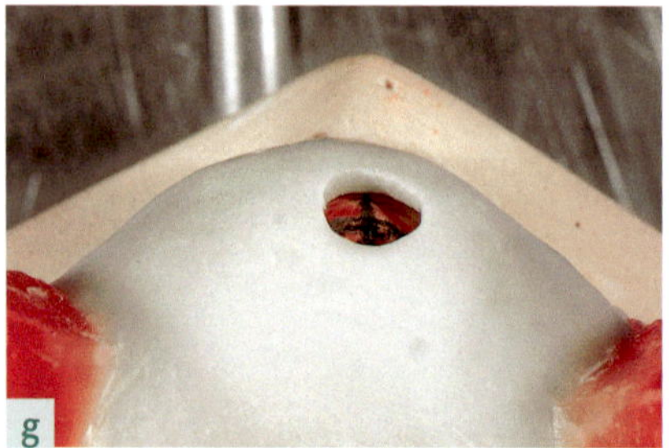
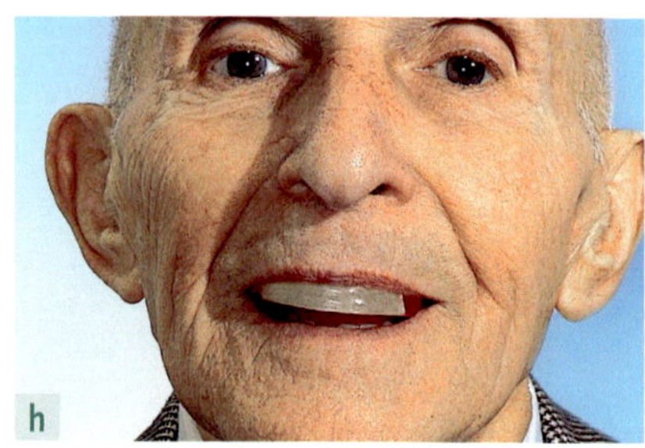
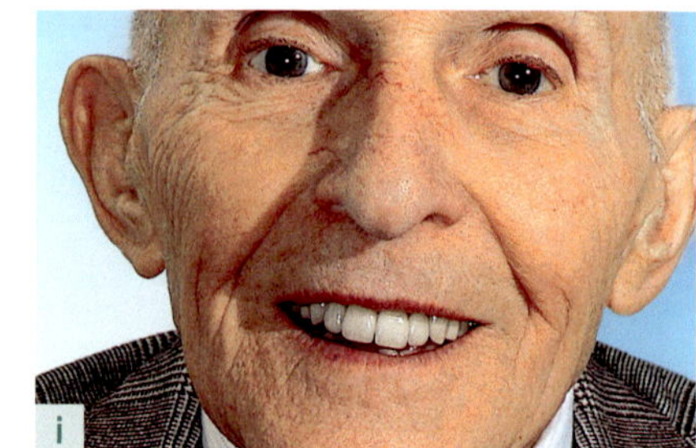

can be useful for the dental technician during preparation of a wax occlusal rim in which the anterior part corresponds approximately to the position of the incisors, in turn facilitating the dentist in positioning the incisors (Fig 3-51).

Positioning maxillary incisors on the vertical plane

The incisal margin of the maxillary teeth should extend about 0.5 mm under the upper lip, and the canines and the first premolars should skim over the lower lip when the mouth is in a half-open position.[84,85] It is opportune to take into consideration that if the upper lip is long, the incisal margin does not appear, whereas with a short lip, a larger portion of the teeth is visible. A reliable parameter is the phonetic one, described for the first time by Robinson[86]: During the pronunciation of the labiodental "f," and "v" the incisal margin of the maxillary incisors should skim over the lower lip. If the "f" sounds like a "v," the teeth are too long.

Positioning the mandibular incisors

The accurate positioning of the mandibular incisors is fundamental to correct support and thus correct phonation. An important parameter for the positioning of both the maxillary and mandibular incisors is the pronunciation of the fricative consonants "s" and "z." The incisal margins should come as close together as possible without touching each other during the pronunciation of these consonants.[87]

Positioning the diatoric teeth according to Gerber

Mounting the diatoric teeth of a complete denture must ensure stability during function. The functional loads must be transmitted perpendicularly on the osteomucosal support, with a stabilizing effect on the denture regardless of the phase of mastication, the morphologic arrangement of the ridges, the maxillomandibular relationship, and the force exercised by the cheeks, lips, and tongue. This method of transmission of the functional loads achieves two favorable conditions: *(1)* During function the dentures are pushed against the respective osteomucosal supports, and the interposed salival film becomes thinner, enhancing the retentive forces; and *(2)* The functional loads that act on the edentulous ridges, mediated by a stable denture, are transmitted across a wider area, favoring conservation of the residual alveolar bone.

The criteria for this method were codified by Gerber in a technique called *multilocularly and independently stable mounting.*[88–91] *Multilocularly stable* requires that every tooth, if functionally loaded, must transmit the loads to the respective osteomucosal support so that the denture is not displaced. *Independently stable* requires that the denture, during function, must offer resistance to dislocation independently of the forces of retention.

This mounting technique is described by Gerber according to the phases of mastication:

- Phase 1: The bolus, while still hard, separates the dental arches.
- Phase 2: The bolus is chopped and the first interdental contacts take place.
- Phase 3: The bolus is swallowed.

Stability in phase 1 of mastication

In the first phase of mastication, the firm bolus separates the dental arches. The mounting is multilocularly and independently stable if the teeth are mounted using the following criteria:
- Compensation of the occlusal inclined planes

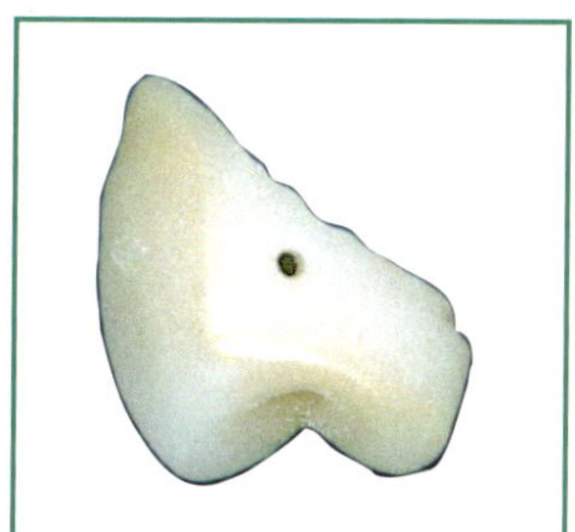

Fig 3-52 Morphology of the sloping buccal and lingual cusp of Condyloform teeth.

- Compensation of the occlusal inclined planes in relation to the morphologic arrangement of the alveolar ridges
- Compensation of the occlusal inclined planes in relation to the incongruence of the ridges, respecting the neutral zone

Compensation of the occlusal inclined planes

Condyloform teeth (Candulator) used to require this type of mounting, ie the occlusal surface of the artificial teeth, in which buccal and palatal/lingual cusp slopes could be distinguished (Fig 3-52). If the palatal/lingual slope is subject to a functional load mediated by the hard bolus, it will tend to transmit it to the inside of the alveolar ridge in a stabilizing action. In contrast, the buccal slope has a displacing effect if subject to a functional load. A stabilizing effect on the denture, in correspondence with a tooth, is obtained when the stabilizing and displacing forces compensate each other and the load is transmitted along the imaginary axis of the artificial tooth, which must ideally correspond to the center of the ridge. The stabilizing or displacing action of the occlusal slopes is influenced by the inclination with which the tooth is mounted. If the tooth is rotated toward the exterior, the stabilizing effect of the palatal/lingual inclined plane prevails; the contrary occurs if the tooth is rotated toward the interior (Fig 3-53). The mandibular premolars and molars of the Condyloform (Fig 3-54) have a buccal wear facet that has a double purpose: *(1)* to reduce the width of the buccal cusp and therefore its displacing action and *(2)* to increase the stabilizing action through its orientation, which is similar to that of the palatal/lingual cusp.

Compensation of inclined occlusal planes in relation to morphologic arrangement of alveolar ridges

The edentulous alveolar ridges often have inclined sagittal and frontal planes. Until the denture stays multilocularly and independently stable during the first phase of mastication, the aforementioned inclinations must be compensated through an appropriate orientation of the occlusal plane. This orientation must ensure that the functional loads are transmitted perpendicularly to the underlying osteomucosal support. For this reason, a careful analysis of the morphology of the edentulous alveolar ridges is necessary. The ridges may be curved on the

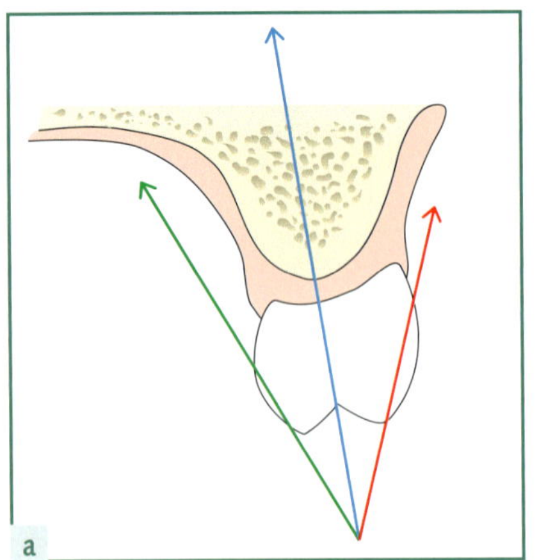 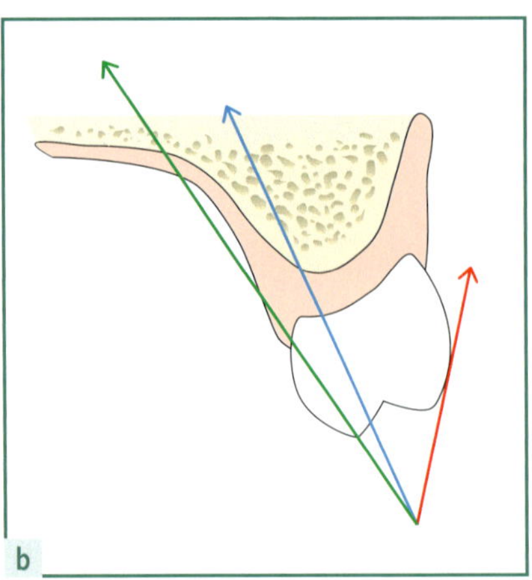 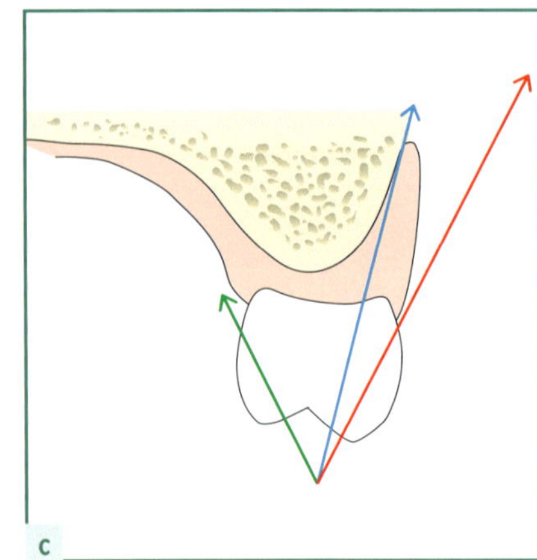

Fig 3-53 Stabilizing and destabilizing influence of a maxilliary posterior tooth depending on its position with respect to the alveolar crest. The tooth perpendicular to the crest *(a)*; rotated buccally *(b)*; rotated lingually *(c)*.

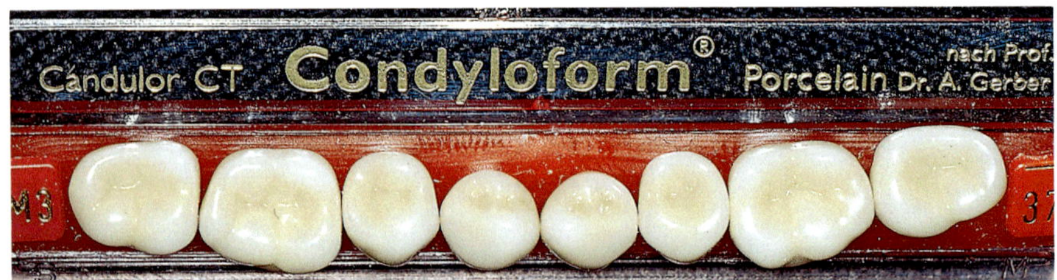

Fig 3-54 Wear facets stabilize the mandibular Condyloform teeth.

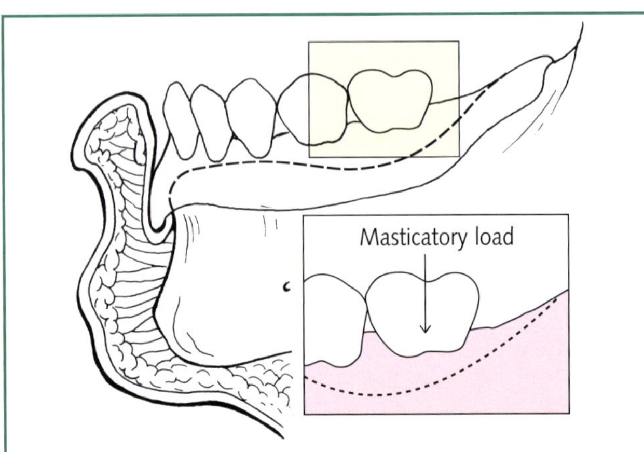

Fig 3-55 Dislocation of the full prosthesis under loading due to the construction of a flat occlusal plane corresponding to use of a curved alveolar crest.

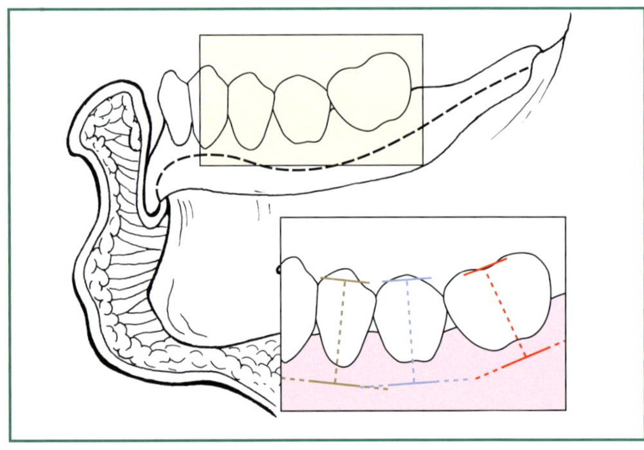

Fig 3-56 Correct preparation of an occlusal plane parallel to the corresponding alveolar crest.

sagittal plane. If in correspondence with a curved ridge a flat artificial occlusal plane is seen, the functional loads will be transferred along an inclined plane, and the denture will tend to be dislocated (Fig 3-55). In the presence of an edentulous alveolar ridge with a curved shape, it is necessary that the occlusal plane follow the same curve to obtain a transmission of the functional loads that is perpendicular to every portion of the underlying alveolar ridge (Fig 3-56). In these conditions the resulting curve of Spee is often accentuated and therefore only apparent in the presence of a very steep sagittal condylar path. In the presence of a flat sagittal condylar path, a curved occlusal plane would cause serious articular interference. In these cases

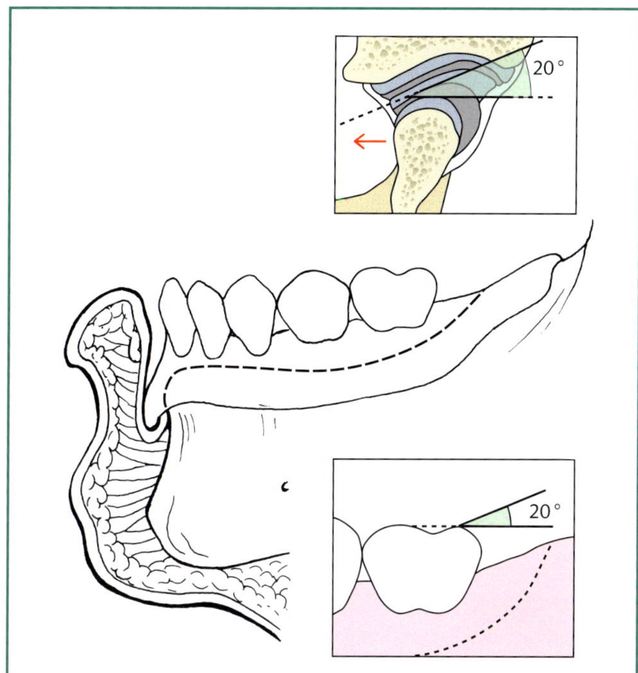

Fig 3-57 With a condylar pathway of 20 degrees at the end of the protruding balance, the occlusal surface is not parallel to a substantial portion of the alveolar crest.

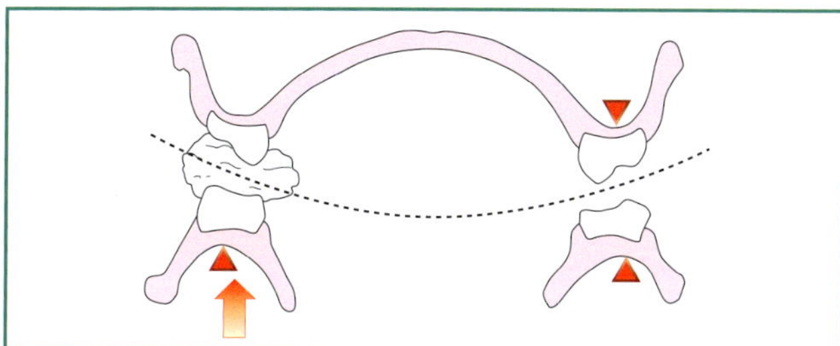

Fig 3-58 Mandibular occlusal surfaces oriented on the frontal plane parallel to the alveolar crest ad linguam. The linear pathway indicates the path of the occlusal plane on the frontal plane. The triangles indicate the summits of the crest.

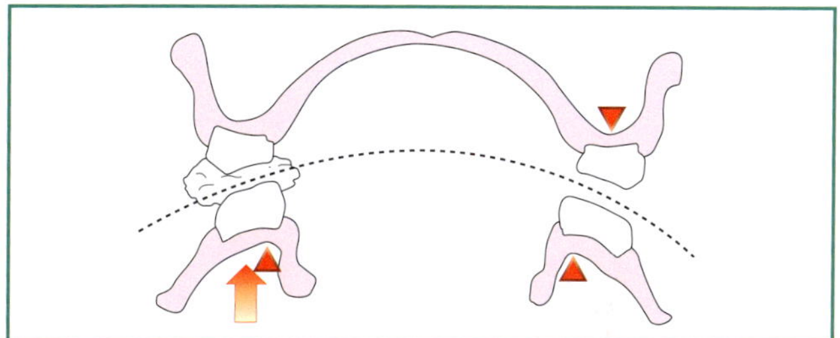

Fig 3-59 Mandibular occlusal surface oriented on the frontal plane, parallel to the course of the alveolar crest ad vestibulum. The linear pathway indicates the path of the occlusal plane on the frontal plane. The triangles indicate the summits of the crest.

it is good practice to fill only the linear portion of the ridge with artificial teeth (Fig 3-57). To achieve correct transmission of the functional loads, the ridges must also be morphologically analyzed on the frontal plane. The development must be analyzed first. For narrow alveolar ridges, occlusal surfaces with a reduced vestibulolingual diameter are indicated (generally only the premolars are used). Furthermore, the presence of inclined planes on ridges with prevalent lingual or buccal development must also be compensated for with adequate orientation of the occlusal surfaces (Figs 3-58 and 3-59).

Compensation of the inclined occlusal planes in relation to the incongruence of the ridges while respecting neutral zones

As noted, the edentulous alveolar ridges tend to resorb. The resorption occurs in a centripetal direction in the maxilla and in a centrifugal direction in the mandible. These different patterns of resorption cause the opposing edentulous ridges to become incongruous on the frontal plane over time. In the completely edentulous mouth, the pattern of resorption also causes a sagittal discrepancy between the jaws: the mandible tends to become more advanced. The incongruence between the edentulous jaws on the frontal and sagittal planes are frequent and often concomitant.

Mounting the teeth in correspondence with the top of resorbed and incongruent ridges often means that good contact with the cheek will not be attained, and tongue movement will be restricted. In theses conditions a space between the cheek on one side and the artificial teeth and external surface of the flange on the other side is created. Food tends to accumulate in this area, and it becomes difficult to push the food from the cheek back between the dental arches. Furthermore, the space between the cheek and the teeth impedes the buccinator muscle from neutralizing the exerted force of the tongue toward the exterior. With this type of mounting, the neutral zone is not respected. On the contrary, trying to mount the artificial teeth in the same position originally occupied by the natural teeth, without considering the compensation of the displacing inclined planes, often has as a consequent transmission of functional loads toward the exterior with respect to the osteomucosal support.

The neutral zone

The natural dental arches are shaped under the influence of genetic factors and the forces of the tongue, lip, and cheek muscles during tooth eruption. The muscular activity is lifelong and continues after the loss of the teeth. In the place of lost

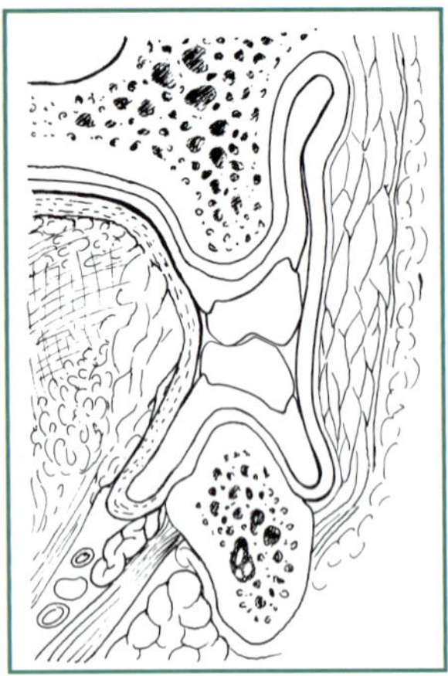

Fig 3-60 Mounting of the teeth, respecting the neutral zone.

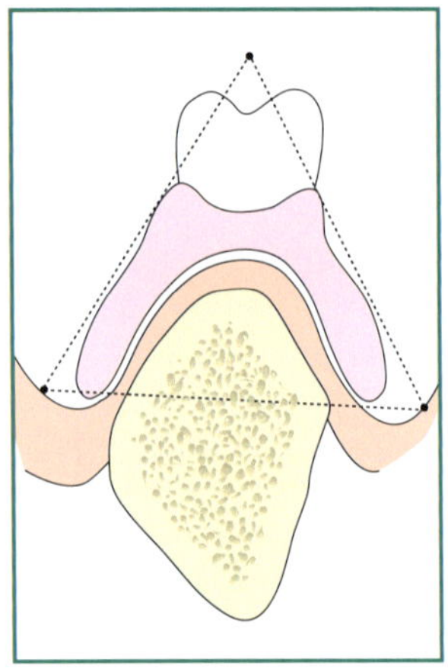

Fig 3-61 Triangular form of the second prosthesis. (From Fish[90].)

teeth, a space forms in the oral cavity, called the *prosthetic space* or the *neutral zone*.[89] This zone can be defined as the area in which the outward forces of the tongue are neutralized by the inward forces of the cheeks and lips during function. Such forces do not act only during mastication but also during speech and swallowing. It is therefore important that the neutral zone be considered when planning artificial teeth and the prosthetic base (Fig 3-60). If not, the denture will be subjected to a continuous horizontal displacing action, which will have repercussions on the edentulous ridges.

In order to receive a stabilizing effect from the muscular forces, the denture saddles must occupy the neutral zone and be able to receive these forces with the correct angulation. According to Fish,[90] in a cross-section at the molar level, a denture must have the form of a triangle, where the apex is the artificial teeth and the base is the peripheral margins of the denture saddle (Fig 3-61). The cheeks and the tongue can exercise their forces on the inclined plane. A force that is exercised on an inclined plane can be subdivided into two components: one that acts in a parallel direction to the inclined plane and one that acts perpendicularly to the inclined plane. If the inclined planes of the prosthetic flanges are modeled correctly and the opposing forces are of equal intensity, the resultant forces are stabilizing.

The artificial teeth must therefore be mounted in the area of the neutral zone. At the same time it is necessary that the functional loads be transmitted perpendicularly to the underlying alveolar ridges independently of their morphology, degree of resorption, and the resulting incongruence. This objective can be reached using the principles of the multilocularly and independently stable setup described in the following section.

Multilocularly and independently stable mounting in maxillomandibular relationships on the frontal plane

The principles are described in relation to common clinical situations.

1. In the presence of congruent, well-shaped edentulous alveolar ridges, from the anatomic point of view there is no difficulty. The setup of the opposing teeth in the center of the respective ridges is easy. The occlusal inclined planes are compensated, and the functional loads are transmitted perpendicularly, with a stabilizing effect on the ridges. The teeth, with the respective prosthetic base, are then located inside the neutral zone (normal occlusion) (Fig 3-62).

2. In the presence of moderately incongruent alveolar ridges (a narrower maxilla), it is possible to keep the maxillary teeth within the neutral zone and at the same time obtain perpendicular transmission of the functional loads on the underlying ridges by inclining them slightly outward. This light rotation enables the displacing action of the buccal cusp to be reduced while the stabilizing action of the palatal cusp is enhanced (reduced occlusion) (Fig 3-63).

3. If the incongruence increases, it is not sufficient to rotate the maxillary teeth outward to obtain the same result described previously. It is also necessary to reduce the buccal cusp by grinding. Often only the fossa is moved when trying to obtain a correct cusp-to-fossa relationship without being constrained to move all the opposing mandibular teeth. The reduction of the buccal cusp improves the transmission of the functional load (minimal occlusion) (Fig 3-64).

4. When the incongruence is such that it cannot be compensated by a reduced or minimal occlusion, it is necessary to resort to the crossbite, where maxillary molars and premolars are moved in a palatal direction. A double disadvantage results, however: The buccal surfaces tend to lose contact with the cheek, and the palatal surface tends to reduce the tongue space. The degree of movement of the maxillary teeth in the palatal direction can be in part reduced by modifying the buccal and palatal cusps. With the remodeling of the buccal cusp, a plane with the same orientation as the occlusal palatal plane is obtained, which therefore has a supplementary stabilizing action (Fig 3-65). Schumman and Palla[92] have shown that with the crossbite, stabilization of the maxillary denture is obtained only if the buccal and palatal cusps are at the same height (Fig 3-66). It is better to avoid this application if there is interference in the biomechanical balance, which is established with the crossbite prosthesis, and difficulty in respecting the neutral zone.

5. In cases of extreme incongruence of the alveolar ridges, it is sometimes necessary to resort to the *cap* setup. To

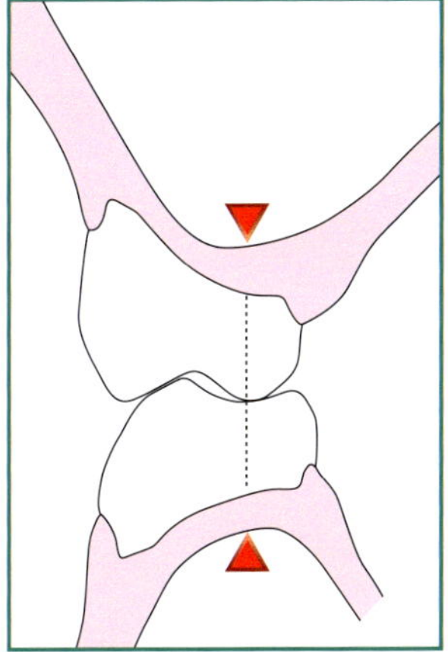

Fig 3-62 Normal occlusion: In the presence of an edentulous crest it is well shaped and congruent.

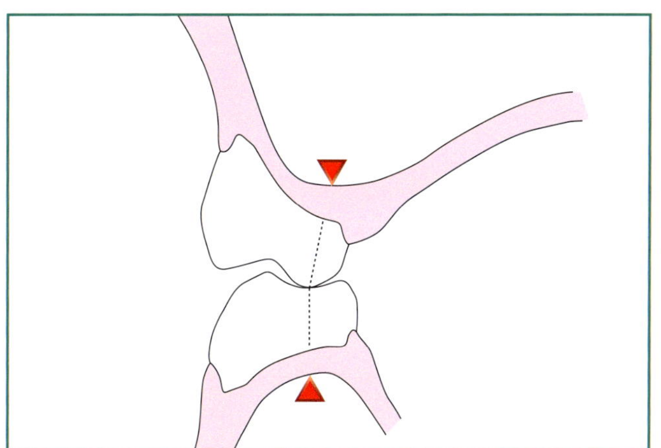

Fig 3-63 Reduced occlusion: In the presence of an edentulous crest it is modified and incongruent. The stabilizing effect is obtained by a slight buccal inclination of the maxillary teeth. The rotated teeth maintain optimal contact with the cheek and do not reduce the tongue space. The resultant drift respects the neutral zone and the transmission of the load to the center of the crest.

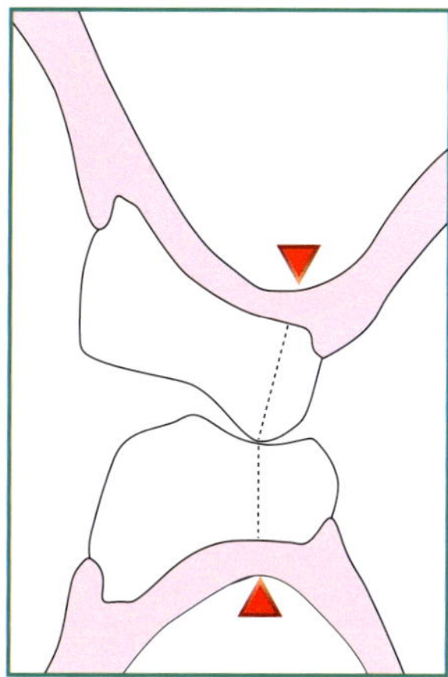

Fig 3-64 Minimal occlusion: In the presence of an incongruent edentulous crest, the stabilizing effect is obtained through rotation of maxillary teeth and grinding of their buccal cusps.

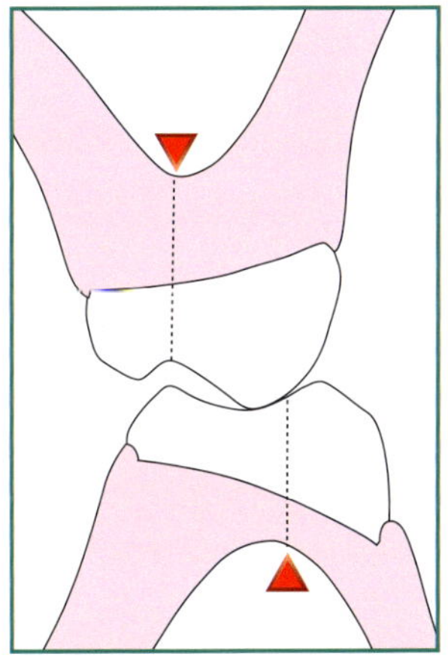

Fig 3-65 Crossbite according to Gerber.[91] Reduction of palatal cusps is recommended to avoid interference during lateral movements.

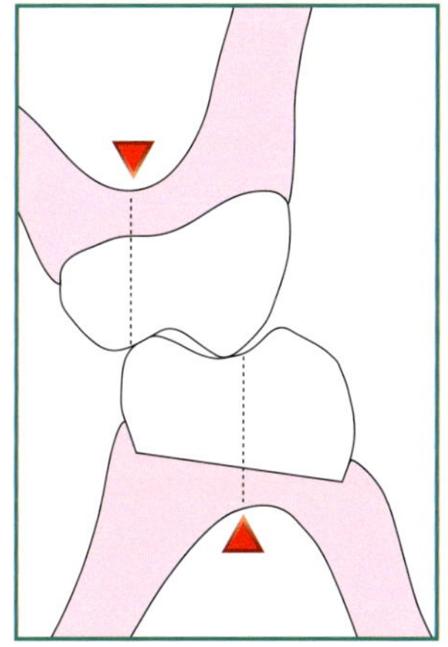

Fig 3-66 Crossbite according to Schumann[92]. The prosthesis is more stable during the first phase of mastication if the buccal and palatal cusps are at the same height.

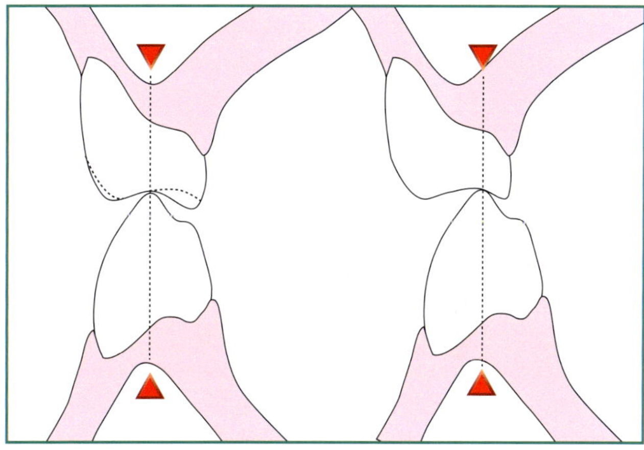

Fig 3-67 In a case where the maxilla is wider that the mandible, the fossae should be moved instead of the maxillary teeth. This example shows the removal of the fossae in the palatal direction and reduction of the sloping of the buccal cusps.

obtain contact with the maxillary teeth, the mandibular occlusal surfaces must be orientated lingually. The forces acting downward therefore have a buccal direction which, in the case of atrophic ridges, often result in displacement. According to Gerber,[91] the cap setup is above all indicated in cases in which the morphology of the mandible has developed in a lingual direction. In these cases the existing parallelism between the occlusal surfaces and alveolar ridges, both oriented lingually, favors the transmission of stabilizing forces. The disadvantage of the cap mounting is the presence of occlusal slopes, which are hyperbalanced in lateral movement because of their lingual inclination.

6. In some cases (eg, class II, deep bite), despite resorption, the mandibular alveolar ridge, particularly in correspondence with the first premolar, is narrower than the maxillary ridge. To avoid moving the maxillary premolar in a palatal direction, only the fossae should be moved. Furthermore, to avoid the displacing effect of the buccal cusp slope, its inclination should be reduced (Fig 3-67).

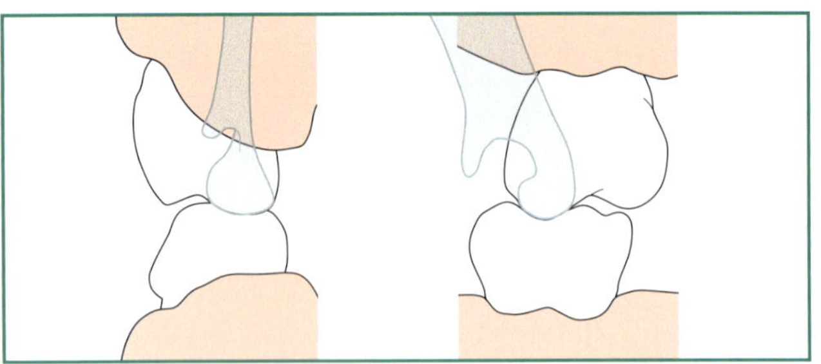

Fig 3-68 Condylar theory of Gerber. The palatal cusp is considered to function like a microcondyle (that is, a pestle) that occludes the fossa of the opposing tooth that acts as a glenoid microcavity (that is, a mortar). *(a)* Frontal view; *(b)* sagittal view.

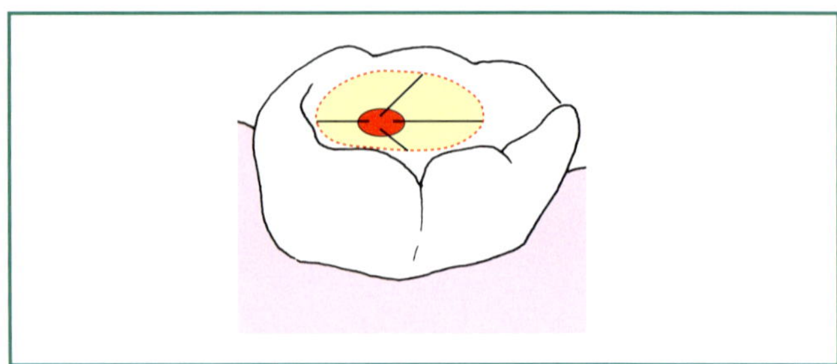

Fig 3-69 Free centric relation obtained by having a pestle of small radius that works in a mortar of a larger dimension.

Stability in phase 2 of mastication

In phase 2 of mastication, as soon as the food is reduced to small pieces, the first interdental contacts occur. These contacts occur frequently in MI and around this position (mesially, distally, buccally, and lingually).[93] The degree of lateral sliding varies from cycle to cycle and depends on the type of occlusion, the degree of abrasion, and the type of food.[94] To avoid displacement of the denture or a mandibular dislocation in the case of a very stable denture, it is necessary that: *(1)* the determination of maxillomandibular relationships on the horizontal plane take into consideration both the correct condyle–articular disc–temporal relationships and the paths of muscular closure and *(2)* the occlusion has freedom around the MI, since the paths of muscular closure are influenced by the position of the head (the dorsal flexion of the head provokes a distal movement of the mandible and vice versa), which is not an evaluable parameter during the determination of the maxillomandibular relationships on the horizontal plane. This freedom around the maximal ICP can be foreseen using the concept of lingualized occlusion when planning Condyloform teeth placement.[95]

The purpose of lingualized occlusion with respect to anatomic occlusion is to simplify the tooth mounting to avoid interferences in phase 2 mastication without penalizing efficiency.

By applying the conventional concept of anatomic occlusion, the buccal and lingual cusps of the opposing teeth come into contact during lateral movements. By applying lingualized occlusion, the number of contacts is considerably reduced. In MI only the lingual cusps of the maxillary posterior teeth come into contact with the central fossae of the mandibular teeth, whereas the buccal cusps do not come into contact. However, there exists only one centric stop for every pair of opposing teeth.

Around the end of the 1950s, Gerber made an important modification to the concept of lingualized occlusion. The interdental relationship at the level of the first premolar was

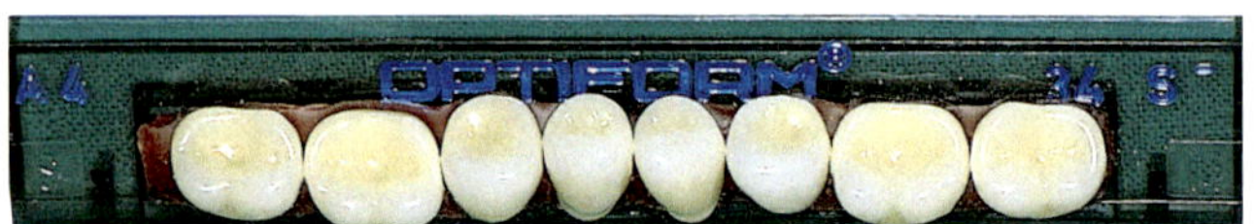

Fig 3-70 Diatoric teeth from Optiform. The ample central fossae require minimal selective grinding.

inverted: the cusp of the first mandibular premolar occludes with the mesial fossa of the first maxillary premolar. As a result the canine and premolar create a scissor effect, which improves masticatory efficiency. The occlusion is of the tooth-to-tooth type. Gerber also introduced the concept of *condylar theory*, according to which the palatal cusp of every tooth is considered a sort of microcondyle, which acts like a pestle and comes into contact with the fossa of the corresponding tooth. The fossa constitutes the mortar and is considered a microglenoid fossa. The pestle and mortar relationships are inverted at the level of the premolar, where the pestle consists of the cusp of the mandibular tooth and the mortar of the fossa of the maxillary tooth (Fig 3-68). With selective drilling, the freedom around the MI is determined through the small radius of the pestle, which contacts a mortar with a bigger radius (Fig 3-69).

In 1987, a series of teeth called Optiform (ENTA BV) were created according to the concept of lingualized occlusion and the condylar theory of Gerber, whereby the fossae of the mandibular teeth are preshaped so that the selective grinding around the centric stop is almost superfluous (Fig 3-70).

Whatever the choice of diatoric teeth, Condyloform or Optiform, after the polymerization but before finishing the prosthetic bodies the contacts in protrusion, retrusion, and lateral movements must take place without interference. Selective grinding allows for eventual corrections of small errors that can occur during transformation of the prosthetic bodies from wax to resin. Through selective grinding it is possible to modify the morphology of the occlusal slopes of the diatoric teeth in rela-

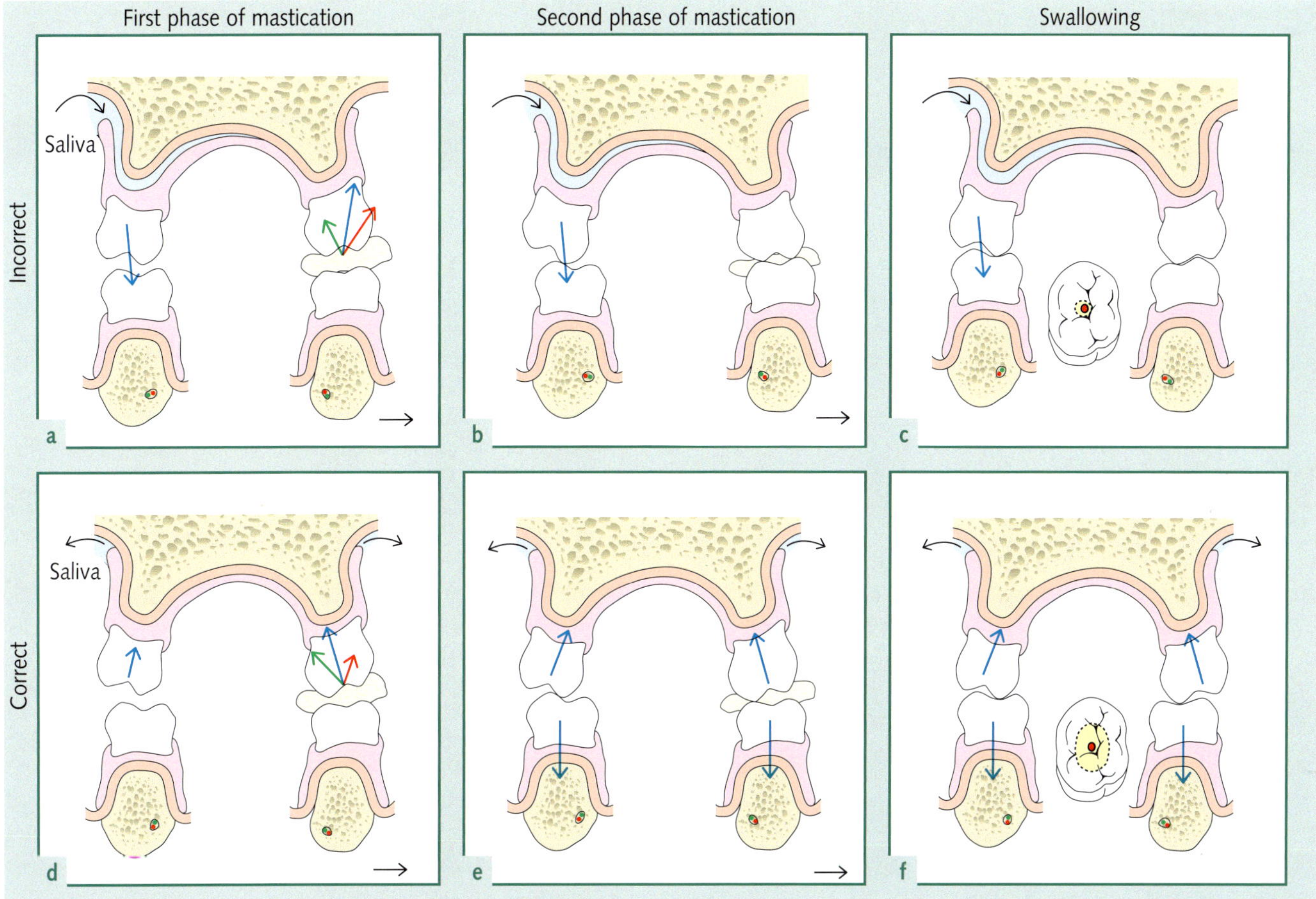

Fig 3-71 *(a)* In the first phase of mastication the bolus separates the dental arches. In this case the displacing forces (red) are greater with respect to the stabilizing forces (green). The displacing force is greater than the forces of adhesion, cohesion, and surface tension. The meniscum is interrupted, and saliva from the outside is attracted, interposing between the prosthetic body and the mucosa, causing the detachment/displacement of the denture. *(b)* In the second phase of mastication the food is mashed and, if unbalanced, interdental contacts occur, and the denture abandons its osteomucosal support. *(c)* The presence of precontacts in ICP provokes detachment of the denture. The area of freedom around the CR is too reduced. *(d to f)* Mistakes have been eliminated, and in the three phases of mastication the denture is pushed against the respective alveolar ridges, the saliva flows out, the interposed saliva film diminishes in thickness, and the retention of the denture increases.

tion to the movements of the articulator. This step ensures that simultaneous contacts are obtained on the working side and the balancing side of all the occlusal slopes of the teeth.

Stability during deglutition

During deglutition, occlusal contacts last longer than they do during mastication[95] (683 milliseconds versus 194 milliseconds). Deglutition occurs hundreds of times during the day and night. Occlusal contacts in deglutition occur in MI; however, contact can come about in a more distal position. It is therefore necessary that between centric occlusion (CO) and CR, no precontact occurs that would provoke an overload. With selective grinding in retrusion carried out on the Condylator, it is possible to eliminate eventual precontacts in the CO-CR path.

Summary

During function, the complete denture keeps in contact with the respective alveolar ridge because of the interaction of retention, stability, and support. An optimum interaction of these factors is obtained, anatomic conditions being equal, through the accuracy of every foreseen step during the manufacturing of the complete denture (impression, determination of the maxillomandibular relationships, and mounting of the teeth). Figure 3-71 summarizes these concepts.

References

1. Hardy IR, Kapur KK. Posterior border seal—Its rationale and importance. J Prosthet Dent 1958;8:386–397. Cat. 7
2. Gerber A, Defabianis E, Mongini F, Preti G. I problemi basilari in protesi totale. Minerva Stomatol 1967;16:689–692. Cat. 7
3. Appelbaum M. Il sigillo palatino posteriore. In: Winkler S. Protesi totale. Padova: Piccin, 1988:171–192. Cat. 7
4. Lye TL. The significance of the fovea palatina in complete denture prosthodontics. J Prosthet Dent 1975;33:504–510. Cat. 4
5. Millsap CH. Posterior palatal seal area for complete denture. Dent Clin North Am 1964;8:663–673. Cat. 7
6. Maurizio A, Spirgi M, Logoz A. La rétention des prothéses totales adjointes supérieures et inférieures: Facteurs physiques et éléments anatomo-physiologiques à exploiter et à respecter. SSO Schweiz Monatsschr Zahnheilkd 1974;84:1063–1081. Cat. 7
7. Douglas JR, Maritato FR. "Open Rest," a new concept in the selection of the vertical dimension of occlusion. J Prosthet Dent 1965;15:850–856. Cat. 4
8. Sears VH. An analysis of art factors in full denture construction. J Am Dent Assoc Dental Cosmos 1938;25:3–12. Cat. 8
9. Monbelli A, Geering AH. Zur aestetischen Wirkung des Zahnersatzes. SSO Schweiz Monatsschr Zahnheilkd 1982;92: 586–596. Cat. 3
10. Hartono R. The occlusal plane in relation to facial types. J Prosthet Dent 1967;17:549–558. Cat. 4
11. Koller MM, Merlini L, Spandre G, Palla S. A comparative study of two methods for the orientation of the occlusal plane and the determination of the vertical dimension of occlusion in edentulous patients. J Oral Rehabil 1992;19:413–425. Cat. 2
12. Bassi F, Deregibus A, Previgliano V, Bracco P, Preti G. Evaluation of the utility of cephalometric parameters in constructing complete denture. Part I: Placement of posterior teeth. J Oral Rehabil 2001;28:234–238. Cat. 2
13. Monteith BD. A cephalometric method to determine the angulation of the occlusal plane in edentulous patients. J Prosthet Dent 1985;54:81–87. Cat. 4
14. Hickey JC, Zarb GA, Bolender CL. Boucher's Prosthodontic treatment for Edentulous Patients, ed 9. St Louis: Mosby, 1985:355. Cat. 7
15. Niswonger ME. Obtaining the vertical relation in edentulous cases that existed prior to extraction. J Am Dent Assoc Dental Cosmos 1938;25:1842–1847. Cat. 9
16. Thompson JR, Brodie AG. Factors in the position of the mandible. J Am Dent Assoc 1942;29:925–941. Cat. 7
17. Thompson JR. The rest position of the mandible and its significance to dental science. J Am Dent Assoc 1946;33:151–180. Cat. 4
18. Cohen MM. Clinical studies in the development of dental height. Am J Orthod 1950;36:917–932. Cat. 8
19. Thompson JR. Concepts regarding function of the stomatognathic system. J Am Dent Assoc 1954;48:626–637. Cat. 7
20. Pound E. Controlling anomalies of vertical dimension and speech. J Prosthet Dent 1976;36:124–135. Cat. 7
21. Ismail YH, George WA, Sassouni V, Scott RH. Cephalometric study of the changes occurring in the face height following prosthetic treatment. I. Gradual reduction of both occlusal and rest face heights. J Prosthet Dent 1968;19:321–330. Cat. 3
22. Lambadakis J, Karkazis HC. Changes in the mandibular rest position after removal of remaining teeth and insertion of complete dentures. J Prosthet Dent 1992;68:74–77. Cat. 3
23. Ismail YH, Sassouni V. Cephalometric study of the changes occurring in the face height following prosthetic treatment. II. Variability in the rate of face height reduction. J Prosthet Dent 1968;19: 331–337. Cat. 4
24. Preiskel HW. Some observations on the postural position of the mandible. J Prosthet Dent 1965;15:625–633. Cat. 4
25. Carlsson GE. An international comparative multicenter study of assessment of dental appearance using computer-aided image manipulation. Int J Prosthodont 1998;18:246–254. Cat. 2
26. Palla S. Registration of maxillo mandibular relationship [in German]. In: Hupfauf L (ed). Total Prothesen, ed 3. München, Baltimora: Urban & Schwarzenberg, 1991:133–194. Cat. 7
27. Modica R. Il ripristino dell'occlusione nell'edentulo. Minerva Stomatol 1968;17:486–531. Cat. 7
28. Tryde G, McMillian DR, Christensen J, Brill N. The fallacy of facial measurements of occlusal height in edentulous subjects. J Oral Rehabil 1976;3:353–358. Cat. 2
29. Ekfeldt A, Jemt T, Mansson L. Interocclusal distance measurement comparing chin and tooth reference points. J Prosthet Dent 1982;47:560–563. Cat. 4
30. Carossa S, Catapano S, Scotti R, Preti G. The unreliability of facial measurements in the determination of the vertical dimension of occlusion in edentulous patients. J Oral Rehabil 1990;17:287–290. Cat. 2
31. Gattozzi JG, Nicol BR, Somes GW, Ellinger CW. Variations in mandibular rest positions with and without dentures in place. J Prosthet Dent 1976;36:159–163. Cat. 2
32. Fish SF. The respiratory associations of the rest position of the mandible. Br Dent J 1964;116:149–159. Cat. 4
33. Burnett CA, Clifford TJ. Closest speaking space during the production of sibilant sounds and its value in establishing the vertical dimension of occlusion. J Dent Res 1993;72:964–967. Cat. 4
34. Silverman MM. Vertical dimension must not be increased. J Prosthet Dent 1952;2:188–197. Cat. 8
35. Geissler PR. Studies of mandibular movements in speech. J Dent 1975;3:256–260. Cat. 4
36. Clémençon R. Das Beruhren in engsten Sprechabstand—Ein Trigger factor? SSO Schweiz Monatsschr Zahnheilkd 1967a;77: 251–254. Cat. 8
37. Clémençon R. Beitrag zur Feineinstellung der Bisshhe. SSO Schweiz Monatsschr Zahnheilkd 1967b;77:425–428. Cat. 8
38. Schierano G, Mozzati M, Bassi F, Preti G. Influence of the thickness of the resin palatal vault on the closest speaking space with complete dentures. J Oral Rehabil 2001;28:903–908. Cat. 2
39. Ichikawa J, Komoda J, Horiuchi M, Matsumoto N. Influence of alterations in the oral environment on speech production. J Oral Rehabil 1995;22:295–299. Cat. 3
40. Tsuchiya M, Lowe AA, Pae EK, Fleetham JA. Obstructive sleep apnea subtypes by cluster analysis. Am J Orthod Dentofacial Orthop 1992;101:533–542. Cat. 2
41. Lowe AA, Ozbek MM, Miyamoto K, Pae EK, Fleetham JA. Cephalometric and demographic characteristics of obstructive sleep apnea: An evalutation with partial least squares analysis. Angle Orthod 1997;67:143–153. Cat. 3

42. Rivera-Morales WC, Mohl ND. Variability of closest speaking space compared with interocclusal distance in dentulous subjects. J Prosthet Dent 1991;65:228–232. Cat. 4

43. Palla S. Occlusal consideration in complete denture. In: McNeill C (ed). Science and Practice of Occlusion. Chicago: Quintessence, 1997:457–468. Cat. 7

44. Kawazoe Y, Hamada T. The role of saliva in retention of maxillary dentures. J Prosthet Dent 1978;40:131–136. Cat. 4

45. Niedermeier W, Hofmann M. Die Beeinflussung der physikalischen Grundhaftung von Totalprothesen durch die Anordnung der künstlichen Zahnreihen. Dtsch Zaharztl Z 1979;34:616–618. Cat. 4

46. Firtell DN, Finzen FC, Holmes JB. The effect of clinical remount procedures on the comfort and success of complete dentures. J Prosthet Dent 1987;57:53–57. Cat. 2

47. Preti G, Bassi F, Barbero P, Lorenzetti M, Valente G. Histological changes in edentulous oral mucosa under implant-supported overdentures. J Oral Rehabil 1996;23:651–654. Cat. 4

48. Garzino M, Ramieri G, Panzica G, Preti G. Changes in the density of protein gene product 9.5-immunoreactive nerve fibres in human oral mucosa under implant-retained overdentures. Arch Oral Biol 1996;41:1073–1079. Cat. 2

49. Schierano G, Bassi F, Gassino G, Mareschi K, Bellone G, Preti G. Cytokine production and bone remodeling in patients wearing overdentures on oral implants. J Dent Res 2000;79:1675–1682. Cat. 2

50. Niedermeier W. Physikalische grundlagen beim halt der totalprothese. Dtsch Zahnarztl Z 1982;37:708–717. Cat. 4

51. Preti G, Gassino G, Lombardi M, Mazzone P. Monitoring of the discrimination threshold for interocclusal thicknesses in rehabilitated edentulous patients. J Oral Rehabil 1994;21:185–190. Cat. 2

52. Schierano G, Arduino E, Bosio E, Preti G. The influence of selective grinding on the thickness discrimination threshold of patients wearing complete dentures. J Oral Rehabil 2002;29:184–187. Cat. 2

53. Lambadakis J, Karkaziz H. Changes in the mandibular rest position after removal of remaining teeth and insertion of complete dentures. J Prosthet Dent 1992;68:74–77. Cat. 3

54. Helkimo M, Ingervall B, Carlsson GE. Variation of retruded and muscular position of mandible under different recording conditions. Acta Odontol Scand 1971;29:423–435. Cat. 4

55. Esposito SJ. Esthetics for denture patients. J Prosthet Dent 1980;44:608–615. Cat. 7

56. Yarbus AL. Eye movements and vision. New York: Plenum Press, 1967. Cat. 7

57. Stein MR. Williams' classification of anterior tooth forms. Am Dent Assoc J 1936;23:1512–1518. Cat. 9

58. Carlsson GE, Wagner IV, Odman P, et al. An international comparative multicenter study of assessment of dental appearance using computer-aided image manipulation. Int J Prosthodont 1998;11:246–254. Cat. 2

59. Lefer L, Pleasure MA. Psychiatric approach to denture patient. Psychosom Res 1962;6:199–207. Cat. 2

60. Hirsch B, Levin B, Tiber N. Effects of patient involvement and esthetic preference on denture acceptance. J Prosthet Dent 1972;28:127–132. Cat. 2

61. McCord JF, Burke T, Roberts C, Deakin M. Perceptions of denture aesthetics: A two-centre study of denture wearers and denture providers. Aus Dent J 1994;39:365–367. Cat. 4

62. Wagner IV, Carlsson GE, Ekstrand K, Odman P, Schneider N. A comparative study of assessment of dental appearance by dentists, dental technicians, and laymen using computer-aided image manipulation. J Esthet Dent 1996;8:199–205. Cat. 3

63. Frush JP, Fisher RD. Dentogenics: Its practical application. J Prosthet Dent 1958;6:914–921. Cat. 9

64. Belser UC. Esthetics checklist for the fixed prosthesis. Part II: Biscuit try-in. In: Scharer P, Rinn LA, Kopp FR (eds). Esthetic Guidelines for Restorative Dentistry. Chicago: Quintessence, 1982;188–192. Cat. 7

65. Lombardi RE. The principles of visual perception and their clinical application to denture esthetics. J Prosthet Dent 1973;29: 358–382. Cat. 7

66. Woodhead C. The mesiodistal diameter of permanent maxillary central incisor teeth and their prosthetics replacements. J Dent 1977;5:93–98. Cat. 4

67. Portalier. Comunicazione personale congresso AIOP 1998. Cat. 9

68. Gerber A. Dominante ästhetische und klinische Probleme des Frontzahnersatzes. Zahnärtliche Rundschau 1960:10. Cat. 7

69. Scotti R, Pera P, Sedran A. Studio clinico-statistico sui rapporti dimensionali tra incisivi centrale e laterali e base e radice del naso. Minerva Stomatol 1988;37:813–817. Cat. 4

70. Bedsford J. Comunicazione personale al congresso the 8th annual convention di Beirut-Levanon, 2000. Cat. 9

71. Merlini C. Face profile improvement: Psychological aspects. In Bassi F, Carossa S, Gassino G, et al. (eds). Advances in Clinical Prosthodontics. Padova: Piccin, 1999:126–146. Cat. 7

72. Frush JP, Fisher RD. Introduction to dentogenic restorations. J Prosthet Dent 1955;5:586–595. Cat. 9

73. Bliss CH. Philosophy of patient education. Dent Clin North Am July 1960:277–292. Cat. 7

74. Curtis TA, Shaw FI, Curtis DA. The influence of removable prosthodontic procedures and concepts on the esthetics of complete dentures. J Prosthet Dent 1987;57:315–323. Cat. 7

75. Atwood DA, Coy WA. Clinical, cephalometric, and densitometric study of reduction of residual ridges. J Prosthet Dent 1971;26: 280–295. Cat. 3

76. Tallgren A. The continuing reduction of the residual alveolar ridges in complete denture wearers: A mixed-longitudinal study covering 25 years. J Prosthet Dent 1972;27:120–132. Cat. 4

77. Bergman B, Carlsson GE. Clinical long-term study of complete denture wearers. J Prosthet Dent 1985;53:56–61. Cat. 4

78. Lambadakis J, Karkazis HC. Changes in the mandibular rest position after removal of remaining teeth and insertion of complete dentures. J Prosthet Dent 1992;68:74–77. Cat. 3

79. Bassi F, Rizzatti A, Schierano G, Preti G. Evaluation of the utility of cephalometric parameters in constructing complete denture. Part II: Placement of anterior teeth. J Oral Rehabil 2001;28:349–353. Cat. 2

80. Harper RN. Incisive papilla-basis of a technique to reproduce the positions of key teeth in prosthodontics. J Dent Res 1948;27: 661–668. Cat. 8

81. Schiffman P. Relation of the maxillary canines to the incisive papilla. J Prosthet Dent 1964;14:469–472. Cat. 4

82 Marxkors R. Die Aufstellung der Frontzähne. ZWR 1975;84: 522–527. Cat. 4

83. Preti G, Pera P, Bassi F. Prediction of the shape and size of the maxillary anterior arch in edentulous patients. J Oral Rehabil 1986;13: 115–125. Cat. 4

84. Sears VH. An analysis of art factors in full denture construction. J Am Dent Assoc Dental Cosmos 1938;25:3–12. Cat. 3

85. Mombelli A, Geering AH. Zur aesthetischen wirkung des zahnersatzes. SSO Schweiz Monatsschr Zahnheilkd 1982;92:586–596. Cat. 7

86. Robinson SC. Physiological placement of artificial anterior teeth. J Can Dent Assoc 1969;35(5):260–266. Cat. 9

87. Silverman MM. The speaking method in measuring vertical dimension. J Prosthet Dent 1953;3:193–199. Cat. 7

88. Gerber A, Defabianis E, Mongini F, Preti G. I problemi basilari in protesi totale. Minerva Stomatol 1967;16:689–692. Cat. 7

89. Beresin VE, Schiesser FJ. The neutral zone in complete and partial dentures. Chicago: Mosby, 1978. Cat. 7

90. Fish W. Using the muscles to stabilize the full lower denture. J Am Dent Assoc 1933;20:2163–2169. Cat. 9

91. Gerber A. Complete denture. IV. The teamwork of complete dentures in chewing-function. Quintessence Int Dent Dig 1974;5: 41–46. Cat. 4

92. Schumann R, Palla S. Untersuchung über den Einfluss der Okklusionsgestaltung auf die Richtung der okklusalen Kräfte beim Kauen in der Totalprothetik. Schweiz Monatsschr Zahnheilk 1986;96: 935–946. Cat. 4

93. Woda A, Vigneron P, Kay D. Nonfunctional occlusal contacts: A review of the literature. J Prosthet Dent 1979;42:335–341. Cat. 7

94. Gibbs CH, Mahan PE, Lundeen HC, Brehnan K, Walsh EK. Occlusal forces during chewing and swallowing as measured with sound transmission. J Prosthet Dent 1981;46(4):443–449. Cat. 3

95. Becker CM, Swoope CC, Guckes AD. Lingualized occlusion for removable prosthodontics. J Prosthet Dent 1977;38:601–608. Cat. 7

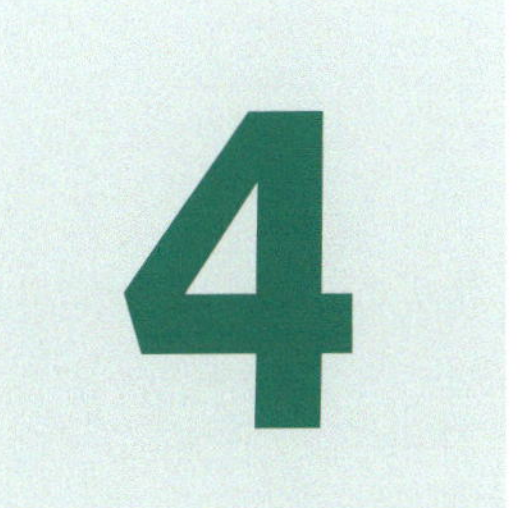

Introduction to Prosthetic Rehabilitation of Edentulous Patients

Prosthetic rehabilitation of the edentulous patient is not only a challenge in terms of technical skill but also in terms of the ability to understand and sympathize with the patient. The success of treatment depends on a complex interaction of psychologic, biologic, and constructive factors.[1–3]

The loss of teeth is a traumatic event, which the psychiatrist Botta[4] described as follows:

> Tooth loss may also affect the person's entire life. . . . [It is necessary] to distinguish between efficiency and attractiveness to characterize the emphasis placed on certain parts of the body. On the subject of attractiveness of different parts of the face, statistics showed dentition to be referred to most often (followed in order by the shape of the nose, the shape of the face, and voice quality). In line with this observation, it can be said that people who have lost their teeth have also lost a source of self-satisfaction. This is a problem of self-image. . . . People who have lost their teeth are disoriented, which is why this loss is their principal concern [...] Having lost teeth, however, they are enormously concerned about the empty space left by the missing teeth and typically express their feelings of loss with the classic complaint 'Oh I wish I still had my teeth!'
> This complaint is an attempt to reconstitute a sort of imaginary possibility, an attempt to avoid a fate which they feel helpless to resist. However, they also appeal to the practitioner to change the course of events. . . . They observe themselves, look at themselves in the mirror, and note how other people see them. . . . If this necessary phase lasts too long, patient-practitioner relationships may suffer, and even lead to conflict."

A patient's reaction to edentulism and the treatment process is individual and unpredictable.[5] Therefore, individualized consideration should be given to the patient's emotional state and concerns. However, the patient's view of the ideal denture may not be what is clinically recommended or even possible. If the satisfaction of the patient is adopted as the exclusive criteria to evaluate the success of a denture, there is a risk that the resulting denture will be incongruous to what is clinically appropriate for the patient. Collett[6] describes the process of "overadaptation" by some patients, for whom check-ups and eventual corrections and modifications become useless. Ideally, prosthetic rehabilitation should satisfy both the patient and the clinician. The clinician must, with respect to the expectations of the patient, satisfy the constructive criteria as well.

Patient Satisfaction and Incorporation of the Complete Denture

The majority of edentulous patients (70% to 80%) are satisfied with their complete denture once they have adapted to it.[7,8] These patients are motivated, have modest expectations, cooperate, and accept advice and instructions. However, a certain percentage of patients are unsatisfied, often because of psychologic problems unrelated to their oral health. The scientific community has undertaken much research concerning this issue but has not reached an unequivocal conclusion.[9–24] More than one author agrees that oral function does not seem to be correlated to the satisfaction of these patients. Satisfaction seems to correlate more with sociopsychologic background.[25,26] The efforts of even the most prepared specialist do not satisfy such patients, who may have exaggerated expectations.

They also may be nervous, depressed, and have impaired neuromuscular coordination, which is necessary for the incorporation of the denture. The causes of this behavior are often attributed to a distorted perception of body image and function, leading to anxiety and depression.[27] Depression is most prevalent in the later years, defined by Klerman[28] as "the age of melancholy." Chamberlain and Chamberlain[29] subjected hundreds of patients with complete dentures to the Beck Depression Inventory (BDI), a semistructured interview that is considered a valid instrument for identifying depression (Box 4-1). The authors ascertained that the majority of patients in the older age groups—in which edentulism is most frequent—

Box 4-1 Beck Depression Inventory (BDI) Questionnaire

This questionnaire is composed of 13 groups of phrases. Carefully read all the phrases in each group and choose the phrase that best describes you now—circle the number next to the phrase you have chosen.

1.
0 = No, I don't feel sad
1 = I feel sad or unhappy
2 = I feel unhappy and sad all the time and I don't know how to change
3 = I am so sad and unhappy that I can't support this

2.
0 = No, I don't feel very pessimistic or discouraged about the future
1 = I feel discouraged about the future
2 = I don't expect anything positive for the future
3 = I feel without hope for the future and things will not get better

3.
0 = No, I don't feel that I am a failure
1 = I feel that I have done bad things to others
2 = If I think of my past, I see only many errors
3 = I feel that as a person (parent, wife, husband…) I am a total failure

4.
0 = No, I am not particularly unsatisfied
1 = I don't enjoy any more the things as in the past
2 = There is nothing that gives me satisfaction anymore
3 = I am unsatisfied with everything

5.
0 = No, I don't feel particularly guilty
1 = Often I feel bad and I don't feel valued
2 = I feel rather guilty
3 = I feel that I am very bad and without any value

6.
0 = No, I don't feel disappointed in myself
1 = I am disappointed in myself
2 = I am disgusted by myself
3 = I hate myself

7.
0 = No, I don't think about hurting myself
1 = I think that it would be better if I were dead
2 = I have made precise plans of killing myself
3 = I would kill myself if I had the possibility

8.
0 = No, I have not lost interest in others
1 = With respect to the past I am less interested in others
2 = I have lost the major part of my intersest in others
3 = I have lost all interest in others and I don't worry about others

9.
0 = I make my decisions as always
1 = I tend to put off making decisions
2 = I have a lot of difficulties in making decisions
3 = I am not able to make any decisions

10.
0 = No, I don't feel worse than in the past
1 = I am worried because I feel old and not attractive
2 = I feel that I have permanent changes in my appearance and am not attractive
3 = I think that I am ugly and revolting

11.
0 = I work well just as always
1 = To start to do something takes me a lot of effort
2 = I have to make a great effort to do anything
3 = I am not able to do anything

12.
0 = No, I am not more tired that usual
1 = I get tired more than I used to
2 = Doing anything makes me very tired
3 = I can't start anything anymore

13.
0 = My appetite is the same as always
1 = My appetite is not as good as before
2 = My appetite is much less than before
3 = I really don't have any appetite for anything.

Patients who score 9 or more can be considered as having a mood disturbance of a depressive type (minor depression, major depression, or an adaptation disturbance) had depressive symptoms (Fig 4-1). Patients who have difficulty adapting to complete dentures can be classified in the following manner[27]:

- Class I: Patients who experience the loss of teeth as a serious limitation to their quality of life and who adapt to the denture physically but not emotionally.
- Class II: Patients who do not adapt to the denture either emotionally or physically and who do not accept the loss of teeth or the denture. They require an enormous amount of attention.
- Class III: Patients who do not wear a denture and who do not ask for help from the clinician. They become chronically depressed and isolate themselves from society.

Compensatory incorporation is a process through which the manufactured denture is integrated into the natural oral structures, is in harmony with the complex functions of the mouth, and is accepted psychologically by the patient.[30]

The incorporation of a denture is important for structural integrity so that the remaining oral structures are kept in good health. An incongruous denture accelerates the deterioration of these structures; moreover, a significant correlation has been shown between pain and occlusal disturbances.[31] Occlusal harmony, on the other hand, preserves both the soft and hard support tissue.[32–34] A correct occlusion allows the patient to discriminate thickness and to modulate mandibular dynamics in such a way that the masticatory load is contained within physiologic limits.[35]

A complete denture can be considered incorporated when it does not separate from the osteomucosal support during function, does not provoke pain, and is accepted by the patient. This result cannot, however, always be guaranteed. Besides psychologic interferences, there may be systemic or local conditions that interfere with the incorporation of the denture. Older patients frequently have systemic illnesses that need pharmacologic treatment. It has been calculated that 55% of medications taken by older patients inhibit salivation,[36] and reduced salivary flow has a negative effect on the retention of the denture and on the health of the supporting tissues.[37,38]

Other conditions that hinder the incorporation of the denture are those that interfere with neuromuscular control, a determining factor in the stability of the denture in terms of resistance to horizontal and rotational dislocating forces. Older patients may have more difficulty controlling dentures neuromuscularly,[39] because of progressive cerebral atrophy. The motor ability and the ability to adapt to the complete denture are not, however, strictly linked to age, nor is aging strictly linked to chronologic age. Thus, there is considerable individual variation in oral motor ability and adaptation capacity.[40]

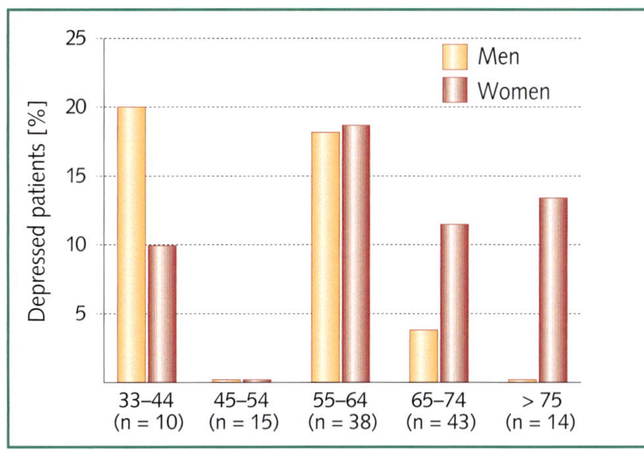

Fig 4-1 Incidence of depression in patients wearing a complete denture by age and sex. (Data from Chamberlain and Chamberlain.[29])

The most frequent local complications are severe atrophy of the maxilla and mandible. Atrophy of the alveolar ridges compromises retention and stability and therefore impedes correct functioning. Furthermore, if the edentulous patient has temporomandibular disorders,[41] incorporation of the denture is more difficult. For example, patients with bruxism have frequent decubitus even when the denture is correctly made.

The degree of compensatory incorporation of the denture therefore depends not only on the quality of the denture but also on the condition of the residual structures of the oral cavity. Recently, the concept of the *prosthetic condition* has been introduced, which combines the quality of the residual alveolar ridges with that of the denture.[42] Some variables of the prosthetic condition have been shown to be significantly correlated to those aspects of the denture that the patients most commonly complain about: esthetics of the maxillary denture, mobility during function, and pain caused by the mandibular denture[43,44] (Fig 4-2). In a study[45] in which dentures with vertical dimension errors, occlusion errors, or with poor retention and stability had been modified or substituted, an increased number of patients perceived improvement in terms of greater comfort while chewing, greater appreciation of foods, and a greater general sense of security.

Guidelines for Prosthetic Rehabilitation of the Edentulous Patient

When dealing with prosthetic rehabilitation of the edentulous patient, the clinician must know how to explore, identify, and interpret the patient's problem and then offer a diagnosis and

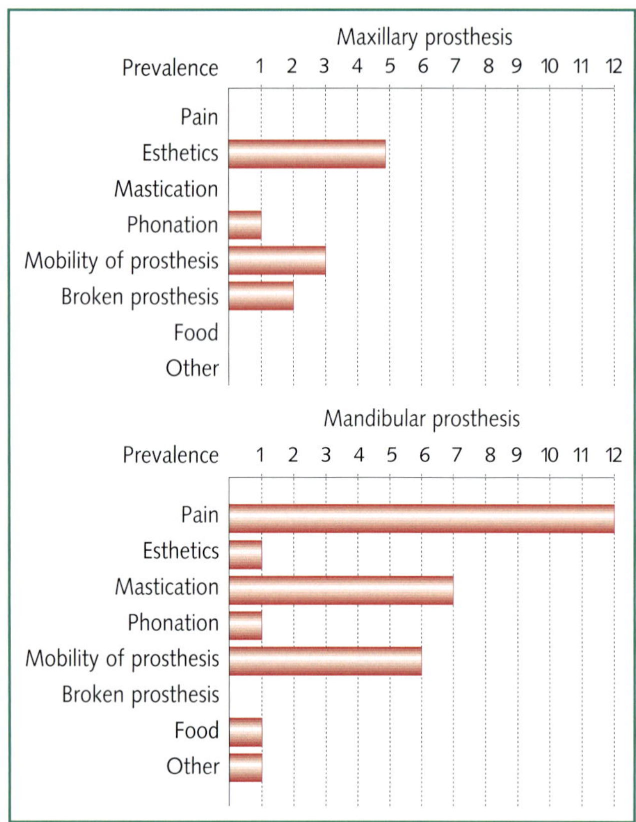

Fig 4-2 Frequency and distribution of complaints about prostheses. (Data from Kotkin H.[44])

solution. Edentulism presents a wide variety of problems that cannot be resolved easily with a unilaterally decided treatment. In a purely indicative manner, the clinician can proceed as follows:

- If the patient has a stable personality and no psychologic problems, and the oral anatomic and functional conditions are acceptable, it is sufficient to apply the constructive principles.
- If the patient has psychologic problems (eg, depression, disturbed moods, personality disorders), it is necessary to refer him or her for psychologic treatment.
- If the anatomic and functional characteristics of the patient do not permit the creation of a stable denture, preprosthetic surgery or implant placement may be necessary.

These problems, considered separately for didactic reasons, may all be present in one patient.

Initial Patient Visit

Patient examination, diagnosis, and treatment planning must follow a strict protocol (Box 4-2).

Approaching the patient: Exploration of the problem

The first moments with the patient should involve establishing a good relationship and creating the basis for reciprocal respect.[46,47] The clinician must know how to ask simple questions and must also know how to listen.[48] Each patient has a history of experience, behavior, aspirations, physical and emotional resources, and capacity for adaptation. All these factors can favor or hinder the relationship between patient and practitioner and the course of treatment.

In this initial phase, besides understanding the patient's sociocultural and psychologic background, it is important to understand his or her preferences and expectations. Many edentulous patients have unrealistic expectations with regard to the esthetic and functional results of complete prosthetic rehabilitation. Bell[49] has pointed out that the clinician should present the patient with a realistic perspective of treatment and its limitations. With this aim in mind, it is useful to provide the information in a sequential manner throughout treatment so that it is better assimilated and understood. It is also important that the information be provided in writing as well.

Generally clinicians are inclined to use one method of dealing with all patients: it may be bossy or totally understanding. This idea that "one approach is valid for all situations" should be renounced, and the clinician should be sufficiently flexible to adapt his or her behavior to each patient. The approach needs to be decided through listening to the messages that

Box 4-2 Guidelines for prosthetic rehabilitation of the edentulous patient

Exploration of the problem	Approach to the patient
Identification of the problem	Case history and clinical examination
Interpretation of the problem and prognosis	Approach, case history, clinical examination
Informing the patient	Personal letter, informed consent
Solution of the problem	Correct constructive principles, psychologic support, preprosthetic surgery, implant anchorage (overdenture)

the patient communicates both literally and unconsciously. Nonverbal communication through body language and facial expression can provide important clues. Knowledge of the patient's personality and attitude toward the clinician and treatment can be used to reduce apprehension and improve the clinical relationship.

Before the medical examination, simple, open questions should be asked. Throughout this interview, the clinician should record the exact words used by the patient to identify positive factors (awareness of the limits of the pathology and prognosis, optimism, faith, and past positive experiences) and negative factors (lack of acceptance of the pathology and prognosis, pessimism, lack of faith, and past negative experiences). The clinician can then help the patient change his or her negative views into positive ones.

The patient should be given a letter summarizing his or her specific problems and their eventual solution. This personal approach can help take away the legal sterility of the formal Agreement to Treatment and improve the clinician-patient relationship. Hirsch and colleagues[50] found that patients actively involved in the various phases of therapy are more satisfied than those who are not involved or whose clinician is too authoritarian. The clinician needs to understand the emotional situation of the patient and adapt his or her behavior. Patients send messages asking for help and reassurance to which the clinician must be sensitive and able to respond adequately. Studies carried out by Corah and colleagues[51] showed that patients who do not have a good dialog with the clinician are less satisfied with their therapy than patients who have a constructive dialog with the clinician.

Considering that the type of approach influences the entire treatment, most authors agree that the clinician must welcome the patient in an equalitarian way and not, for example, standing over the the patient sitting in the dental chair or from behind an enormous desk in a presidential armchair. After putting the patient at ease, the clinician must allow the patient to explain his or her problems, the reason for the visit, and any expectations he or she might have. Open questions allow a more articulated reply and aid in passing from exploration of the problem to its identification. The attitude of the patient toward accepting the therapy can be assessed during this process.

This equalitarian manner toward the patient should be the same in all cases, regardless of the clinical situation: dentate patient, partially edentulous patient who has had previous treatment, totally edentulous patient who has never been treated, and totally edentulous patient who has had previous treatment. Patients who have had different rehabilitation experiences require different clinical considerations.

Dentate patients

One of the most difficult situations is when a patient with partial edentulism has to have the remaining teeth removed. In these cases, it is best to avoid extracting all of the teeth in one sitting; it is better to resort to a provisional partial denture that allows the patient to adapt both psychologically and functionally. When these patients first come under observation, they are often in a situation that is so compromised, with diffuse and localized pain and reduced masticatory function, that the move to a denture can be seen as a liberation. Very often the perceived mutilation of tooth extraction can be mitigated by the positive esthetic results that can be obtained with the immediate delivery of a denture. From the psychologic point of view, these patients are experiencing difficulties and are in need of professional support. In these cases, the approach toward the patient is even more important. The clinician must emphasize the positive aspects of resolving the problem rather than its negative aspects. Whatever is explained before treatment makes the patient's acceptance easier and improves his or her opinion of the clinician. Whatever is explained afterward, on the other hand, may be interpreted as an excuse for mistakes made. Some simple questions are useful, such as "Do you know someone with a denture?" If the answer is "yes," then ask, "How does he or she like it?" "What sort of limitations does he or she have?" and "What does he or she expect from the denture?"

Partially edentulous patients who have already been treated

These patients are more likely to adapt psychologically and clinically to the complete denture because they have known that they are probable candidates for a while. Without doubt, much depends on the number of teeth substituted and on the extension of the prosthetic base. Even for these patients, the transition to a complete denture must be gradual to reduce discomfort as much as possible.

Totally edentulous patients who have never been treated

These patients represent one of the most difficult challenges for the clinician because of the inherent psychologic problems, which are themselves in close relationship with the motivational obstacles to treatment. Very often, these patients are pressured by family members to get dentures. It is opportune to ask questions, such as "Why have you decided to seek treatment?" and "What do you expect from the denture?" It is difficult to convince them of the advantages of rehabilitation, because they are often convinced that they chew well and do not feel it necessary from an esthetic point of view. Showing consideration for their difficulties, even by simply underlying aspects which, although of minor importance from a therapeutic point of view, are important motivational factors for them: "A thin, light denture will silence those nagging family members."

Totally edentulous patients who have already been treated

If the patient already wears a complete denture, avoid making negative comments about the work carried out previously. By this time, the patient may perceive his or her complete denture as a part of his or her own body even if has not been done correctly. It is helpful to remember that when a denture is placed at a young age, the neuromuscular system adapts itself. It is very important, in this case, to understand the motives that have prompted the patient to request a new denture in order to formulate a treatment plan that can satisfy all or a part of his or her expectations.

A special subcategory of these patients is the "collector of prostheses," who arrives with a bag full of previous dentures, comparing them and pointing out the good points and the defects of each one. Each denture is identified with the person responsible. In these cases it is difficult to establish whether the patient is chronically unsatisfied or whether he or she has become this way because of unsuited prosthetic rehabilitations. These patients very often lay the blame for their problems on the dentures, which have been poorly prepared, and on the "dentists who did not want to follow my instructions on how to construct or adjust the denture."[52] In these cases a correct approach is difficult. It is important not to concede to the presumption of being the best in order not to become the object of their collection. Professional psychologic support can be useful in these cases.

It is important to create a good relationship with the patient. However, it is just as important not to create a parent-child relationship. When everything is finished, the patient may look for excuses to go back to the dental clinic to receive those attentions he or she has missed at home.

Case history and clinical examination

The first visit must not be a mere collection of information but must serve as a comparison between the information provided by the patient and the objective facts gathered by the clinician. During the initial interview and the clinical examination, the clinician's experience plays a fundamental role in identifying all of the factors that can influence the treatment in order to formulate a correct prognosis and so avoid possible failure. To obtain a predictable result, therefore, it is important to proceed to a brief evaluation of the conditions of the patient's general and oral health, of the existent denture, of the patient's

expectations, and of his or her psychologic condition.[53] In this phase, the use of a patient dental record is important to create an outline of the situation and to ensure the possibility of re-evaluating the case at a later date.[52,54]

The patient's visit is divided into different phases:

1. General medical history
2. Dental history
3. Prosthetic history
4. Objective examination of previous dentures
5. Objective examination of the oral cavity

The medical history includes a family history and a pathologic history to investigate for systemic illnesses, which are of concern in totally edentulous patients (Box 4-3). Edentulism can be associated with neurologic conditions, pathology of salivary glands, and bone and hormone syndromes. It is also important to be aware of the pharmacologic therapies that patients may be undergoing, since many medications for geriatric illnesses reduce salivation as an adverse effect. This symptom can also be a consequence of radiotherapy.

The dental history (Box 4-4) documents previous disease, trauma, neoplastic pathology, and surgical and radiation treatment of the oral cavity. The patient should be asked what caused the loss of teeth, whether it came about gradually or not, whether it was caused by disease or trauma, and whether the lost teeth were substituted one by one or all at once. The patient will adapt less easily to a complete denture if the loss of teeth was rapid or if the loss was gradual but the teeth were not replaced.

Box 4-3 Systematic illness that can influence prosthetic rehabilitation

Neurologic conditions	Parkinson disease
	Hemiparesis
	Cranial nerve deficit
	Myasthenia gravis
	Alzheimer disease
	Muscular dystrophy
	Myotomy
Salivary gland pathology	Sjögren syndrome
	Mikulicz syndrome
Bone and metabolic maladies	Paget disease of bone
	Acromegaly
	Multiple myeloma
	Osteoporosis
	Secondary hyperthyroidism
	Cushing syndrome
	Diabetes mellitus

When obtaining the prosthetic history (Box 4-5), it is important to know how long the patient has been totally edentulous and how much time passed between becoming edentulous and the first restoration. If a long time has passed, morphologic and functional alterations will have taken place (hypertrophy of the musculature of the tongue, hyperkeratosis of the lingual mucosa, and loss of vertical dimension), which are unfavorable prognostic factors.

The patient with a complete denture in place should be asked about the process of obtaining the denture, for example, whether he or she started out with combined prostheses or whether a complete denture was placed immediately. From a prognostic point of view, gradual rehabilitation is more favorable because it allows the patient to adapt better to having a foreign body in the oral cavity. Patients with complete dentures should also be asked whether it has been relined or whether adhesives were used (in the latter case the patient probably has not had regular check-ups).

After this stage of questioning, an objective examination of the previous denture should be done (Box 4-6). The esthetic conditions of the denture are evaluated by observing whether the teeth-face harmony has been respected (Fig 4-3) as far as form, dimension, and color of the maxillary incisors are concerned. Ask the patient about his or her concept of esthetics, whether teeth that are similar to those of a natural set of teeth are preferred or those that are very white and regular.

Stability (Fig 4-4) is tested by putting digital pressure on each premolar and molar after having moved aside the cheek from the opposite side to eliminate the effect of stabilization caused by the muscles. The denture should be stable during this test. Compare this information with the subjective impressions of the patient.

Can the patient correctly pronounce words containing "s,"

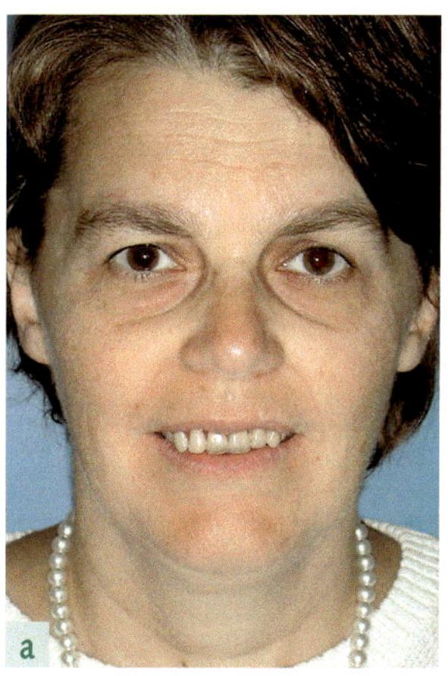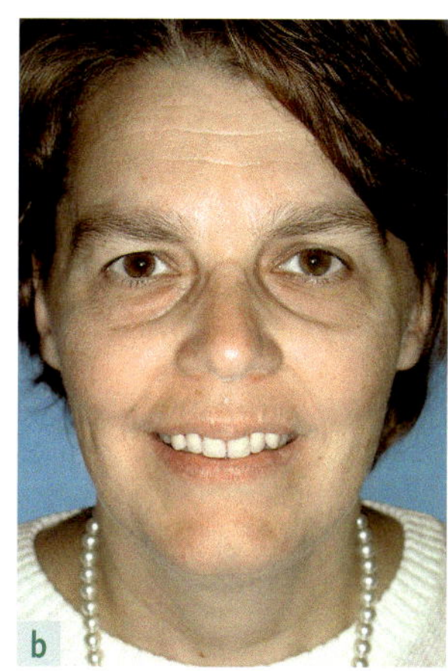

Fig 4-3 *(a)* Patient with a nonharmonious dentofacial balance. *(b)* The same patient with a new prosthesis.

"f," and "ee" (Fig 4-5)? It is important to remember that some pronunciation defects can be due to dialect or old age.

The interocclusal rest space (Fig 4-6), which is 1 to 3 mm on average but can vary from 0 to 10 mm, and the vertical dimension should be checked (Fig 4-7). The exact extension of the prosthetic body and the eventual presence of decubitus should be verified (see chapter 7) and the possibility of conditioning the tissues evaluated.

The objective examination of the oral cavity (Box 4-7) serves to evaluate the state of the anatomic structures to identify the favorable and unfavorable prognostic elements (Box 4-8).

The state of health of the remaining groups of teeth should be examined (Fig 4-8), the presence of caries or periodontal lesions evaluated, and an appropriate plan of treatment defined. When possible, it is advisable to maintain residual teeth, devitalizing them and reducing them to the gingival level

Box 4-4 Dental history

Previous dental disease and traumas
Cause of tooth loss
Timeline of tooth loss

Box 4-5 Prosthetic history

Timeline of becoming edentulous and the first restoration
Type of prostheses used previously
Use of relining or adhesive pastes
Overall impression of previous prostheses

Box 4-6 Examination of previous dentures

Esthetics
Stability
Phonation
Interocclusal rest space
Vertical dimension
Distal extension
Decubitus
Necessity of soft tissue conditioning

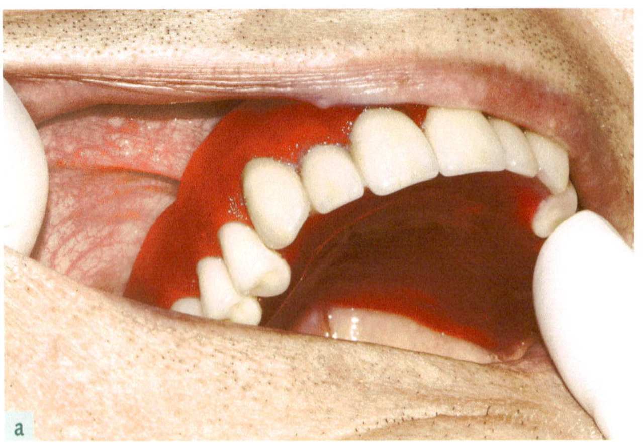

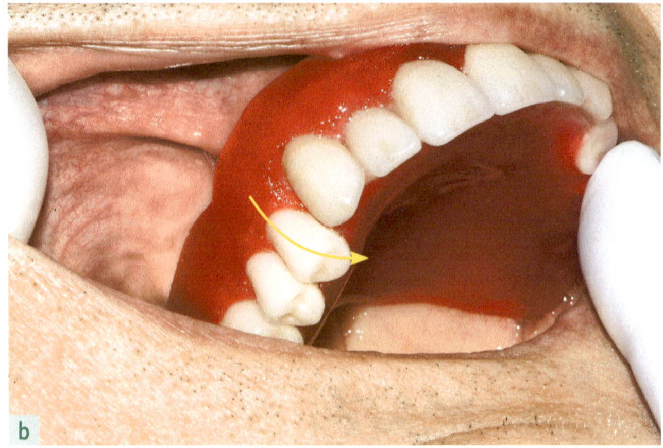

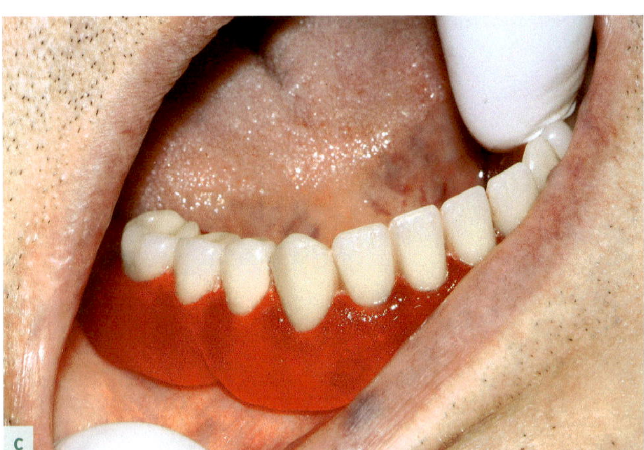

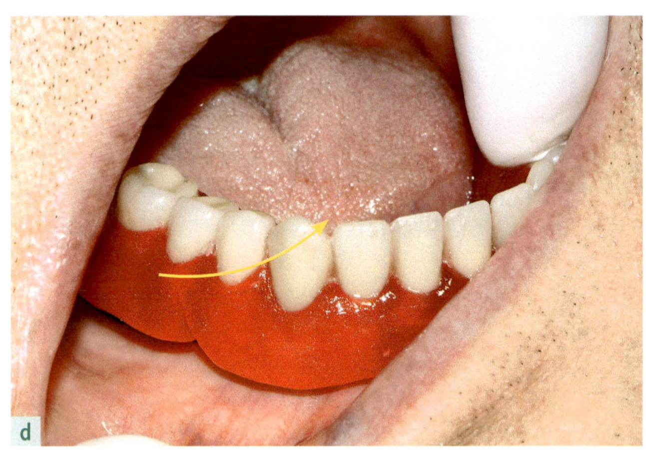

Fig 4-4 Positive digital pressure to test stability of a denture.

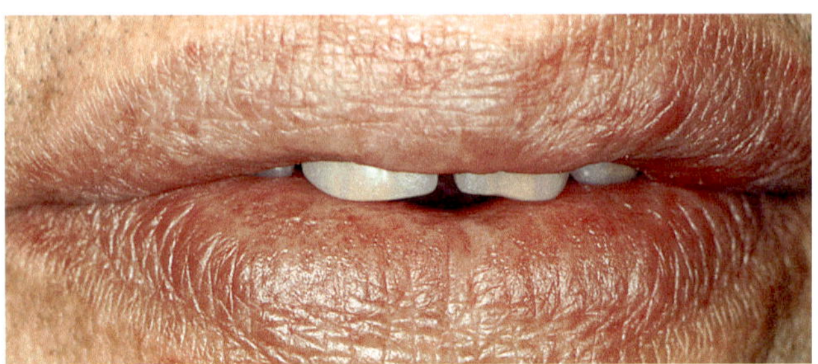

Fig 4-5 Patient pronouncing labiodental sounds to evaluate the position of the maxilary incisors.

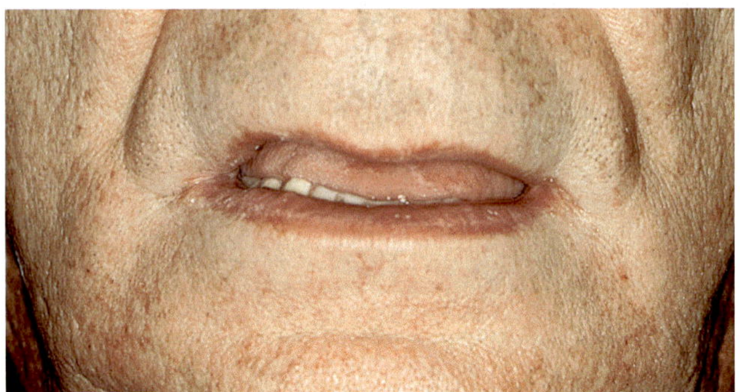

Fig 4-6 Evaluation of the interocclusal rest space.

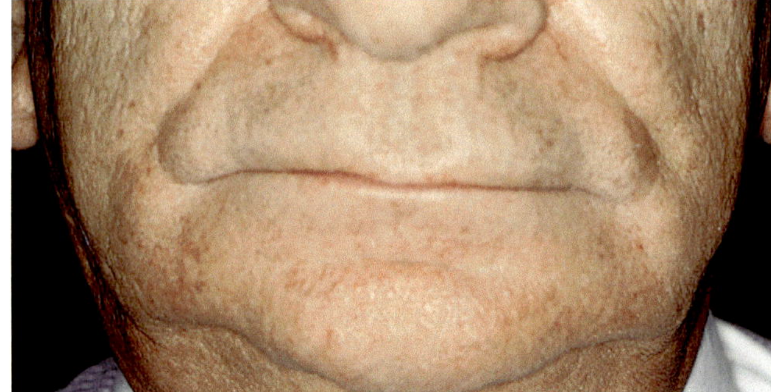

Fig 4-7 Vertical dimension too low.

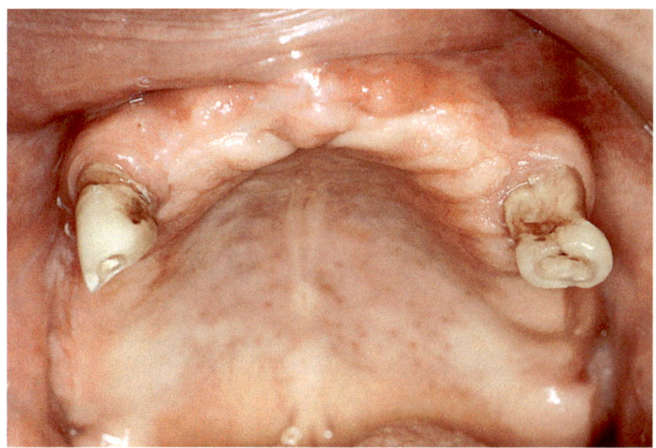

Fig 4-8 Remaining dentition to be maintained if possible.

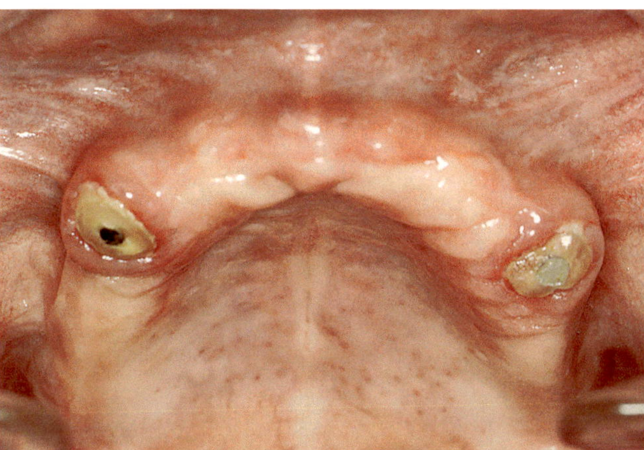

Fig 4-9 Remaining teeth devitalized and reduced to the gingival level in a patient with poor hygiene.

(Fig 4-9); these residual teeth reduce postextraction osseous resorption, conserve some periodontal tissue, and can facilitate adaptation to the complete denture, acting as anchors for an overdenture.

The quantity and quality of the saliva should also be evaluated. Reduced salivation represents a negative prognostic factor; the opposite can be said for viscous saliva, with a normal or abundant flow. To evaluate the viscosity of the saliva, a digital test is performed (Fig 4-10), taking into account the fact that the viscosity can be altered by psychologic and pharmacologic factors.

The examination proceeds with an evaluation of the tongue's dimensions, position, and the degree of cleanliness. Macroglossia is apparent when the patient can touch the point of the chin with the point of the tongue, when there is hypertrophy of the muscles of the floor of the mouth, and when the tongue shows the imprint of teeth in the dentate patient. The position of the tongue can be observed during pronunciation of "a" as

Box 4-7 Examination of oral cavity

• Remaining teeth	• Mandible
• Saliva	• Mucosa
• Tongue	• Frena
• Maxilla	

Box 4-8 Prognostic factors

Favorable
- Residual teeth
- Early replacement of extracted teeth
- Viscous and abundant saliva
- Trophic mucosa and a large bend of attached gingiva
- High-attached, thin, and mobile frenula
- Thick U-shaped crests
- Congruent antagonist crests
- Monolateral hypertrophic tuberosity
- Fixed piriform eminence
- Rectilinear soft palate
- Mandible can be manipulated

Unfavorable
- Rapid loss of teeth
- Lack of teeth replacement
- The patient has not been treated for a long period
- Limited and watery saliva
- Hypertrophic mucosa
- Low-attached, fan-shaped, and thick frena
- Reabsorbed, V-shaped crests
- Undeveloped tuberosity
- Palatine torus
- Mobile piriform eminence
- Intermediate soft palate
- Pleated mucosa

Extremely unfavorable
- Negative attitude
- No previous partial prosthesis
- Macroglossia with retracted tongue
- Atrophic mucosa
- Knife-edge fluctuating crests
- Incongruent antagonist crests
- Atrophic tuberosity
- Curtain-shaped soft palate
- Knife-edge or painful mylohyoid ridges
- Prominent genal apophysis
- Superficial neurovascular structures
- Mandible cannot be manipulated

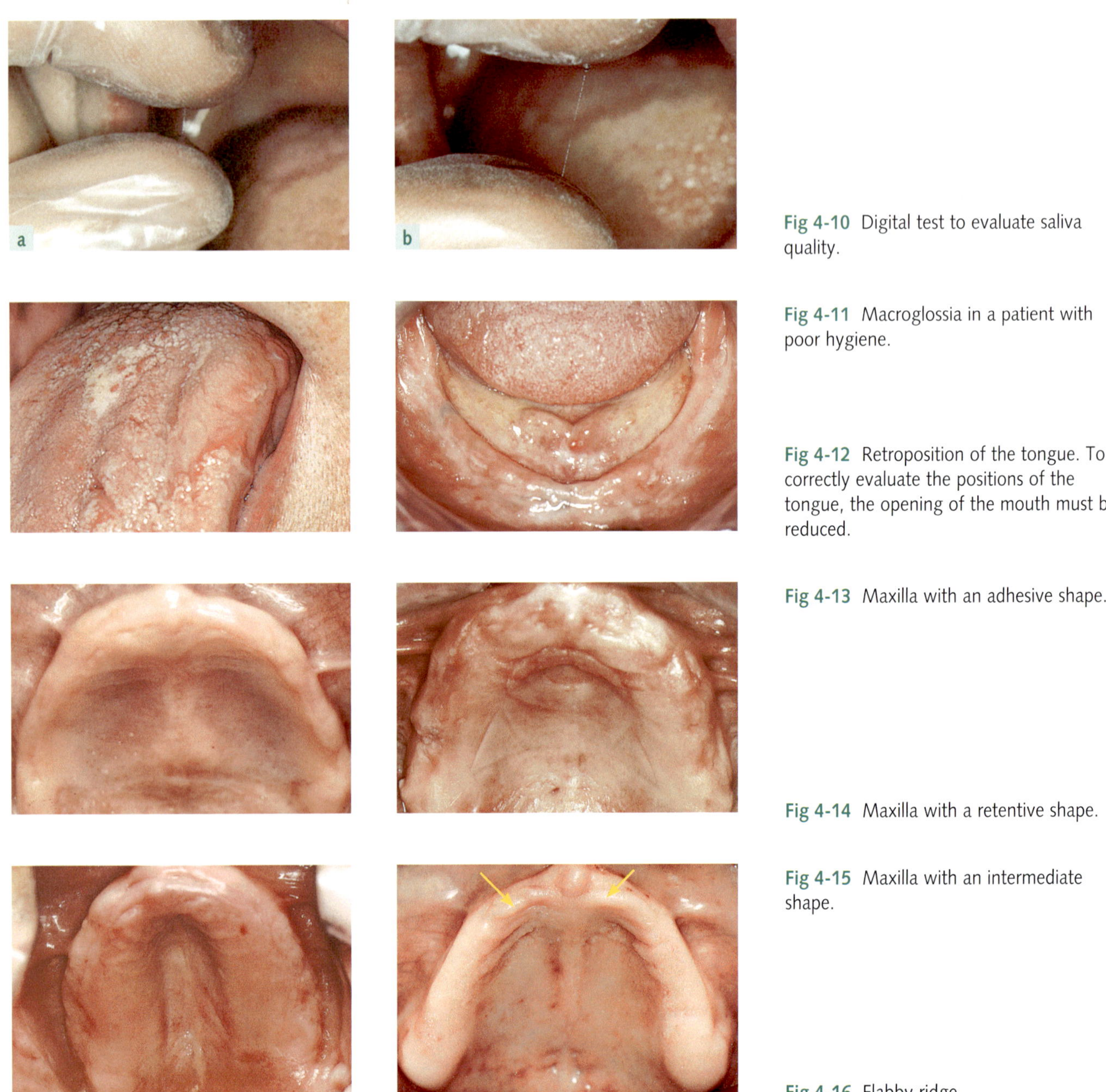

Fig 4-10 Digital test to evaluate saliva quality.

Fig 4-11 Macroglossia in a patient with poor hygiene.

Fig 4-12 Retroposition of the tongue. To correctly evaluate the positions of the tongue, the opening of the mouth must be reduced.

Fig 4-13 Maxilla with an adhesive shape.

Fig 4-14 Maxilla with a retentive shape.

Fig 4-15 Maxilla with an intermediate shape.

Fig 4-16 Flabby ridge.

in "cat." The tongue should be flattened on the floor of the mouth and should touch the inferior part of the alveolar ridge with its tip. Frequently the position of the tip is not in contact with the alveolar ridge (retropositioned) because of the early loss of premolars and molars that have not yet been substituted. Both macroglossia (Fig 4-11) and retropositioning (Fig 4-12) are considered unfavorable prognostic factors, because they alter the balance between the forces exercised by the tongue, the oral floor, and the cheeks. The maxilla is analyzed on its shape, alveolar ridges, tuberosities, tori, and soft palate. The shape can

be adhesive or retentive, with various situations in between (Figs 4-13 to 4-15). It is important to analyze the ridges—their level of resorption, morphology, and the presence of unstable tissue (flabby ridges) (Fig 4-16). Flabby ridges form as a result of substitution of the osseous tissue with fibrous tissue. These ridges most frequently correspond with the incisive bone in patients with a complete maxillary denture and a removable partial mandibular denture anchored to the incisors and canines.

The maxillary tuberosities are important structures for the stability of a complete denture. A hypotrophic tuberosity (Fig

Fig 4-17 Hypotrophic tuberostiy.

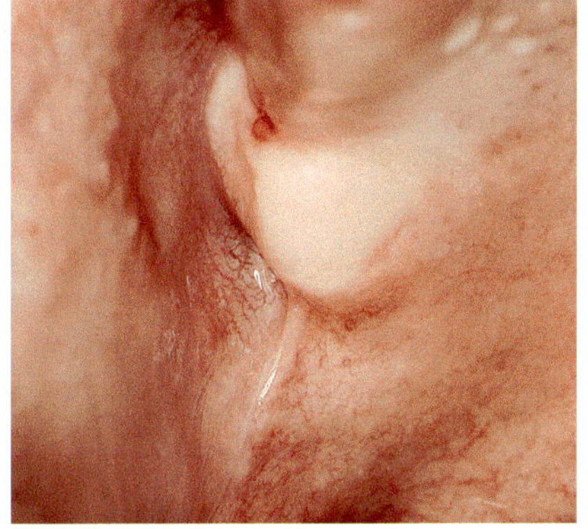
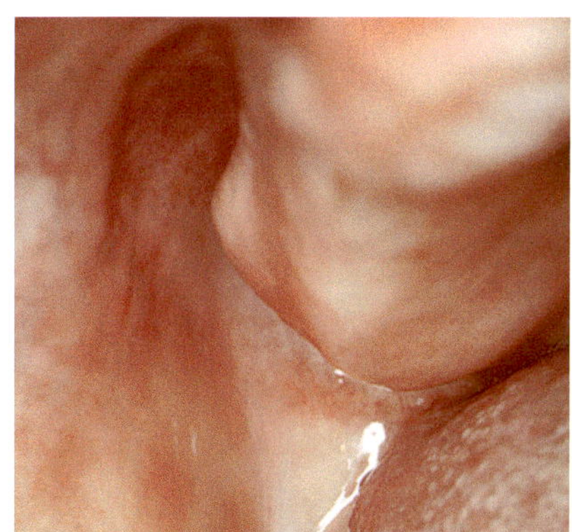

Fig 4-18 Hypertrophic tuberosity.

Fig 4-19 Knife-edge ridge.

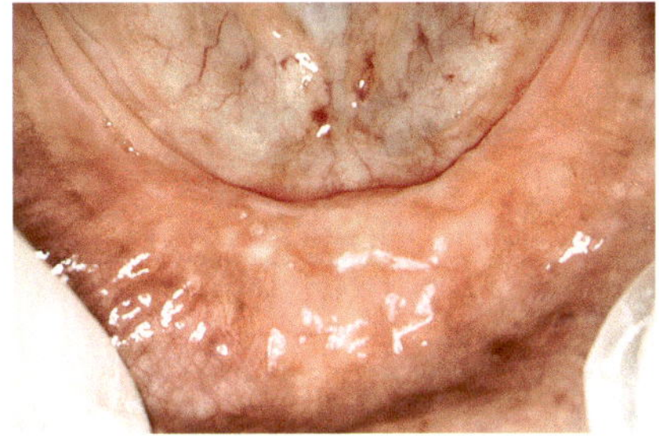
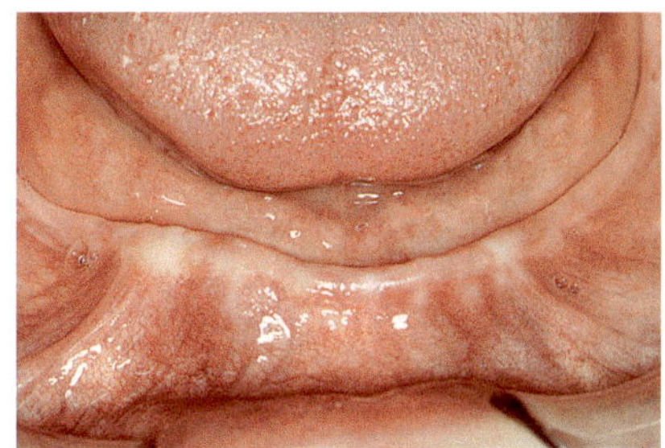

Fig 4-20 Rounded ridge.

Fig 4-21 Squared ridge.

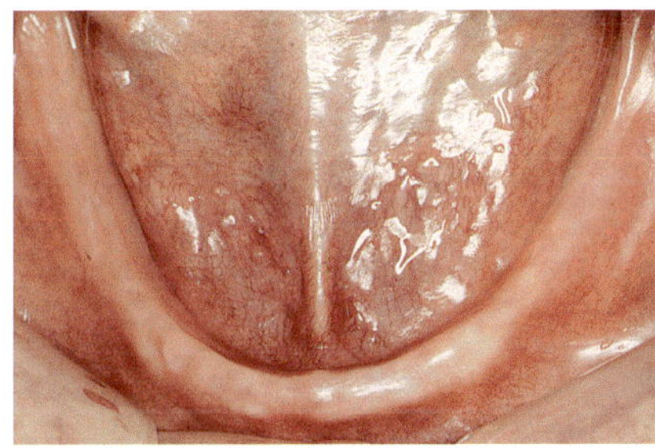
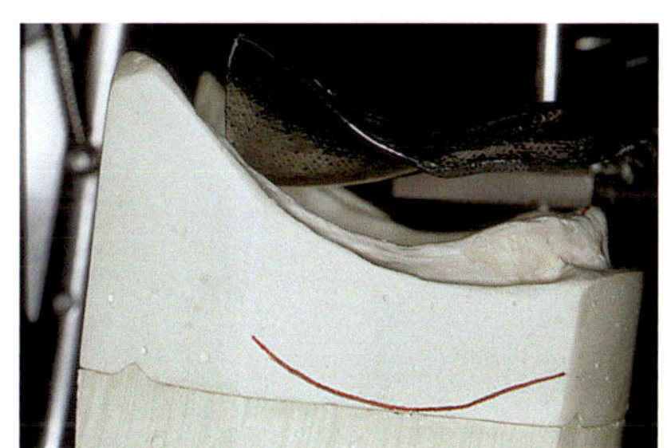

Fig 4-22 The trace of movement of the ridge on the sagittal curvilinear plane.

4-17) is a negative factor, whereas a hypertrophic and undercut tuberosity can be used to increase the stability of the denture when it is on one side only. In this case the patient must be taught how to correctly insert the denture (Fig 4-18). If both tuberosities are hypertrophic and undercut, one of them must be surgically remodeled.

If the lingual torus is overdeveloped, it must be reduced with preprosthetic surgery.

Finally, it is necessary to evaluate the movement of the soft palate, which can be straight (favorable factor), intermediate, or fluctuating (unfavorable factor) (Fig 3-4).

In the mandible the alveolar ridges can be knife-edge (Fig 4-19), round (Fig 4-20), or square (Fig 4-21). The knife-edge ridge is the most unfavorable, and the most favorable is the square ridge. It is also necessary to evaluate the movement: a very curved movement is a negative factor (Fig 4-22).

The retromolar pad represents a good area of stability and support for the denture if it is fixed to the osseous planes.

The mylohyoid ridge is evaluated by palpation. When it is segmented or painful it must be surgically remodeled; if this is not possible, the area of the prosthetic body that corresponds to the mylohyoid ridge must be made of soft resin (see chapter 9).

The congruency of the two ridges on the frontal plane and whether they are parallel on the sagittal plane need to be determined. Their incongruence is a negative prognostic factor.

Regarding the mucosa of the oral cavity, it is favorable when it is trophic and unfavorable when it is atrophic or hypertrophic. It is necessary to look for eventual mucosal creases (Figs 4-23 and 4-24) by evaluating whether they are distendable by stretching them with a finger.

As far as the frena are concerned (Figs 4-25 and 4-26), low insertion and a fan shape are considered unfavorable conditions.

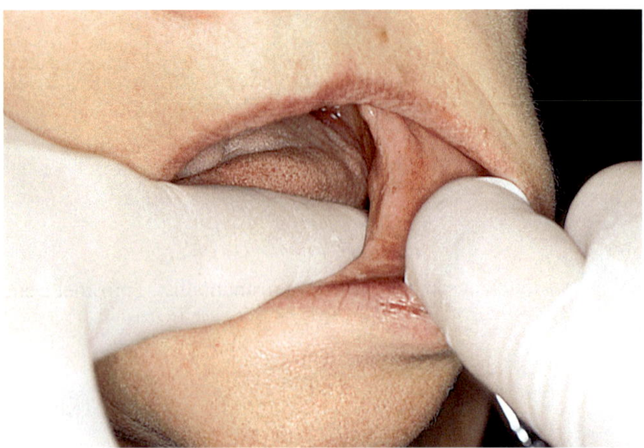

Fig 4-23 Technique to relax the mucosal folds. The same result must be obtained with the impression.

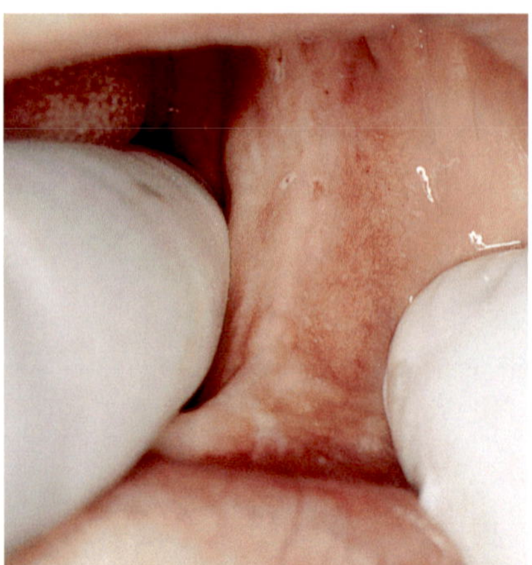

Fig 4-24 Technique to relax the mucosal folds (detail).

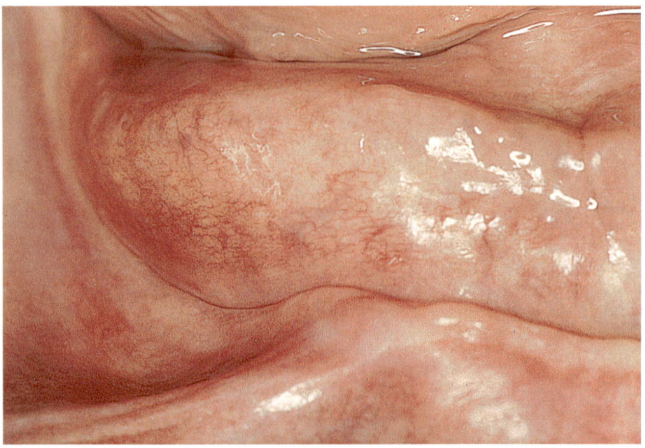

Fig 4-25 Fan-shaped thick frena at a low position.

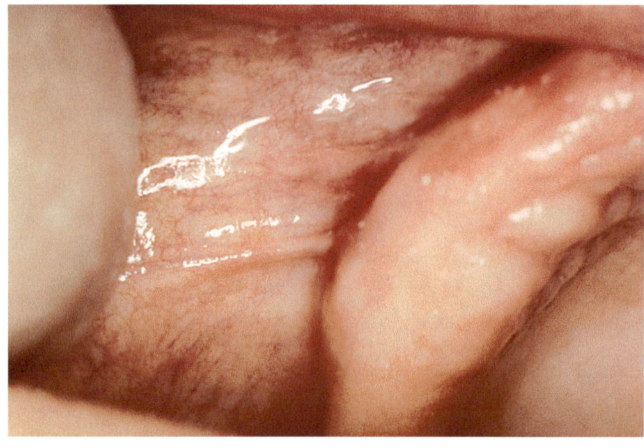

Fig 4-26 Thin and nonmobile frena at a high position.

Finally, the manipulability of the mandible, the capacity of the patient to carry out movements of protrusion and laterality, and the muscular tone are checked. Patients who have a mandible that is difficult to manipulate and who have difficulty in carrying out eccentric movements need particular care in the assessment of the maxillomandibular relationships.

Summary

The approach, case history, clinical examination, and interpretation of the problem allow the clinician to evaluate the real possibilities of satisfying the patient with prosthetic rehabilitation. At this point it is advisable to summarize the prognosis in a personal letter for the patient.

References

1. Langer A, Michman J, Seifert I. Factors influencing satisfaction with complete dentures in geriatric patients. J Prosthet Dent 1961;11:1019–1031. Cat. 3.
2. Lindquist TJ, Ettinger RL. Patient management and decision making in complete denture fabrication using a duplicate denture procedure: A clinical report. J Prosthet Dent 1999;82:499–503. Cat. 8
3. Carlsson GE. Clinical morbidity and sequelae of treatment with complete dentures. J Prosthet Dent 1998;77:17–23. Cat. 7
4. Botta JM. Living without teeth: A psychological approach. In: Bassi F, Carossa S, Gassino G, et al (eds). Advances in Clinical Prosthodontics. Padova: Piccin, 1998:147–150. Cat. 7
5. van Waas MA. Determinants of dissatisfaction with dentures: A multiple regression analysis. J Prosthet Dent 1990;64:569–572. Cat. 4
6. Collett HA. Motivation: A factor in denture treatment. J Prosthet Dent 1967;17:5–15. Cat. 7

7. Palmqvist S, Soderfeldt B, Arnbjerg D. Subjective need for implant dentistry in a Swedish population aged 45-69 years. Clin Oral Implants Res 1991;2:99–102. Cat. 4

8. Jonkman REG, Marinus AJ, van Waas DDS, Kalk W. Satisfaction with complete immediate dentures and complete immediate overdentures. A 1 year survey. J Oral Rehabil 1995;22:791–796. Cat. 1

9. Carlsson GE, Otterland A, Wennstrom A. Patient factors in appreciation of complete dentures. J Prosthet Dent 1967;17:322–328. Cat. 4

10. Bergman B, Carlsson GE. Review of 54 complete denture wearers. Patients' opinions 1 year after treatment. Acta Odontol Scand 1972;30:399–414. Cat. 4

11. Lefer L, Pleasure MA. A psychiatric approach to the denture patient. J Psychosom Res 1962;6:199–207. Cat. 2

12. Bolender CL, Swoope C, Smith DE. The Cornell Medical Index as a prognostic aid for complete denture patients. J Prosthet Dent 1969;22:20–29. Cat. 4

13. Hirsch B, Levin B, Tiber N. Effects of patient involvement and esthetic preference on denture acceptance. J Prosthet Dent 1972;28:127–132. Cat. 2

14. Hirsch B, Levin B, Tiber N. Effects of dentist authoritarianism on patient evaluation of dentures. J Prosthet Dent 1973;30:745–748. Cat. 2

15. Silverman S, Silverman SI, Silverman B, Garfinkel L. Self-image and its relation to denture acceptance. J Prosthet Dent 1976;35:131–141. Cat. 4

16. Smith M. Measurement of personality traits and their relation to patient satisfaction with complete dentures. J Prosthet Dent 1976;35:492–503. Cat. 4

17. Guckes AD, Guckes D, Smith D, Swoope CC. Counseling and related factors influencing satisfaction with dentures. J Prosthet Dent 1978;39:259–267. Cat. 3

18. Manne S, Mehra R. Accuracy of perceived treatment needs amoung geriatric denture wearers. Gerodontology 1983;2:67–71. Cat. 4

19. Yoshizumi TD. An evaluation of factors pertinent to the success of complete denture service. J Prosthet Dent 1964;14:866–878. Cat. 4

20. Berg E. The influence of some anamnestic, demographic, and clinical variables on patient acceptance of new complete dentures. Acta Odontol Scand 1984;42:119–127. Cat. 4

21. Berg E, Ingebretsen R, Johnsen TB. Some attitudes towards edentulousness, complete dentures, and cooperation with the dentist. A study of denture patients attending a dental school. Acta Odontol Scand 1984;42:333–338. Cat. 3

22. Berg E, Johnsen TB, Ingebretsen R. Social variables and patient acceptance of complete dentures. A study of patients attending a dental school. Acta Odontol Scand 1985;43:199–203. Cat. 4

23. Berg E, Johnsen TB, Ingebretsen R. Psychological variables and patient acceptance of complete dentures. Acta Odontol Scand 1986;44:17–22. Cat. 4

24. Magnusson T. Clinical judgment and patient's evaluation of complete dentures 5 years after treatment. A follow-up study. Swed Dent J 1986;10:29–35. Cat. 4

25. Pera P, Bassi F, Schierano G, Appendino P, Preti G. Implant anchored complete mandibular denture: evaluation of masticatory efficiency, oral function and degree of satisfaction. J Oral Rehabil 1998;25:462–467. Cat. 1/3

26. Boretti G, Bickel M, Geering AH. A review of masticatory ability and efficiency. J Prosthet Dent 1995;74:400–403. Cat. 7

27. Friedman N, Landesman HM, Wexler M. The influence of fear, anxiety, and depression on the patient's adaptive responses to complete dentures. Part 1. J Prosthet Dent 1987;58:687–689. Cat. 4

28. Klerman GL. Affective disorders. In: Nicholi AM (ed). Harvard Guide to Modern Psychiatry. ed 1. Cambridge, MA: Belknap Press, 1978:253.

29. Chamberlain BB, Chamberlain KR. Depression: A psychologic consideration in complete denture prosthodontics. J Prosthet Dent 1985;53:673–675. Cat. 4

30. Rovera GC. Comunicazione personale. Cat. 9

31. Firtell DN, Finzen FC, Holmes JB. The effect of clinical remount procedures on the comfort and success of complete dentures. J Prosthet Dent 1987;57:53–57. Cat. 1

32. Lytle RB. The management of abused oral tissues in complete denture construction. J Prosthet Dent 1957;7:27–42. Cat. 7

33. Lytle RB. Complete denture construction based on a study of the deformation of the underlying soft tissues. J Prosthet Dent 1959;9:539–551. Cat. 8

34. Lytle RB. Soft tissue displacement beneath removable partial and complete dentures. J Prosthet Dent 1962;12:34–43. Cat. 2

35. Schierano G, Arduino E, Bosio E, Preti G. The influence of selective grinding on the thickness discrimination threshold of patients wearing complete dentures. J Oral Rehabil 2002;29:184–187. Cat. 3

36. Kreher JM, Graser GN, Handelman SL. The relationship of drug use to denture function and saliva flow rate in a geriatric population. J Prosthet Dent 1987;57:631–638. Cat. 4

37. Stanitz JD. An analysis of the part played by the fluid film in denture retention. J Am Dent Assoc 1948;37:168–172. Cat. 6

38. Edgerton M, Tabak LA, Levine MJ. Saliva: A significant factor in removable prosthodontic treatment. J Prosthet Dent 1987;57:57–66. Cat. 7

39. Brill N, Tryde G, Schubeler S. The role of learning of denture retention. J Prosthet Dent 1960;10:468–475. Cat. 8

40. Muller F, Hasse-Sander I. Experimental studies of adaptation to complete dentures related to aging. Gerodontology 1993;10:23–27. Cat. 3

41. Lundeen TF, Scruggs RR, McKinney MW, Danie SJ, Levitt SR. TMD symptomology among denture patients. J Craniomandib Disord 1990;4:40–45. Cat. 4

42. De Baat C, van Aken AAM, Mulder G, Kalk W. "Prosthetic condition" and patient's judgment of complete dentures. J Prosthet Dent 1997;78:472–478. Cat. 4

43. Brunello DL. Mandikos MN. Construction faults, age, gender and relative medical health: Factors associated with complaints in complete denture patients. J Prosthet Dent 1998;79:545–554. Cat. 4

44. Kotkin H. Diagnostic significance of denture complaints. J Prosthet Dent 1985;53:73–77. Cat. 4

45. Garrett NR, Kapur KK, Perez P. Effects of improvements of poorly fitting dentures and new dentures on patient satisfaction. J Prosthet Dent 1996;76:403–413. Cat. 3

46. Carlsson GE, Otterland A, Wennstrom A. Patient factors in appreciation of complete dentures. J Prosthet Dent 1967;17:322–328. Cat. 4

47. van Waas MA. The influence of clinical variables on patients' satisfaction with complete dentures. J Prosthet Dent 1990;63:307–310. Cat. 3

48. Hoffman W, Bomberg TJ, Hatch RA, Benson BW. Complete dentures [review]. Quintessence Int 1985;5:349–355. Cat. 7

49. Bell DH Jr. Prosthodontic failures related to improper patient education and lack of patient acceptance. Dent Clin North Am 1972;16:109–118. Cat. 4

50. Hirsch B, Levin B, Tiber N. Effects of patient involvement and esthetic preference on denture acceptance. J Prosthet Dent 1972; 28:127–132. Cat. 3

51. Corah NL, O'Shea RM, Bissell GD. The dentist-patient relationship: Perceptions by patients of dentist behaviour in relation to satisfaction and anxiety. J Am Dent Assoc 1985;111:443–446. Cat. 3

52. Budtz-Jørgensen E. The edentulous patient. In: Owal B, Kayser AE, Carlsson GE (eds). Prosthodontics: Principles and Management Strategies. London: Mosby-Wolfe, 1996. Cat. 7

53. Berg E. Acceptance of full dentures. J Int Dent 1993;43:299–306. Cat. 7

54. Appleby RC, Ludwig TF. Patient evaluation for complete denture therapy. J Prosthet Dent 1970;24:11–17. Cat. 4

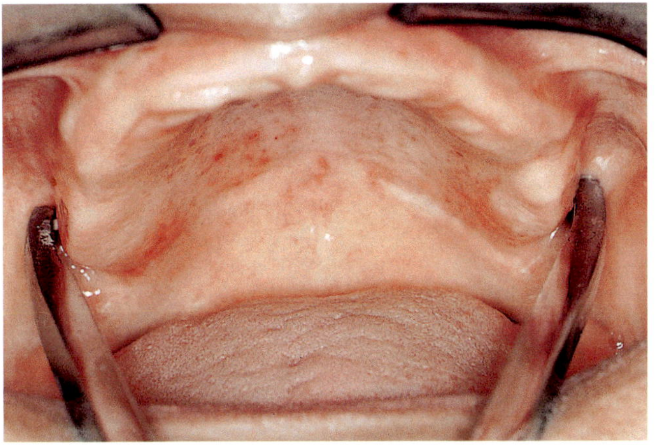

Fig 1 Sizing for stock impression tray using blunt calipers. The reference measurement is the distance between the external surfaces of the maxillary tuberosities.

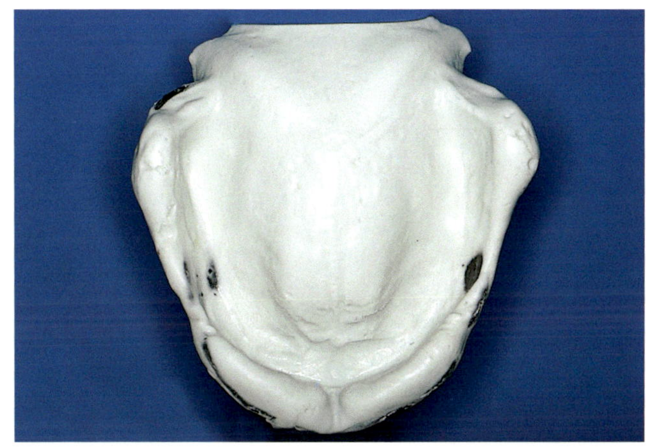

Fig 2 Alginate impression. Any imperfections (eg, margins too thick or areas of compression) can be corrected by relining with fluid alginate.

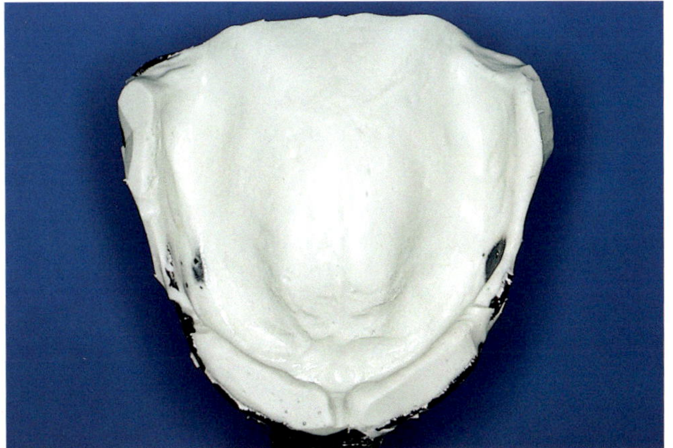

Fig 3 With a scalpel remove any excess that impedes the replacement of the impression tray in the patient's mouth. Margins that are too thick can be sliced thinner and beveled to about 45 degrees.

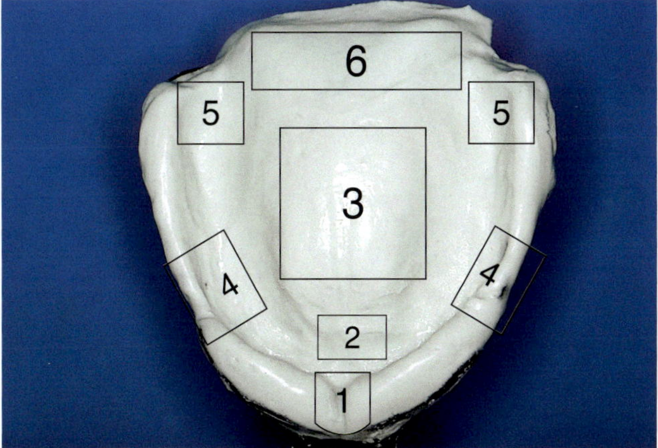

Fig 4 Relined impression. The following characteristics must be visible: (1) labial frenum, (2) interincisor papilla, (3) hard palate, (4) lateral frena, (5) maxillary tuberosities, and (6) the line between the hard and soft palate.

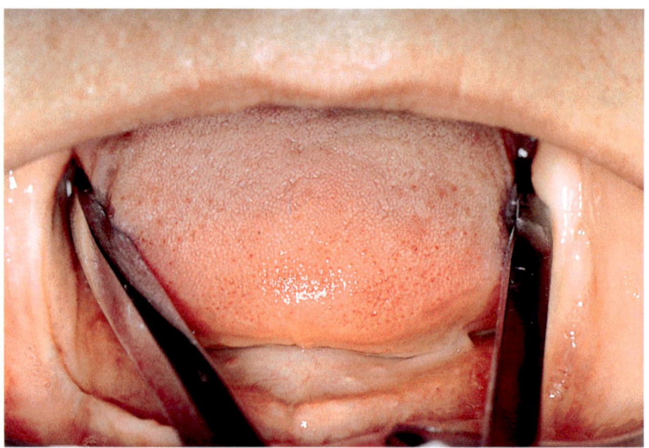

Fig 5 The reference distance for a mandibular impression tray is between the internal surfaces of the mandibular tuberosities.

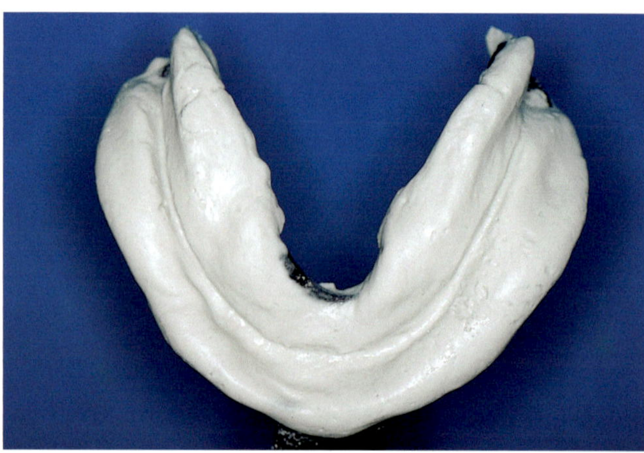

Fig 6 Alginate impression. In the mandible the alginate must be denser (20% less water that the amount indicated by the manufacturer) to fill the mucosal folds and conform to the underlying bone structure.

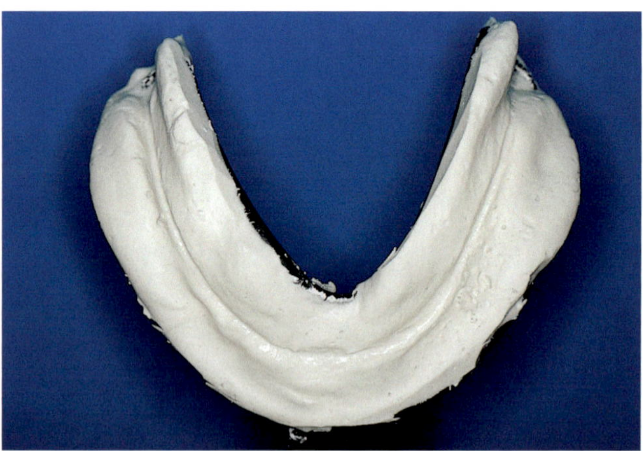

Fig 7 Modified impression before relining.

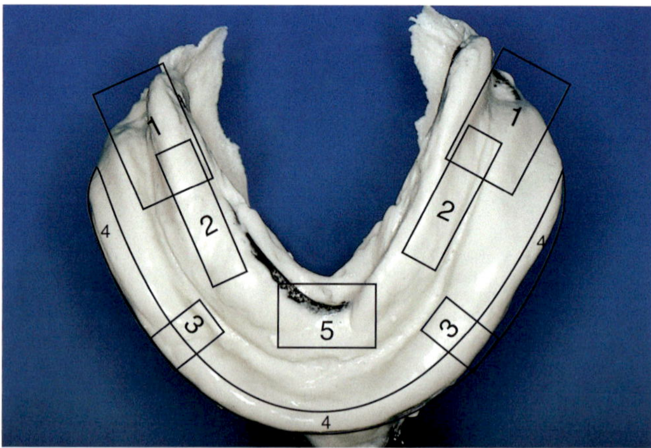

Fig 8 The relined impression. The following characteristics must be visible: (1) piriform eminences, (2) mylohyoid ridge, (3) buccal frena, (4) vestibule, and (5) anterior sublingual area.

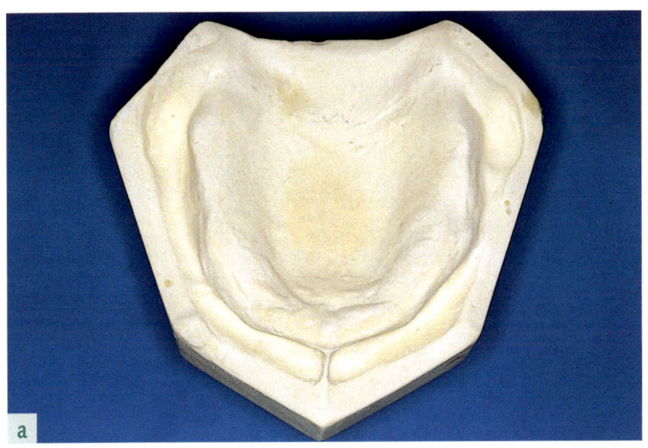

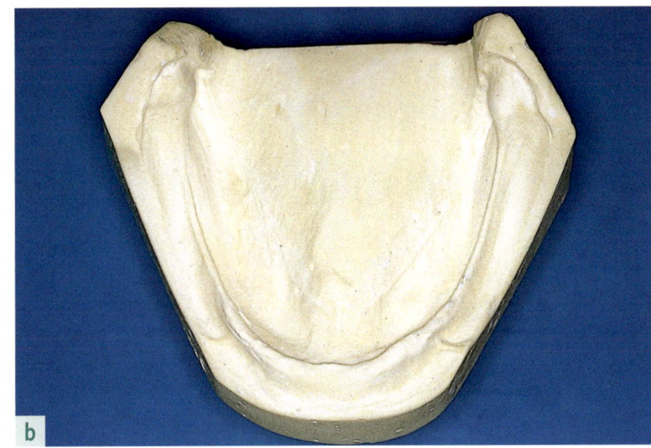

Fig 9 *(a)* First plaster cast of the maxilla using recommended plaster for hard casts (type 3). *(b)* First plaster cast for the mandible.

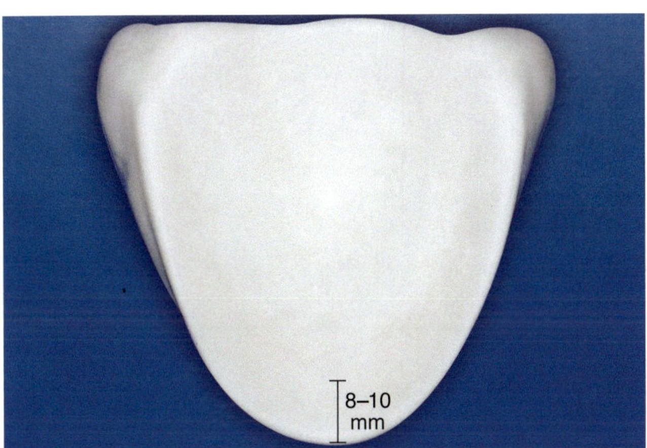

Fig 10 External surface of a custom maxillary impression tray. The handle must be positioned anteriorly at the area of the incisors and canines, 8 to 10 mm from the interincisive papillae.

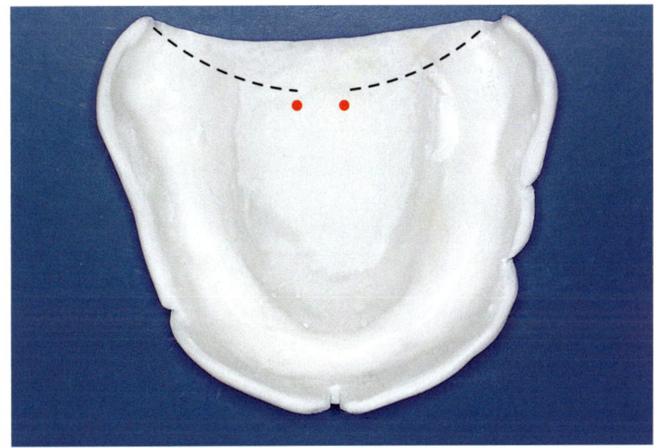

Fig 11 The impression tray must reproduce the dimensions of the definitive prosthesis. The materials used for the borders must be supported by the resin of the impression tray. The area between the hard and soft palates must extend beyond the fossae.

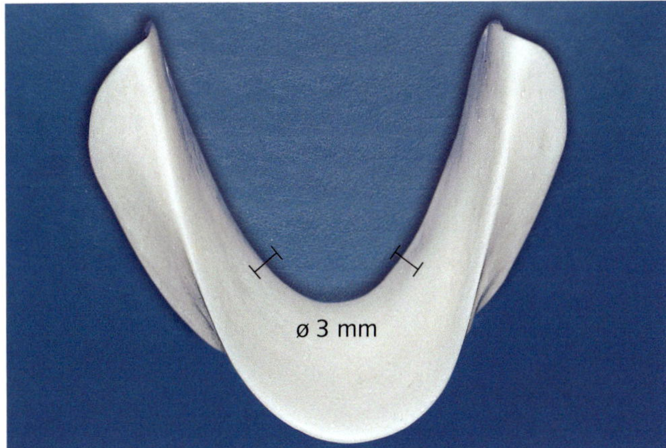

Fig 12 Exterior surface of a custom mandibular impression tray. The handle must be in the shape of a shield to accommodate the lip. In the anterior sublingual area the border must have a dimension of 3 mm.

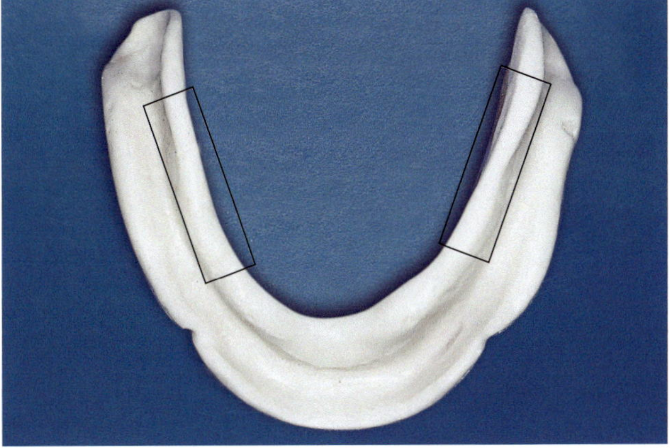

Fig 13 Lateral sublingual area of the mandibular impression tray. The impression tray must extend beyond the mylohyoid ridge by 3 to 4 mm. The musculature of the oral floor is thus lowered, favoring the distension of the mucosal folds and conforming to the underlying bone structure.

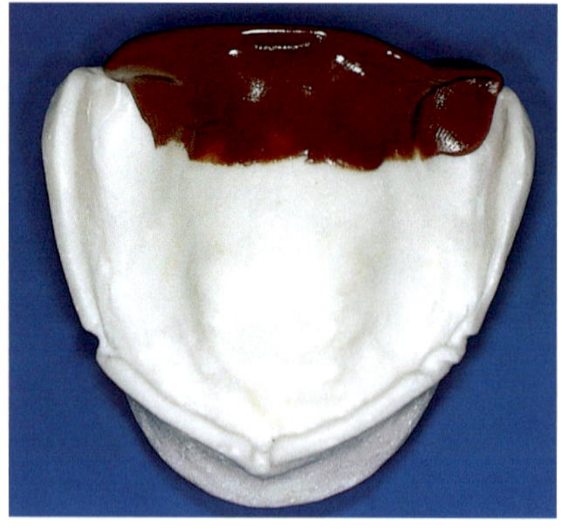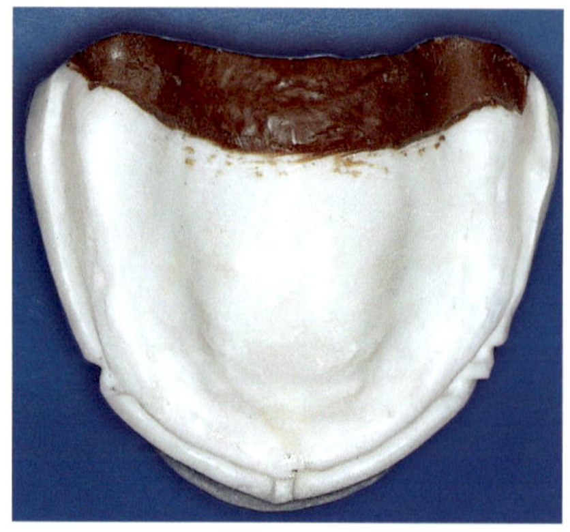

Fig 14 Sequence for making the maxillary borders using thermoplastic paste (Kerr). The posterior border is made first, to establish the position of the impression tray.

Fig 15 The thermoplastic paste is then trimmed with a scalpel to remove any excess.

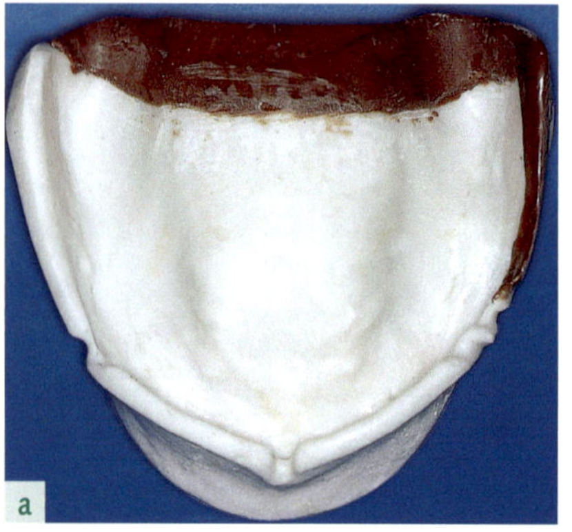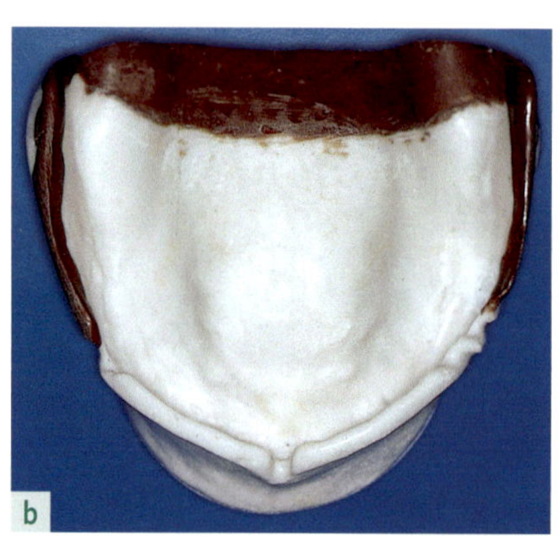

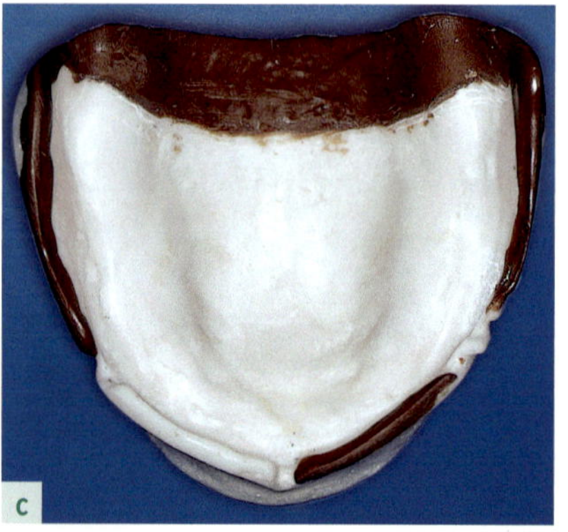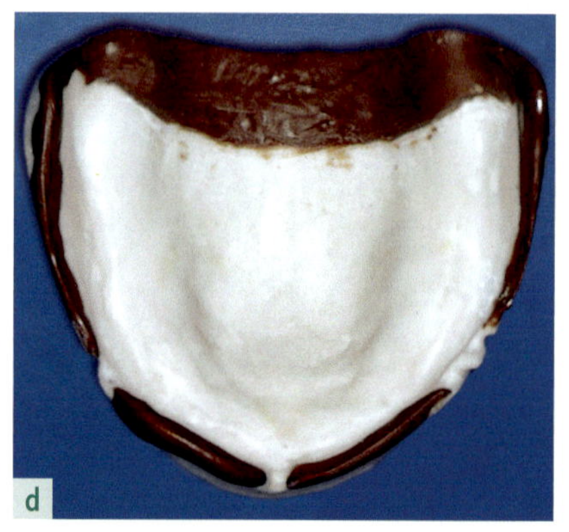

Fig 16 (a to d) Trimming the border must be done symmetrically to maintain the correct position of the impression tray. The thermoplastic border paste must be in contact with the mucosa and adequately support the perimaxillary tissues.

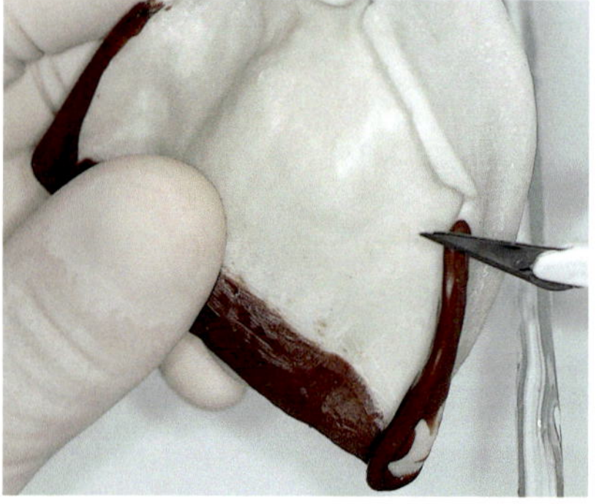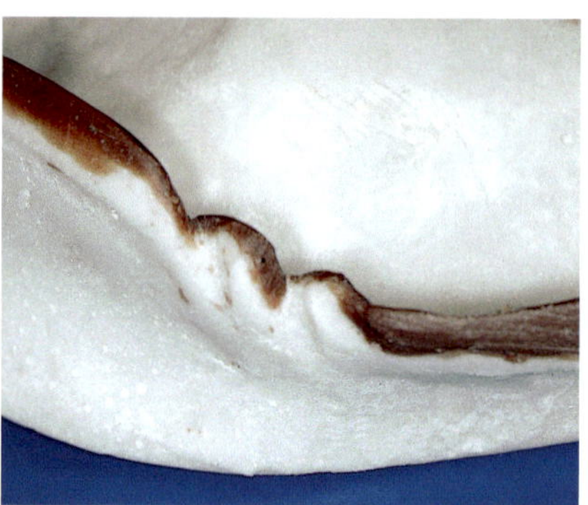

Fig 17 Margins are beveled to about 45 degrees to take advantage of the support of the perimaxillary muscular fibers that cover the bone surface with the same inclination.

Fig 18 Details of the position of the frena. Note the elliptic morphology.

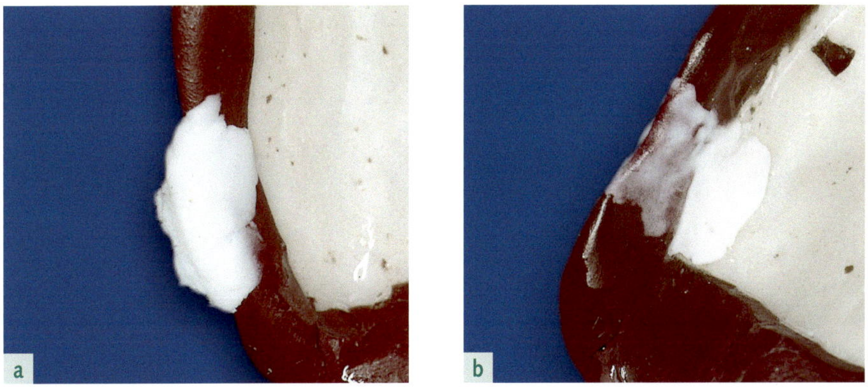

Fig 19 Using disclosing wax, check the contact of the mucosa with the border before taking the mucostatic impression. *(a)* The revealing paste is too dense. *(b)* Correct contact of the impression tray with the mucosa.

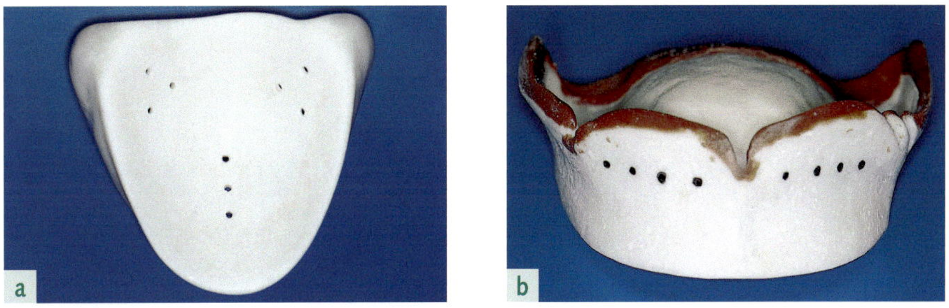

Fig 20 *(a and b)* Position of defluxion holes. The holes serve to avoid the compression of the impression material in the areas of the minor salivary glands, tori, and the edentulous maxillary crest from premolar to premolar.

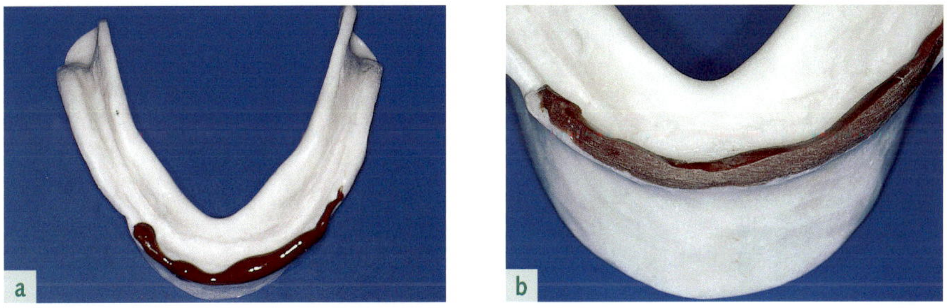

Fig 21 *(a and b)* The sequence for finishing the mandibular border starts with the anterior labial flange to establish the position of the impression tray.

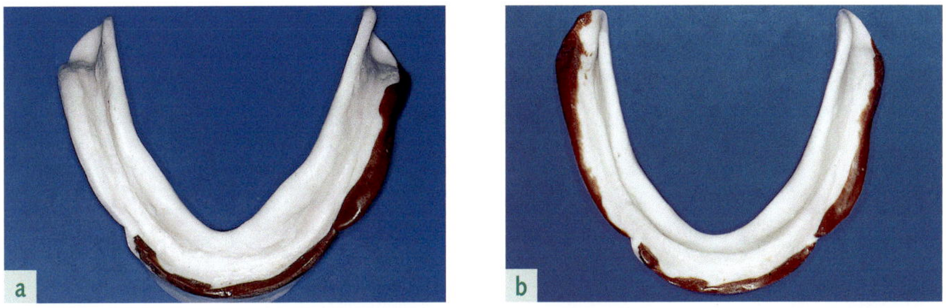

Fig 22 *(a and b)* Progressive symmetric trimming of the border in the posterior buccal regions.

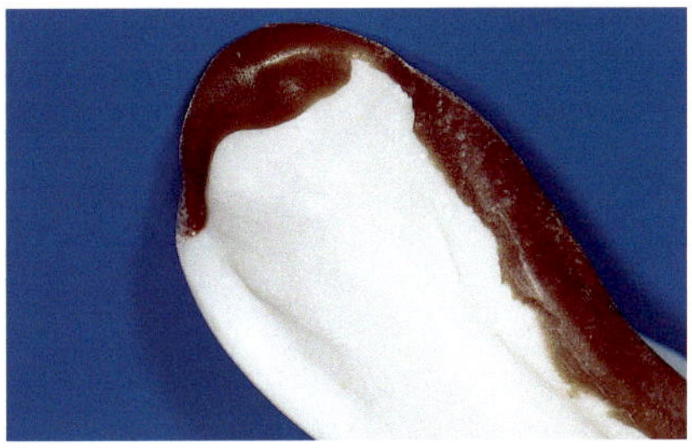

Fig 23 All of the piriform eminence must be included in the impression even if the tissues are mobile with respect to the plane of the underlying bone.

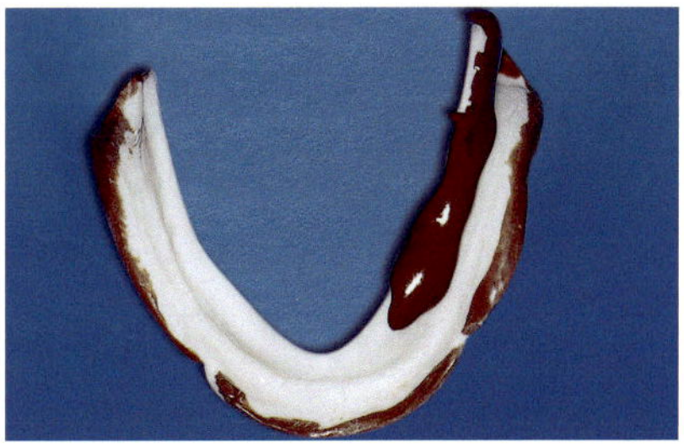

Fig 24 Sufficient thermoplastic paste is deposited on the lateral sublingual margin.

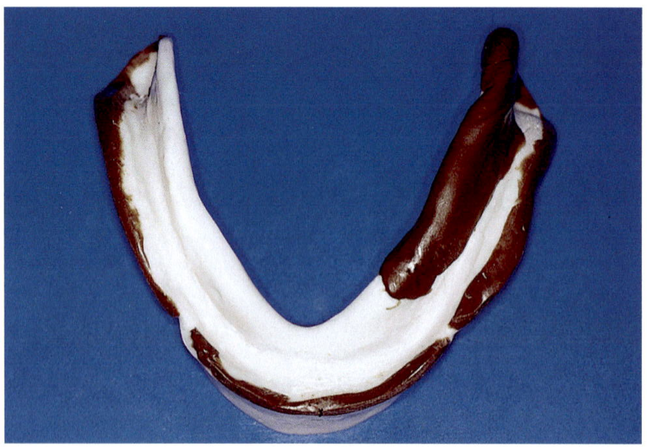

Fig 25 Sufficient material permits the distension of the mucosal folds on the oral floor and on the lingual surface of the mandible.

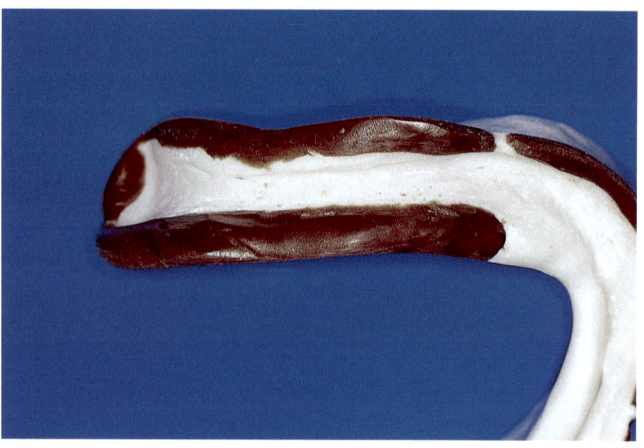

Fig 26 Excess thermoplastic paste will cause compression and must be removed. The mylohyoid ridge must be visible.

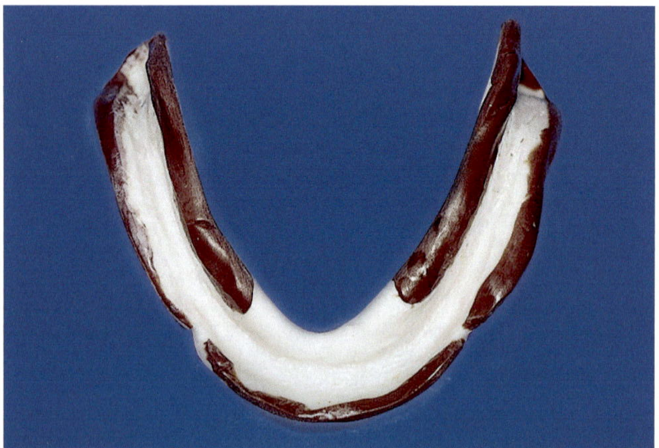

Fig 27 Progressive symmetric trimming of the border in the lateral sublingual region.

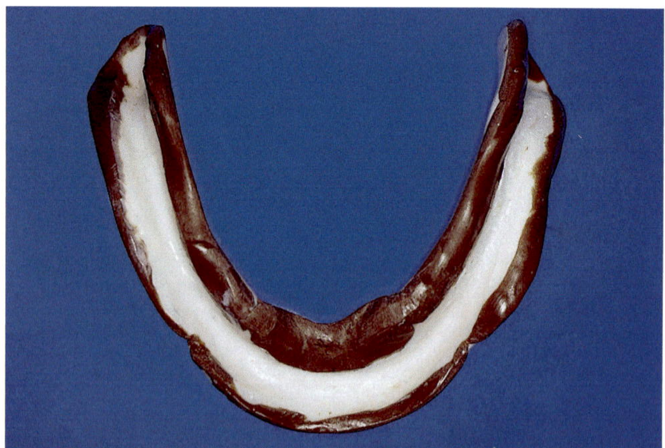

Fig 28 Trimming of the impression tray in the anterior sublingual sulcus. This margin must be rounded and must moderately compress the area.

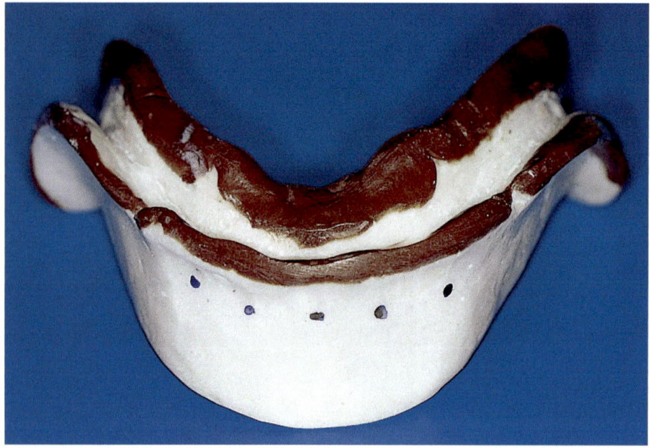

Fig 29 Holes of defluxation on the anterior labial flange. It is not necessary to resorb the holes in the mandible.

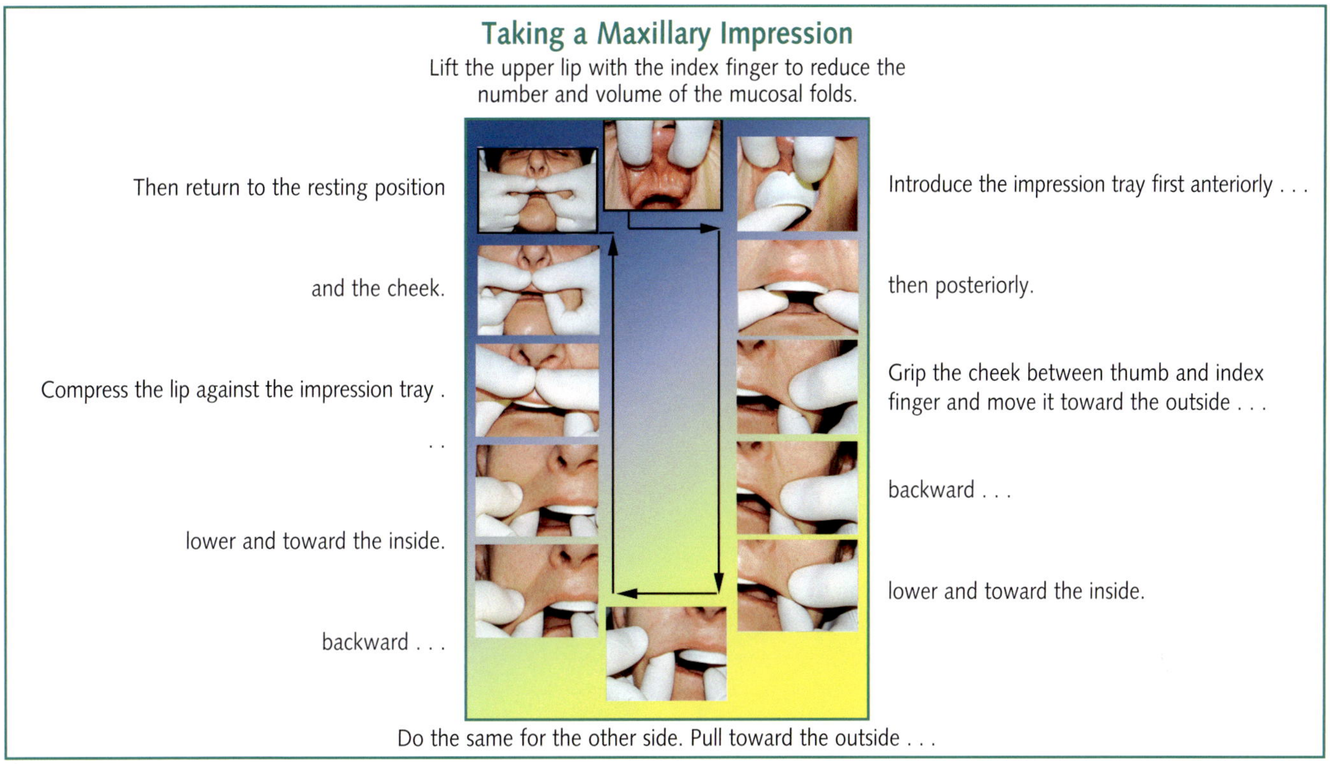

Taking a Maxillary Impression

Lift the upper lip with the index finger to reduce the number and volume of the mucosal folds.

Then return to the resting position

and the cheek.

Compress the lip against the impression tray . . .

lower and toward the inside.

backward . . .

Introduce the impression tray first anteriorly . . .

then posteriorly.

Grip the cheek between thumb and index finger and move it toward the outside . . .

backward . . .

lower and toward the inside.

Do the same for the other side. Pull toward the outside . . .

Fig 30 Sequence of movements during maxillary impression taking.

Taking a Mandibular Impression

Lift the lower lip and introduce the impression tray into the mouth first anteriorly then posteriorly.

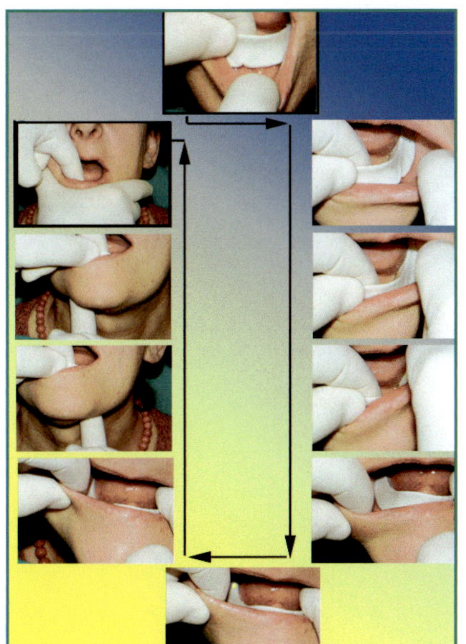

Then assume the resting position.

then to the right.

With the index finger push the floor of the mouth first to the left . . .

upward.

Grip the cheek with the index finger and the thumb and move it toward the outside . . .

backward . . .

upward.

Repeat the movement on the opposite side, moving the cheek toward the outside . . .

backward . . .

Fig 31 Sequence of movements during mandibular impression taking.

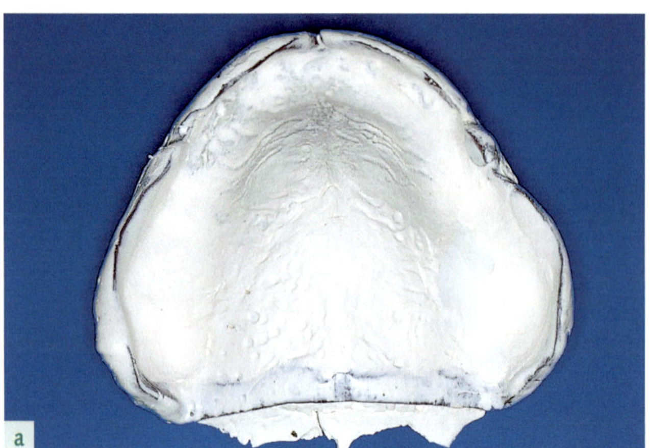 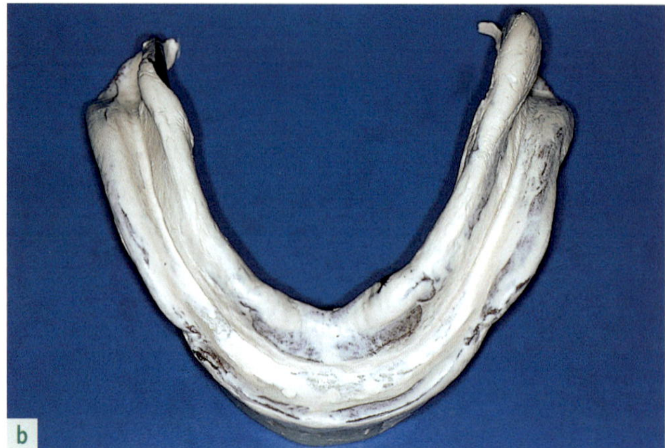

Fig 32 *(a and b)* Impressions with zinc oxide–eugenol paste. The patient should remove the old prosthesis at least 24 hours before the definitive impression is made.

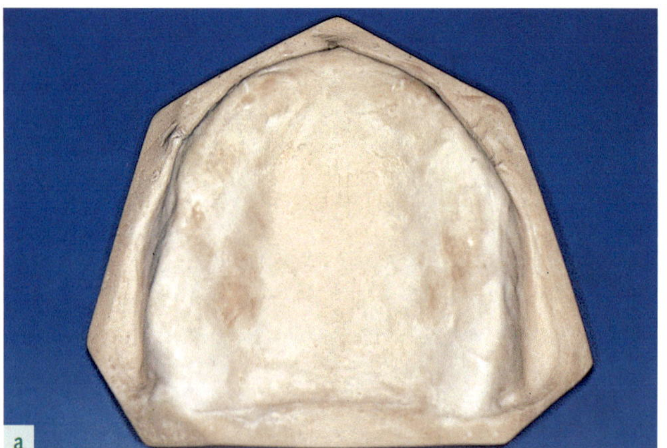 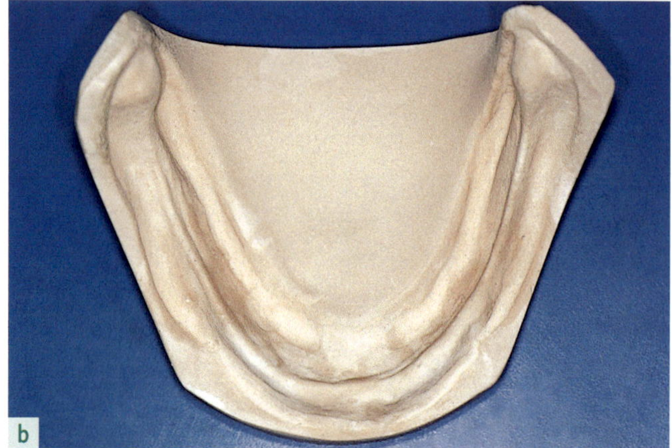

Fig 33 *(a and b)* Master casts for maxilla and mandible. The plaster should be extra hard but not of low expansion, as is used for fixed dentures. The minimum expansion must compensate for the polymerization contraction of the acrylic resin.

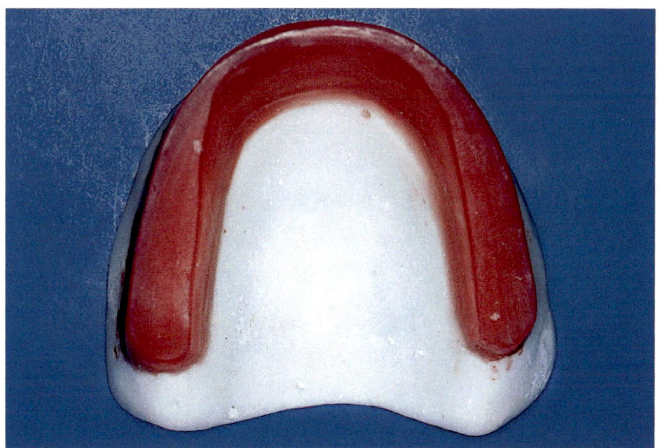

Fig 34 Maxillary occlusion registration base. The morphology of the wax rim must simulate the position of the teeth. The thickness of the wax must simulate the anterior incisal margins and the posterior occlusal surfaces.

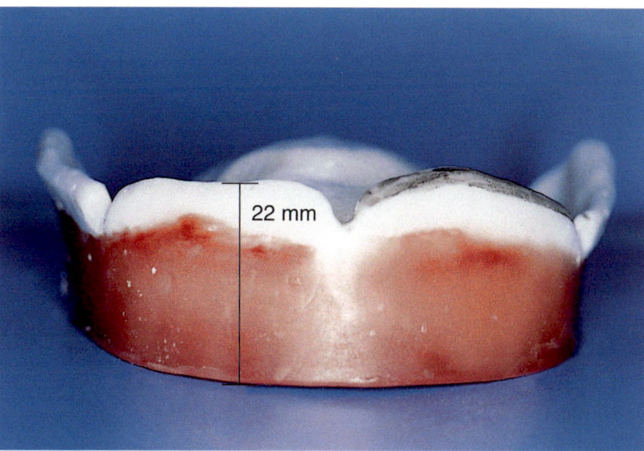

Fig 35 Height of the wax rim in the labial region measured at the depth of the fornix is 22 mm.

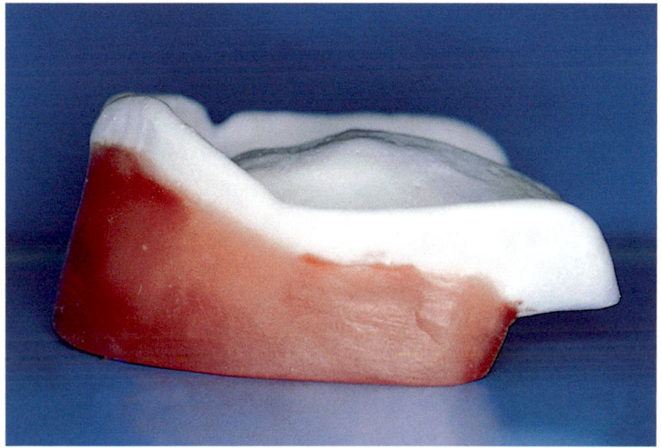

Fig 36 Height of the wax rim in the posterior region.

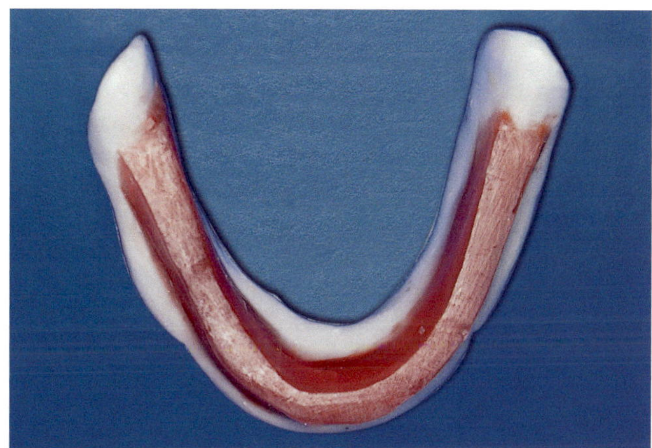

Fig 37 Mandibular occlusion registration base. The wax rim must be modeled to allow the clinician to adapt the cast for neutral zones.

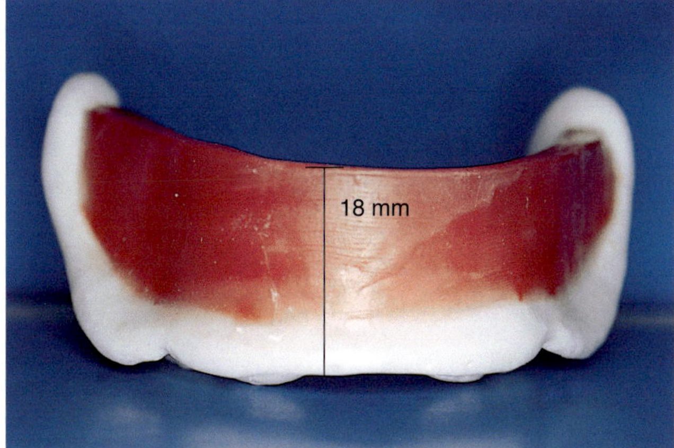

Fig 38 Height of the wax rim in the labial region measured at the depth of the fornix is 18 mm.

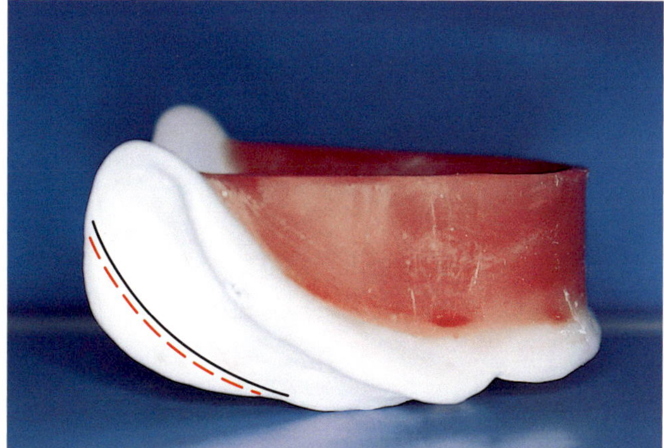

Fig 39 Height of the wax rim in the posterior region must reach the superior third of the piriform eminence. The sublingual flange must be shortened and not extend beyond the mylohyoid ridge more than 0.5 to 1.0 mm.

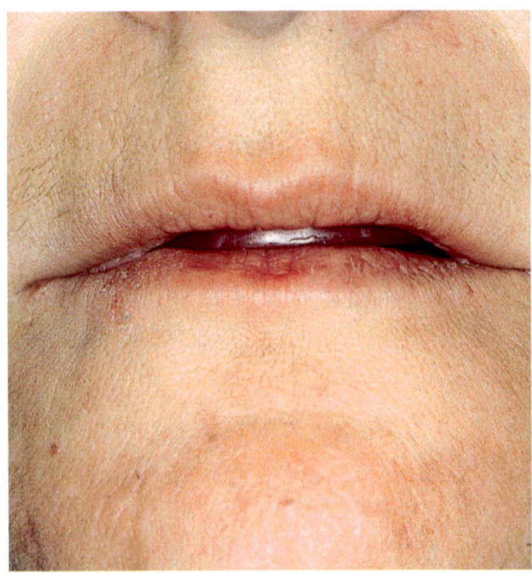

Fig 40 Maxillary wax rim in the anterior region must show below the lip by about 1 mm when the mouth is in the open-rest position.

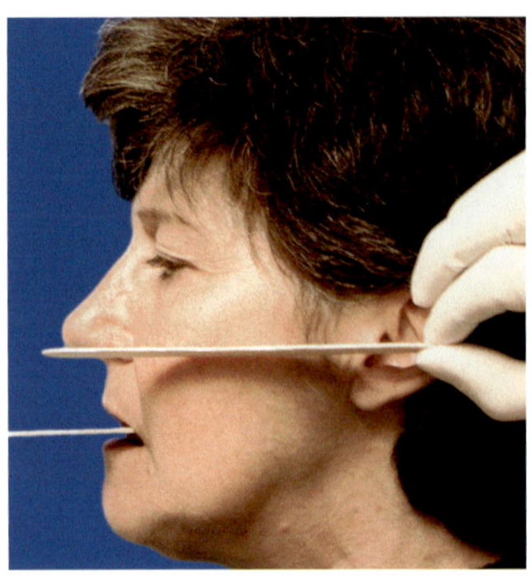

Fig 41 The maxillary wax rim on the sagittal plane must be parallel to the cutaneous plane that goes from the inferior margin of the ala of the nose to the inferior portion of the tragus.

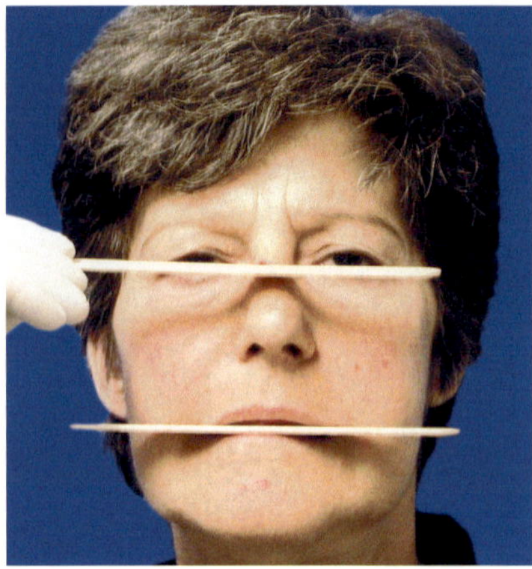

Fig 42 In the posterior region, the wax rim must be parallel to the line between the pupils.

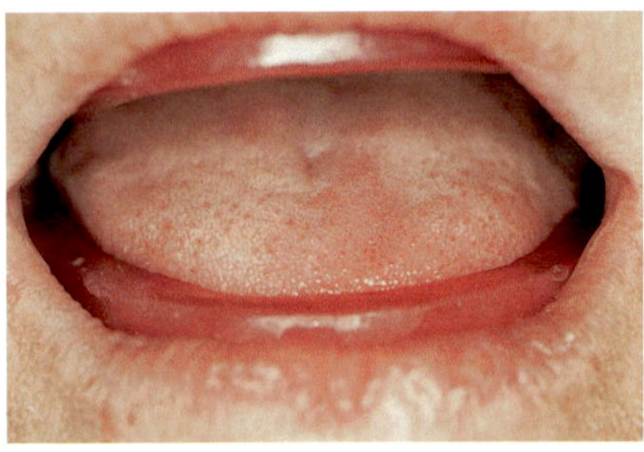

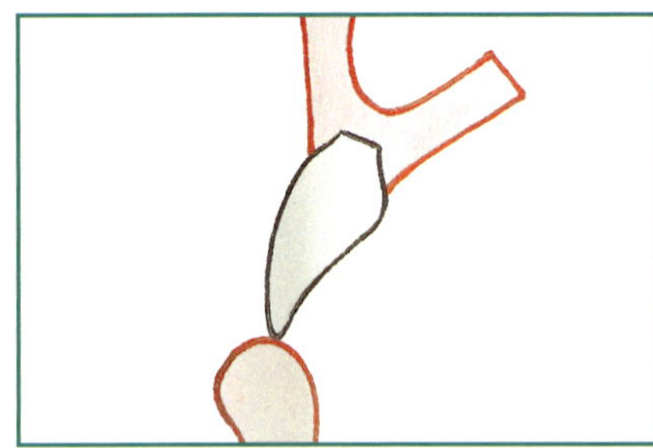

Fig 43 The wax rim of the mandibular occlusal registration base must be adapted to the plane of the maxillary wax rim, with the tongue as the equator.

Fig 44 The maxillary wax rim must touch the wet line of the inferior lip to simulate the position of the incisors during the pronunciation of "F".

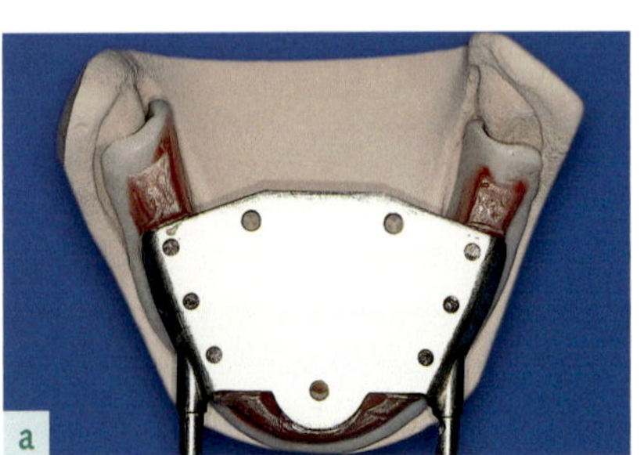

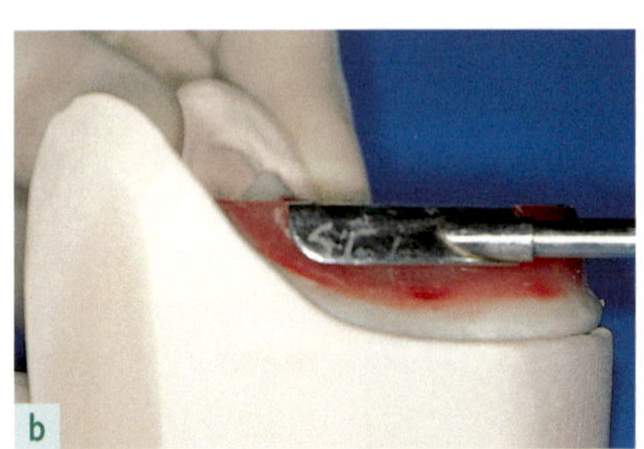

Fig 45 *(a and b)* First phase of extraoral registration: placing of the registration plate. It is important to insert it in the wax rim so that its thickness is part of the plane of registration of the vertical dimension of occlusion (VDO).

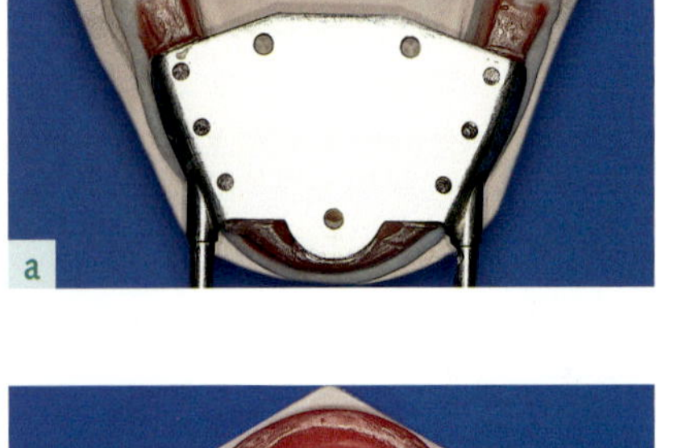

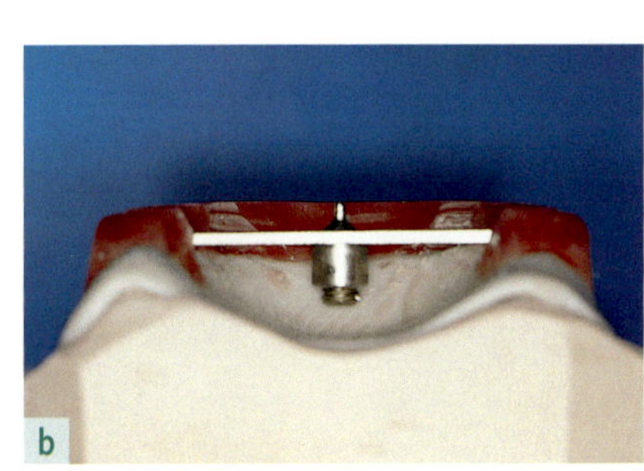

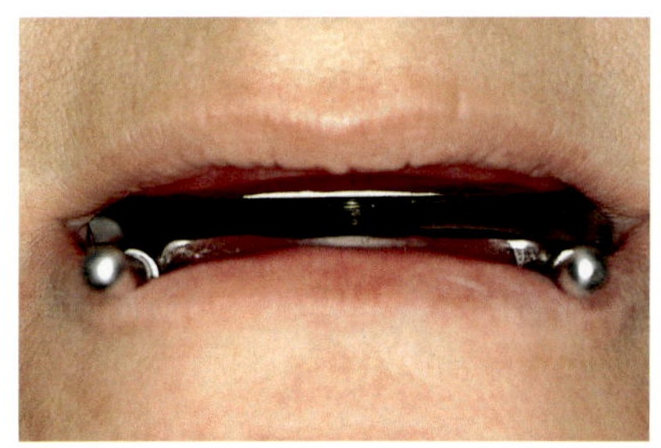

Fig 47 Remove the wax that is over the butterfly plate so that during protrusion and lateral movements there is no interference.

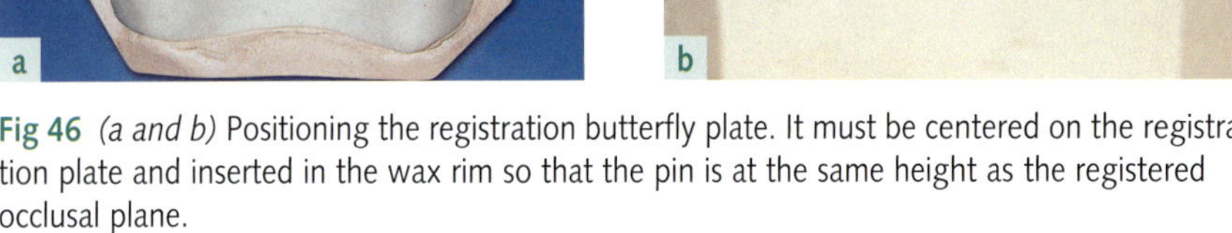

Fig 46 *(a and b)* Positioning the registration butterfly plate. It must be centered on the registration plate and inserted in the wax rim so that the pin is at the same height as the registered occlusal plane.

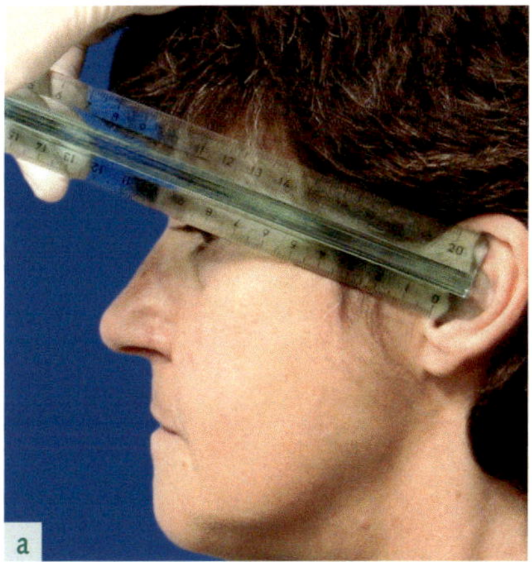
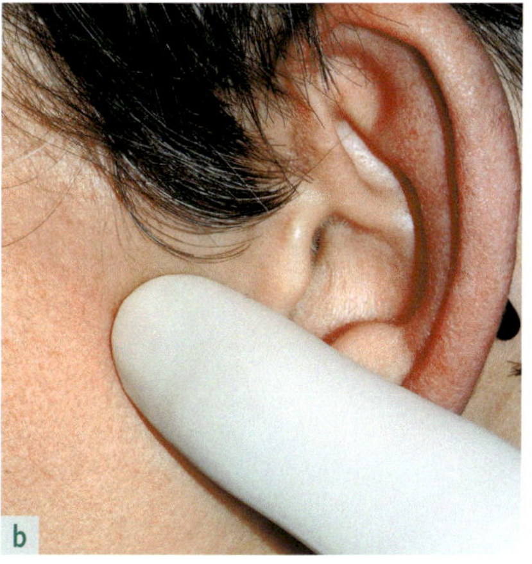

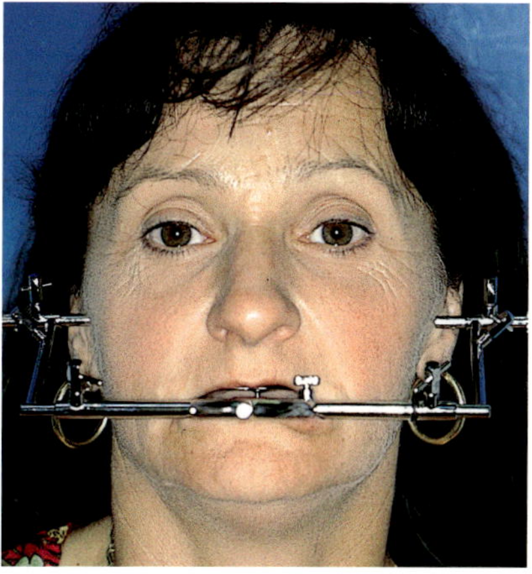

Fig 48 Marking the position of the mandibular hinge axis using measuring and palpation methods. *(a)* The supposed axis is identified on the tragus-cantus 11 to 13 mm anterior to the tragus. *(b)* The lateral pole of the condyle can be palpated while the patient opens and closes the mouth. Draw the line of the axis on the patient with a dermatologic pen.

Fig 49 Kinematic facebow in place. Ask the patient to assume a position of maximum retrusion (not forced). Make the pencils coincide with the marks made on the skin.

Fig 50 The "clock rule" is another way to verify that the registered positions are correct. Ask the patient to make a small opening and closing movement and look for any small movements of the pencils. If during these movements the two pencils rotate, the registered position is correct.

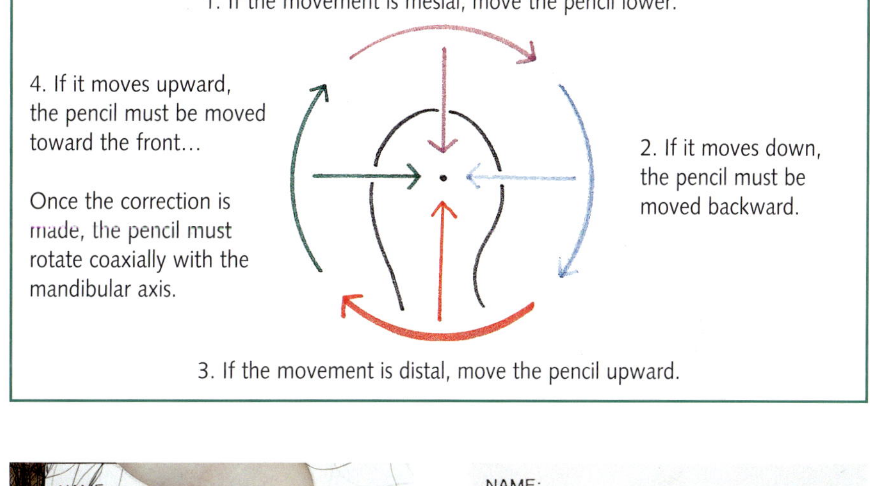

Fig 51 *(a and b)* Graphic recording of the sagittal condyle trajectory. The reference axis must be parallel to the registration card placed between the skin and the pencil. Record three tracings of protrusion and draw the corresponding tangents to the functional trace. The angle measurement is the mean of the inclination of the three tangents with reference to the occlusal plane.

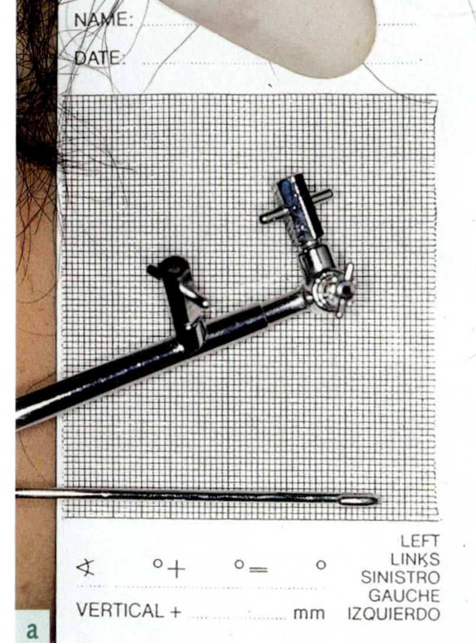

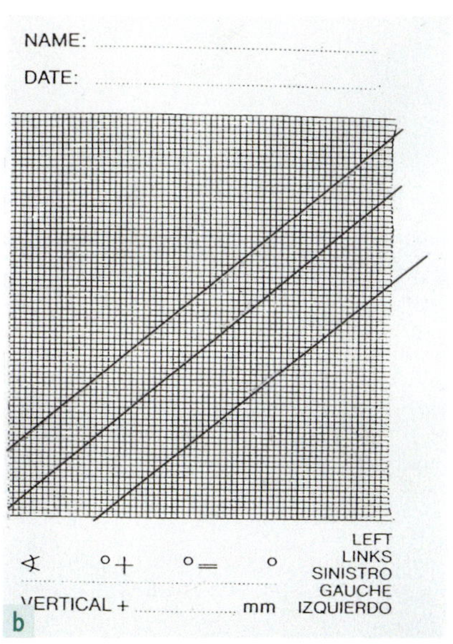

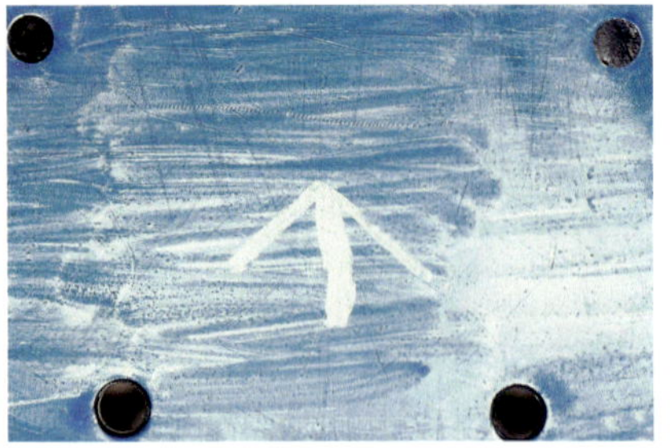

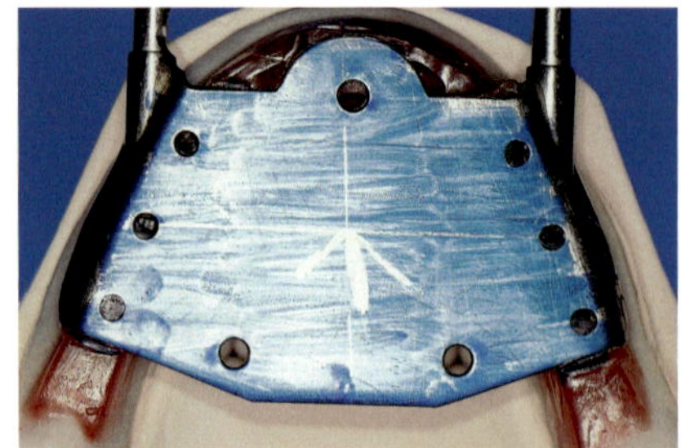

Fig 52 Remove the kinematic facebow, place a felt pen in the registration plate, and ask the patient to make protrusive, retrusive, and lateral movements. These will result in a gothic arch tracing.

Fig 53 Then draw a line through the apex of the gothic arch.

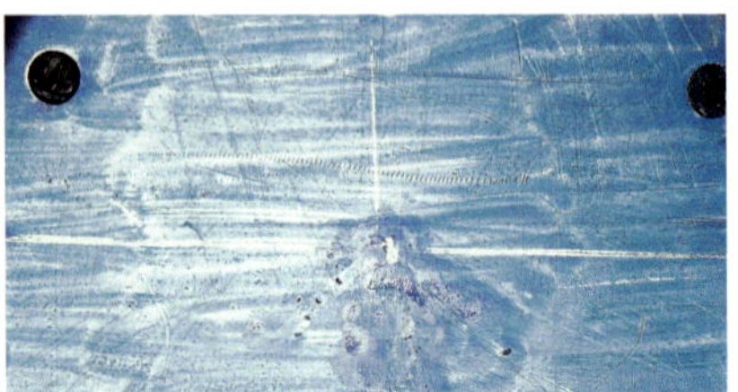

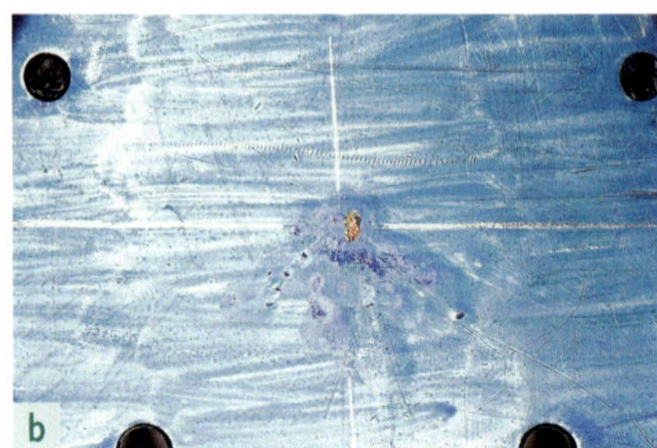

Fig 54 (a and b) Erase the gothic arch, leaving the cross lines. The neuromuscular center is registered by asking the patient to make small, rapid opening and closing movements. This measurement may coincide with the apex of the gothic arch but is normally 0.5 mm distal to the apex of the arch.

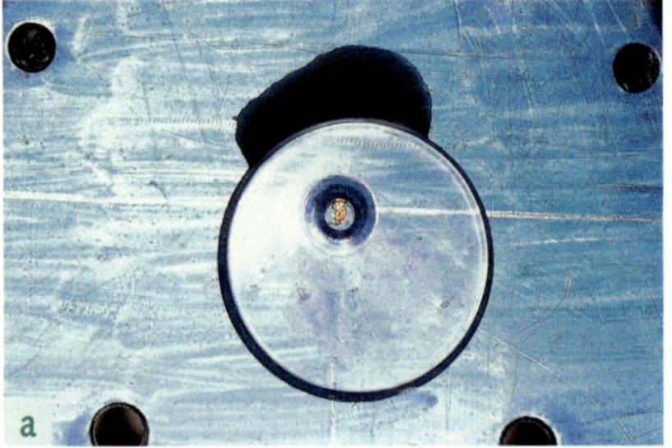

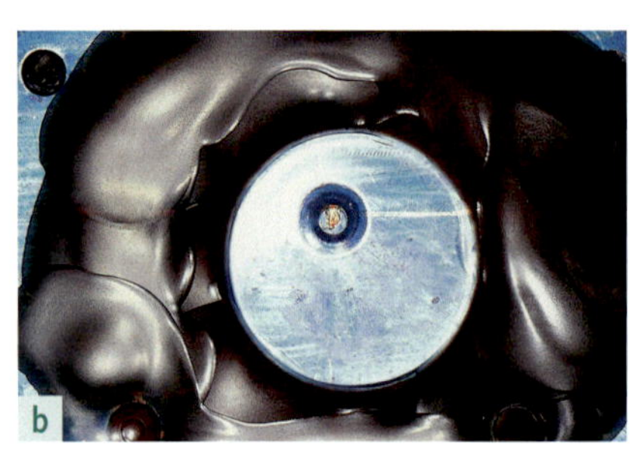

Fig 55 (a and b) Application and fixation of a plastic disc perforated in the *therapeutic position*. A neuromuscular center more than 2 mm from the apex of the gothic arch indicates a muscular disturbance and requires, over time, a new registration to adapt the system (it is also necessary to check that this measurement is not an artifact).

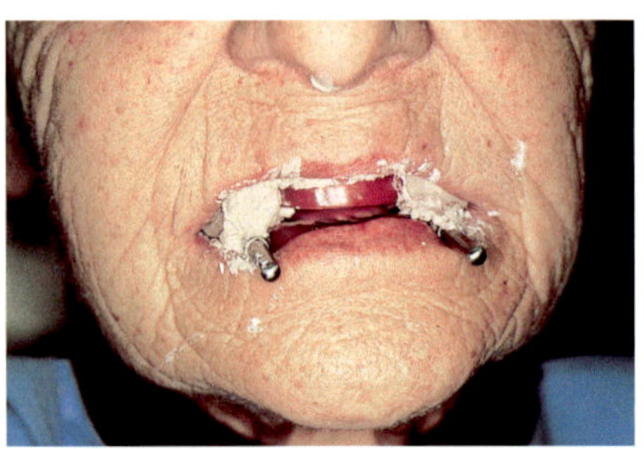

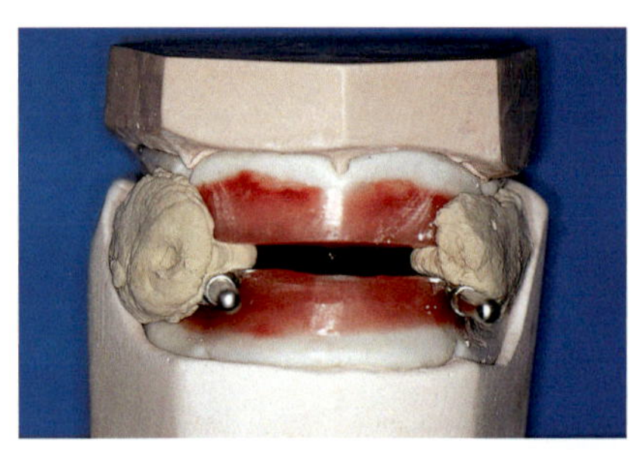

Fig 56 Ask the patient to close the mouth so that the pin is inserted into the perforation in the plastic disc. This position is then blocked using plaster wedges.

Fig 57 The master cast is then blocked in the therapeutic position using the plaster wedges prepared in the mouth.

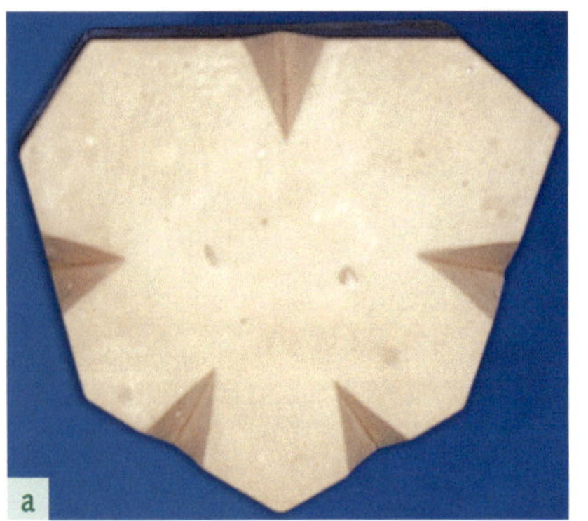

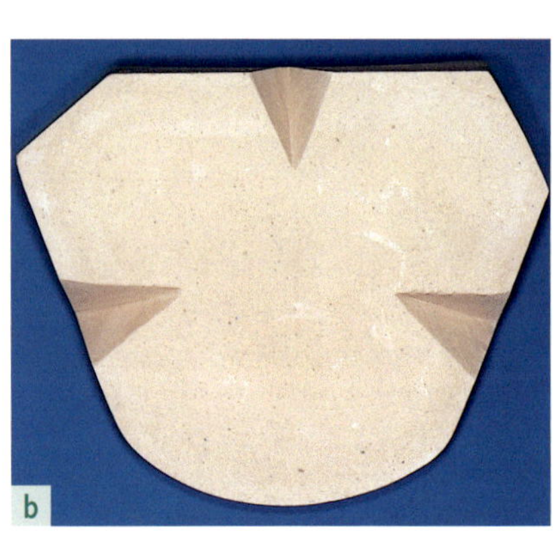

Fig 58 (a and b) On the base of the master casts, three-dimensional gutters are made that permit the separation of the casts from their respective bases.

Fig 59 Transfer the mandibular master cast to the articulator. The pencils used to trace the trajectory of the sagittal condyle are then substituted with the appropriate metal points. The reference rods of the facebow must be parallel to the work plane.

Fig 60 *(a to c)* Possible relationships between anatomic and the mechanical articulation after the extraoral registration. Because of the anatomic variation among patients, there are frequent cases in which the red spots do not coincide with the hinge axis of the articulator. Therefore, the areas within the concentric rings around the mechanical condyle are considered acceptable compromises. The operator must fix the left and right points within the circle of the same color (the colored circles were included to demonstrate use of the mechanical articulator) with simple movements of the stand in the anteroposterior and superoinferior directions.

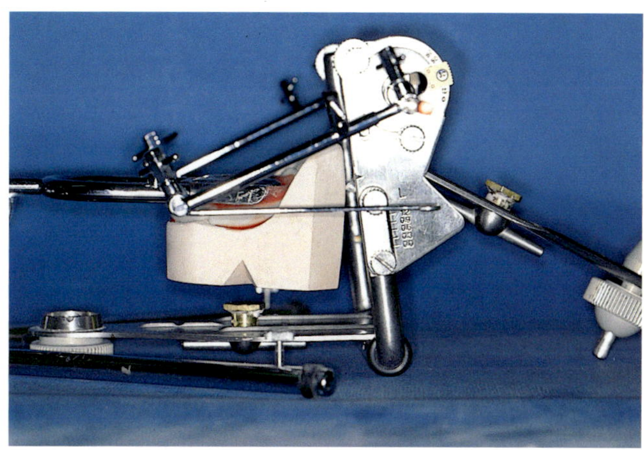

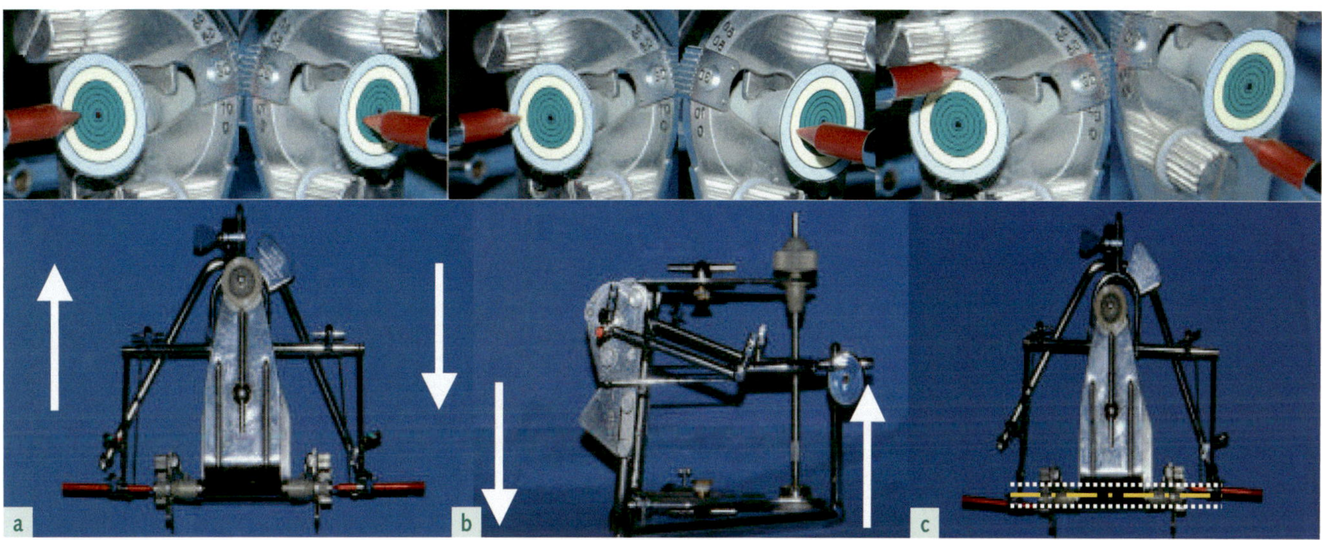

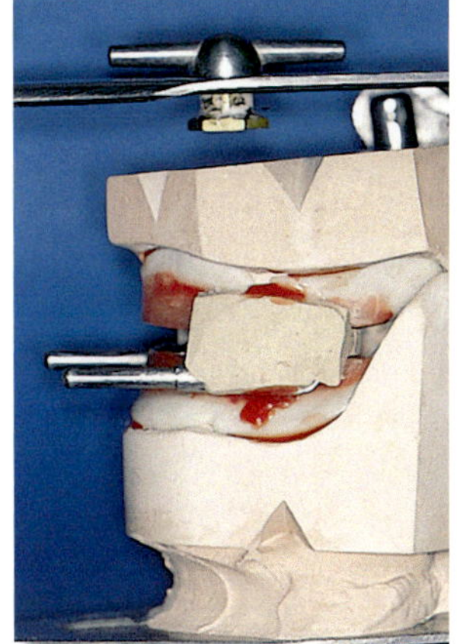

Fig 61 Mandibular cast is blocked with low-expansion plaster (type 4).

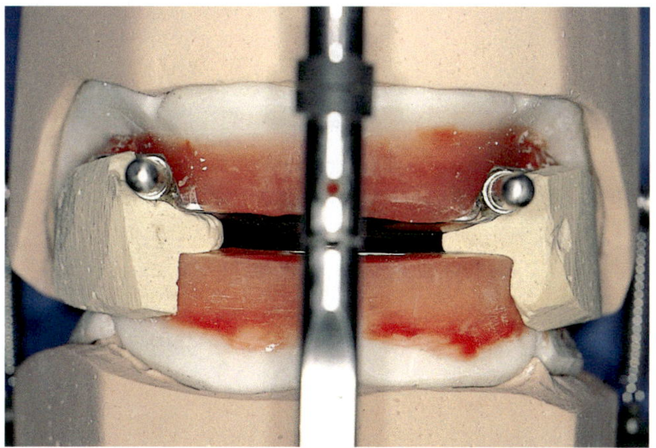

Fig 62 Blocking the maxillary cast and refinishing the base of both casts.

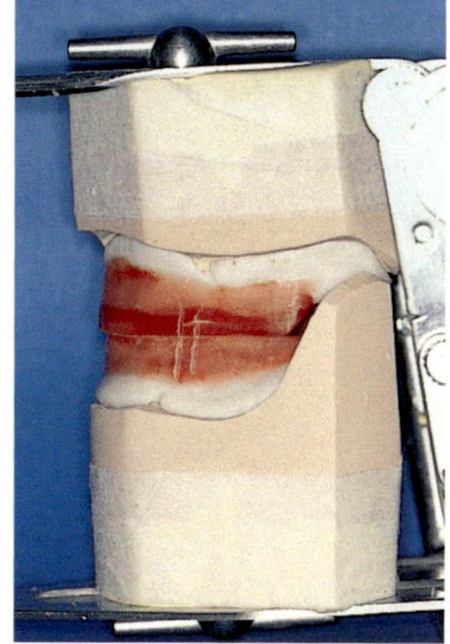

Fig 63 The maxillary rim is refinished first, taking advantage of the baseplate backing of the mandible, and then the mandibular rim is refinished, adapting it to that of the maxilla.

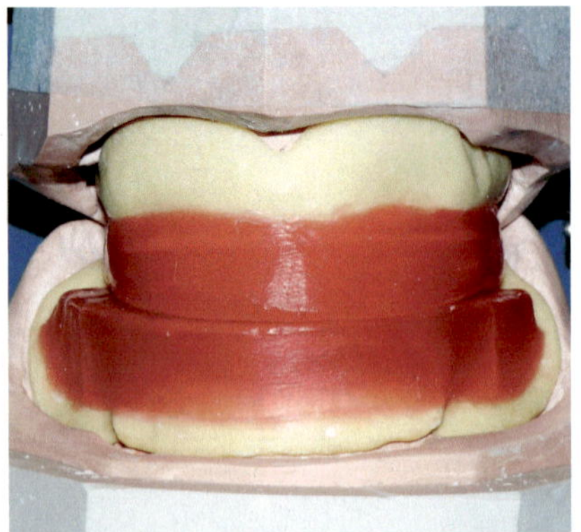

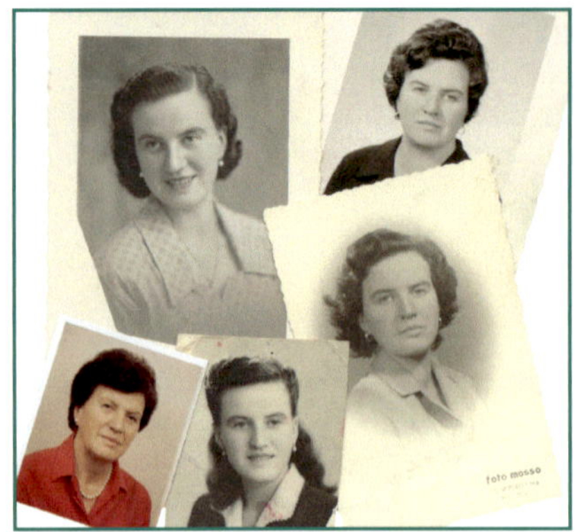

Fig 64 Baseplates for occlusal registration in the articulator. Check the vertical dimensions in centric occlusion in the patient's mouth and then proceed with mounting the incisors and canines.

Fig 65 Photographs of the patient before loss of teeth assist the restoration of dentofacial harmony.

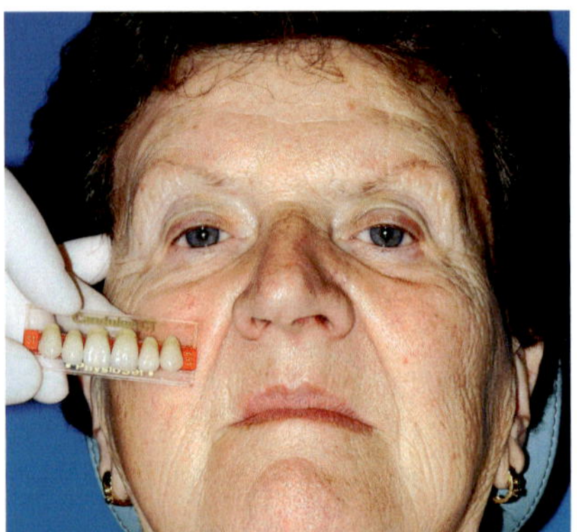

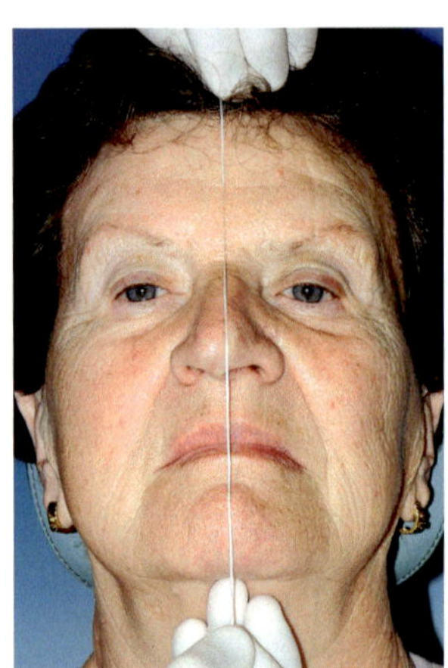

Fig 66 Choose the shape and color of the teeth directly on the patient. The choice is based on the color of the skin and the morphology of the face. Dark skin and hair require gray tones, and pink skin and blond hair, pinkish tones.

Fig 67 Line of symmetry is registered on the patient's face and then transferred to the wax rim.

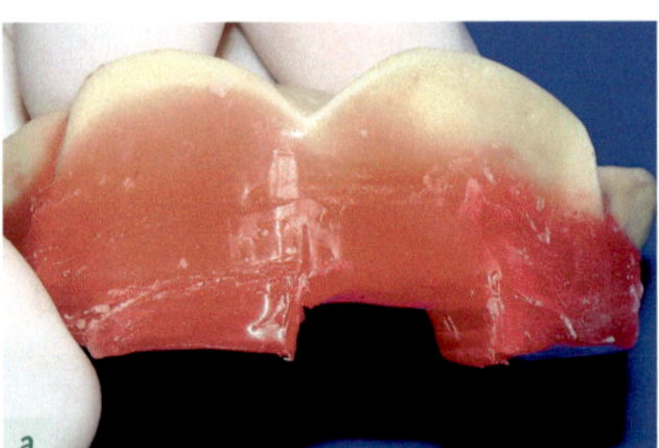

a

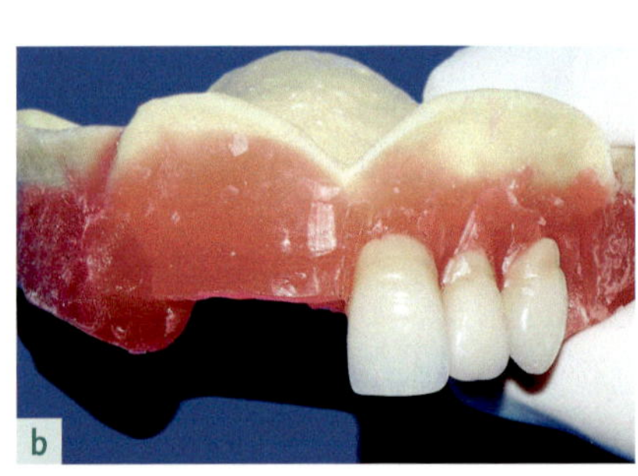

b

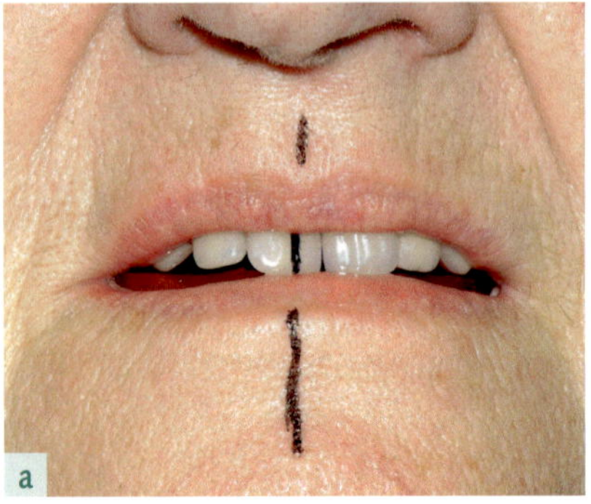

c

Fig 68 *(a to c)* Mounting sequence. The wax rim must be removed on one side only. The other side is used as a guide for mounting the first three teeth. Complete mounting of the contralateral teeth is then carried out, using the teeth already in position as a guide.

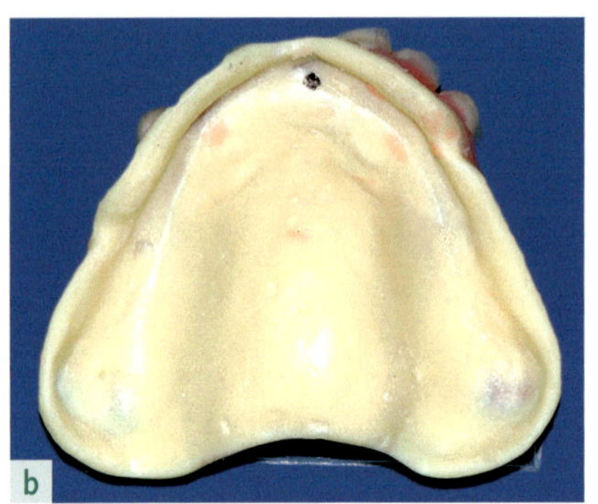

a

b

Fig 69 *(a)* The interincisive line does not coincide with the line of symmetry of the face. *(b)* The left-side teeth have been mounted too close to the palate (note their position compared with the interincisive papilla indicated with a dot).

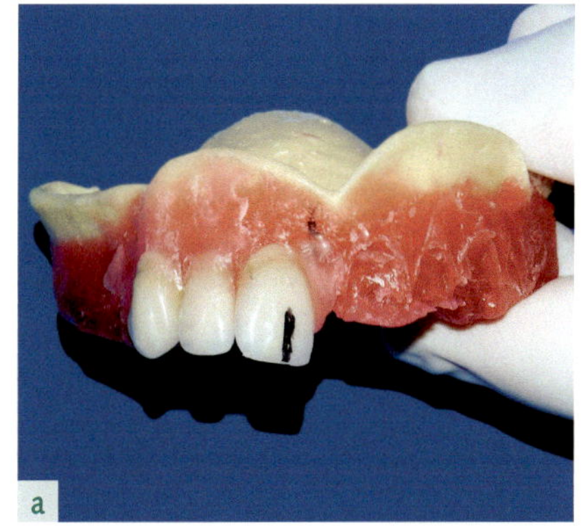

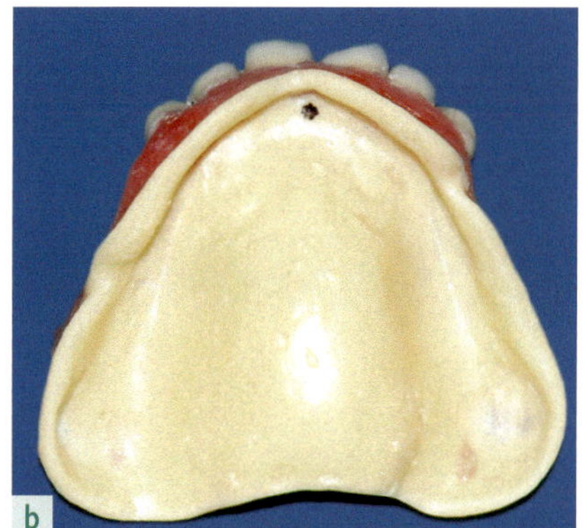

Fig 70 *(a and b)* Errors on the frontal plane are corrected so that the interincisive line coincides with the line of symmetry of the face. On the sagittal plane, the anteroposterior position of the teeth is now correct with respect to the interincisive papilla.

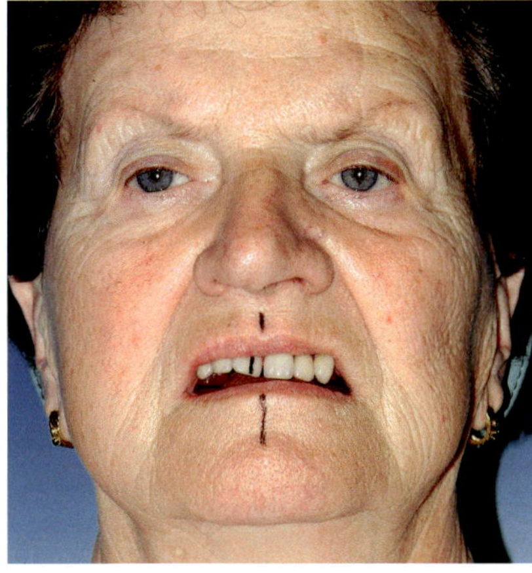

Fig 71 The corrections made to the prosthesis are checked.

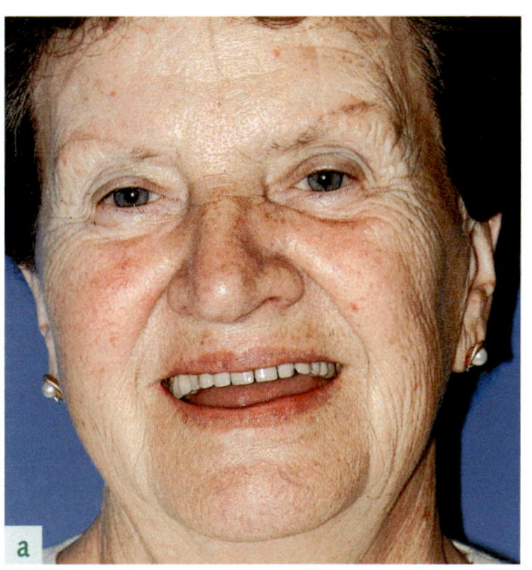

Fig 72 Comparison of the old prosthesis *(a)* with the new one *(b)*. Note that the new prosthesis has restored the esthetics and the physiognomy.

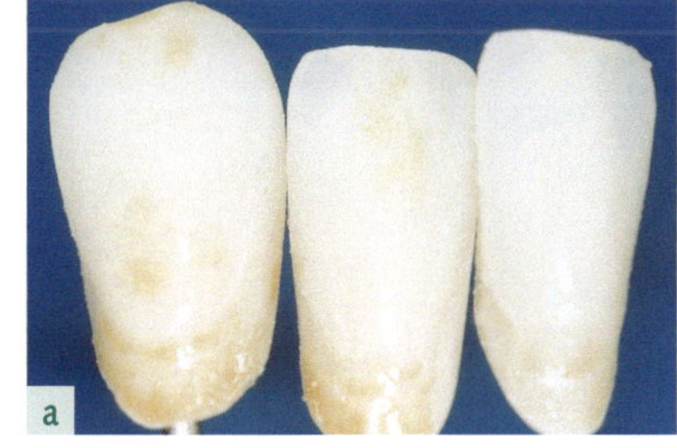

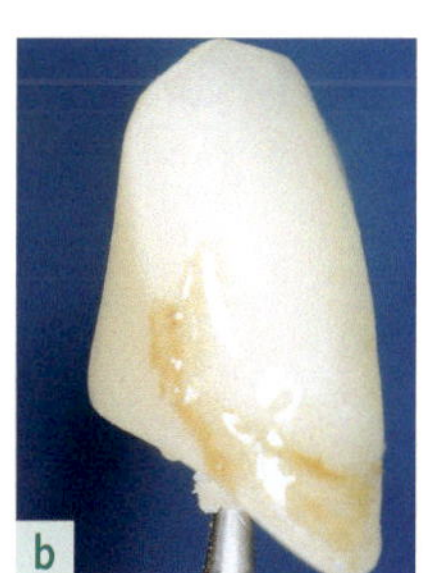

Fig 73 *(a and b)* Manufactured teeth for prostheses must be considered semifinished products—the form and color can be modified. Always discuss these choices with the patient, who may not always appreciate modifications.

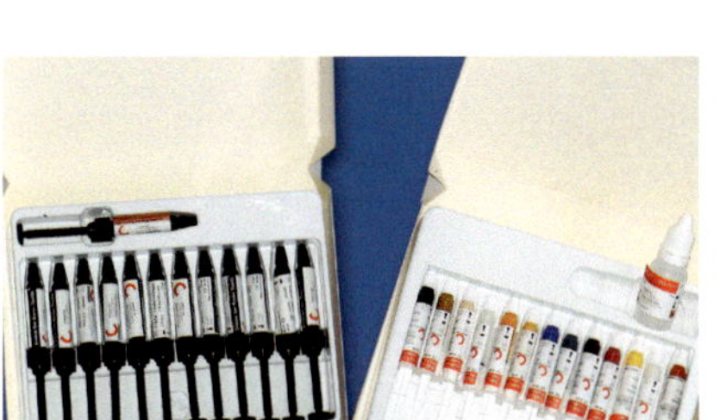

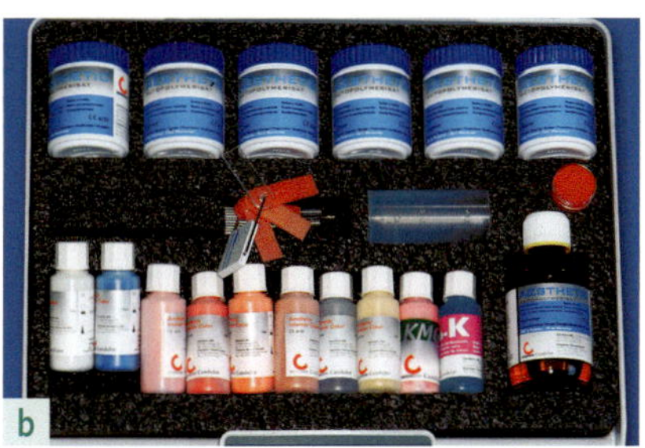

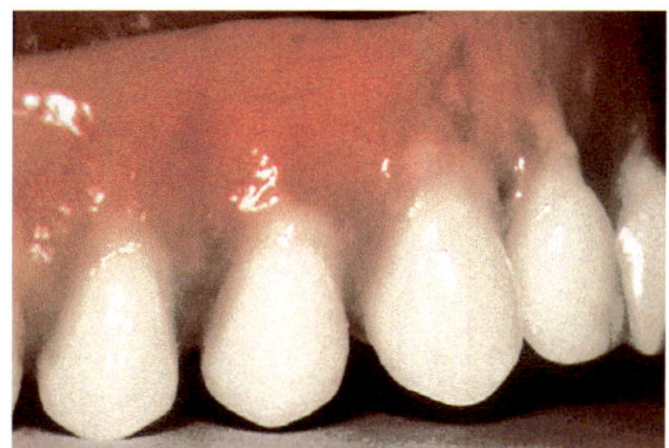

Fig 74 *(a and b)* Kits showing the colors available for customizing teeth in resin ceramic as well as prosthetic bases.

Fig 75 Coloring the prosthetic base is particularly useful for smiles that show the gingiva.

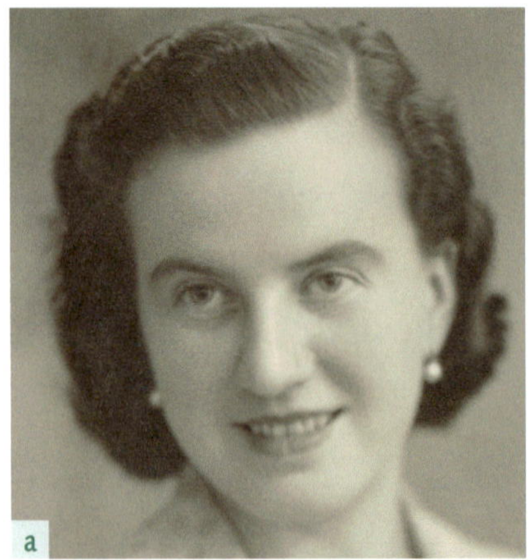
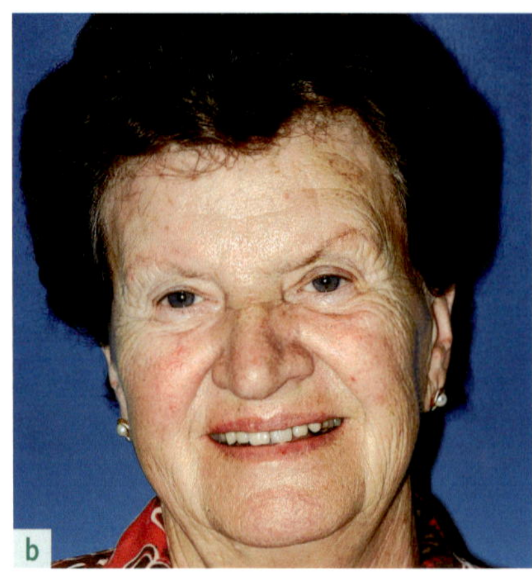

Fig 76 Comparison between a photo of the patient when she was younger *(a)* and the esthetic result obtained with the new prosthesis *(b)*. The dentofacial harmony has been restored, giving a satisfactory esthetic result.

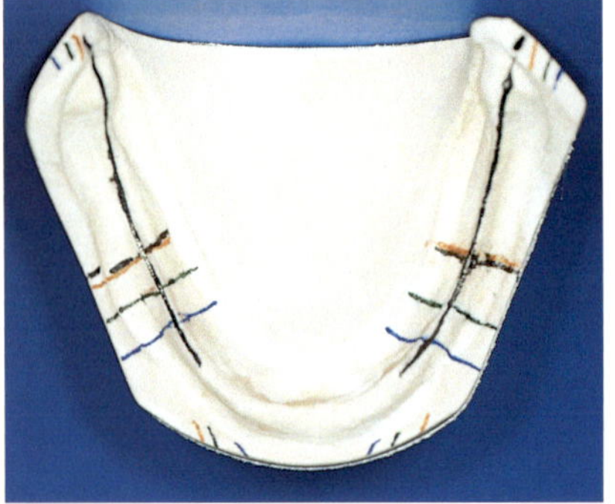

Fig 77 Mounting the premolars and posterior teeth must be preceded by careful analysis of the edentulous crest. It is useful to draw the future positions of the teeth on the mandibular master cast with different identifiable colors.

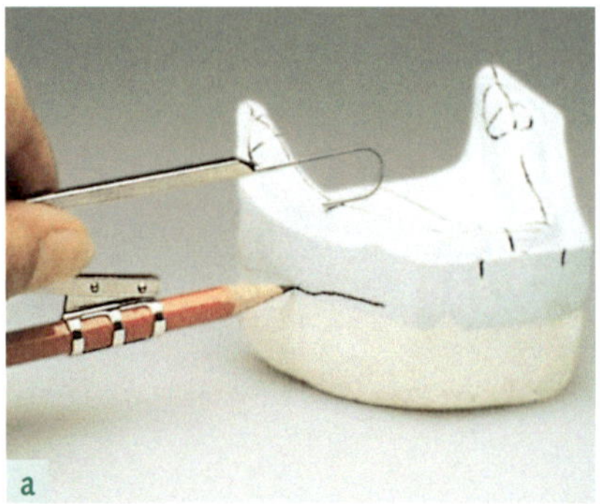

Fig 78 *(a and b)* Using the appropriate caliper (Condylator Service), it is possible to transfer the shape of the edentulous crest onto the master cast. This will permit verification that the occlusal plane is parallel with the shape of the crest during mounting.

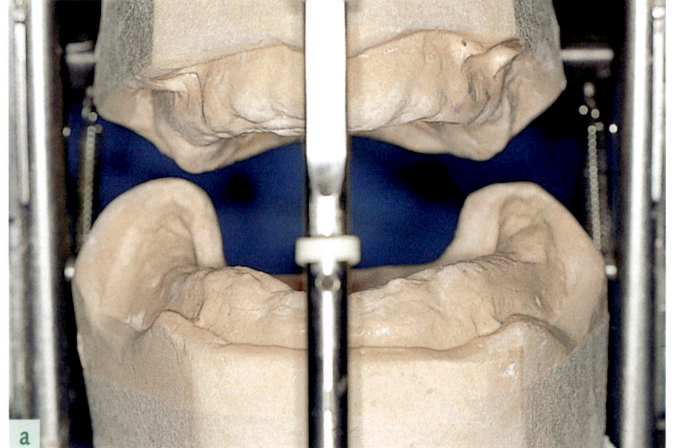
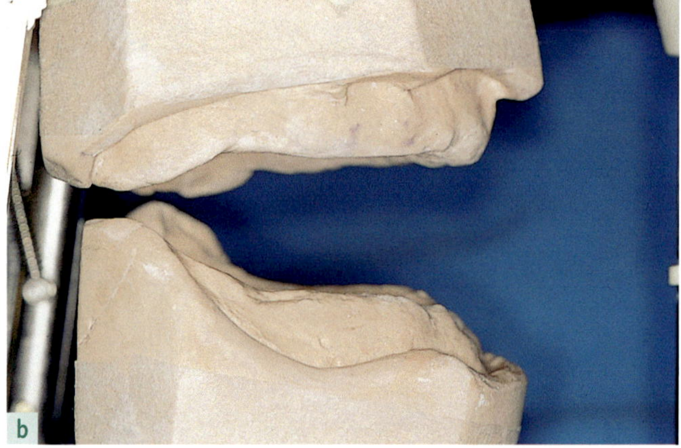

Fig 79 *(a and b)* Evaluation of the congruence of the two arches on the frontal and sagittal planes. The different modes of resorption between the maxilla and mandible can create diverse situations of spatial discrepancy that will determine the type of mounting.

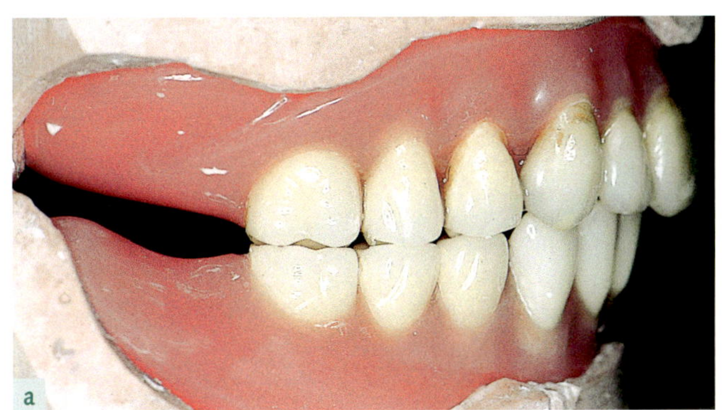
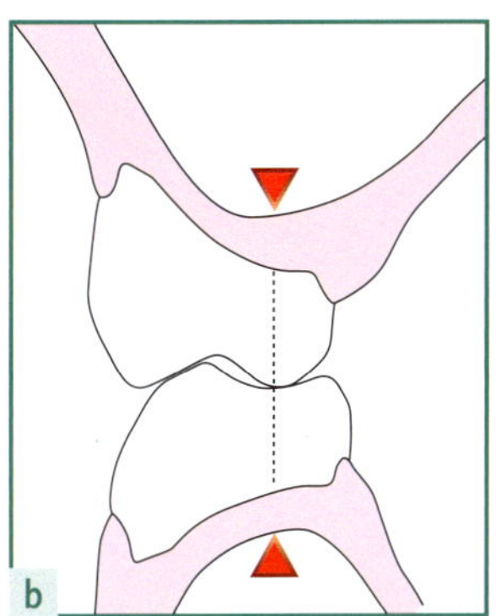

Fig 80 *(a and b)* When the discrepancy on the frontal plane is nonexistent or minimal, a normal occlusion is chosen.

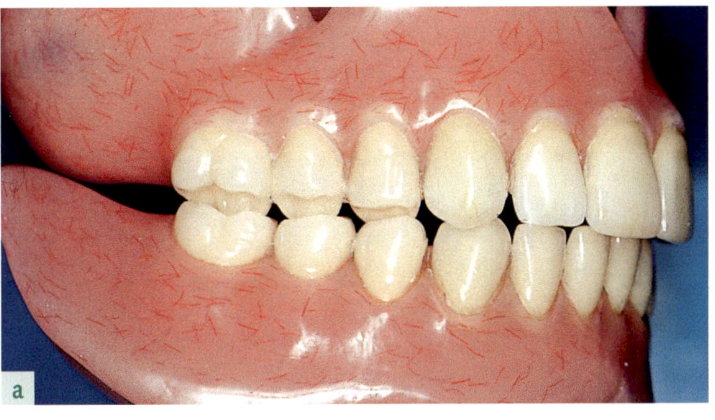
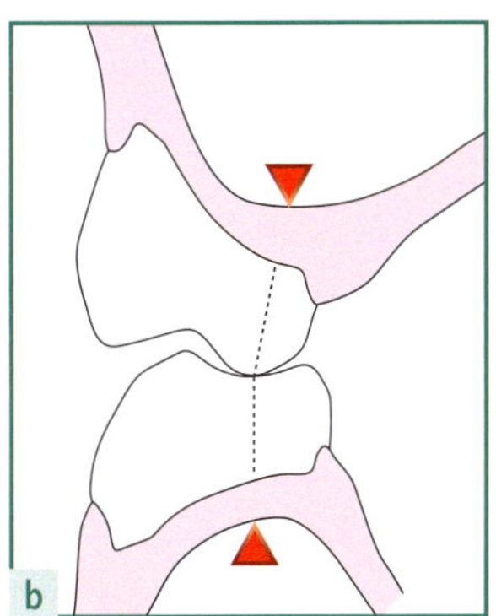

Fig 81 *(a and b)* When the discrepancy is noticeable, a reduced occlusion should be chosen.

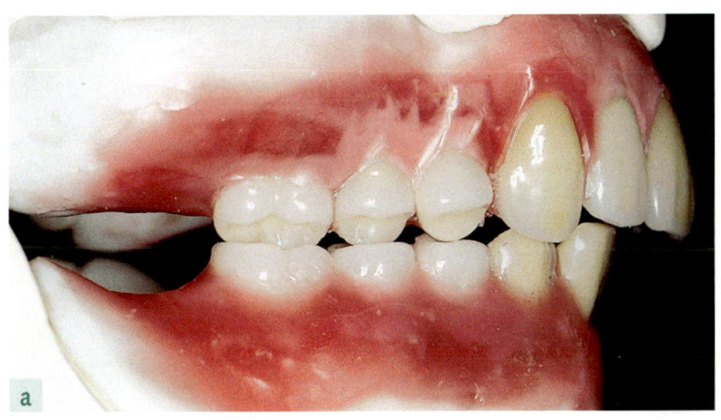
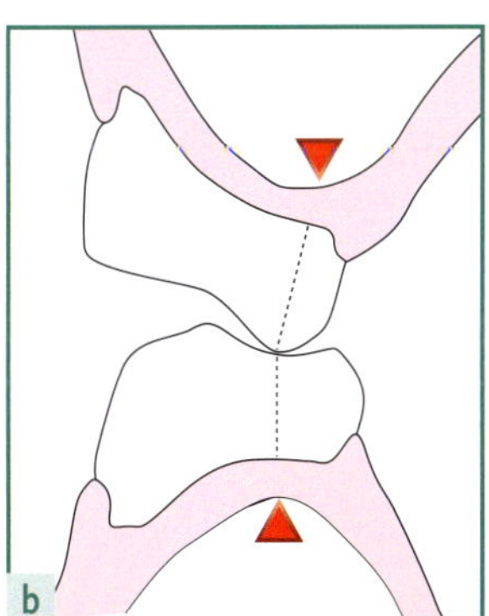

Fig 82 *(a and b)* For a very large discrepancy, a minimum occlusion is chosen.

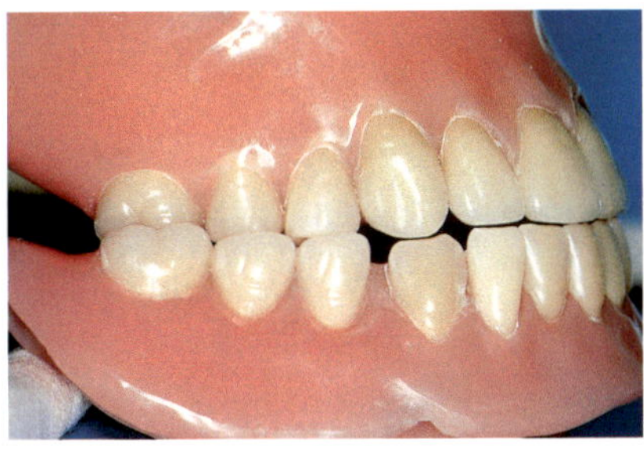
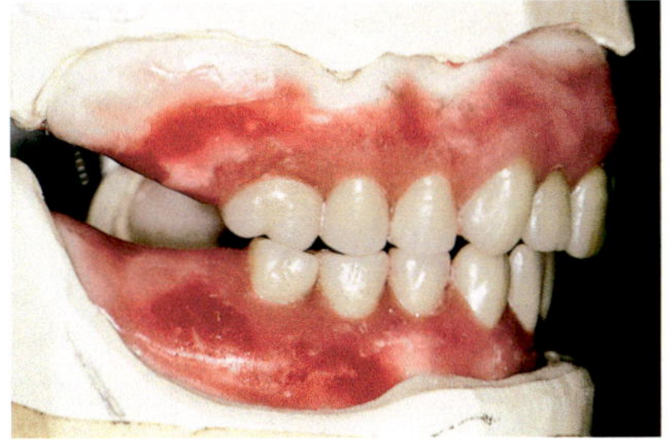
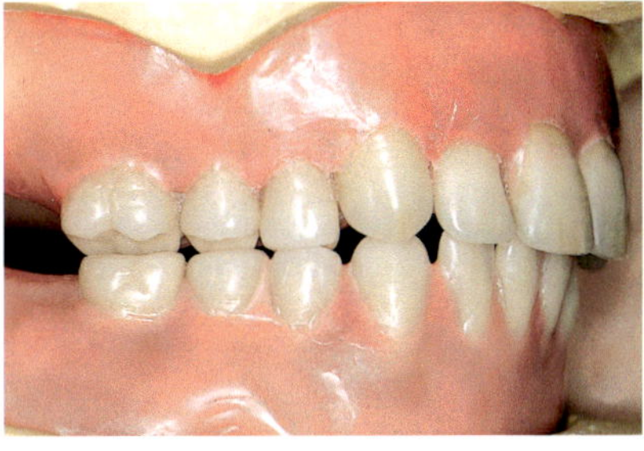

Fig 83 An obvious incongruence between the maxilla and mandible can only be resolved with a crossed mounting, where the buccal cusps of the maxillary teeth substitute the lingual cusps in their function of pestle.

Fig 84 In case of a flat sagittal path or an edentulous crest that is very curved in the posterior, a reduced arch with three premolars is used. This method limits the occlusal plane to the straight portion of the crest.

Fig 85 The three types of mounting (normal, reduced, and minimal occlusion) can coexist in the same mounting, to obviate a case of diverse grades of incongruence in the same patient.

71

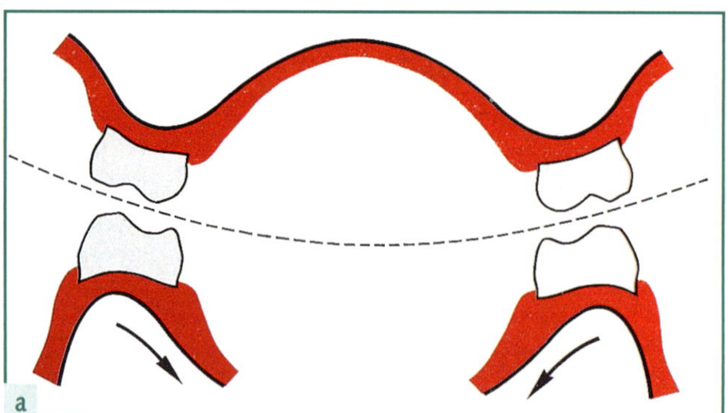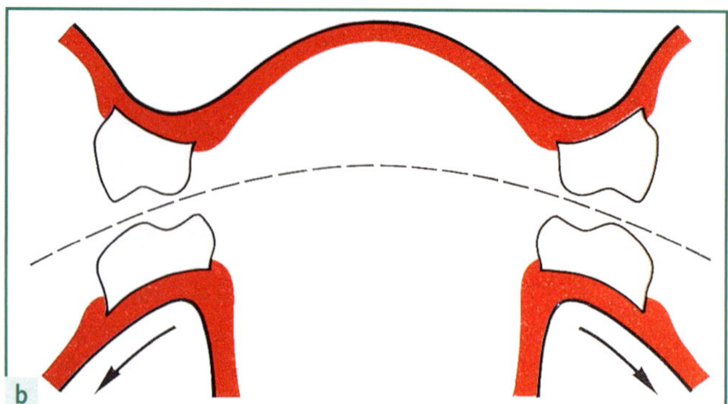

Fig 86 On the frontal plane, the mandibular edentulous crest may have a predominant buccal or lingual slope. To ameliorate the stability of the prosthesis, the mandibular teeth can be mounted with the occlusal plane parallel to the predominant slope. If the slope most used is the lingual, the mounting is *ad linguam (a)*. If the slope most used is buccal, the mounting is *ad vestibulum (b)*. Although these techniques improve the stability, they present balancing problems during selective grinding.

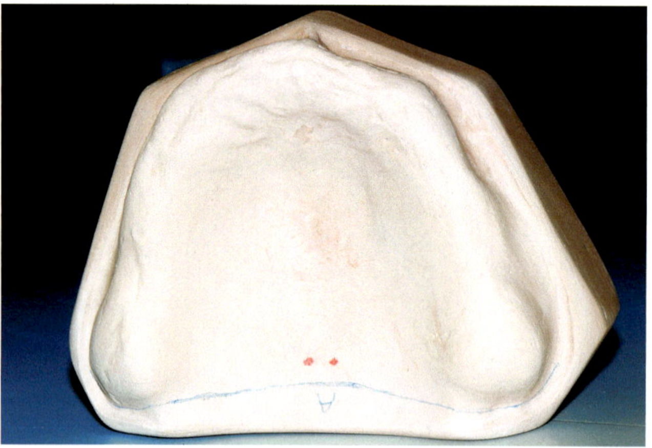

Fig 87 To determine the position of the transition between the hard and soft palate, line "A" is marked directly on the maxillary master cast and strictly dependent on the conformation of the soft palate.

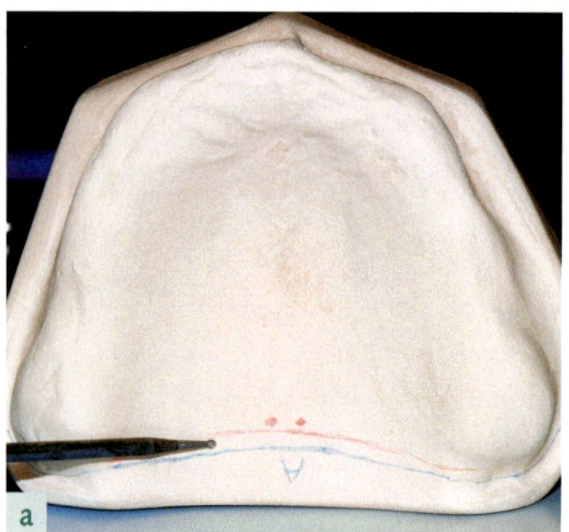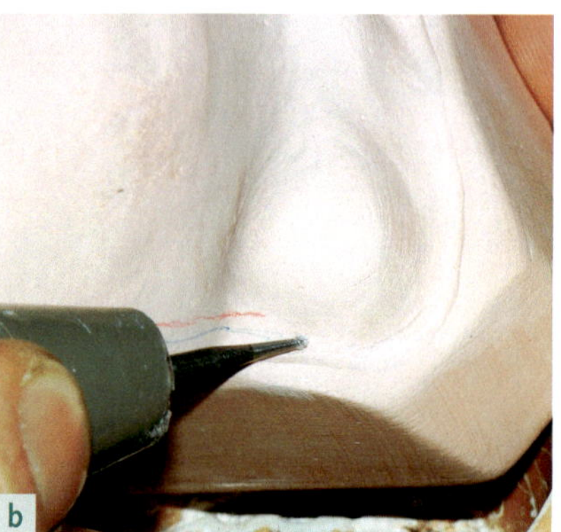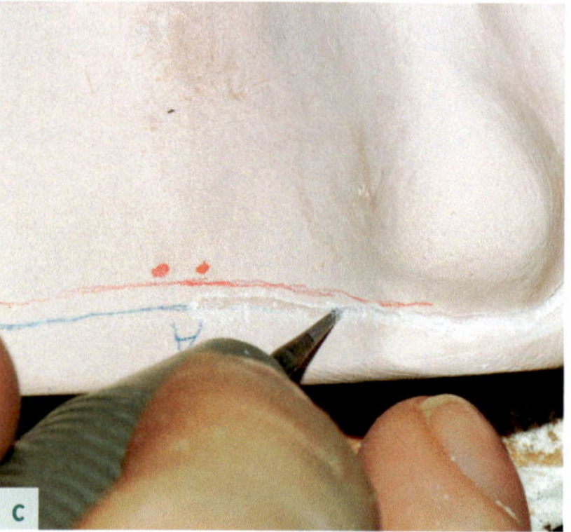

Fig 88 *(a to c)* Preparation sequence of the sulcus with a rose bur. The depth of the sulcus is greatest on the "A" line (1 mm) and gradually diminishes toward the fossae.

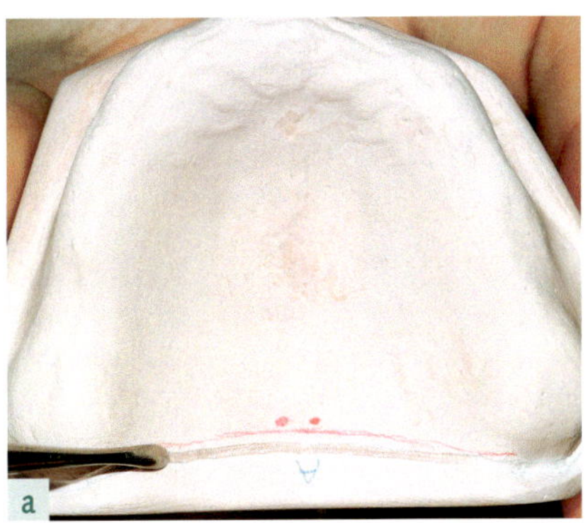 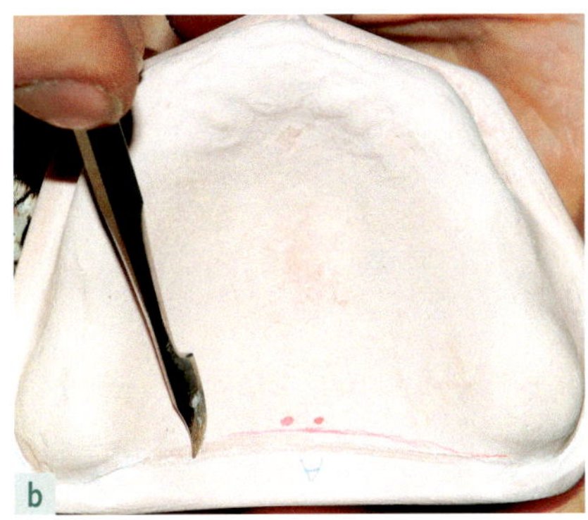 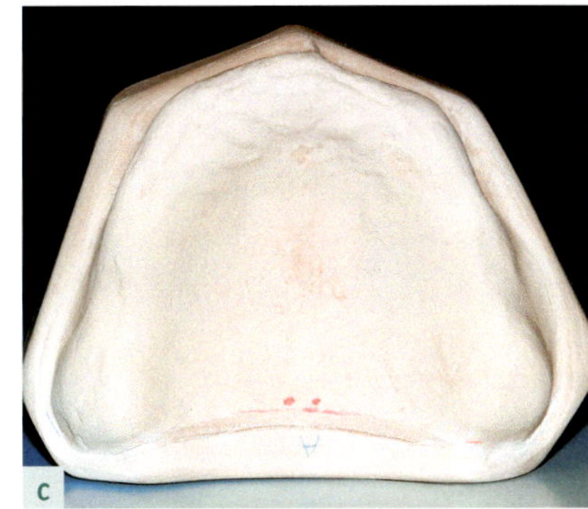

Fig 89 *(a to c)* With a cutting spatula the sulcus is finished so that the compression is gradual. With this preparation, any possible contractions of the resin during polymerization or small touch-ups in this zone will not influence retention.

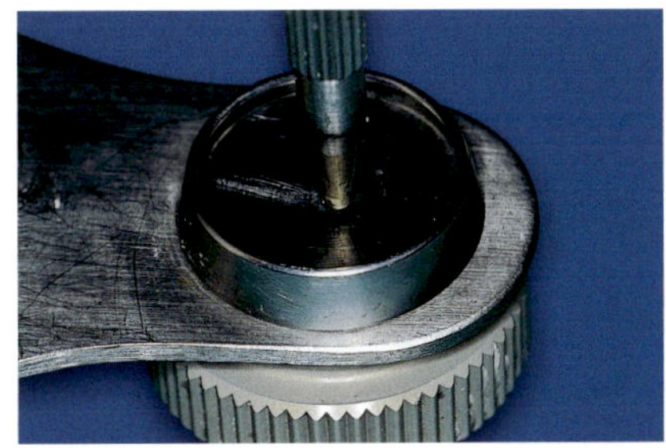

Fig 90 Once the polymerization is completed, the prosthesis is repositioned in the articulator. Small vertical discrepancies around the incisive vertical rod resulting from the polymerization process may result with the prosthesis in maximal intercuspidation, slightly detached from the disk.

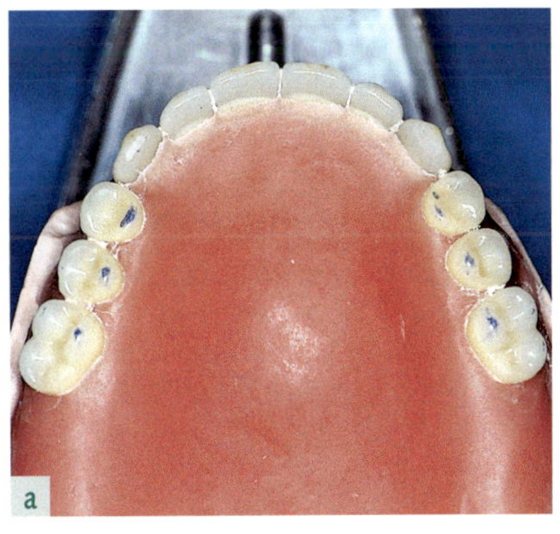 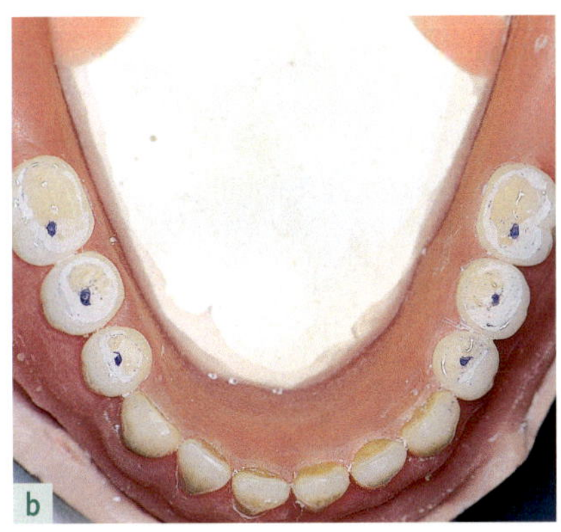 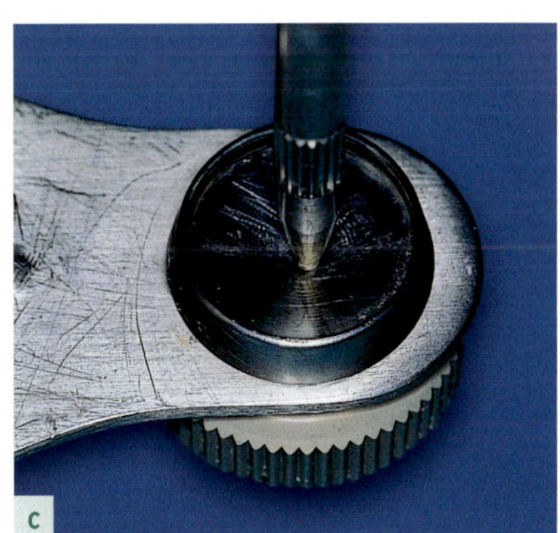

Fig 91 *(a to c)* The first selective grinding is to re-establishes the registered VDO, relocating the centric stop on all posterior teeth. After this process, the incisive vertical rod must touch the disk. If in some teeth the centric stop is missing after grinding, they must be removed and replaced in the resin in the correct position.

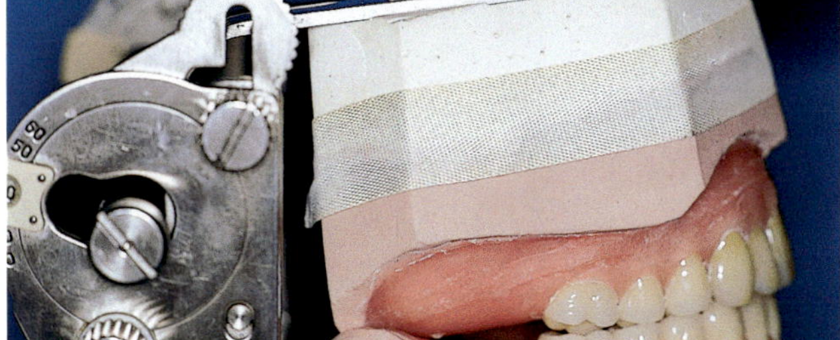

Fig 92 Opening of the ring nut of the mechanical condyle to permit the movements of laterality and protrusion.

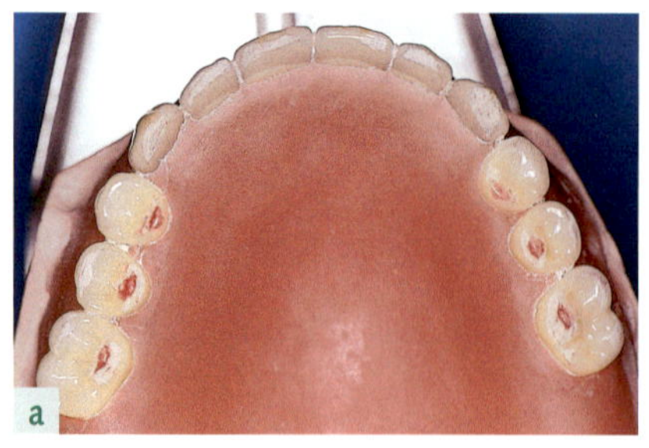

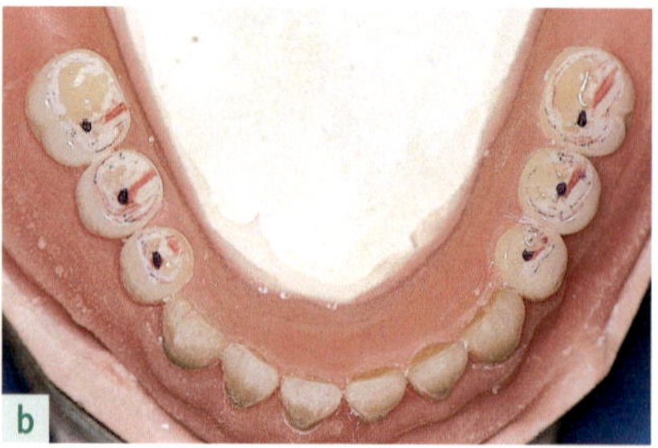

Fig 93 *(a and b)* The lateral contacts (either left or right) are touched up with the appropriate bur. At the same time, sliding contacts must be obtained either on the working side or on the balancing side without interference.

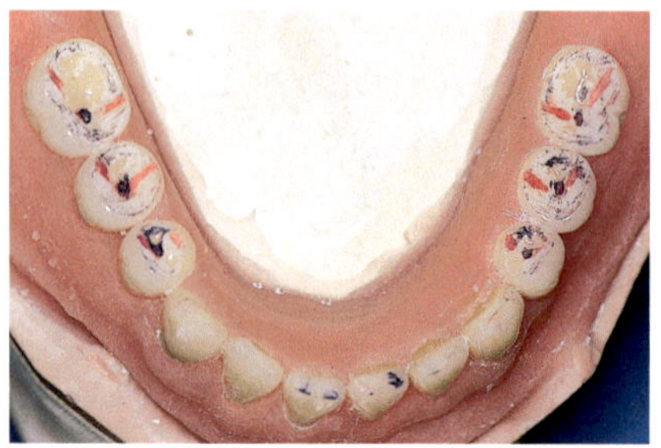

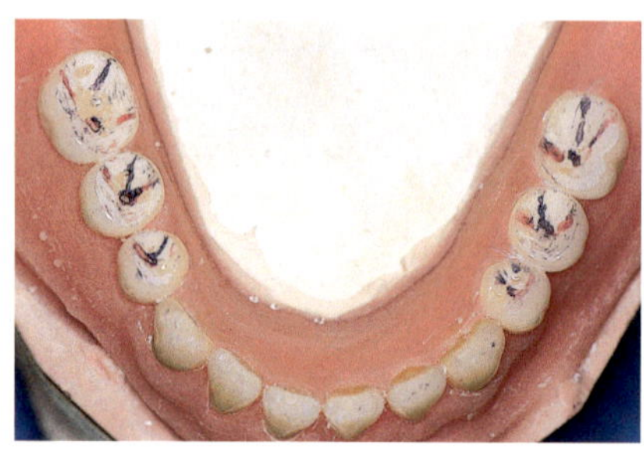

Fig 94 Checking the contacts on the other side must be completed in the same manner.

Fig 95 Grinding in protrusion is always made with the condyle ring nut open, using the same system as for controlling laterality.

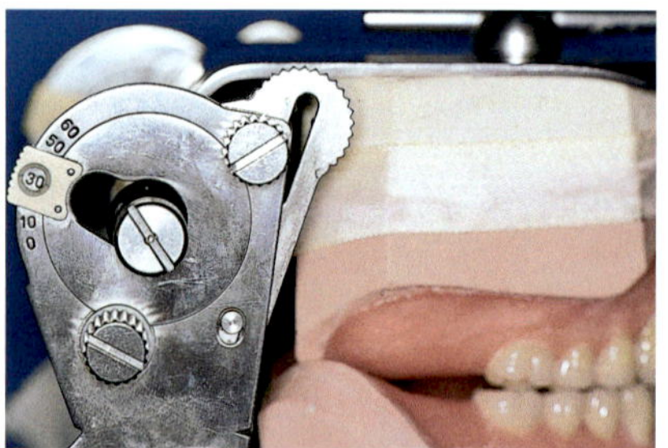

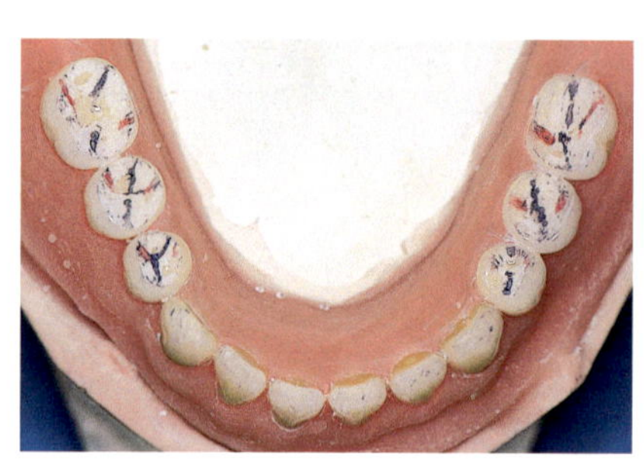

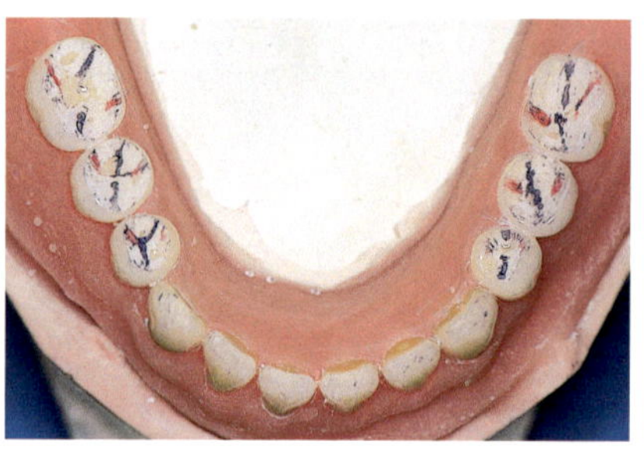

Fig 96 The Condylator allows a slight movement of retrusion with the forward movement of the condyle ring-nut.

Fig 97 It is then possible to touch up the small interferences in retrusion.

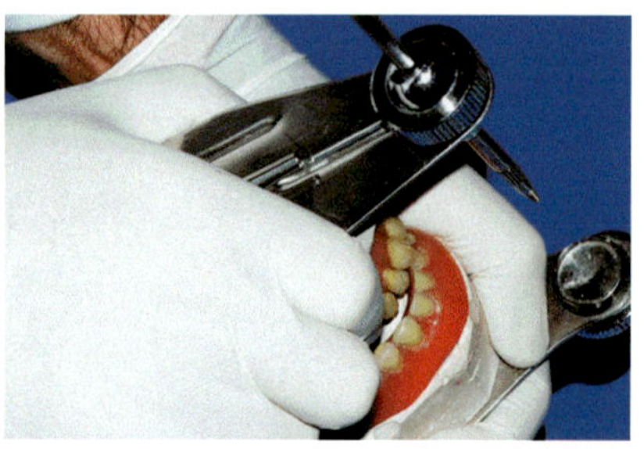

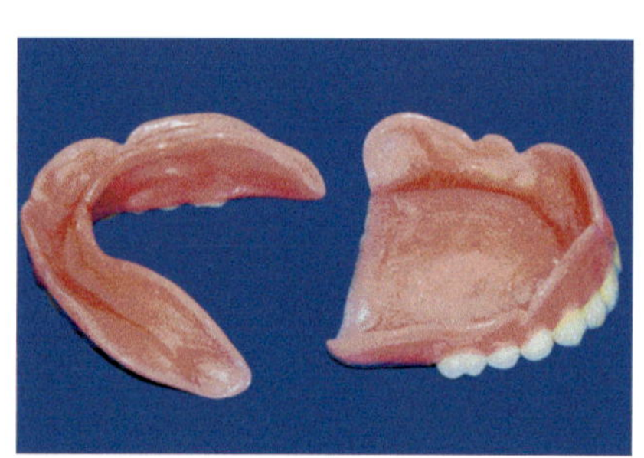

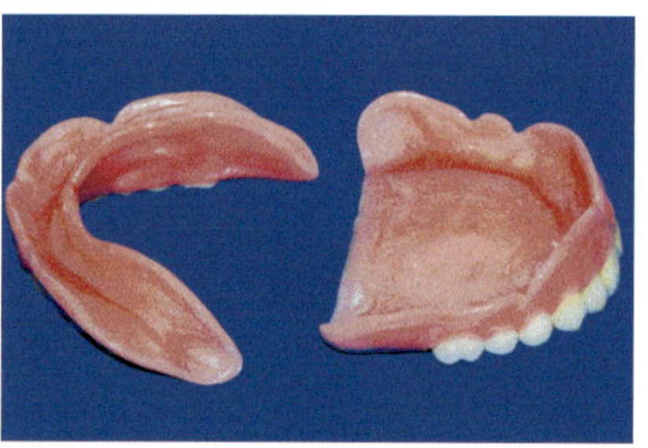

Fig 98 To render the sliding movements uniform at the completion of selective grinding, an abrasive paste made of petroleum jelly and carburundum powder is used. Rotary clockwise and counterclockwise movements are used with moderate pressure to complete the selective milling.

Fig 99 Prosthesis ready for adapting in the mouth.

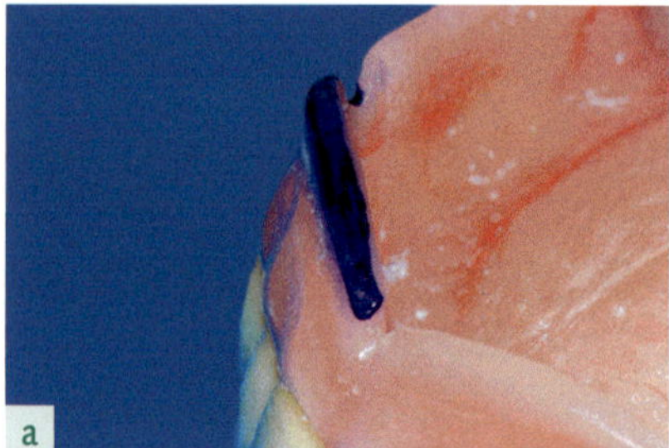

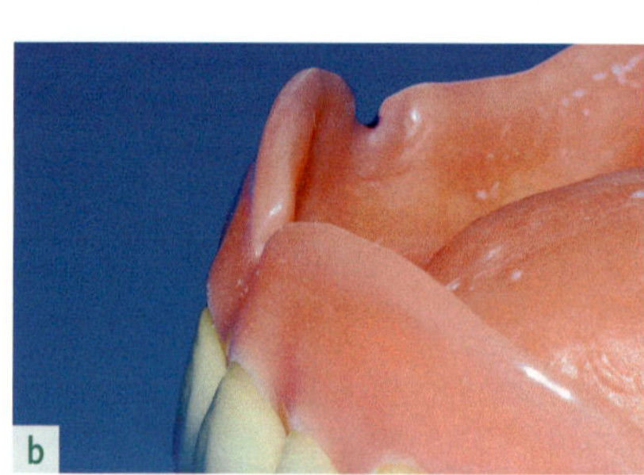

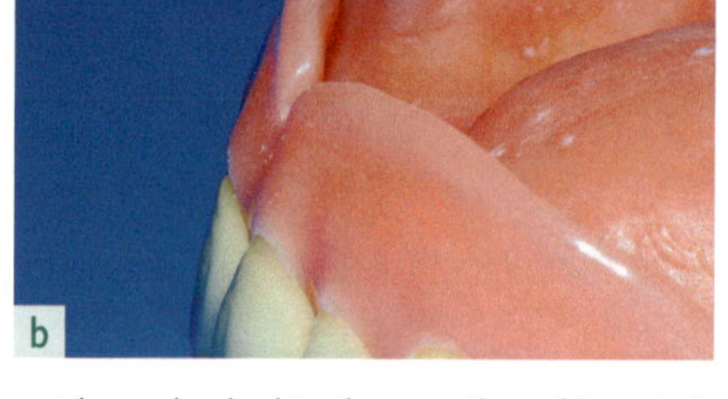

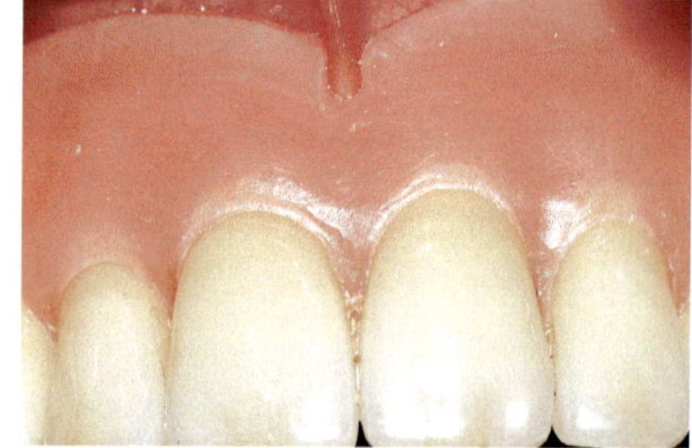

Fig 100 *(a and b)* The margins of the prosthesis must be rechecked in the mouth and beveled to 45 degrees.

Fig 101 The maxillary median frenum must be accommodated without functionalization.

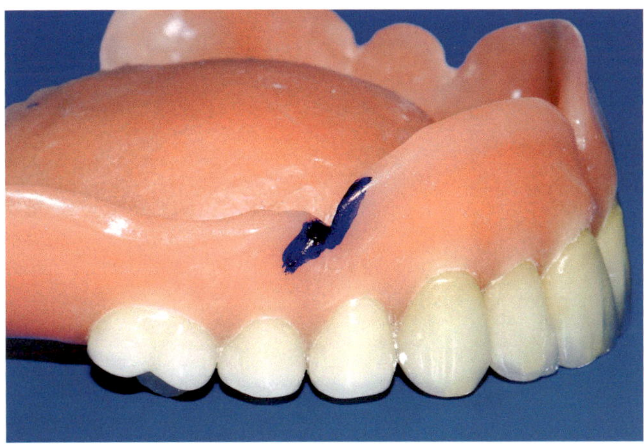

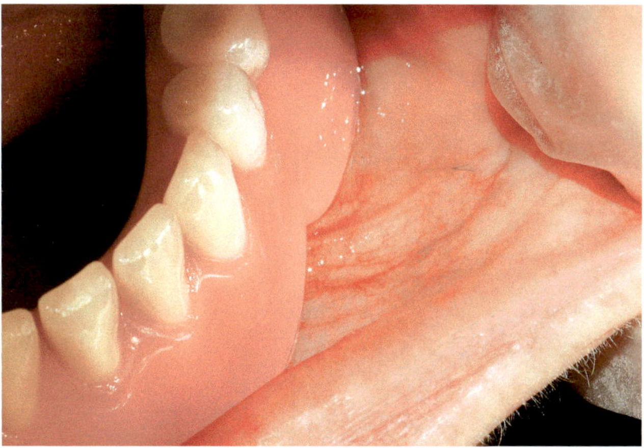

Fig 102 The lateral maxillary frena must be accommodated, taking into account their elliptic path.

Fig 103 The lateral mandibular frena must be accommodated using the same technique as for the maxillary frena.

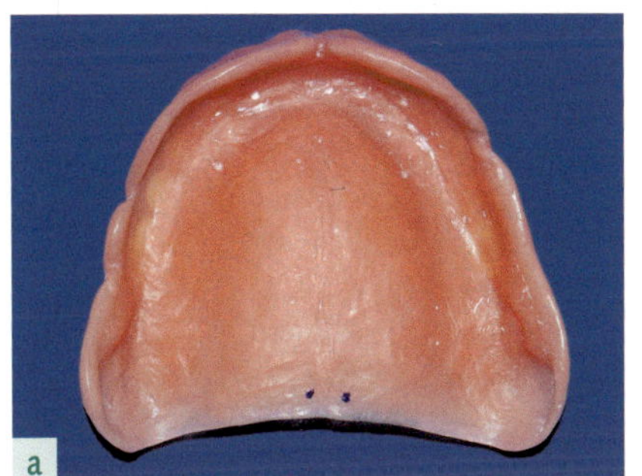

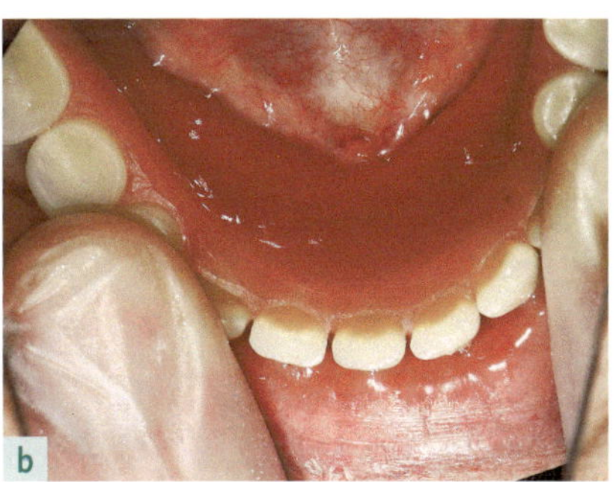

Fig 104 *(a)* The posterior margin of the maxillary prosthesis often does not coincide with the anatomic limits of the fossae. *(b)* In the anterior sublingual region, the mandibular prosthesis must occupy the entire sublingual sulcus area, taking care not to cover the openings of the salivary glands.

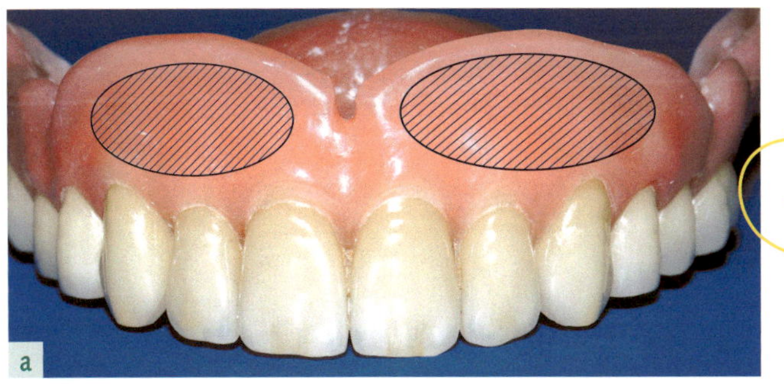

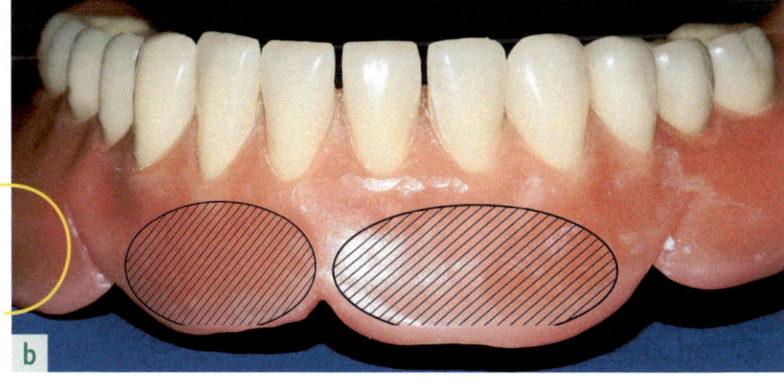

Fig 105 *(a and b)* The orbicular muscles of the lips must be accommodated by means of grooves in the anterior flange of the prosthesis.

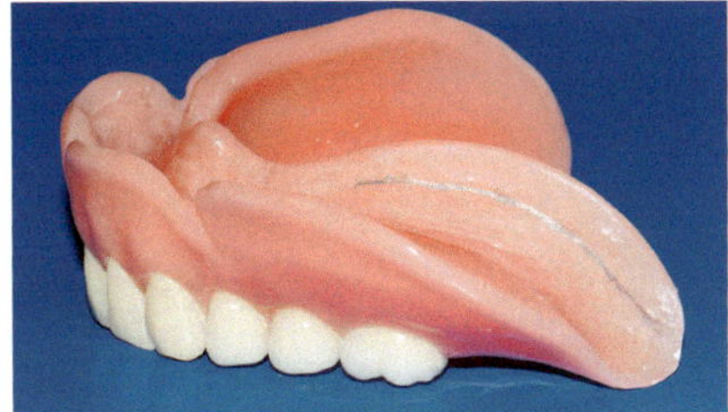

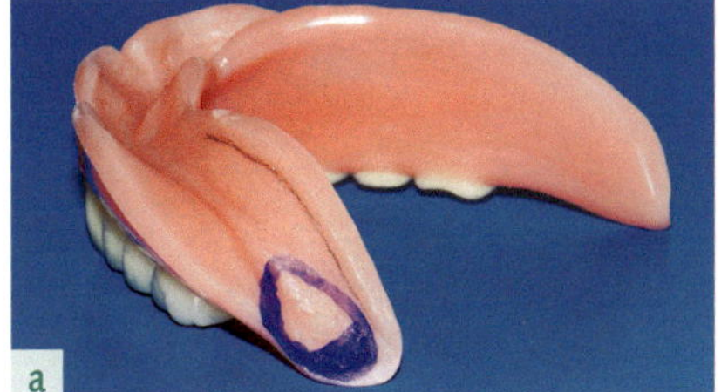

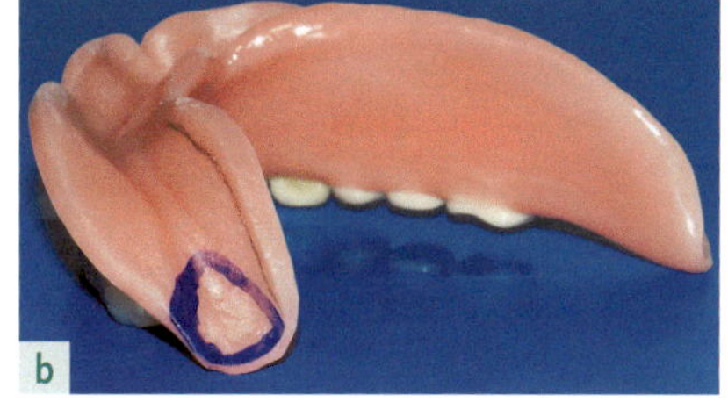

Fig 106 The body of the mandibular prosthesis in the lateral sublingual areas must be shortened so as to cross the mylohyoid ridge by 0.5 to 1.0 mm.

Fig 107 *(a and b)* The prosthesis must cover the piriform eminences only if the mucogingival tissues that cover them are fixed to the underlying bony plane. If these tissues are mobile, the eminences are only half covered.

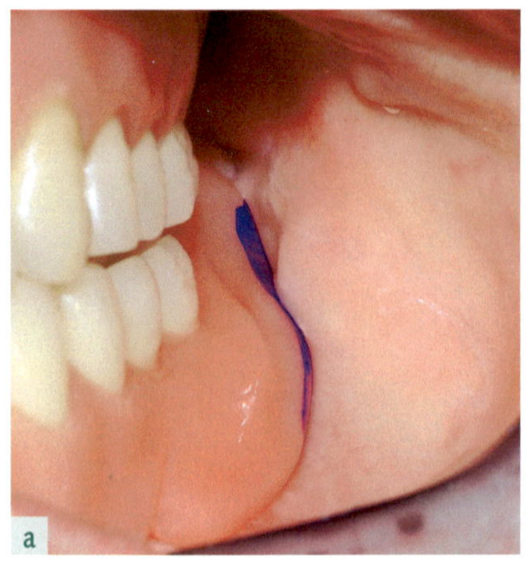 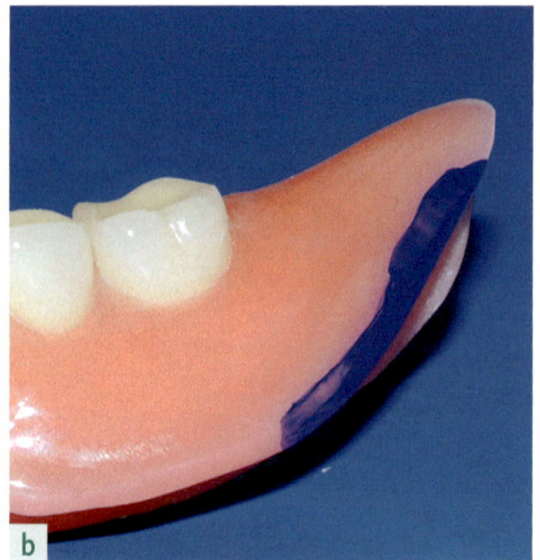 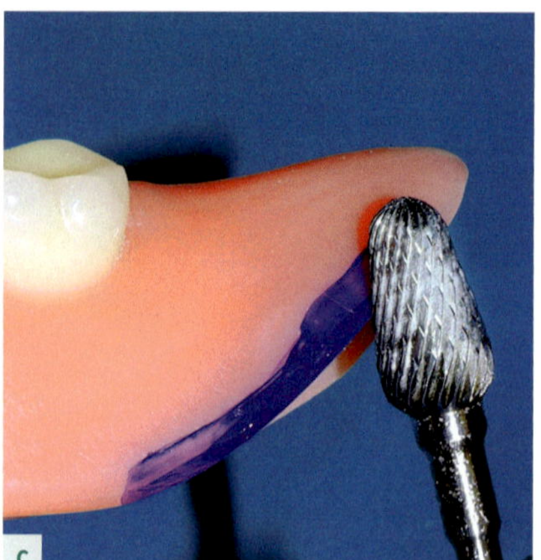

Fig 108 *(a to c)* Correction in the masseter zone.

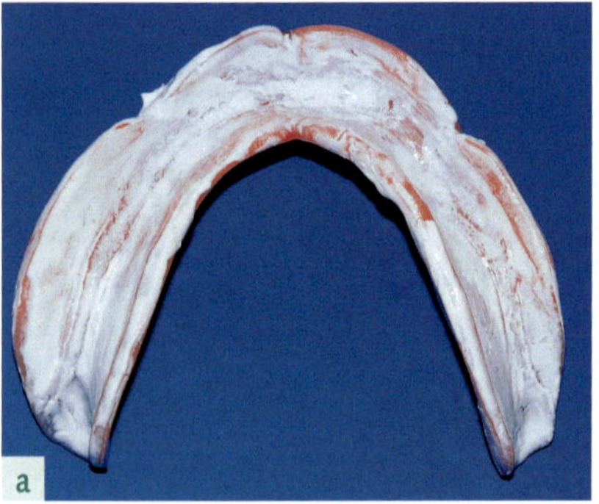 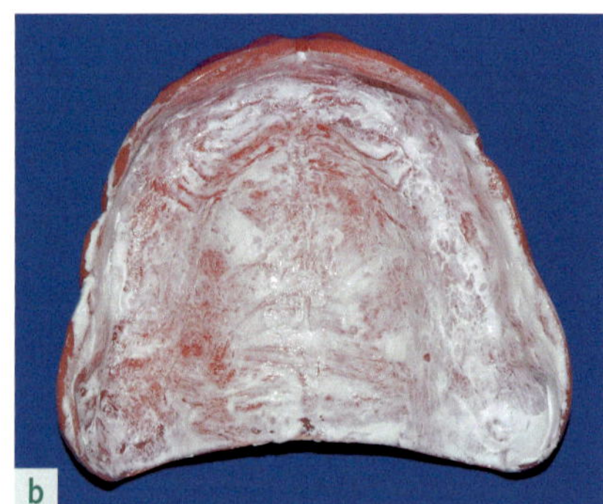

Fig 109 *(a and b)* The use of pressure-revealing paste permits the identification of possible areas of compression that may cause decubitus.

Treatment of Single-Arch Edentulism

Single-arch edentulism refers to edentulism in one arch that is opposed by an arch with natural teeth or by a fixed or removable partial denture. The mounting of the posterior teeth may be problematic in this case.

The rehabilitation technique is illustrated by a case of maxillary edentulism with natural teeth in the opposing arch. The same techniques can be applied to mandibular edentulism. Maxillary edentulism will be the form most frequently seen in the immediate decades.[1]

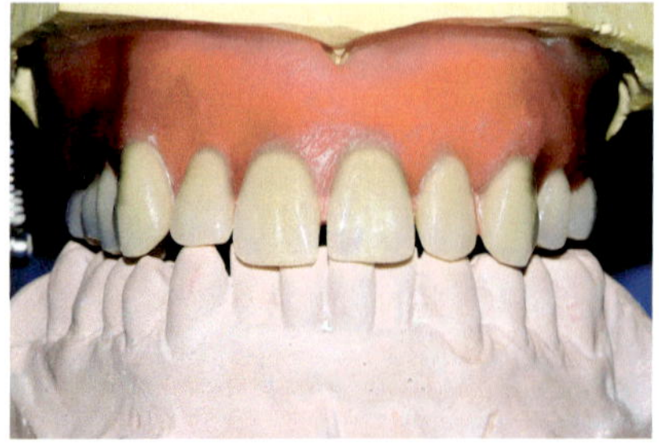 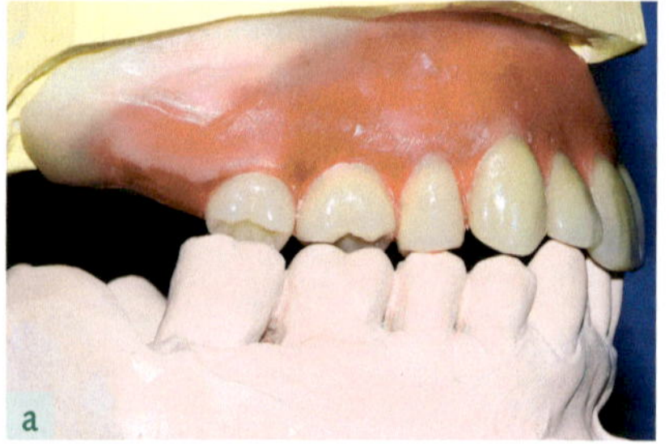 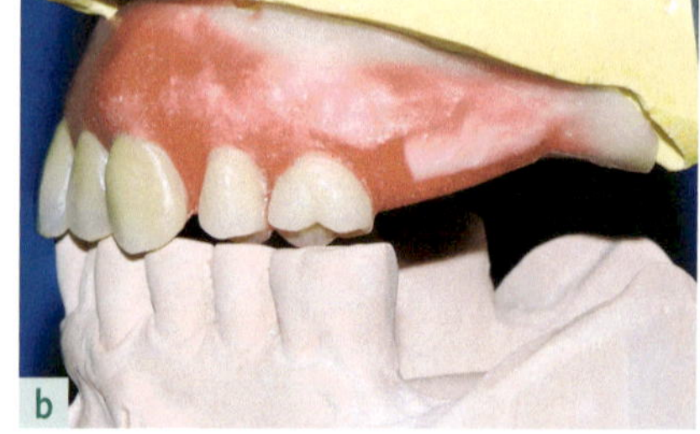

Fig 110 Frontal view of the incisors, canines, and posterior teeth on an articulator.

Fig 111 *(a and b)* Lateral view of the posterior teeth. To obtain optimal pestle-mortar contacts, it may be necessary to modify the occlusal surfaces of the opposing cast. In this phase, selective grinding should be prepared.

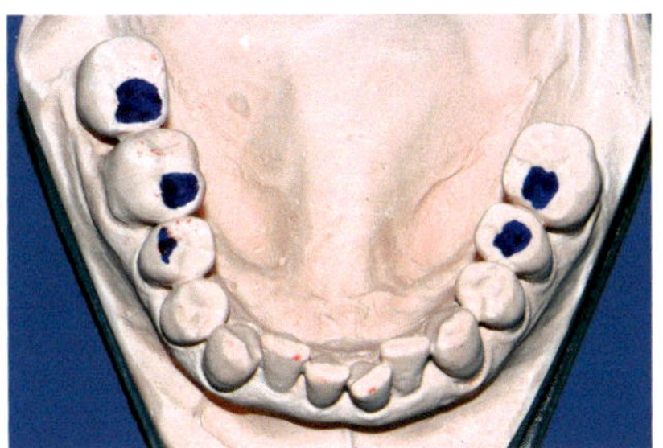

Fig 112 With a felt-tip pen, the modifications should be made on the opposing study cast.

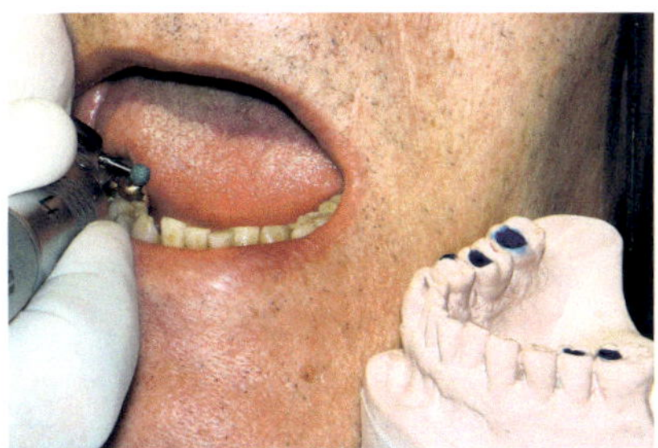

Fig 113 The modifications made on the study cast must be accurately transferred to the mouth using targeted enamel contouring.

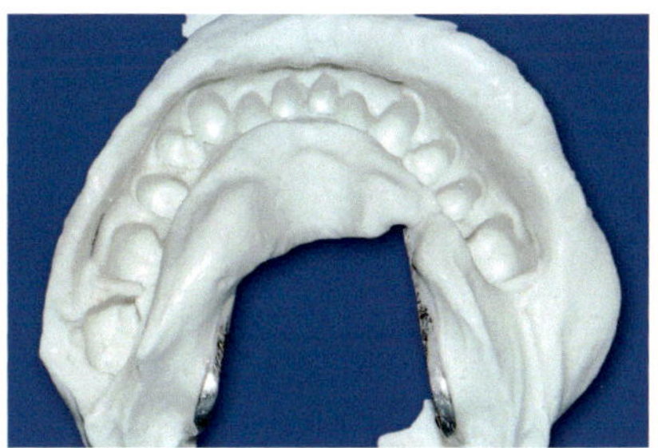

Fig 114 From the modified cast, an impression of the mandibular arch is taken.

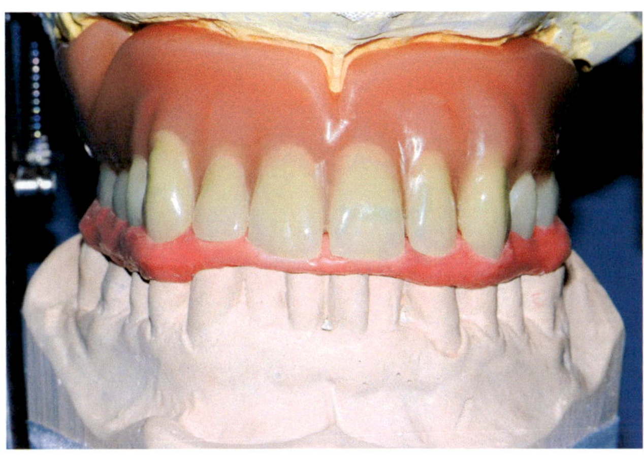

Fig 115 The new cast is then repositioned in the articulator, using a transferring wax cast made from the preceding cast. Small modifications to the load on the maxillary teeth can then be made.

Follow-up

After delivering the prosthesis, it is necessary to follow up with the patient periodically The orofacial system will undergo continual changes (eg, resorption of the edentulous alveolar crest, alterations of the neuromuscular equilibrium), the most important of which will manifest after 2 months of wearing the prosthesis.[2] Patients who in their initial visit revealed difficulties during manipulation of the mandible and in making the movements of protrusion and laterality will manifest the first changes after a few weeks.

During the constructive phase of the prosthesis, identification of occlusal relationships in some patients cannot be considered definitive. They must therefore be checked, with necessary corrections made after 2 months (or after a few weeks for patients with neuromuscular problems) and successively at periodic follow-up. Some patients may not adhere to the follow-up schedule. If they regularly use adhesive paste to compensate for any problems, for example, they may not feel the need to follow up.

During the follow-up, the precision of the prosthetic base must be checked, as well as the occlusal relationships and the health of the oral and perioral tissues. The precision of the base may be assessed by making a rotational movement on the horizontal plane or using pressure-revealing materials. If the prosthesis is mobile, and an area of compression and incongruity with respect to the morphology of the oral tissues is identified, the prosthetic body should be relined.

A test using a shimstock foil strip between the arches allows evaluation of the congruity of the prosthesis and the correctness of the occlusal relationships. The shimstock foil strip, with a thickness of 8 mm, must be folded until the patient becomes aware of its thickness. The incapacity to discriminate and perceive thicknesses less than 100 mm indicates the need to verify the adaptation and to proceed with relining the prosthesis.[2,3]

Every time the prosthesis is relined, it is necessary to reregister the occlusal relationships. If the occlusal incongruence is slight, selective grinding can be performed; however, in some cases, it is necessary to remount one or more groups of teeth.

A patient with a full prosthesis may also experience pathologic alterations of the mucosa. In cases of candidiasis, pharmaceutical intervention is needed.

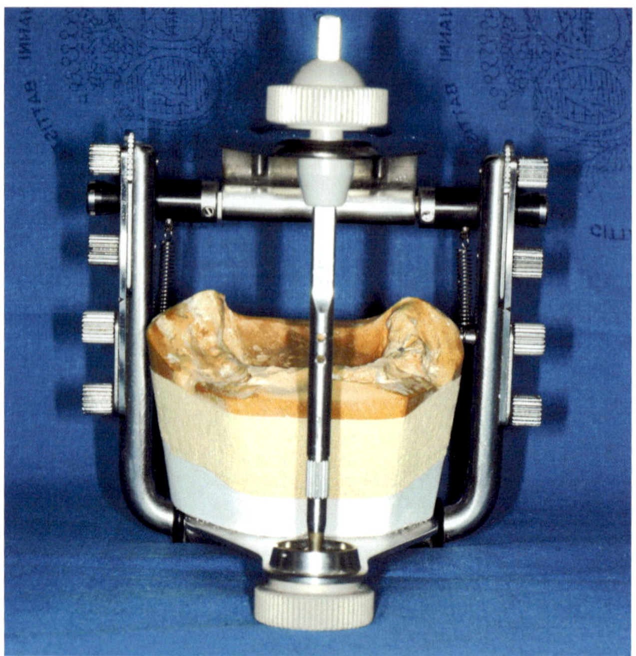

Fig 116 Mandibular cast mounted in the articulator. After giving the prosthesis to the patient, at least one of the two casts mounted in the articulator should be saved to avoid another extraoral registration.

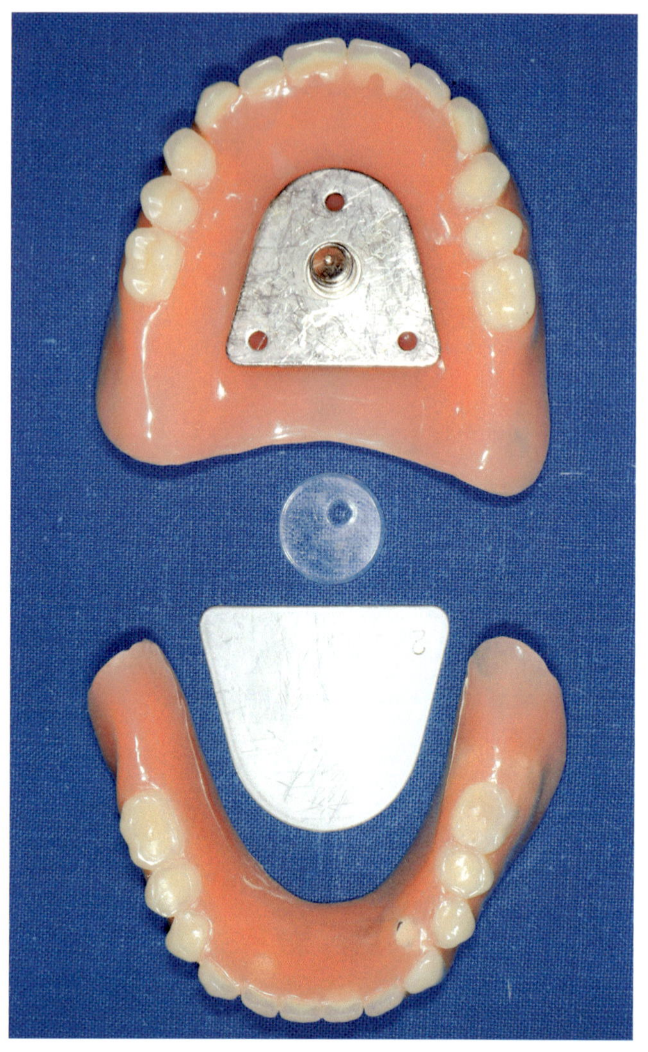

Fig 117 A set of instruments for intraoral registration for a complete prosthesis. The post inserted in the plate enables a rigid connection to be made with the maxillary prosthesis. Metal plates of various dimensions are available for the mandibular prosthesis.

Fig 118 (a and b) A metal plate locked into the mandibular prosthesis. The thermoplastic paste must create a secure supporting balcony to avoid movement of the plate during the clinical registration phase.

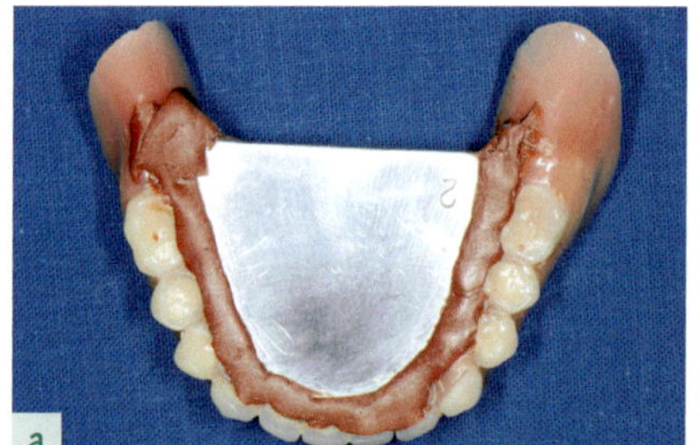

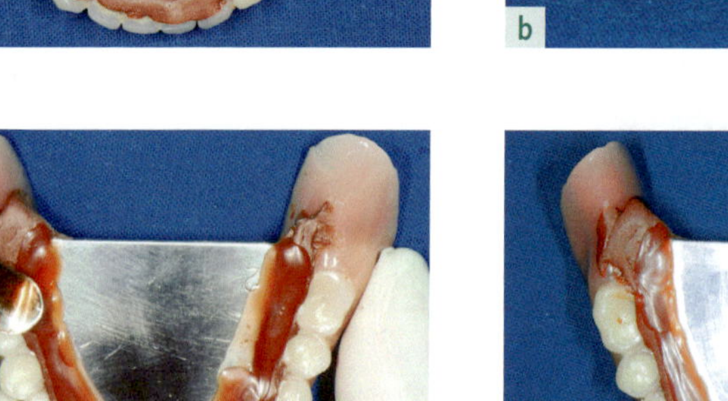

Fig 119 (a and b) To improve adhesion of the metal to the thermoplastic paste, a sticky wax is added to the margin of the plate.

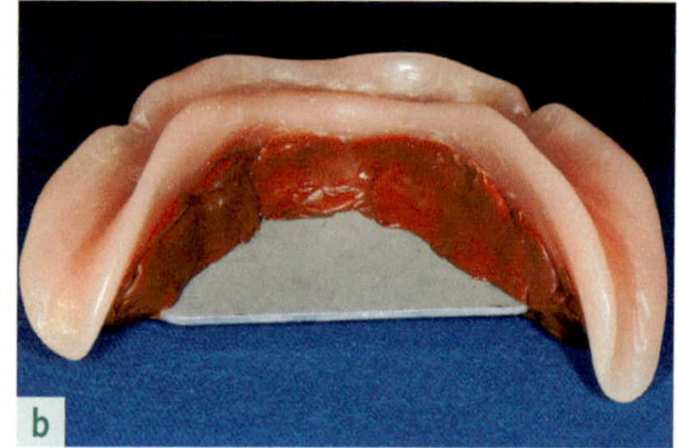

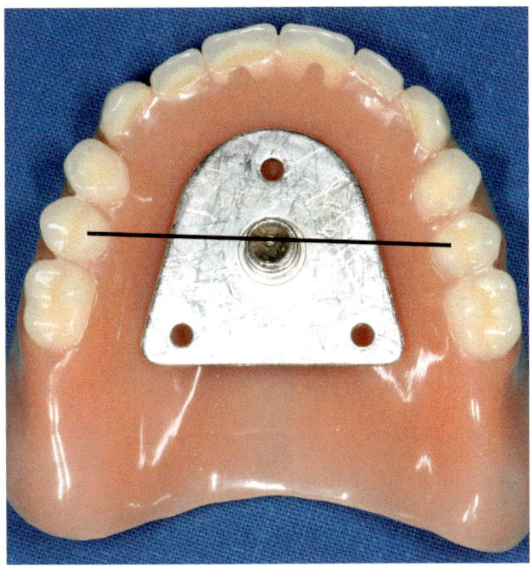

Fig 120 Use the line passing between the palatal cusps of the second premolars as a guideline to position the supporting post.

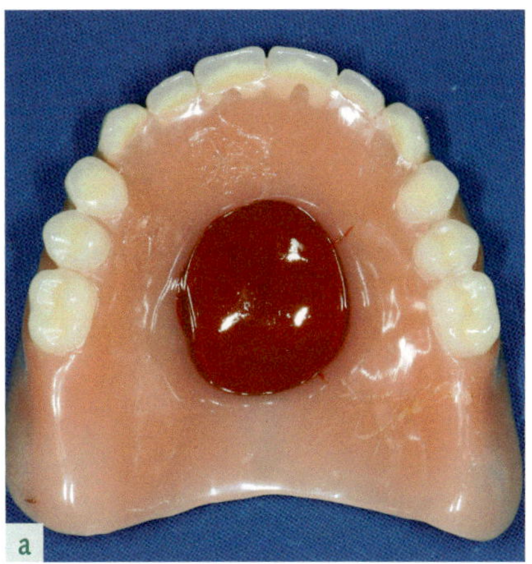

Fig 121 *(a and b)* The post is attached with an abundant quantity of thermoplastic paste.

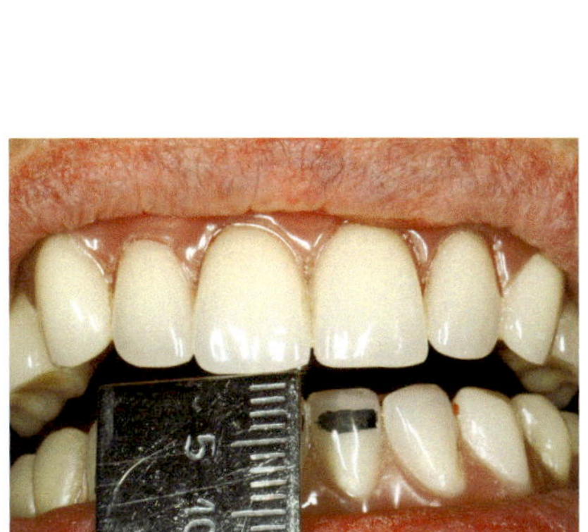

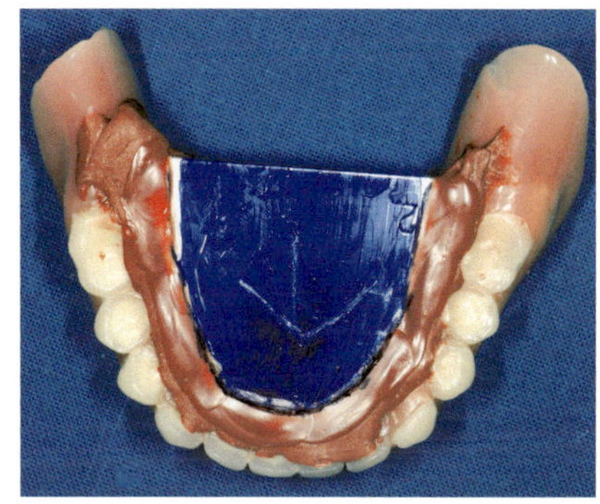

Fig 122 Color the mandibular plate with a felt-tip pen. To avoid interference during the movements, the registration must be made while increasing the VDO.

Fig 123 The height must be calculated and transferred to the articulator using a correcting factor. The height in millimeters must be multiplied by 1.3. The dimension obtained will be the height that is imposed on the incisive axis.

Fig 124 The movements of protrusion and laterality will designate the gothic arch tracing.

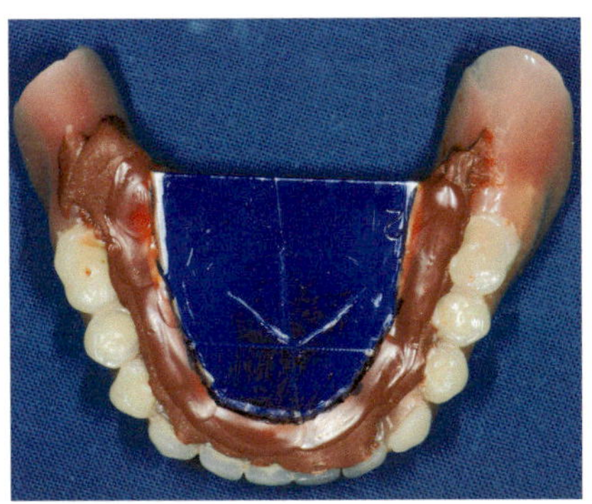

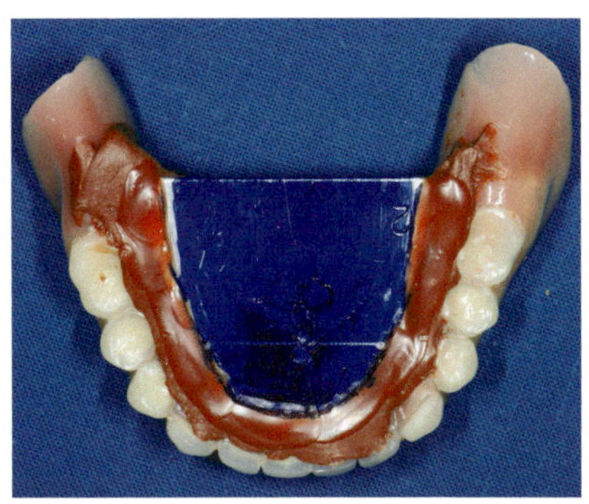

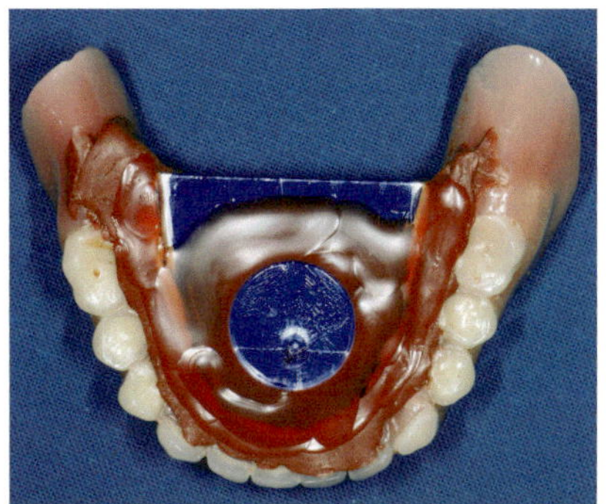

Fig 125 Creation of a referral system to identify the apex of the gothic arch. The gothic arch can then be erased to determine the neuromuscular center.

Fig 126 Identification of the neuromuscular center.

Fig 127 Blocking the therapeutic position with a disk of Plexiglas and gluing wax.

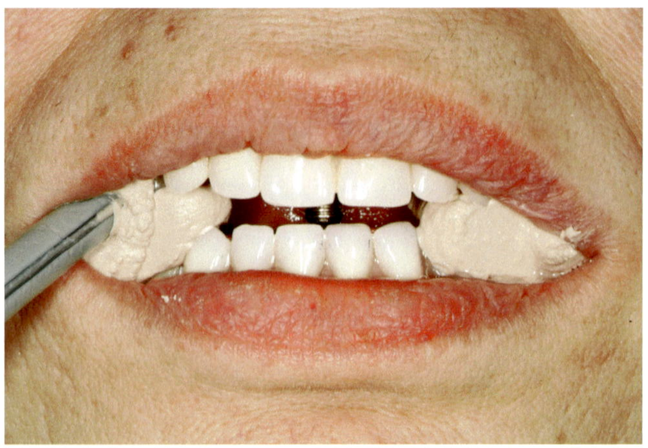

Fig 128 Preparing the plaster blocking indices.

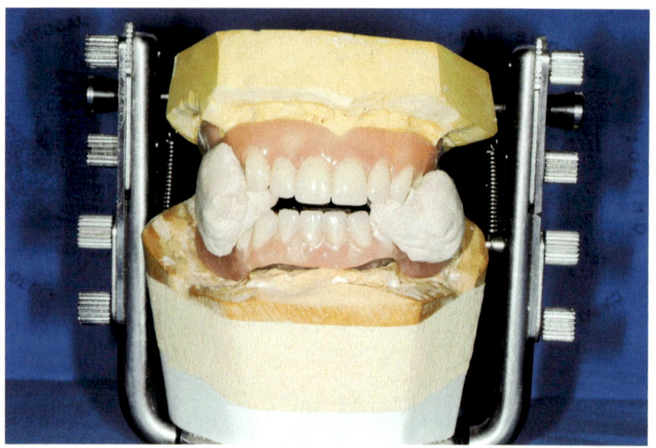

Fig 129 Transfer to the articulator and blocking the maxillary cast.

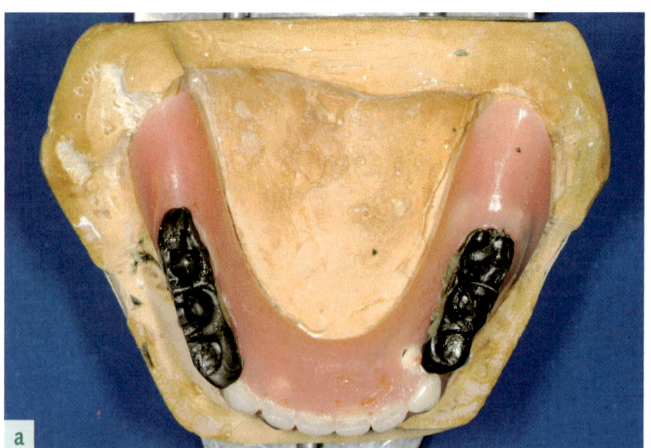

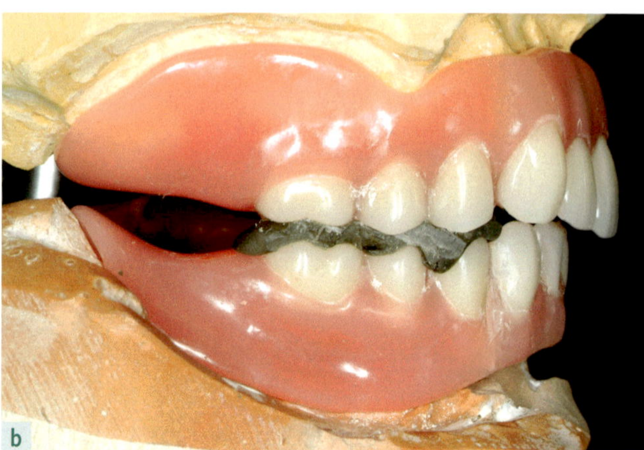

Fig 130 Before selective grinding or remounting of the teeth, it is advisable to check the registration position using indices of thermoplastic paste. If the patient easily finds the occlusal position corresponding to the registered one, then proceed with the chosen modifications and place the finished prosthesis in the patient's mouth.

References

1. Selin LW. The future of dentistry. J Am Dent Assoc 2001;132: 1667–1677. Cat. 4
2. Pera P, Bassi F, Schierano G, Appendino P, Preti G. Implant anchored complete mandibular denture: Evaluation of masticatory efficiency, oral function and degree of satisfaction. J Oral Rehabil 1998;25:462–467. Cat. 2
3. Schierano G, Ardunio E, Bosio E, Preti G. The influence of selective grinding on the thickness discriminations threshold of patients wearing complete dentures. J Oral Rehabil 2002;29: 184–187. Cat. 2

Oral Mucosal Diseases in Patients with Removable Dentures

The edentulous patient is often middle-aged or older and therefore may have cardiovascular, gastrointestinal, or metabolic (eg, diabetes mellitus) problems that can influence oral health directly or through pharmacologic treatment. It has also been hypothesized that the oral mucosa undergoes age-related modifications, in particular a reduction in thickness and cellular turnover and an increase in permeability, but no definitive supporting data exist.[1] Furthermore, many pathologies of the oral mucosa (eg, oral lichen planus, pemphigoid of the mucous membrane, and squamous cell carcinoma) are more frequent among those aged 70 to 80 years, and such patients often need a removable denture.

Partial or complete loss of teeth both reflects and causes changes in general and oral health. For example, edentulism causes reduction of the dimensions and tonus of the pharyngeal muscles, in turn causing a reduction in sensitivity and alterations of the masticatory cycles, among other effects.[2,3] Furthermore, various changes in the oral mucosa can be a direct consequence of a removable denture. These changes include prosthetic stomatitis, angular cheilitis, prosthetic hyperplastic fibrosis, traumatic ulcers (decubitus),[4] and contact allergies.

The prevalence of oral mucosal lesions in patients with a removable denture is not clear despite published findings (Table 5-1). Various factors may offer an explanation:

- Heterogeneity of the sample analyzed (patients in the hospital, in nursing homes, or in retirement communities who are edentulous or partially dentate or who have complete or partial dentures)
- The relatively low sample numbers
- Different diagnostic criteria used to define the various pathologies
- Diverse studies were directed toward observing specific diseases (eg, prosthetic stomatitis or precancerous lesions, and oral cancers)
- Lack of studies considering the influence of age, sex, nonessential habits, oral hygiene, and condition of the denture

Table 5-1 Distribution of alterations of mucosa in geriatric patients[*]

	Jorge et al[5] N = 350†	Dorey et al[6] N = 200‡	Fleishman et al[7] N = 456§	Samaranayake et al[8] N = 147†	Carrassi et al[9] N = 294†	MacEntee et al[10] N = 255¶
Prosthetic stomatitis	20	135	11	19	23.5	30
Angular cheilitis	9	7.5	7	25	1	4
Fibrotic hyperplasia	12	1.5	1.3	5	1.4	6
Traumatic ulcer	–	5	3	0	1	1
Leukoplakia	3	10	–	–	6	2
Lichen planus	–	1	–	–	–	–
Carcinoma	1	0.5	–	–	1	–
Total	59	48	NR	45	47	43

*Only studies with internationally accepted diagnostic criteria and that have similarities are presented. Data are given as percentage.
† Geriatric patients in a hospital care residence.
‡ All patients were edentulous.
§ Geriatric patients (no other information).
¶ Geriatric patients (older than 70 years) randomly selected from an electoral list in Vancouver, BC.

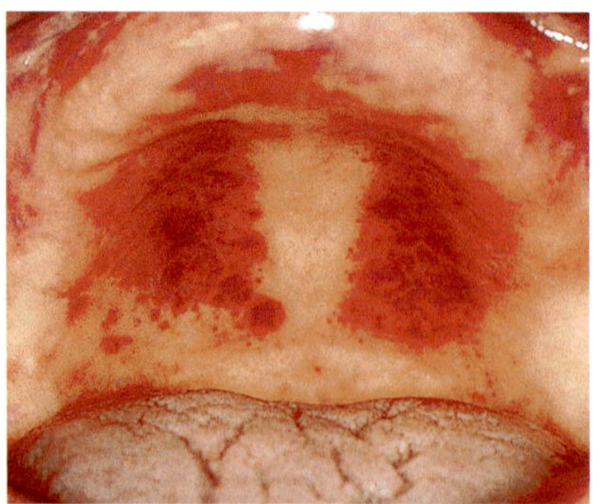

Fig 5-1 Prosthetic stomatitis type 1.

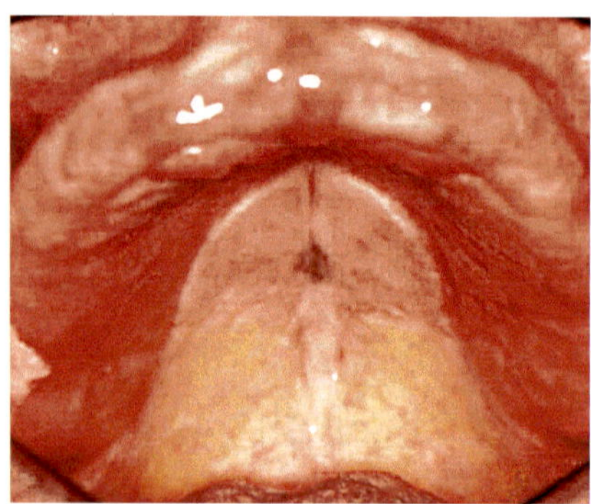

Fig 5-2 Prosthetic stomatitis type 2.

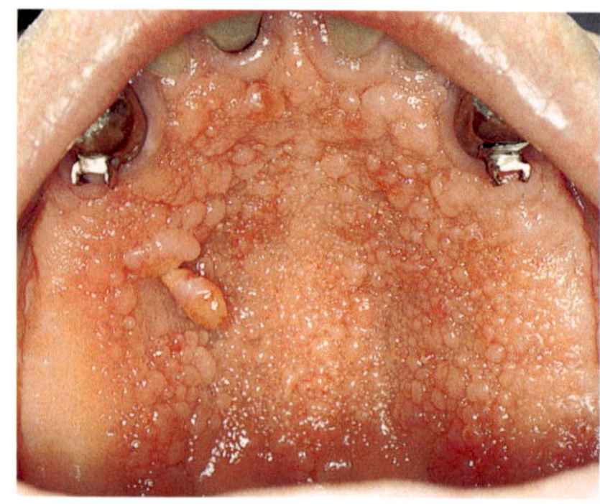

Fig 5-3 Prosthetic stomatitis type 3.

As a consequence, comparisons between different studies are difficult and often do not represent the population of a given geographic area.[11] At the moment, it is not known whether these pathologies present variations that are racial, sex-based, or whether they are linked to immunogenetic factors, among other variables.

Taking these various premises into consideration, prosthetic stomatitis is probably the oral mucosal disease most frequently found in edentulous patients with dentures, followed by angular cheilitis, fibrosis hyperplasia (which may also be referred to as *epulis fissuratum*[12]), and traumatic ulcers.

Prosthetic Stomatitis

This condition is characterized by chronic inflammation and is frequently found in patients wearing dentures. Three clinical varieties of prosthetic stomatitis can be distinguished[13,14]:

1. Type 1: Localized erythema (Fig 5-1)
2. Type 2: Extended erythema occurring only in areas covered by a denture (Fig 5-2)
3. Type 3: Papillary hyperplasia of the area at the base of the denture (Fig 5-3)

Although types 1 and 2 do not show a site preference, type 3 is almost exclusively found in the central part of the palate.[15]

Epidemiology

The prevalence of prosthetic stomatitis varies in published surveys from 11% to 30% of the patients analyzed (see Table 5-1). It is often associated with angular cheilitis,[16] and in 28% to 70% of cases it is associated with the presence of symptoms such as dry mouth, alterations in taste, and a burning sensation.[15,17] There does not seem to be significant differences in the prevalence of prosthetic stomatitis by sex[15] and age.[10]

Etiology

Among the etiologic factors, the colonization of the denture by bacterial plaque or, more frequently, by *Candida albicans* and related species, prosthetic trauma, and an allergic reaction to the resin (usually monomers) have been hypothesized. Undoubtedly the pre-eminent etiologic factor is a *Candida* infection.[15,17] Further, because intraepithelial invasion of the hyphae of *C albicans* does not occur in these cases,[16,18] its extracellular proteases are thought to support the inflammatory process.[19] The adhesion of the organism to the prosthetic material is probably linked to its hydrophobic nature.[20] Predisposing factors for *Candida* infection are wearing the denture constantly, poor hygiene, incongruence of the prosthetic body, a diet rich in carbohydrates, diabetes, hypothyroidism, hyperparathyroidism, iron and folate deficiency, reduced salivary flow, prolonged immunosuppressive antibiotics, and immunodeficiency (eg, human immunodeficiency virus 1 [HIV-1] infection).[18]

Diagnosis

The diagnosis is mostly clinical. Periodic acid-Schiff (PAS) staining does not show hyphae or mycelium but it can show the presence of spores in prosthetic stomatitis.[18] A tampon culture of the affected tissue and of the internal surface of the denture can be useful.[18] A quantitative determination of *Candida* can help the diagnosis,[4] even if Borromeo and colleagues[21] did not show differences in the concentration of *Candida* in patients with and without dentures, and McCullough et al[22] suggested that specific numbers of colonies are not able to differentiate the ill from the healthy. In 50% of the population it is normal to find 1,000 CFUs /mL, whereas in infected patients, 4,000 to 20,000 CFUs/mL are found.[18]

If a possible allergy to methylmethacrylate is found, epicutaneous patch tests should be done,[23] particularly in subjects with previous allergic manifestations.

Fig 5-4 Low-level angular cheilitis (type 3).

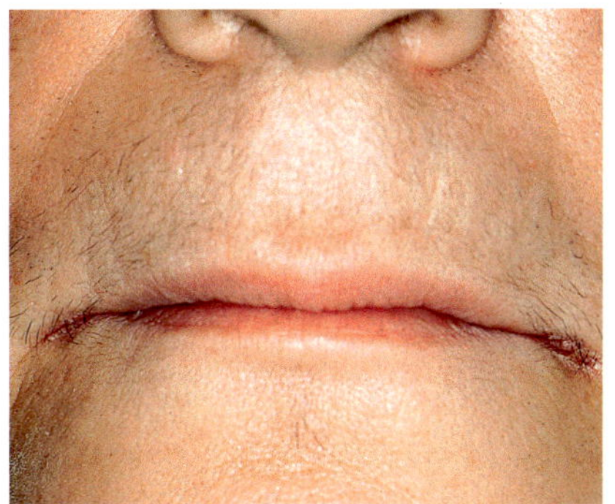

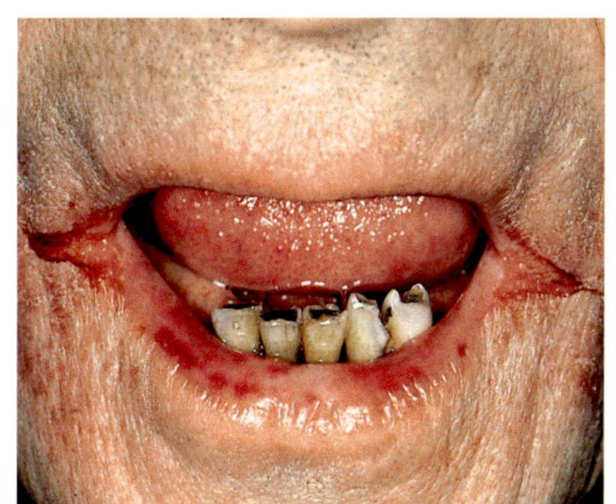

Fig 5-5 Severe angular cheilitis with ulceration (type 3).

The differential diagnosis includes burns, reactions to medications (permanent erythema), pernicious anemia, red lesions of lichen planus, and discoid lupus erythematosus.[18] Differential diagnosis is important between erythroplakia and a precancerous lesion, which also appears as a red mark with a velvety aspect. It is generally not prominent or depressed in relation to the surrounding mucosa, is commonly localized on the soft palate or on the floor of the oral cavity, and is rarely found on the hard palate. If in doubt, however, a biopsy is necessary.

Treatment

The etiologic agent found determines the treatment; nevertheless, preventive measures such as regular brushing of the denture and its removal during the night to keep it dry[24,25] are useful. It is also necessary to evaluate the elimination of eventual predisposing factors. In immunocompetent patients with *Candida* infection, it is advisable to prescribe topical antimycotics (miconazole oral gel, three applications per day; or nystatin suspension, three rinses per day), to eliminate the surface layer of resin on the denture, and to apply conditioning materials and immerse the denture in hypochlorite, nystatin, or chlorhexidine for 1 hour per day. Note that chlorhexidine can have an antagonistic reaction with nystatin. Epithelial hyperplasia of the palate (type 3) must also be treated surgically (by scalpel, electrosurgery, or laser). In immunocompetent patients, systemic antimicrobial therapy with fluconazole can sometimes, although rarely, be necessary (50 mg per day for 14 days or 100 mg for 3 days and 50 mg for the following 8 days).

In the case of an allergy, after identifying the allergen, resurfacing of the prosthetic base with a different material (to which the patient is not hypersensitive) generally resolves the problem.

Angular Cheilitis

Originally named *Perlèche* by Leimastre in 1886,[26] angular cheilitis is characterized by lesions in the commisures of the mouth, including erythema, fissures with possible bleeding, and symmetric cutaneous crusts. In 1986, Ohman and colleagues[26] proposed a clinical classification in ascending order of seriousness:

1. Type 1 (mild): Lesions confined to commisural mucosal edges with the presence of erythema and fissurization (Fig 5-4)
2. Type 2 (moderate): Lesions that extend to the surrounding skin
3. Type 3 (severe): Lesions with ulcerations and suppuration (Fig 5-5)

Epidemiology

This condition is a clinical manifestation relatively common in elderly edentulous patients with removable dentures, present in 1% to 25% of cases (see Table 5-1).

Etiology

Angular cheilitis is usually caused by a *C albicans* infection,[27,28] and most patients have associated prosthetic stomatitis. It is even possible to isolate *Staphylococcus aureus*[29] and/or *Streptococcus* organisms[30] in cultures from the lesions. Other possible causes are iron deficiency, severe vitamin deficiency (primarily of the group B),[31–34] malabsorption (eg, Crohn disease), diabetes,[35] HIV infection[36] or other immune system defects, antibiotic therapy,[36] and decrease in vertical dimension of the oral cavity.[37]

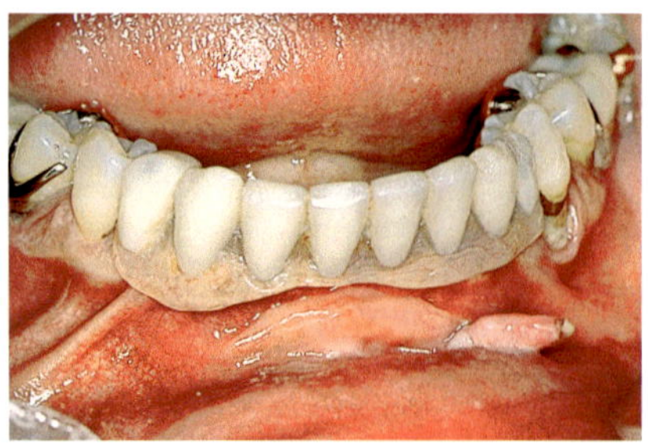

Fig 5-6 Prosthetic fibrotic hyperplasia. The prosthesis is partial incongruent in the inferior area, and has provoked fibrotic hyperplasia.

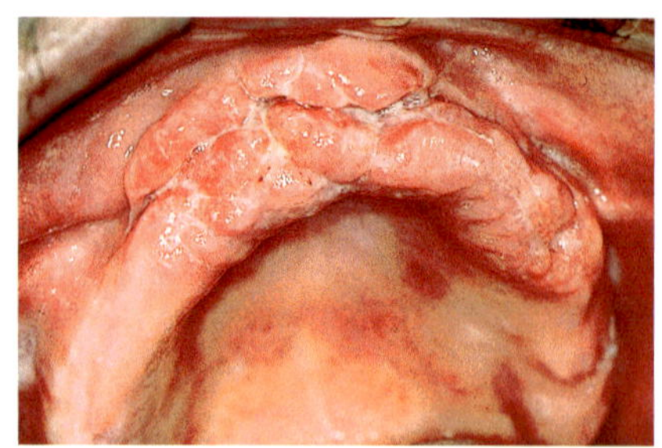

Fig 5-7 Prosthetic fibrotic hyperplasia before surgical removal.

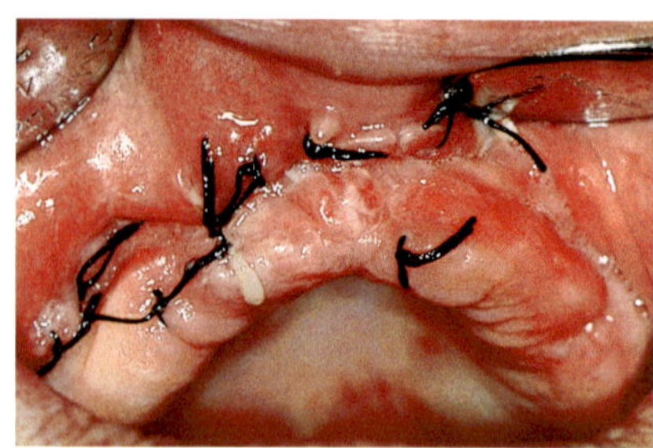

Fig 5-8 After the surgical removal of the prosthetic fibrotic hyperplasia in Fig 5-7.

Diagnosis

Hematochemical screening and the use of strips for bacterial and fungal culturing may be necessary.

Treatment

The predisposing factors should be eliminated and the prosthetic stomatitis treated. The angular stomatitis should be treated with topical antimycotics such as miconazole oral gel, three applications per day. The vertical dimension will need to be corrected. Also, the patient should be instructed to improve oral hygiene and the cleanliness of the denture body. Any traumatizing factors should be eliminated.

Prosthetic Hyperplastic Fibrosis

The prosthetic hyperplastic fibrosis, also called *prosthetic fibroma, hyperplasty from prosthetic trauma,*[5] or *epulis fissuratum,*[13] is usually found near the sulcus as an asymptomatic mass with a smooth surface of a normal color, parallel to the alveolar ridge. It can be fissured from the margin of the prosthetic flange. In general, it is associated with removable dentures, especially in the anterior region (Figs 5-6 to 5-8).

Epidemiology

This condition is common in elderly patients or middle-aged patients who have poorly made removable dentures. The prevalence varies from 1% to 12% (see Table 5-1).

Etiology

The compression of the prosthetic flange causes chronic irritation and a hyperplastic response.

Diagnosis

In general, the diagnosis is easy if the lesion is clearly related to the denture. If the lesion is ulcerated, it can sometimes, but rarely, resemble a carcinoma.

Treatment

Usually, removing the denture leads to clinical improvement but not to complete healing. Therapy consists of the surgical removal of the hyperplastic tissue and modification or substitution of the removable denture.

Allergy: Contact Toxic Stomatitis

Polymers based on polymethylmethacrylate were introduced into oral prosthetic practice in 1936[38] and since then have been used universally, rapidly substituting vulcanite.

Polymethylmethacrylate, which is polymerized by heat, is not an allergen. However, its monomer methylmethacrylate is a powerful allergen; furthermore, prosthetic bases in resin contain different additives that have considerable sensitizing powers,[39,40] and the metals contained in the alloys used in removable partial dentures can also be the cause of allergic reactions.[41] In most cases, a local reaction may occur, but systemic allergies occur in only a few cases.[42] Signs and symptoms can be limited to oral burning and/or itching without evident signs, or can include clinical aspects of prosthetic stomatitis eventually accompanied by edema (Fig 5-9). In some rare cases, dermatitis or diffuse itching or asthmatic phenomena are noted. Hypersensitivity must then be distinguished from the chemical irritation caused by high levels of residual monomer.[43]

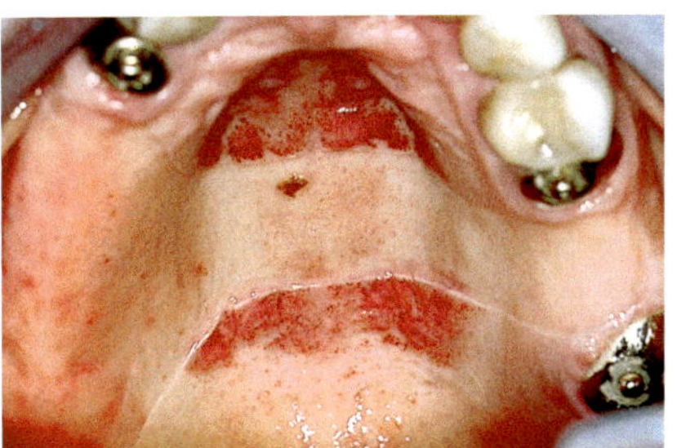

Fig 5-9 Contact stomatitis.

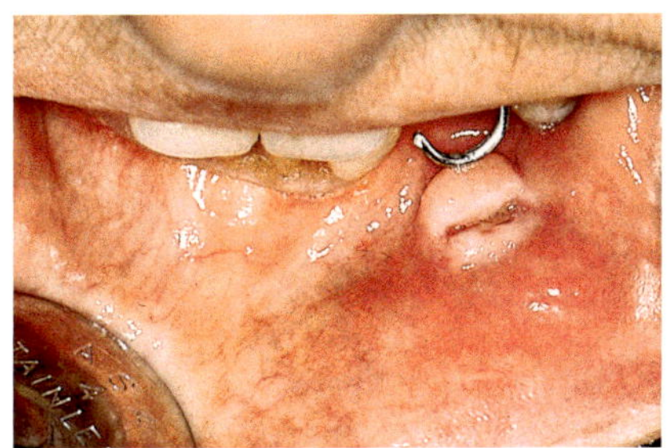

Fig 5-10 Traumatic ulcer.

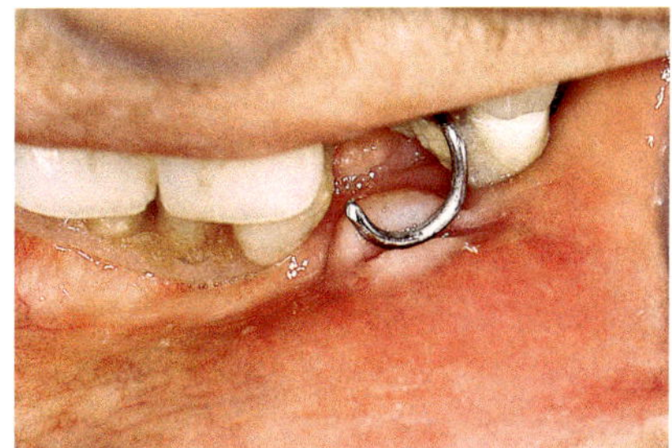

Fig 5-11 Traumatic ulcer. Note the anatomic correspondence between the traumatic agent and the ulcer.

Epidemiology

Cases of hypersensitivity to resin or to alloys commonly used for the manufacture of removable dentures are considered rare,[39] although the epidemiologic information on the topic is scarce. In a review of the literature on this topic, comprising works published from 1940 to 1980, Kaaber[40] estimated that there are no more than 150 to 200 cases of possible allergic reactions to prosthetic polymer acrylics. Many diagnoses of allergy do not appear to be very well substantiated,[44] and prosthetic stomatitis from *Candida*, burning mouth syndrome, and simple prosthetic traumas can be confused with hypersensitive reactions.[45–47] The chemical polymerization systems introduced in 1975[48] have, theoretically, increased the risk of sensitization because there are more unstable polymerization products with a content of monomer residues 5 to 11 times higher than that obtained with heat polymerization and with a similar level of formaldehyde released.[49,50] Nevertheless, reported cases of hypersensitivity do not seem to have significantly increased. It is possible that the relatively rare allergic manifestations from oral contact are caused by various factors, such as saliva, which dilutes the antigens and eliminates them before they penetrate the oral mucosa or the high vascularization of the mucosa, which rapidly removes absorbed antigens, and its reduced keratinization, which makes the formation of allergen-antibody complexes with proteins of keratinic origin difficult.[51]

Etiology

Reactions from contact with acrylics and/or metals that make up removable dentures are generally of type IV (cell-mediated) or type III (immunocomplex-mediated) hypersensitivity.[42] The allergens can be methylmethacrylate; formaldehyde, which is released during polymerization[50]; benzoyl peroxide, which starts the process of polymerization[52]; plastifiers such as dibutyl phthalate; hydroquinone[53]; and coloring agents.[39,40,42]

Reactions from oral contact with (cold) relining resins have also been noted.[54] Metals contained in the alloys for removable partial dentures, such as stellite (chromium-cobalt-molybdenum) can also cause allergic reactions.[41,55] In particular, nickel, cobalt, and chromium not only cause local manifestations, such as stomatitis or gingivitis, but also eczema and dermatitis without oral lesions.[41]

Diagnosis

Allergy from intraoral contact can be diagnosed if there is a clear temporal relationship between exposure to a suspected allergen and the beginning of signs and symptoms. Epicutaneous tests (patch tests) are among the most used laboratory tests. The agents to be tested are contained in little discs of aluminum, called *Finn chambers*, that are applied using an adhesive, generally on the skin of the back, and left in place for at least 48 hours. A positive result is identified by the presence of an inflammatory reaction. Not all patients with contact allergic reactions have a positive reaction to the patch test, however. A certain level of experience is necessary to distinguish a true positive reaction from that of mere irritation. Another important cause of variability is the concentration of the allergen to be tested.[39] These tests can also cause sensitization to an antigen.

Other immunologic tests,[39] such as the lymphocyte transformation test and the migration-inhibitory factor test, have the advantage of being made in vitro and therefore cannot cause sensitization. Nevertheless, none of these tests is sufficiently sensitive and specific. Likewise, an oral biopsy does not often show a definitive reaction in patients with suspected contact allergies, although an inflammatory infiltrate containing many eosinophils and/or plasma cells is compatible with a hypersensitivity reaction. Analysis of the constituents of the denture, through chromatography, for example, could be of importance.

Treatment

The management of oral contact lesions varies from palliative treatment of the symptoms to the removal of the allergen. Fundamentally, it consists of identifying the causal agent and removing it. In the case of allergies to metals contained in the common alloys used for the manufacture of removable partial dentures, alloys of a titanium base can be used.[55] In recalcitrant cases, strong topical cortisone can be useful, such as clobetasol propionate 0.05% in a cream preparation or 4% in a hydroxyethyl cellulose gel in equal quantity.

Traumatic Ulcers

Ulcerations due to prosthetic trauma are found in 1% to 5% of edentulous patients (see Table 5-1) and usually appear within a few days of the insertion of a new denture.[4] The ulcers are usually small, painful, and often surrounded by a white hyperkeratosis halo, are soft to palpation, and correspond anatomically to the cause of the trauma (Figs 5-10 and 5-11). All traumatic ulcers heal within 7 to 10 days once the cause has been eliminated. In the case of persistence, a biopsy is imperative to exclude the possibility of a carcinogenic nature. Therapy with chlorhexidine rinses can be useful to prevent eventual superinfections.

Other Lesions

Patients who wear removable dentures are usually in the geriatric age group. Therefore, these patients are more commonly prone to erosive bullous diseases of the oral mucosa (eg, lichen planus, pemphigoid of the mucous membrane, and pemphigo vulgaris), autoimmune diseases (eg, Sjögren syndrome), oral precancerosis (eg, leukoplakia and erythroplakia), and squamous cell carcinoma (see Table 5-1). Although many of these illnesses can create complications or sometimes make a removable denture at least temporarily impossible, according to current knowledge, none of these illnesses seems to have an etiopathogenetic relationship with the presence of removable dentures.

References

1. Winning TA, Townsend GC. Oral mucosal embryology and histology. Clin Dermatol 2000;18:499–511. Cat. 7
2. Garzino M, Ramieri G, Panzica G, Preti G. Changes in the density of protein gene product 9.5-immunoreactive nerve fibres in human oral mucosa under implant-retained overdentures. Arch Oral Biol 1996;41:1073–1079. Cat. 1
3. Mantecchini G, Bassi F, Pera P, Preti G. Oral stereognosis in edentulous subjects rehabilitated with complete removable dentures. J Oral Rehabil 1998;25:185–189. Cat. 3
4. Budtz-Jorgensen E. The edentulous patient. In: Owal B, Kayser AE, Carlsson GE (eds). Prosthodontics: Principle, and Management Strategies. London: Mosby-Wolfe, 1996. Cat. 7
5. Jorge J Jr, de Almeida OP, Bozzo L, Scully C, Graner E. Oral mucosal health and disease in institutionalized elderly in Brazil. Community Dent Oral Epidemiol 1991;19:173–175. Cat. 4
6. Dorey JL, Blasberg B, MacEntee MI, Conklin RJ. Oral mucosal disorders in denture wearers. J Prosthet Dent 1985;53:210–213. Cat. 4
7. Fleishman R, Peles DB, Pisanti S. Oral mucosal lesions among elderly in Israel. J Dent Res 1985;64:831–836. Cat. 4
8. Samaranayake LP, Wilkieson CA, Lamey PJ, MacFarlane TW. Oral disease in the elderly in long-term hospital care. Oral Dis 1995;1:147–151. Cat. 4
9. Carrassi A, Berardinelli R, Weinstein R, Strohmenger L, De Stefano L. Prevalence of oral mucosal lesions in a sample of the elderly in the city of Milan. Mondo Odontostomatol 1983;25:39–47. Cat. 4
10. MacEntee MI, Glick N, Stolar E. Age, gender, dentures and oral mucosal disorders. Oral Dis 1998;4:32–36. Cat. 4
11. MacEntee MI, Scully C. Oral disorders and treatment implications in people over 75 years. Community Dent Oral Epidemiol 1988;16:271–273. Cat. 4
12. Cutright DE. The histopathologic findings in 583 cases of epulis fissuratum. Oral Surg Oral Med Oral Pathol 1974;37:401–411. Cat. 4
13. Newton AV. Denture sore mouth. Br Dent J 1962;112:357–360. Cat. 7
14. Budtz-Jorgensen E, Bertram U. Denture stomatitis. II. The effect of antifungal and prosthetic treatment. Acta Odontol Scand 1970;28:283–304. Cat. 1
15. Stohler C. Etiology and occurrence of denture stomatitis. A review of literature. Schweiz Monatsschr Zahnmed 1984;94:187–194. Cat. 7
16. Cawson RA. Chronic oral candidiasis and leukoplakia. Oral Surg Oral Med Oral Pathol 1966;22:582–591. Cat. 4
17. Budtz-Jorgensen E, Bertram U. Denture stomatitis. I. The etiology in relation to trauma and infection. Acta Odontol Scand 1970;28:71–92. Cat. 2
18. Farah CS, Ashman RB, Challacombe SJ. Oral candidosis. Clin Dermatol 2000;18:553–562. Cat. 7
19. Reichart PA, Philipsen HP. Patologia Orale. Milano: Masson, 1999. Cat. 7
20. Radford DR, Challacombe SJ, Walter JD. Denture plaque and adherence of Candida albicans to denture-base materials in vivo and in vitro. Crit Rev Oral Biol Med 1999;10:99–116. Cat. 7
21. Borromeo GL, McCullough MJ, Reade PC. Quantitation and morphotyping of Candida albicans from healthy mouths and from mouths affected by erythematous candidosis. J Med Vet Mycol 1992;30:477–480. Cat. 2

22. McCullough MJ, Ross BC, Reade PC. Candida albicans: A review of its history, taxonomy, epidemiology, virulence attributes, and methods of strain differentiation. Int J Oral Maxillofac Surg 1996;25:136–144. Cat. 7

23. Kaaber S. Allergy to dental materials with special reference to the use of amalgam and polymethylmethacrylate. Int Dent J 1990; 40:359–365. Cat. 7

24. Lombardi T, Budtz-Jorgensen E. Treatment of denture-induced stomatitis: A review. Eur J Prosthodont Restor Dent 1993;2:17–22. Cat. 7

25. Stafford GD, Arendorf T, Huggett R. The effect of overnight drying and water immersion on candidal colonization and properties of complete dentures. J Dent 1986;14:52–56. Cat. 2

26. Finnerud CW. Perleche: A clinical and etiological study of 100 cases. Arch Dermatol 1929;20:454–488. Cat. 3

27. Ohman SC, Dahlen G, Moller A, Ohman A. Angular cheilitis: A clinical and microbial study. J Oral Pathol 1986;15:213–217. Cat. 3

28. MacFarlane TW, Helnarska SJ. The microbiology of angular cheilitis. Br Dent J 1976;140:403-406. Cat. 4

29. MacFarlane TW, McGill JC, Samaranayake LP. Antibiotic sensitivity and phage typing of Staphylococcus aureus isolated from non-hospitalized patients with angular cheilitis. J Hosp Infect 1984;5:444–446. Cat. 3

30. Dias AP, Samaranayake LP. Clinical, microbiological and ultrastructural features of angular cheilitis lesions in Southern Chinese. Oral Dis 1995;1:43–48. Cat. 4

31. Rose JA. Aetiology of angular cheilosis. Iron metabolism. Br Dent J 1968;125:67–72. Cat. 2

32. Rose JA. Folic-acid deficiency as a cause of angular cheilosis. Lancet 1971;2:453–454. Cat. 2

33. Dreizen S, Levy BM. Histopathology of experimentally induced nutritional deficiency cheilosis in the marmoset (Callithrix jacchus). Arch Oral Biol 1969;14:577–582. Cat. 5

34. Burton JF. Angular cheilitis and iron deficiency. N Z Dent J 1969;65:258–261. Cat. 8

35. Ritchie GM, Fletcher AM. Angular inflammation. Oral Surg Oral Med Oral Pathol 1973;36:358–366. Cat. 7

36. McKendrick AJ. Denture stomatitis and angular cheilitis in patients receiving long-term tetracycline therapy. Br Dent J 1968;124:412–417. Cat. 1

37. Lantz HJ. Angular chelitis caused by over-closure of the jaws and avitaminosis. Bull Phila Cty Dent Soc 1968;34:13–16. Cat. 7

38. Schmidt A. History of methacrylates in stomatology. Zahntechnik (Berl) 1978;19:436–444. Cat. 7

39. Devlin H, Watts DC. Acrylic 'allergy'? Br Dent J 1984;157:272–275. Cat. 7

40. Kaaber S. Allergy to dental materials with special reference to the use of amalgam and polymethylmethacrylate. Int Dent J 1990;40:359–365. Cat. 7

41. Brendlinger DL, Tarsitano JJ. Generalized dermatitis due to sensitivity to a chrome cobalt removable partial denture. J Am Dent Assoc 1970;81:392–394. Cat. 8

42. Barclay SC, Forsyth A, Felix DH, Watson IB. Case report—Hypersensitivity to denture materials. Br Dent J 1999;187:350–352. Cat. 8

43. Austin AT, Basker RM. Residual monomer levels in denture bases. The effects of varying short curing cycles. Br Dent J 1982;153:424–426. Cat. 6

44. Turrell AJW. Allergy to denture base materials—Fallacy or reality. Br J Dent 1966;120:415–422. Cat. 9

45. Weaver RE. Goebel WM. Reactions to acrylic resin dental prostheses. J Prosthet Dent 1980;43:138–142. Cat. 4

46. Ali A, Bates JF, Reynolds AJ, Walker DM. The burning mouth sensation related to the wearing of acrylic dentures: An investigation. Br Dent J 1986;161:444–447. Cat. 4

47. Nyquist G. Study of denture sore mouth. Acta Odontol Scand 1952;10(suppl 9):13–17. Cat. 7

48. Becker CM, Smith DE, Nicholls JI. The comparison of denture-base processing techniques. Part I. Material characteristics. J Prosthet Dent 1977;37:330–338. Cat. 6

49. Austin AT, Basker RM. Residual monomer levels in denture bases. The effects of varying short curing cycles. Br Dent J 1982;153:424–426. Cat. 6

50. Ruyter IE. Release of formaldehyde from denture base polymers. Acta Odontol Scand 1980; 38: 17–27. Cat. 6

51. De Rossi SS, Greenberg MS. Intraoral contact allergy: A literature review and case reports. J Am Dent Assoc 1998;129:1435–1441. Cat. 7

52. Smith DC. The acrylic denture base—The peroxide concentration in dental polymers. Br Dent J 1959;107:62–67. Cat. 6

53. Torres V, Mano-Azul AC, Correia T, Soares AP. Allergic contact cheilitis and stomatitis from hydroquinone in an acrylic dental prosthesis. Contact Dermatitis 1993;29:102–103. Cat. 8

54. Zaki HS, Ketzan KJ, Carrau RL. Hypersensitivity of temporary soft denture liners: A clinical report. J Prosthet Dent 1995;73:1–3. Cat. 8

55. Kononen M, Rintanen J, Waltimo A, Kempainen P, Titanium framework removable partial denture used for patient allergic to other metals: A clinical report and literature review. J Prosthet Dent 1995;73:4–7. Cat. 7/8

6

Constructive Principles of the Provisional Prosthesis

Patients who have to endure multiple extractions for therapeutic reasons, such as periodontal disease diagnosed at a late stage (Fig 6-1), organ transplantation, and radiotherapy for neoplasms of the head and neck, would undoubtedly prefer the extracted teeth to be immediately substituted.[1] The reasons for this request are esthetic, functional, and psychologic.

A provisional prosthesis is also important for therapeutic reasons. The presence of a prosthesis slows down the processes of postextraction resorption of the bone. The masticatory forces and those exercised by the cheeks, lips, and tongue are not able to act directly on the osseomucosal support with a prosthesis in place to mediate the forces.

The provisional removable prosthesis must be prepared before the residual teeth of the patient are extracted. The potential problems associated with planning and constructing a provisional prosthesis must first be addressed, however.

Most authors have given more importance to the esthetic aspect of provisional prostheses than to the functional and psychologic aspects and to the maintenance of the residual structures.[2,3] At the same time, most complications reported in the literature are of an esthetic and functional nature[2] and are often linked to the clinician's decision to remove all of the patient's teeth in one sitting. With this approach, the clinician is not able to evaluate the esthetic and functional results of the provisional prosthesis, and the patient does not have sufficient time to adapt to it. The provisional complete prosthesis must always be planned, and an immediate partial prosthesis should be used to initially substitute only the premolars and the molars.

It is good practice to help the patient understand that the esthetic and phonetic results of the provisional prosthesis may not be satisfactory, that time is necessary to satisfy these objectives, and that there is a possibility that not all of the negative factors will be eliminated. However, the provisional removable prosthesis is advisable for all patients who need to have teeth extracted (Box 6-1).

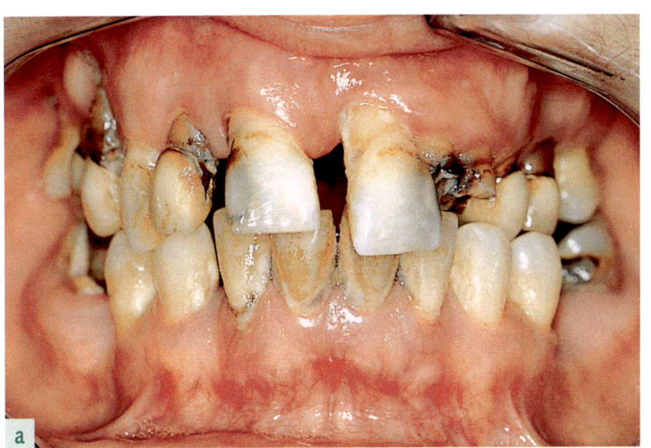
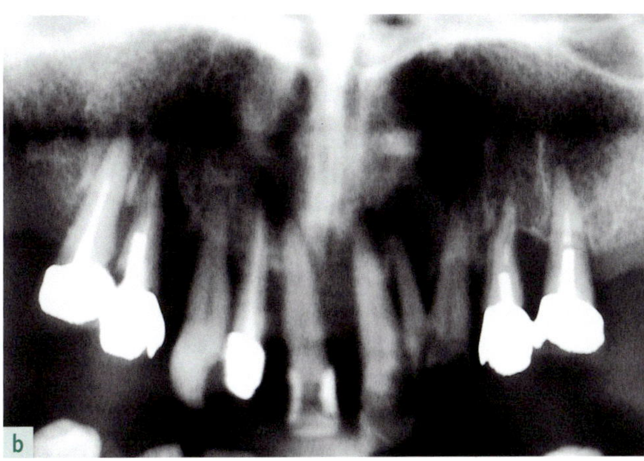

Fig 6-1 (*a and b*) Clinical and radiographic images of a patient with severe periodontal disease.

Box 6-1 Advantages and disadvantages

Advantages
- Esthetic problems are avoided.
- Cheeks and lips are supported.
- Correct height of the face is conserved.
- Tissues are protected.
- Postoperative pain is reduced.
- Healing of the soft tissues is favored.
- Patient's adaptation to the prosthesis is facilitated.
- Tongue cannot get used to occupying the future space of the definitive prosthesis.
- The form and position of the patient's teeth, in particular, the incisor group, can be recreated based on this guide.
- Residual structures are conditioned and preserved.

Disadvantage
- A greater number of check-ups are necessary during healing, with consequent increase in cost.

Preparation Procedure

Preparation for the provisional restoration must follow a strict protocol.[4–10]

1. All posterior teeth that do not have an opposing tooth are extracted (Fig 6-2).
2. The residual teeth are scaled to obtain an improvement in the oral ecosystem and a reduction in gingival inflammation, which is important for subsequent tissue healing.
3. A preliminary impression of both jaws is taken, and the diagnostic casts are prepared (Fig 6-3): Normal stock impression trays can be used, being careful to modify them with wax to extend the impression on the soft tissues. It is advisable to place extra wax at the center of the palate of the impression tray to allow for the most even distribution of impression material in all regions. If necessary, wax can also be inserted into the interdental spaces to avoid accidental avulsion. Once the diagnostic casts are obtained, it is possible to proceed to a preliminary analysis of the residual structure and to evaluate the need to surgically correct the osseous undercut. The remaining teeth must be analyzed and eventually modified to improve retention of the provisional prosthesis.
4. Individual impression trays are constructed on diagnostic casts, taking care to eliminate the undercuts often caused by the malpositioning of the teeth.
5. The definitive impression is taken and the master casts are constructed.

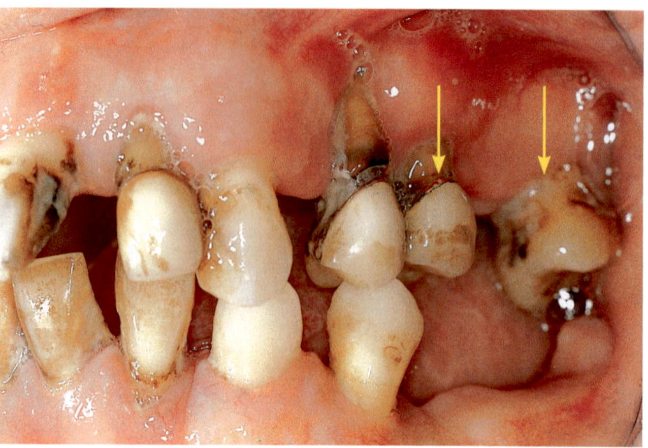

Fig 6-2 Teeth that could be removed before construction of a provisional prosthesis *(arrows)*. Neither of these teeth contributes to the maintenance of the vertical dimension of occlusion.

6. Registration of the maxillomandibular relationships is accomplished. Resin bases with wax rims are used. Once the bases with the rims have been clinically tested, the wax is heated, and the patient is asked to occlude the teeth to obtain the intercuspal position. In cases in which the vertical dimension of occlusion must be modified, it is necessary to use on the facial arc.
7. The casts are mounted in the articulator (Fig 6-4) and the provisional prosthesis is prepared. In the laboratory, the technician eliminates the teeth to be extracted on the cast (Fig 6-5), and one by one they are substituted with the artificial teeth in order to best reproduce their position.
8. The waxup and construction of the prosthesis follows (Fig 6-6): After positioning all of the teeth on the cast, proceed to the waxup of the buccal flange of the prosthetic body, taking care to leave space between the flange and the cast in case of edema or the need to reline materials postextraction. Provisional partial prostheses are supported by metal retainers on the residual teeth.
9. The residual teeth are extracted (Fig 6-7), and the prepared prosthesis is adapted: The surgical phase consists of extraction of the residual teeth and, if necessary, the remodeling of the osseous or fibromucosal structures. It is important that the patient not remove the prosthesis in the first 24 hours after the extraction. To prevent postextraction edema, the tissues must be compressed. Removing and repositioning the prosthesis will also provoke pain. The compression of the prosthesis on the tissues also diminishes the possibility of hemorrhage. Adaptation to the prosthesis of the underlying crests is obtained with the use of soft relining materials (see chapter 7), which allow a better congruency between the prosthetic bases and the osseo-

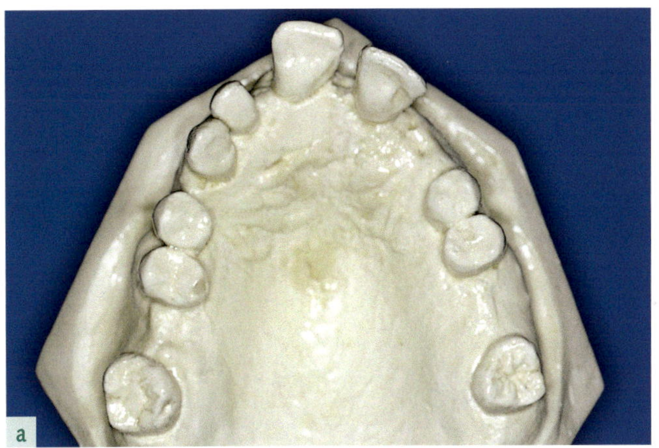

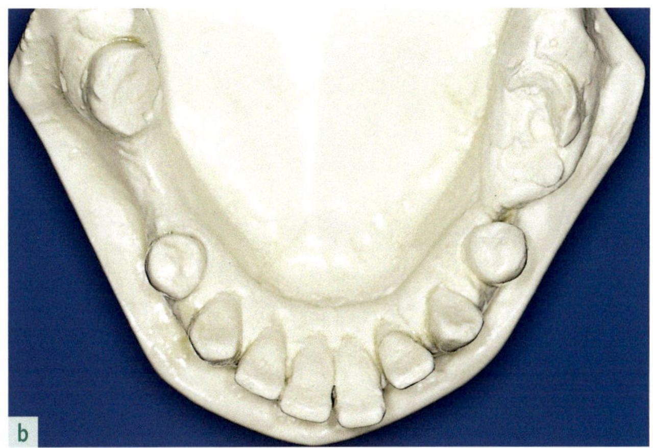

Fig 6-3 Preliminary casts that allow for analysis of the undercut are useful for the retention of the provisional prosthesis, the construction of an individual immpression tray, and for communication with patients.

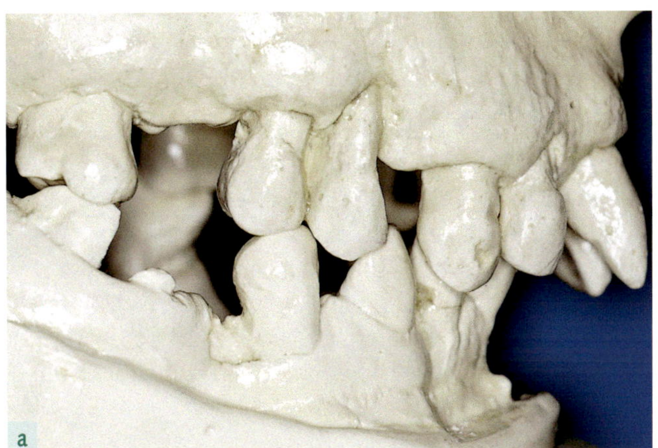

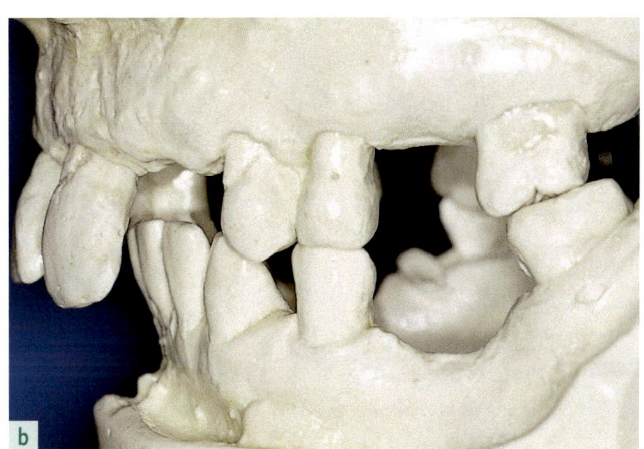

Fig 6-4 Lateral views of the casts in the articulator.

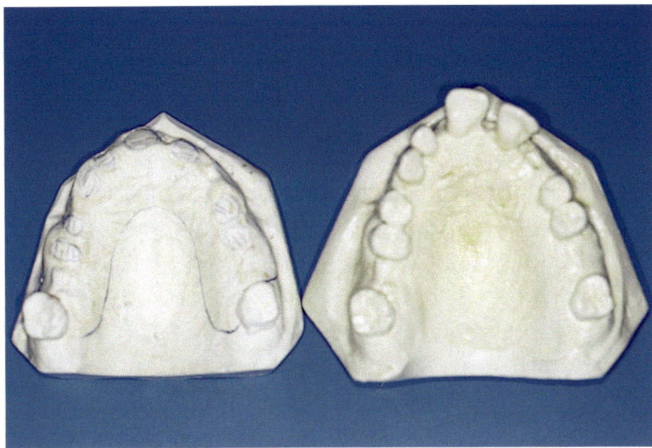

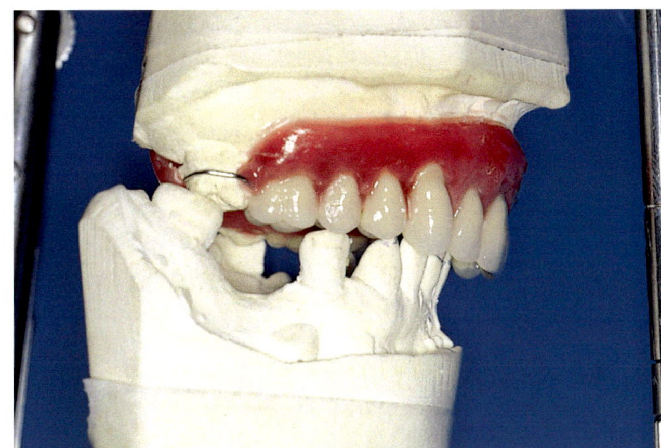

Fig 6-5 Removing the teeth after the impression is mounted in the articulator.

Fig 6-6 Lateral view of the mounting and the waxing of the prosthesis in the articulator.

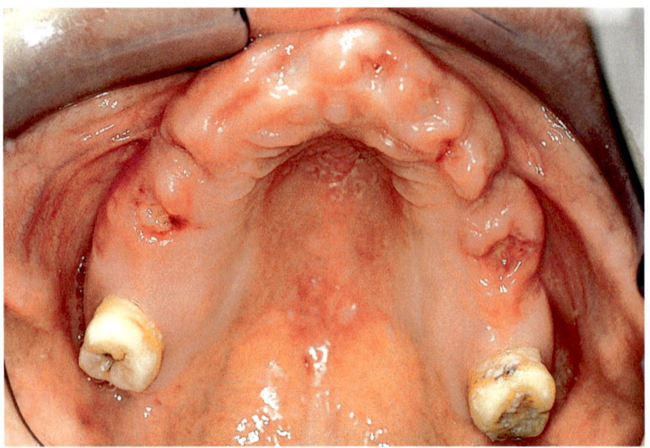

Fig 6-7 Healing of the alveolar crest after multiple extractions. Immediate use of the provisional prosthesis accelerates the healing process.

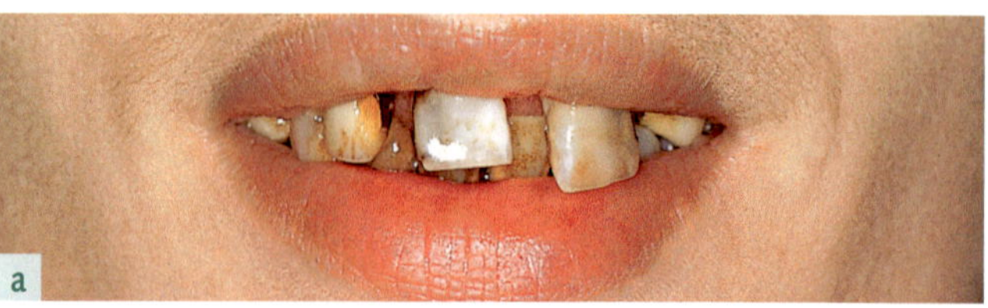

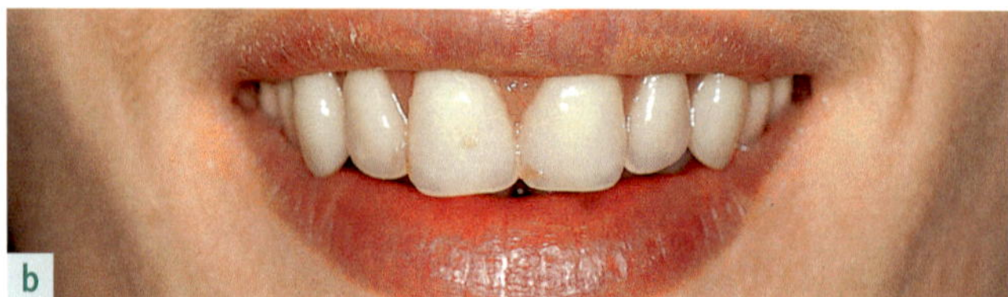

Fig 6-8 Completing the functional esthetic cast serves as the base for preparing the construction of the definitive prosthesis. Esthetic and functional problems can be discussed with the patient in order to understand how the expectations of the patient can be satisfied.

mucosal support and mitigate the pain caused by compression. After a few days, when resorption of the edema has taken place, anterior adaptation of the prosthesis is necessary.

10. Instructions for patients: It is important to make the patient understand that, after the extraction, the bone and the mucosa undergo inevitable size and shape modifications that make it necessary to readapt to the provisional prosthesis a number of times. The clinician must be available to check any decubitus or difficulty in retention and stability of the prosthesis.

11. Modifications to the provisional prosthesis (eg, modification of the flange or addition of teeth) due to more extractions must be made the same day in which the extractions are undertaken.

When the patient receives the provisional prosthesis, he or she needs to be reassured and informed of both the potential and the limitations of the new prosthesis (Fig 6-8).

Restoration of the Preexisting Prosthesis

If a patient is wearing a prosthesis that requires restoration, it must be modified following the constructive principles discussed in the preceding paragraphs so that it can be used temporarily during the construction phases of the new prosthesis. The most common clinical conditions for which a restoration

is required can be classified as (1) inadequate extension of the prosthetic body, (2) occlusal alterations, and (3) localized compressions.

The restoration must maintain the health of the supporting tissues; ensure extension and adaptation of the prosthesis to the underlying tissues to guarantee sufficient retention, stability, and support for the prosthesis; and facilitate adaptation of the neuromuscular system to a new vertical dimension of occlusion, a new position of the teeth, and a new extension of the prosthetic body.

To fulfill these objectives, the clinical phases can be divided as follows:

1. The evaluation of inadequate extension of the prosthetic body must take into consideration areas that are too wide, too small, or too sharp to avoid traumatizing the supporting tissues.[11,12] Particular attention must be given to the placement of the frena. If the prosthetic margins are too small, the prosthesis should be relined with traditional acrylic resin.[11,12]

2. Changes in occlusion cause prosthetic instability, which affects the health of the mucosa. Before treating the mucosal lesions, the relationship between the teeth and the supporting crest and the maxillomandibular relationships on the horizontal plane need to be evaluated. It is often necessary to resort to an occlusal registration by mounting the prosthesis in an articulator to carry out an indirect occlusal analysis.

The preexisting occlusion can be modified in the following ways:

- Self-polymerizing resin if the teeth are resin
- Autopolymerizing resin if the teeth are ceramic
- Selective grinding when possible

Another condition that is frequently observed is the sliding of the inferior prosthesis forward, upward, and toward the opposite side to which it functionally touches. This phenomenon is due to teeth that are mounted distally at the deepest point in a very curved edentulous crest. These teeth should be eliminated.[11,12]

The most common alteration of the vertical dimension[11,12] is a conspicuous decrease. If this reduction is equal to or less than 1 mm, it can be increased in a single sitting using conditioning materials directly on the prosthesis and then sanding it. If the loss is greater than 2 mm, it is opportune to carry out progressive increases of 1 to 1.5 mm per week.[11,12]

The localized areas of compression are identified using a pressure revealer (eg, Fit Checker, GC America). The material is applied to the inside of the prosthetic base, which is then placed in the mouth and kept in place with light pressure. Once the material has hardened, the prosthesis is extracted from the oral cavity, and the points at the prosthetic base are checked. Such areas represent the areas of greatest compression and have to be remodeled. The same operation is repeated until the material assumes a uniform thickness.

A prosthesis that is restored can be relined with conditioning materials to prepare the mucogingival tissues for the first impression.

References

1. Granados JI. Immediate denture using patient's existing dentition. J Prosthet Dent 1979;41:228–231. Cat. 8
2. Passamonti G. Immediate denture prosthesis. DCNA 1964:781–800. Cat. 7
3. Quaranta M, Scaramella F, Fratto G. La terapia immediata dell'edentulismo totale. Dental Cadmos 1985;10:39–44. Cat. 8
4. Walsh JF, Walsh T, Griffiths R. An immediate denture technique to reproduce labial alveolar contour. J Prosthet Dent 1977;37:222–225. Cat. 8
5. Guevara PA, Elstner ET Jr. The chair-side transitional denture. J Prosthet Dent 1976;36:226–231. Cat. 8
6. Chalifoux PR. Transitional denture technique. J Prosthet Dent 1978;40:682–685. Cat. 8
7. McCartney JW. The transitional immediate complete denture. J Prosthet Dent 1978;40:593–595. Cat. 8
8. Oliver LT, Smith RA, Wolfe HE, Koblitz FF. Immediate denture processing with a fluid resin. J Prosthet Dent 1975;34:216–220. Cat. 8
9. LaVere A, Krol AJ. Immediate denture service. J Prosthet Dent 1973;29:10–15. Cat. 7
10. Langenwalter EM, Jordan RD, Espinoza O. Fabrication of provisional complete denture. J Prosthet Dent 1987;58:246–248. Cat. 8
11. Pound E. Conditioning of denture patients. J Am Dent Assoc 1962;64:461–468. Cat. 8
12. Klein IE, Lennon CA. A comprehensive approach to tissue conditioning for complete dentures. J Prosthet Dent 1984;51:147–151. Cat. 8

7

Conditioning Supporting Tissues

When the mucosa has been altered by inflammatory states or mechanical trauma caused by incongruous dentures, conditioners lining the denture allow for functional recovery of the mucosa.[1–3] Conditioners may be used in the pretreatment phases, in particular for the treatment of problems associated with prosthetic stomatitis. Dentures that are not suitable for mucosal support can provoke stomatitis, angular cheilitis, fibrotic degeneration of the residual alveolar ridges, hyperplasia of the mucosa related to prosthetic margins, and trauma.[3]

At the moment the mechanical stimulus is eliminated, the soft oral tissues tend to return to their normal state. In conditions of heightened stress, the tissues lose their resilience and capacity to recuperate. Such changes are caused by histologic alterations, such as the reduction of the keratinized layers due to bacterial superinfections, candidiasis, and inflammation.[4–10] The length of recuperation is influenced by the age and general health of the patient. In young patients the mucosa usually returns to a normal state quicker and more completely than in older patients.[11]

Tissue conditioners are made by mixing a powder and liquid to form a viscous compound. When applied to the inner surface of the resin base of the denture, the mixture undergoes gelation, thereby adapting to the form of the residual ridges. Such materials, used over short periods of time, improve masticatory function[12] and contribute to the functional recovery of the altered oral mucosa, in part because of the presence of bacteriostatic compounds.[13,14]

Biomechanics of the Supportive Tissues: Viscoelastic Behavior

During function, the mucosa of an edentulous patient wearing a complete denture is cyclically compressed between two hard surfaces—the osseous ridge and the prosthetic body. The fibromucosal support has a discrete capacity to physiologically adapt to stress, owing to its own viscoelastic characteristics.[11,15]

The basis of this behavior is a redistribution of the tissue fluids between the areas of major and minor loading (Fig 7-1).

To explain viscoelastic behavior, it is helpful to refer to certain physical models.[16] The first of these is elastic deformation (Fig 7-2), represented by an elastic spring, in which the application of a force produces an immediate modification of shape, and the removal of the force brings about a complete and immediate renewal of the original shape.

The second model is that of viscous deformation (Fig 7-3), represented by a hydraulic damper or a piston that moves fluid in a hollow cylinder. By applying a constant force, the piston maintains a uniform linear movement. The time during which the forces are applied becomes an important element in evaluating the movement of the piston. When the force is removed, there is no return to the original position.

Three possible combinations of the models described above have been proposed to explain viscoelastic behavior:

1. In the Maxwell model (Fig 7-4), the spring and the damper are positioned in series. The application of a force causes the spring to lengthen immediately, followed by a slow

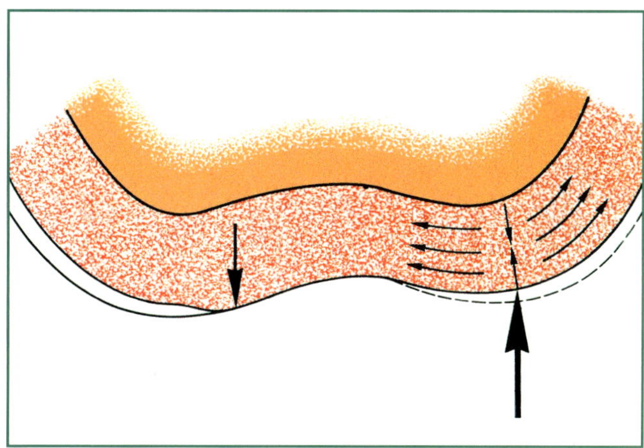

Fig 7-1 Viscoelastic adaptation of the supporting fibrous mucosa to the load, with redistribution of the tissue fluids.

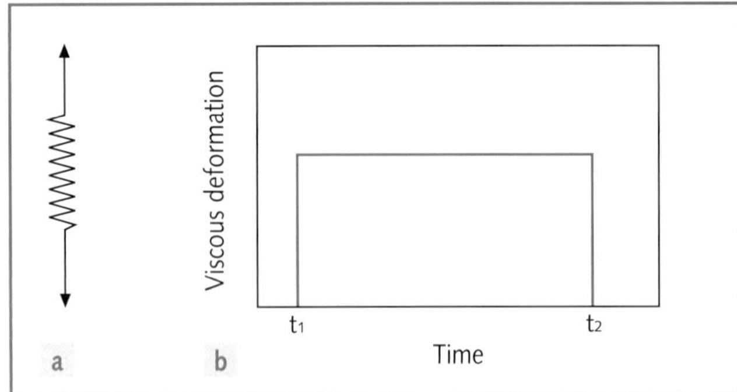

Fig 7-2 Mechanical model of ideal elastic behavior: *(a)* A perfectly elastic spring. *(b)* Graph showing the ideal mechanical model: Instant application to the spring of a constantly maintained force at time t_1 provokes an immediate and constant deformation of the spring itself. Removal of the force at t_2 results in an immediate and complete return to the original shape/position.

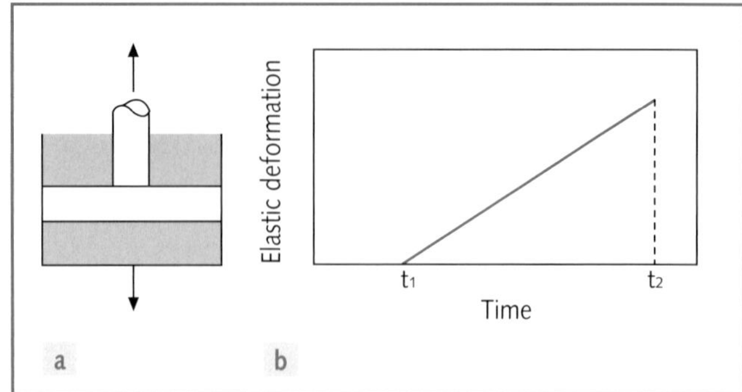

Fig 7-3 Mechanical model of ideal viscous behavior: *(a)* Diagram of a hydraulic damper. *(b)* Graph of the ideal mechanical model: The instantaneous application of a constant force to the damper at time t_1 causes a linear, uniform, and continuous movement till time t_2, after which the force is removed and there is not a return to the original starting position.

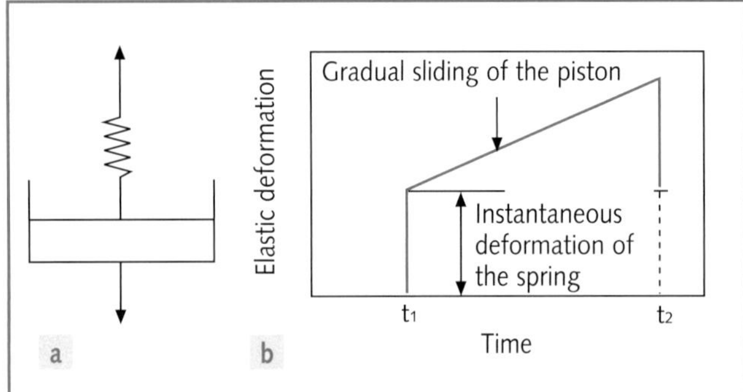

Fig 7-4 Ideal mechanical model of viscoelastic behavior according to Maxwell: *(a)* Diagram of the elastic spring and the hydraulic damper combined in series. *(b)* Graph of the ideal mechanical model: At time t_1 (instanteous application of a force maintained constantly) an instantaneous lengthening of the spring occurs, followed by a slower lengthening of the damper. At time t_2, (removal of the force) the spring recovers its original form instantly, while the damper remains deformed.

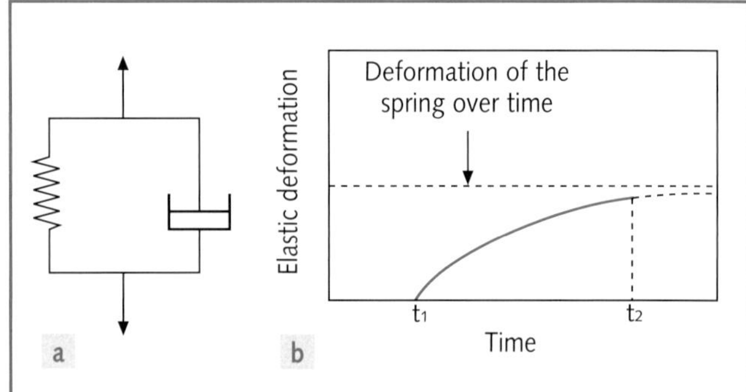

Fig 7-5 Ideal mechanical model of viscoelastic behavior according to Voigt: (a) Diagram of a spring and hydraulic damper, combined in parallel. (b) Graph of the ideal mechanical model: At time t_1 (instantaneous application of constant force) a rapid initial deformation followed by a slower and gradual movement toward a stable situation occurs. If at time t_2 the force is instantaneously removed, an initial rapid return occurs, followed by a slower recovery phase.

lengthening of the damper. When the force is removed, the spring returns instantly to its original form, while the damper remains deformed.

2. The Voigt model (Fig 7-5) is nothing more than the combination in parallel of the two previous elements. When the applied force is constant, a deformation occurs, followed by a slower and more gradual shifting toward a balanced situation. Removing the force produces a rapid initial recovery caused by the elastic component, followed by a phase of slower recovery, caused by the viscous component.

3. In the universal model (Fig 7-6), which considers the Maxwell and Voigt models together, the application of a force determines the lengthening of the spring of the Maxwell system, followed by a slow deformation caused by

the action of the Maxwell damper, which is associated with the deformation obtained with the Voigt model. When the force is removed, there is an immediate return of an elastic type, linked to the Maxwell spring and followed, through the action of the Voigt model, by a gradual recovery, which concludes with a permanent deformation caused by the Maxwell damper.

The universal model better explains the behavior of the mucosa when it is subjected to loading; in-depth analysis has shown viscoelastic characteristics (Fig 7-7) in such a situation.[11] When a load equal to 10 g/mm^2 is applied to the supportive mucosa, an initial instantaneous elastic deformation equal to 30% to 40% of the initial thickness takes place. If the force is applied for 10

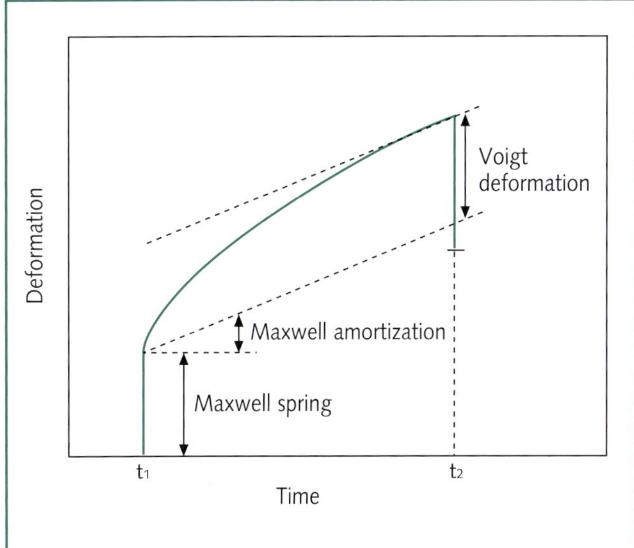

Fig 7-6 Graph of the universal model (Maxwell's and Voigt's models combined in series).

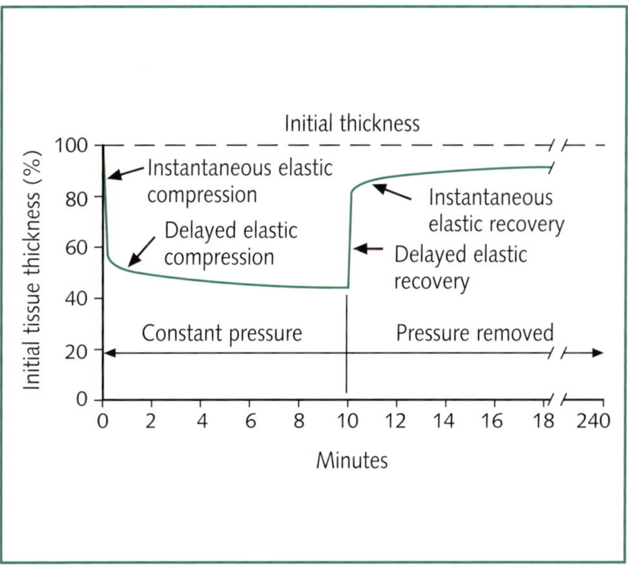

Fig 7-7 Graph of the typical behavior of supporting oral mucosa under 10 minutes of a load with constant pressure. Once the load is removed, the mucosa regains 90% of its original form in 8 minutes.

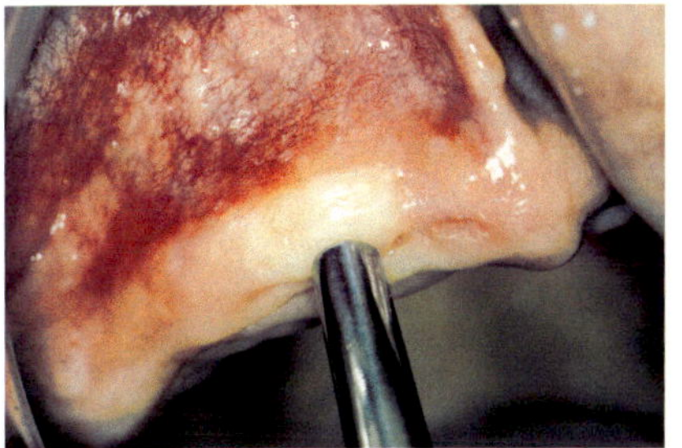

Fig 7-8 Application of two different types of loads to the supporting mucosa: One prolonged (10 minutes) and the other, instantaneous and intense.

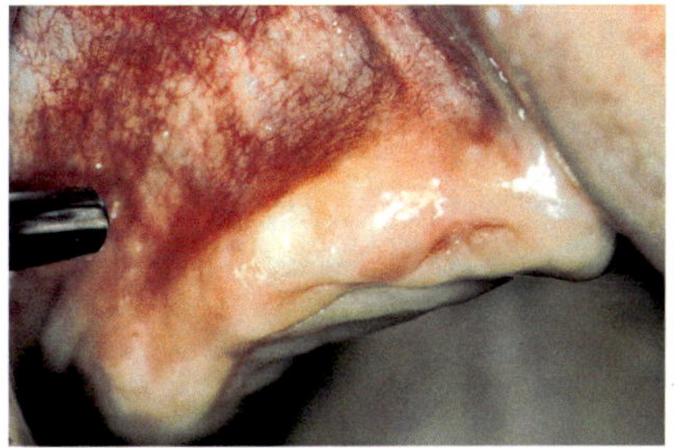

Fig 7-9 Once the prolonged load is removed, a remaining ischemic area can be seen, a consequence of the more stable deformation of the viscoelastic type.

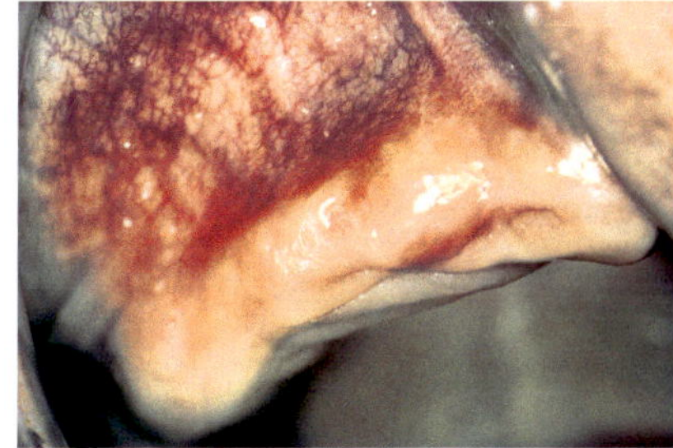

Fig 7-10 Once the instantaneous load is removed, the mucosa shows dimensional recovery of the more elastic type.

minutes, a deformation equal to 50% to 60% is obtained (Figs 7-7 and 7-8).On removal of the forces, most of the deformation undergoes an immediate elastic return, followed by a slow recovery of the remainder over the following 2 hours (Figs 7-7 to 7-9).

It is important to note that the degree of deformation and the time necessary for recovery are not so much related to the intensity of the force applied but more to its duration. A longer-lasting deformation is produced when a force of low intensity is applied over a long period of time, as happens, for example, during parafunctional activity. The deformation is shorter when a force of heightened intensity is applied for only a short period of time, as occurs during masticatory cycles[11] (Figs 7-8 to 7-10).

If the stresses are modest, no damage results, and the relationship between the prosthetic body and the mucosa are optimized during function. If the stress is too intense, as occurs with an incongruous denture, the adapting modifications are more marked and are no longer spontaneously recoverable; after the removal of the pathogenic stimulus a period of recovery is needed. Kydd[11] demonstrated that mucosal deformations linked to a low-intensity load take just a few minutes to return to normal conditions in young subjects, while they take several hours in elderly subjects (Fig 7-11). Most authors[4,5,8–11,15] agree that it is sufficient to remove the denture for at least 72 hours, combined with a soft diet and gum massages, to recuperate the normal morphology of the soft tissues. Often the patient does not accept such a prescription, which would affect his or

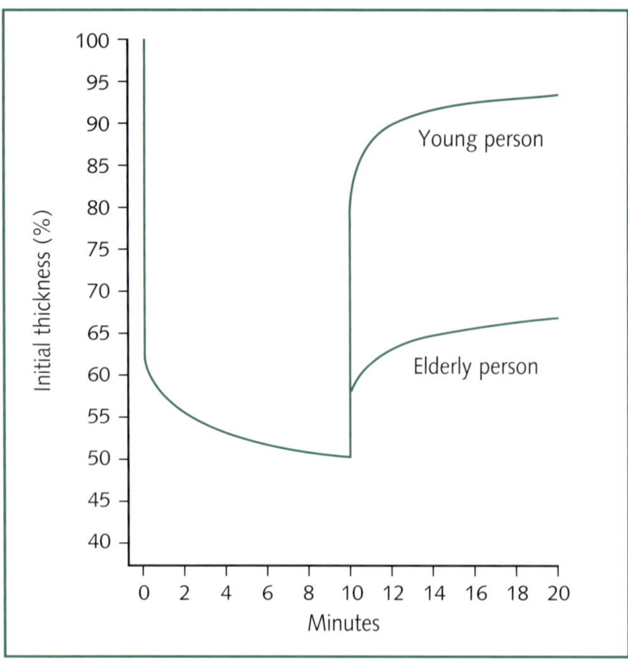

Fig 7-11 Graph of the variation in function of the age of the person and the thickness of the supporting oral mucosa after a constant load (5 g/mm^2).

her social life. In such cases, conditioners can be inserted in the pre-existent denture to allow efficient morphologic recovery.

Composition and Behavior of Conditioning Materials

The conditioners are linear amorphous polymers provided as a powder and liquid, which are then mixed together. The powder is made up of polymethacrylates, the polymers of which can be made up of various combinations of polyethylmethacrylate (PEMA) and other copolymers such as polymethylmethacrylate or polymethacrylate.[3,17] Generally the liquid consists of single or associate aromatic ethanol esters, such as butylphthalate or butyl phthalylglycolate, which serve as plasticizers and aromas.

The gelation activated by mixing the powder and liquid is a process linked to the solubilization of the polymeric molecules because of the aromatic esthers, and is accelerated by the presence of ethanol. Monomeric components, which are responsible for the chemical polymerization reaction,[18] are not present. When the powder and liquid are mixed together, the PEMA dissolves in the solvent. At first such a process gives rise to a very fluid material, which then increases in viscosity as the ethanol and plasticizing aromatic esthers penetrate the acrylic

polymer. After 2 to 3 minutes, the material becomes sufficiently viscous to be introduced into the oral cavity and reaches the final stage of gelation in 15 to 20 minutes.

Conditioners with a shorter gelation time offer better clinical handling characteristics in terms of application to the denture, removal from the oral cavity, and finishing.[3] Once this process has been completed, the product shows a typical viscoelastic behavior.[3] Under constant loading it initially shows rapid deformation, which recovers immediately. A progressive, slower adaptation follows as a result of the readaptation of the internal tensions of the material.

Conditioners differ in composition and structure (eg, weight and dimensions of the particles of powder, content of ethanol, and type of plasticizer), which influence the characteristics of gelation and the viscoelastic properties[19-22] (Table 7-1). In virtue of such properties, the conditioning materials behave differently according to the type of stress to which they are subjected. An instantaneous loading causes the conditioner to assume an elastic behavior, and a continual functional stress causes it to assume a viscoelastic behavior.

Tissue conditioners must possess a heightened elastic capacity, a proper level of viscosity, and stability in terms of structure and physical properties over time. By deforming under a load and returning to the initial state as soon as the force stops, conditioners reduce the stress on the oral mucosa, thus facilitating the healing process. The action of the conditioners therefore changes with respect to the type of load the denture is subjected to. In response to impact during mastication, they deform and then go back to their former shape. In conditions of functional resting, when subjected to the action of modest loading, the gel distributes itself plastically, adapting itself to the changes in the

Table 7-1 Conditioning materials and their relative gelation times

Materials	Manufacturer	Gelation (sec)
COE Comfort	GC America	490
FITT	Kerr Sybron Dental Specialties	100
Fit Softer	Sankin Industry	230
GC Soft Liner	GC Dental Industrial	150
Hydro-cast	Kay See Dental Manufacturing	255
Hi-Soft	Shofu	1150
Softone	Harry J. Bosworth	160
Sr-Ivoseal	Ivoclar	105
Shofu tissue conditioner	Shofu	170
Visco-gel	Dentsply	580

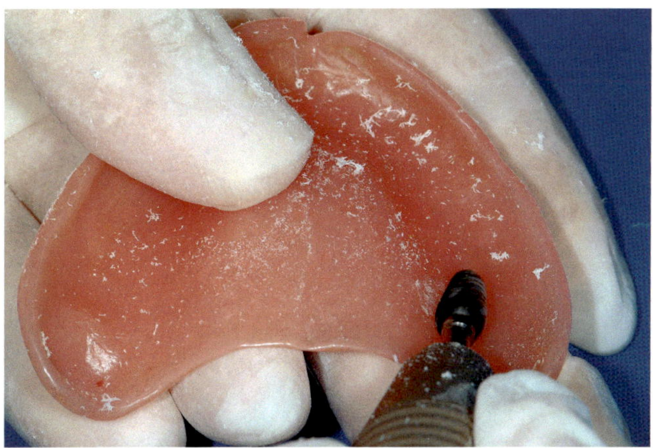

Fig 7-12 Roughening of the denture in the area where the conditioning material will be applied.

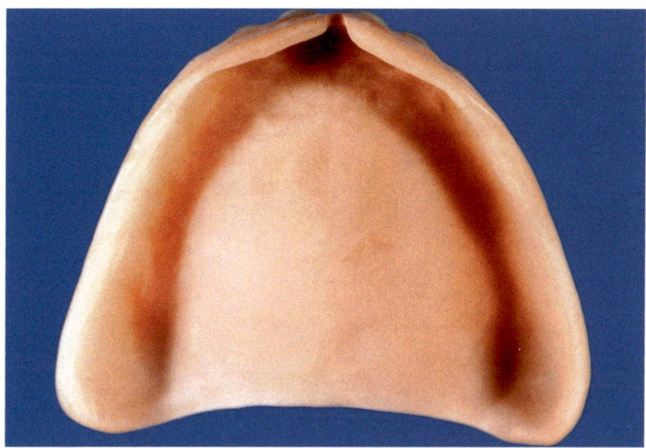

Fig 7-13 Sanding of the roughened surfaces.

tissue morphology. The slow plastic distribution of these materials represents the most useful phase in their application.

Unfortunately, in the oral cavity, the physical properties of these materials gradually change within a few days because of the loss of ethanol, the absorption of water, and the progressive loss of the plasticizing materials. The loss of ethanol begins immediately after the immersion of the material in a water-containing medium and continues until it has almost totally disappeared; at the same time, the polymer itself absorbs water from the environment. First there is an increasing hardening when ethanol release prevails over water absorption, followed by a level of relative softening when the process of water absorption increases. The hardening then continues progressively when the absorption of water reaches a balance, while the ethanol and the plasticizer are continually released.

Furthermore, because of their porous surface structure, these materials are subject to colonization by bacteria and *Candida albicans*.[23,24] Elderly people or patients with reduced or defective immune resistance can also encounter infections of *Staphylococcus aureus* and *Pseudomonas aeruginosa*. To eliminate the risk of infection, studies both in vitro and in vivo have been carried out concerning the addition of bacteriostatic compounds, such as chlorhexidine,[25] antimycotics,[26] (eg, nystatin, miconazole, ketoconazole), microwave treatment,[27] and the use of substances that release metallic ions, such as silver. These last compounds, in contrast with the antimycotics, have shown an antimicrobic effect both on *C albicans* and on the bacteria responsible for hospital-acquired respiratory tract infections without compromising the physical properties of the conditioning material.[13] The period of release of the metallic ions is lengthened by about a month and generally extends well beyond the period of physical degradation of the conditioning material.[14]

Technique

First phase: Preparation of the prosthetic body

Before applying the conditioner, it is necessary to correct the imperfections in the prosthetic body that are responsible for the mucosal alterations,[28–30] eliminating an important cofactor in the prosthetic stomatitis[31–35] and thus obtaining a proper-fitting denture.

Once the mechanical defects have been repaired, the denture must be prepared to receive the conditioner.[36–39] The maxillary and mandibular dentures must be treated in different appointments, beginning with the least stable, to benefit from the stabilizing action of the opposing arch. The tissue-bearing surface of the prosthetic body is roughened using an appropriate bur to eliminate about 1 mm of thickness (Fig 7-12) and successively sanding the surface (Fig 7-13). In some cases it may be necessary to make a series of five to six holes on the vestibular plate to create an outlet for the excess material to avoid dislocation of the prosthetic body during insertion.[30]

Second phase: Relining with the conditioner

The areas of the dentures on which the conditioning material is not to be applied must be covered with an appropriate protective liquid (Fig 7-14). The components of the conditioning material are then mixed until the desired consistency is obtained (Fig 7-15). The power-liquid ratio varies in relation to the final consistency desired. With a ratio of 2:1, a somewhat elastic consistency is obtained. If a more fluid mixture is necessary, the ratio should be 1.5:1.[38]

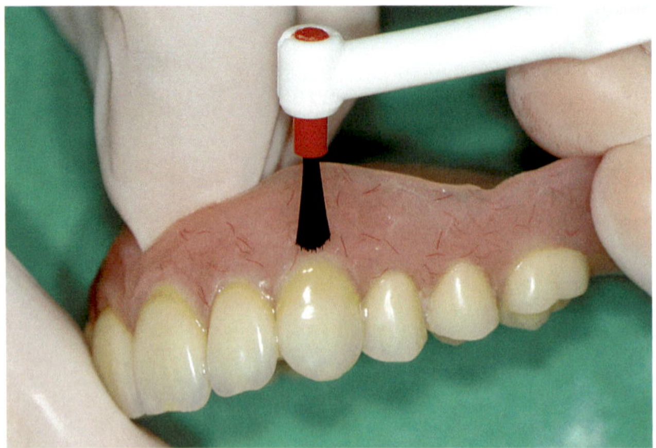

Fig 7-14 Application of a separating liquid.

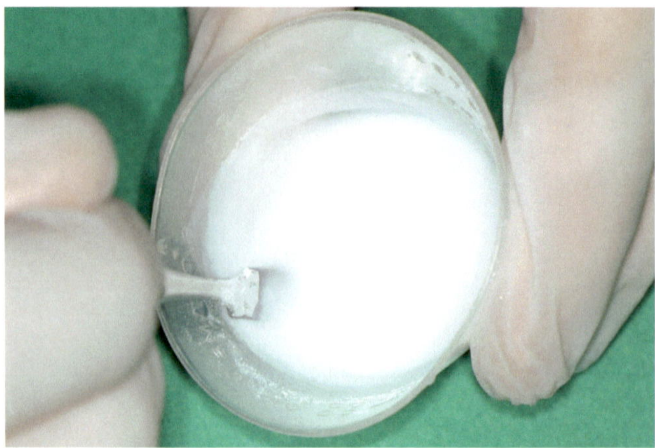

Fig 7-15 Mixing of the components of the conditioner.

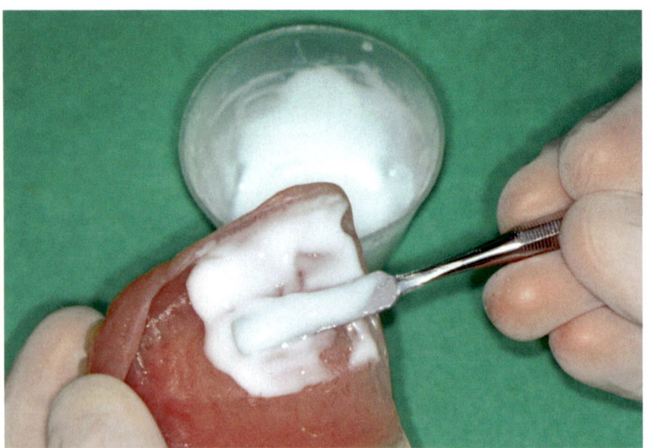

Fig 7-16 Application of the conditioner.

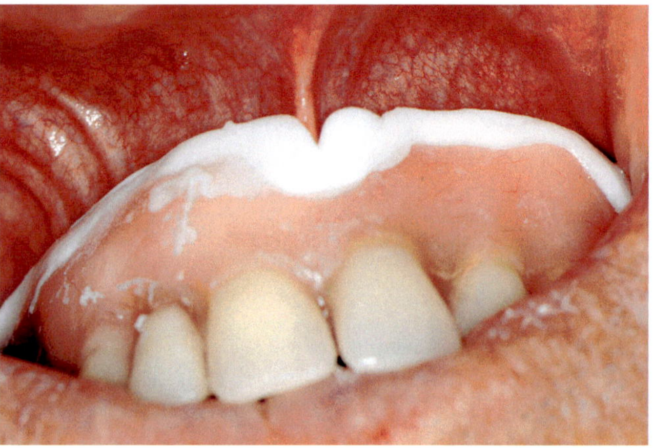

Fig 7-17 Placement of the denture with the conditioner in the oral cavity.

Once mixed, an initial quantity of conditioner is placed inside the denture while it is still fluid to obtain better adhesion to the bur-roughened areas (Fig 7-16). The viscosity must be allowed to increase slightly before the rest of the material is added. It should not run down from the prosthetic margin. In 2 to 3 minutes the material becomes sufficiently viscous to be introduced into the oral cavity, and in 15 to 20 minutes it gels completely. During this period, the patient is asked to maintain light occlusal contact, as occurs during swallowing, warning him or her not to clench the teeth. Some authors[1,39] ask patients to read or speak in a loud voice for 10 minutes to better adapt the new material to these functional movements (Fig 7-17).

Once gelation has taken place, the denture is removed from the oral cavity, and the internal surface inspected to identify eventual areas of overload. These areas, where the base shows through, are reduced with a bur and relined with new conditioner. If extended areas of the base show through, this could mean that at the moment of insertion the material was still too fluid or that the patient exerted too much pressure during the setting period.[30] In this case also, relining with new conditioner is necessary. When a uniform layer is obtained (Fig 7-18), the excess is removed with a scalpel blade that has been warmed over a flame (Fig 7-19).

Given the rapid decline of the physical properties of these materials, they can be substituted every 3 to 4 days at least three to four times,[1,38] until the supportive tissues have healed.

If the conditioning materials are not renewed for a long time, hygiene will be compromised. The patient must be instructed to keep the denture and the mouth scrupulously clean. The surface of the conditioner must be brushed gently. The prosthetic body should be carefully washed in tepid water, using a soft brush and a medicated detergent (eg, betadine). When

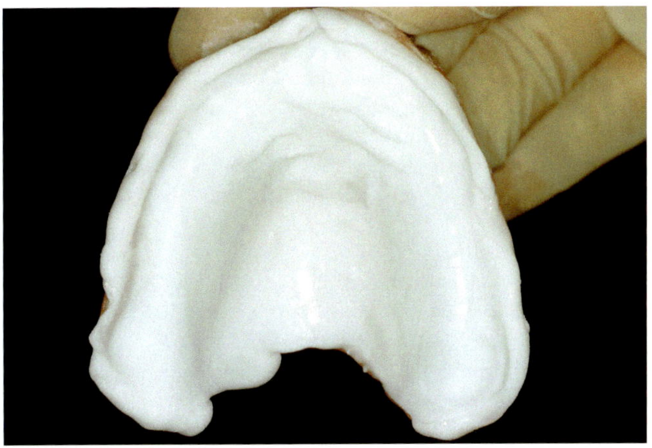

Fig 7-18 Example of a correctly relined denture. The layer of conditioner is uniform and sufficiently thick.

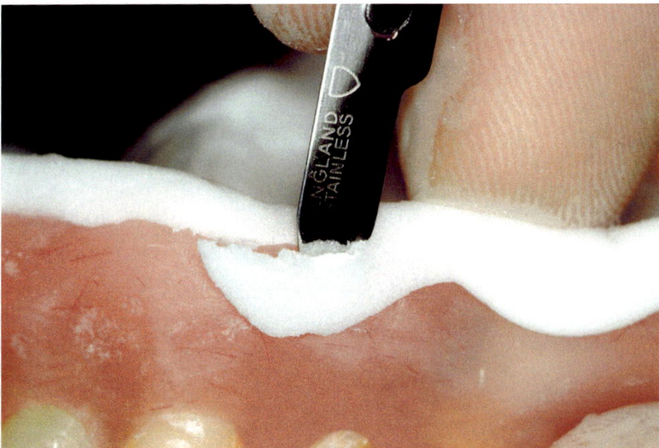

Fig 7-19 Removal of the excess conditioning material with a heated scalpel blade.

the denture is not in the oral cavity, such as at night, it must be kept in water. Some authors[25,26] advise the addition of antiseptic solution (eg, chlorhexidine) or antimicotics (eg, nystatin) to diminish the bacterial and fungal loads that tend to accumulate over time in the porous, rough material.[40]

References

1. Jagger DC, Harrison A. Complete dentures—The soft option. An update for general dental practice. Br Dent J 1997;182:313–317. Cat. 7

2. Murata H, Hamada T, Djulaeha E, Nikawa H. Rheology of tissue conditioners. J Prosthet Dent 1998;79:188–199. Cat. 6

3. McCord JF, Grant AA. Pre-definitive treatment: Rehabilitation prostheses. Br Dent J 2000;188:419–424. Cat. 7

4. Stig G. The effect of complete dentures on the gum tissues. A histological and histopathological investigation. Acta Odontol Scand 1958;16:1–6. Cat. 3

5. Kapur K, Shklar G. The effect of complete dentures on alveolar mucosa. J Prosthet Dent 1963;13:1030–1037. Cat. 3

6. Dorey JL, Blasberg B, MacEntee MI, Conklin RJ. Oral mucosal disorders in denture wearers. J Prosthet Dent 1985;53:210–213. Cat. 4

7. Miller EL. Clinical management of denture-induced inflammations. J Prosthet Dent 1977;38:362–365. Cat. 7

8. Jones PM. Complete dentures and the associated soft tissues. J Prosthet Dent 1976;36:136–149. Cat. 7

9. Pendleton EC. Changes in the denture supporting tissues. J Am Dent Assoc 1951;42:1–15. Cat. 4

10. Razek MK, Shaaban NA. Histochemical and histopathologic studies of alveolar mucosa under complete dentures. J Prosthet Dent 1978;39:29–36. Cat. 2

11. Kydd WL, Daly CH. The biologic and mechanical effects of stress on oral mucosa. J Prosthet Dent 1982;47:317–329. Cat. 7

12. Hayakawa I, Takahashi Y, Morizawa M, Kobayashi S, Nagao M. The effect of fluorinated copolymer coating agent on tissue conditioners. Int J Prosthodont 1997;10:44–48. Cat. 8

13. Ueshige M, Abe Y, Sato Y, Tsuga K, Akagawa Y, Ishii M. Dynamic viscoelastic properties of antimicrobial tissue conditioners containing silver-zeolite. J Dent 1999;27:517–522. Cat. 6

14. Matsuura T, Abe Y, Sato Y, Okamoto K, Ueshige M, Akagawa Y. Prolonged antimicrobial effect of tissue conditioners containing silver-zeolite. J Dent 1997;25:373–377. Cat. 6

15. Picton DC, Willis DJ. Viscoelastic properties of the periodontal ligament and mucous membrane. J Prosthet Dent 1978;40:263–272. Cat. 5

16. Craig RG, Ward ML. Restorative Dental Materials ed 10. St. Louis: Mosby, 1997. Cat. 7

17. Braden M. Tissue conditioners. I. Composition and structure. J Dent Res 1970;49:145–148. Cat. 7

18. Graham BS, Jones DW, Sutow EJ. Clinical implications of resilient denture lining material research. Part II: Gelation and flow properties of tissue conditioners. J Prosthet Dent 1991;65:413–418. Cat. 7

19. Murata H, Murakami S, Shigeto N, Hamada T. Viscoelastic properties of tissue conditioners—Influence of ethyl alcohol content and type of plasticizer. J Oral Rehabil 1994;21:145–156. Cat. 6

20. Jones DW, Sutow EJ, Graham BS, Milne EJ, Johnston DE. Influence of plasticizer on soft polymer gelation. J Dent Res 1986;65: 634–642. Cat. 6

21. Parker S, Braden M. Formulation of tissue conditioners. Biomaterials 1990;11:579–584. Cat. 6

22. Jones DW, Hall GC, Sutow EJ, Langman MF, Robertson KN. Chemical and molecular weight analyses of prosthodontic soft polymers. J Dent Res 1991;70:874–879. Cat. 6

23. Wright PS. Observations on long-term use of a soft-lining material for mandibular complete dentures. J Prosthet Dent 1994;72: 385–392. Cat. 2

24. Radford DR, Challacombe SJ, Walter JD. Denture plaque and adherence of Candida albicans to denture-base materials in vivo and in vitro. Crit Rev Oral Biol Med 1999;10:99–116. Cat. 7

25. Addy M. In vitro studies into the use of denture base and soft liner materials as carriers for drugs in the mouth. J Oral Rehabil 1981;8:131–142. Cat. 6

26. Truhlar MR, Shay K, Sohnle P. Use of a new assay technique for quantification of antifungal activity of nystatin incorporated in denture liners. J Prosthet Dent 1994;71:517–524. Cat. 6

27. Baysan A, Whiley R, Wright PS. Use of microwave energy to disinfect a long-term soft lining material contaminated with Candida albicans or Staphylococcus aureus. J Prosthet Dent 1998;79:454–458. Cat. 6

28. Olsson K, Bergman B. A comparison of two prosthetic methods for the treatment of denture stomatitis. Acta Odontol Scand 1971;29:745–753. Cat. 3

29. Pound E. Conditioning of denture patients. J Am Dent Assoc 1962;64: 461–468. Cat. 7

30. Klein IE, Lennon CA. A comprehensive approach to tissue conditioning for complete dentures. J Prosthet Dent 1984;51:147–151. Cat. 7

31. Love WD, Goska FA, Mixson RJ. The etiology of mucosal inflammation associated with dentures. J Prosthet Dent 1967;18:515–527. Cat. 4

32. Stohler C. Etiology and occurrence of denture stomatitis. A review of literature. Schweiz Monatsschr Zahnmed 1984;94:187–194. Cat. 7

33. Budtz-Jorgensen E, Bertram U. Denture Stomatitis. I. The etiology in relation to trauma and infection. Acta Odontol Scand 1970;28: 71–92. Cat. 2

34. Yemm R. Stress-induced muscle activity: A possible etiologic factor in denture soreness. J Prosthet Dent 1972;28:133–140. Cat. 2

35. Klein IE, Miglino JC. Uses and abuses of the tissue treatment materials. J Prosthet Dent 1966; 16: 5–12. Cat. 2

36. Wilson HJ, Tomlin HR, Osborne J. The assessment of temporary soft materials used in prosthetics. Br Dent J 1969;126:303–306. Cat. 6

37. Travaglini EA, Gibbons P, Craig RG. Resilient liners for dentures. J Prosthet Dent 1960;10:664–672. Cat. 6

38. McCarthy JA, Moser JB. Mechanical properties of tissue conditioners. Part I: Theoretical considerations, behavioral characteristics, and tensile properties. J Prosthet Dent 1978;40:89–97. Cat. 6

39. Wilson HJ, Tomlin HR, Osborne J. Tissue conditioners and functional impression materials. Br Dent J 1966;121:9–16. Cat. 6

40. Nikawa H, Iwanaga H, Hamada T, Yuhta S. Effects of denture cleansers on direct soft denture lining materials. J Prosthet Dent 1994;72:657–662. Cat. 6

8

Denture Adhesives

The use of adhesives in complete dentures can be justified when it is not possible to obtain sufficient retention and stability and when implants are not an option because of the patient's economic situation, health, or age.

Indications
Stabilization during clinical procedures

Adhesives can be used during the recording of maxillomandibular relationships and during phonetic checks to guarantee the stability of the base. In cases of rapid osseous resorption they can immediately improve the adaptation of provisional dentures until they are relined or renewed.[1]

Clinical and pathologic conditions

Adhesives are recommended for significant osseous resorption, unfavorable anatomic conditions in patients for whom preprosthetic surgical interventions are not recommended, reduced salivary flow, and those with conditions related to limited neuromuscular control, such as myasthenia gravis, muscular dystrophy, Parkinson disease, Alzheimer disease, and tardive dyskinesia, involving the mouth, face, and tongue.[2] Patients who need prosthetic rehabilitation in situations of reduced retention after orofacial surgery can also benefit from these adhesives.[1] Studies have demonstrated that regular use of adhesives reduces chronic inflammation of the mucosa caused by mobility of the denture and thus reduces the risk of osseous resorption.[3,4]

In a study[3] of 111 patients who were wearing dentures, it was shown that the increased stability and retention provided by the regular use of adhesives reduces inflammation. At the end of the 6-month study period, nearly all subjects—even those who initially had prosthetic stomatitis—had normal mucosal tissue. The most significant results were found in the subgroup with poorly adapted, more mobile dentures. Other authors[5–7] have reported that adhesives do not cause irritation and osseous resorption. Rather, these products seem to have a cushioning effect, whereby the prosthetic load is distributed across the tissues more regularly. These studies contradict the widespread opinion held by dental practitioners that the use of adhesives can contribute to tissue irritation resulting in osseous resorption.

All responders to a questionnaire distributed to 17 prosthodontic professors from 17 North American universities[8] agreed that adhesives were beneficial in various pathologic conditions or clinical procedures. They also agreed on the importance of correctly educating patients on their use. Fifty percent of the respondents claimed that the use of adhesives improves adaptation of the immediate dentures in the phase following insertion.

Contraindications

It has been shown that the use of adhesives can have a negative effect if the clinician is then less careful during the rehabilitation phases, or if the adhesives are used to correct errors in the planning and execution of the preparation of the prosthesis.[2,8,9] Furthermore, adhesives may give patients a false sense of security, making them less likely to follow up with check-ups after the completion of the therapy.[8]

Adhesives are not recommended for patients who are allergic to one or more of the components, nor should they be used by patients who are not able to correctly use the product.[1]

Adhesives and Candidiasis

It has been shown that there is a relationship between candidiasis and prosthetic stomatitis; it is therefore important to verify whether adhesives support or inhibit this fungus. There is a widespread opinion among clinicians that *Candida* can be encouraged by the use of adhesives.[8] Research on this argument has reached contrasting results, however.

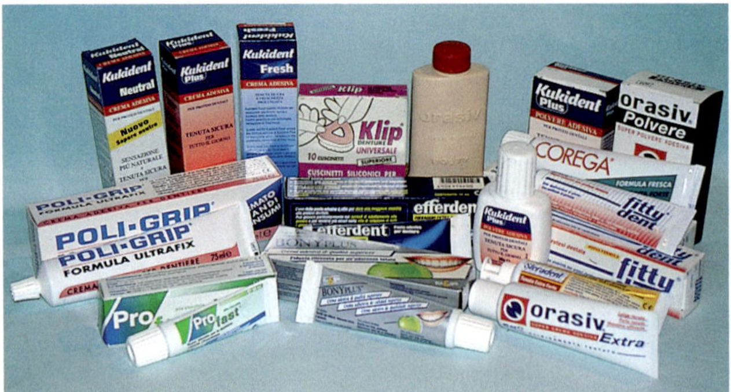

Fig 8-1 Common adhesives for complete dentures.

In one study[10] the effects of a solution of sugar and four adhesives on the development of *Candida albicans*, *Streptococcus mitis*, or *Neisseria pharingis* were analyzed. All of the adhesives supported the growth of the first two organisms, and no growth medium could be found to inhibit their growth. The antimycotic effect of an adhesive associated with amphotericin on 52 patients with prosthetic stomatitis was studied.[7] Clinical and microbiologic analysis of the experimental and control placebo groups revealed no statistically significant effect.

However, the conclusions of a more recent in vitro study on the pH variations induced by adhesives in the growth media of *Candida* were to the contrary. It was demonstrated that the adhesives produced an inhibitory effect on the growth of the fungus. Their presence increased the pH of the culture, diminishing the acid production responsible for the adhesion of the *Candida*. Furthermore, these products contain components such as hexachlorophene, sodium tetraborate, and ethanol, which have an antimicrobic effect.[11]

Because research on the argument is scarce and the results obtained are contrasting, a closer examination of the relationship between the use of the adhesives and the onset of *Candida* is needed.

Composition

The constituents of modern adhesives for dentures can be divided into three categories:
1. Adhesive substances: Karaya rubber, steel, pectin, gelatin, methylcellulose, hydroxyl methylcellulose, sodium carboxymethylcellulose, and synthetic polymers (eg, polyethylene)
2. Antibacterial agents: Hexachlorophene, sodium tetraborate, ethanol
3. Additives, plasticizers, and humidifying agents

Adhesives can be purchased as a powder or as a prepared paste (Fig 8-1). The powders used to make adhesives contain vegetable substances, such as karaya or acacia, which become viscous when mixed with water. Adhesives pastes contain polymers, such as methylcellulose, which have adhesive properties.[1]

Ideal Characteristics

The ideal adhesive should:

■ Be nontoxic, nonirritant, and biocompatible
■ Discourage growth of microorganisms
■ Have no odor or taste
■ Be easy to apply and remove
■ Maintain their adhesive capacity for 12 to 16 hours

Most patients prefer the paste because it is easier to remove and its effect lasts longer.[1]

Mechanism of Action

The greater viscosity of adhesives provides greater retention and stability than saliva.[1] Furthermore, in the presence of water, the material increases in volume and is therefore able to compensate for an incorrect adaptation of the denture by filling the spaces between the denture and the mucosa.[2]

In 1967 a fundamental study[12] showed that the increase in denture retention provided by adhesives was statistically significant. A more recent study[4] confirmed a significant increase in the retention and stability of maxillary dentures during mastication, deglutition, and phonation. The results were the same for old and incorrectly adapted dentures as for new and more precise ones. The efficacy was shown to begin immediately after application and remained almost constant for 8 hours.

Some studies[4,12,13] have found that the use of adhesives enables patients to chew harder food substances. Mastication tests of different food substances confirmed that the number of dislocations decreased significantly in patients using adhesives, and consequently masticatory capacity and comfort[14] increased even for those with incongruous dentures.[15]

References

1. Adisman IK. The use of denture adhesives as an aid to denture treatment. J Prosthet Dent 1989;62:711–715. Cat. 7
2. Shay K. Denture adhesives. Choosing the right powders and pastes. J Am Dent Assoc 1991;122:70–76. Cat. 7
3. Tarbet WJ, Grossman E. Observations of denture-supporting tissue during six months of denture adhesive wearing. J Am Dent Assoc 1980;101:789–791. Cat. 3
4. Grasso JE, Rendell J, Gay T. Effect of denture adhesive on the retention and stability of maxillary dentures. J Prosthet Dent 1994;72:399–405. Cat. 2
5. Grasso JE. Denture adhesives: Changing attitudes. J Am Dent Assoc 1996;127:90–96. Cat. 7
6. Kelsey CC, Lang BR, Wang RF. Examining patients' responses about the effectiveness of five denture adhesive pastes. J Am Dent Assoc 1997;128:1532–1538. Cat. 3
7. Scher EA, Ritchie GM, Flowers DJ. Antimycotic denture adhesive in treatment of denture stomatitis. J Prosthet Dent 1978;40:622–627. Cat. 1
8. Slaughter A, Katz RV, Grasso JE. Professional attitude toward denture adhesives: A Delphi Technique survey of academic prosthodontists. J Prosthet Dent 1999;82:80–89. Cat. 9
9. Chew CL, Boone ME, Swartz ML, Phillips RW. Denture adhesives: Their effects on denture retention and stability. J Dent 1985;13:152–159. Cat. 4
10. Stafford GD, Russel C. Efficiency of denture adhesives and their possible influence on oral microorganisms. J Dent Res 1971;50:832–836. Cat. 2
11. Makihira S, Nikawa H, Satonobu SV, Jin C, Hamada T. Growth of Candida species on commercial denture adhesives in vitro. Int J Prosthodont 2001;14:48–52. Cat. 6
12. Kapur KK. A clinical evaluation of denture adhesives. J Prosthet Dent 1967;18:550–558. Cat. 2
13. Tarbet WJ, Silverman G, Schmidt NF. Maximum incisal biting force in denture wearers as influenced by adequacy of denture-bearing tissues and the use of an adhesive. J Dent Res 1981;60:115–119. Cat. 2
14. Tarbet WJ, Boone M, Schmidt NF. Effect of a denture adhesive on complete denture dislodgement during mastication. J Prosthet Dent 1980;44:374–378. Cat. 2
15. Neill DJ, Roberts BJ. The effect of denture fixatives on masticatory performance in complete denture patients. J Dent 1972;1:219–222. Cat. 1

9

Unfavorable Anatomic Conditions

Anatomic limitations encountered in patients seeking prosthetic rehabilitation can sometimes be resolved with preprosthetic surgery or with the use of special technical devices.

Minor Preprosthetic Surgery

In the edentulous patient, preprosthetic surgery aims to improve the support structures for the complete denture. In patients who have been edentulous for a long time, the anatomic conditions of the residual alveolar ridges may be altered to such an extent that the stability of the denture during function cannot be guaranteed. In the past, resorting to preprosthetic surgery was a widespread practice, and major surgical intervention, such as vestibuloplasty, tuberplasty, and oral floor plastic surgery was often resorted to. The results of these procedures were often disappointing both for the surgeon and the patient.[1]

Today extensive preprosthetic surgery often involves increasing the volume of the alveolar ridges to allow for the placement of osseointegrated implants. Besides guaranteeing stability of the denture, implants are long lasting and counter osseous resorption by stimulating the bone for its maintenance. Implants thus fulfill the functional and esthetic requirements for patient satisfaction.

In this chapter minor preprosthetic surgery and technical expedients as an alternative to surgery will be considered.

Minor preprosthetic surgery includes:

- Frenotomy
- Removal of the torus
- Treatment of flabby ridges
- Increasing vestibular depth
- Deepening of the fornix with tissue grafts
- Reduction of a hypertrophic tuberosity

Frenotomy

The frena are folds of mucosal membrane that run from the fornix to the top of the edentulous ridge. Some frena can interfere mechanically with a prosthesis, dislocating it and compromising proper functioning of the denture. If it is necessary to remove a hypertrophic maxillary median frenum, Z-plasty is advised[2] (Figs 9-1 to 9-4). For hypertrophic lateral frena, surgery to increase the depth of the vestibule in combination with a tissue graft is advised.

Removal of tori

The tori are exostoses found primarily in the center of the hard palate in the maxilla and bilaterally in the mandible in correspondence with the lingual wall in the canine-premolar region. The removal of a torus palatinus is necessary when it acts as a fulcrum and negatively affects the posterior palatal seal or the stability of the denture. After creating a full mucoperiosteal flap, the procedure can be performed with bone scalpels or osteotomy burs, accompanied by abundant irrigation[2] (Figs 9-5 to 9-8). The mucosa on the torus mandibularis is generally thin and subject to chronic irritation because of the prosthetic flange (Figs 9-9 and 9-10). Therefore, surgical removal of mandibular tori is indispensable for complete denture wearers.

Treatment of flabby ridges

Fibrous hypertrophy of the crestal tissue, typically found in long-standing edentulous patients, is referred to as a flabby ridge. Hypertrophy is the consequence of repeated mechanical trauma associated with a chronic inflammatory process, which induces resorption of the bone. Fibrous tissue then takes the place of the resorbed bone. Flabby ridges are most frequently found in the anterior region of the edentulous ridge of the maxilla or in the knife-edge atrophic ridge of the mandible.

Surgical removal of flabby ridges does not always produce favorable results, especially in cases in which there is little

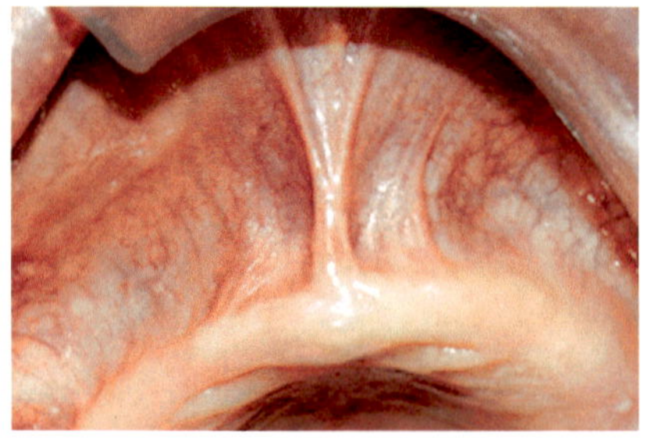

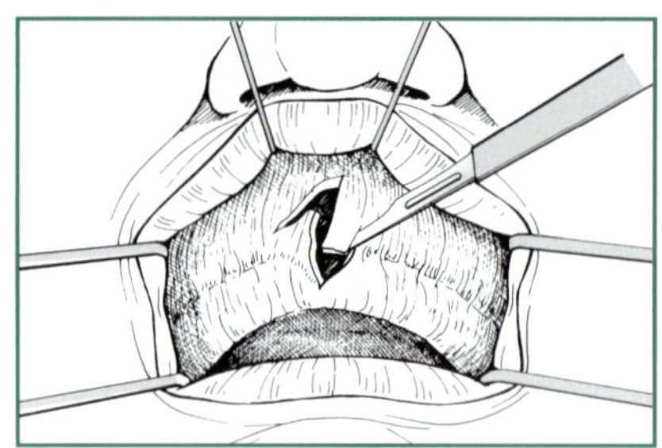

Fig 9-1 Maxillary hypertrophic frena.

Fig 9-2 Diagram of the Z-shaped incision.

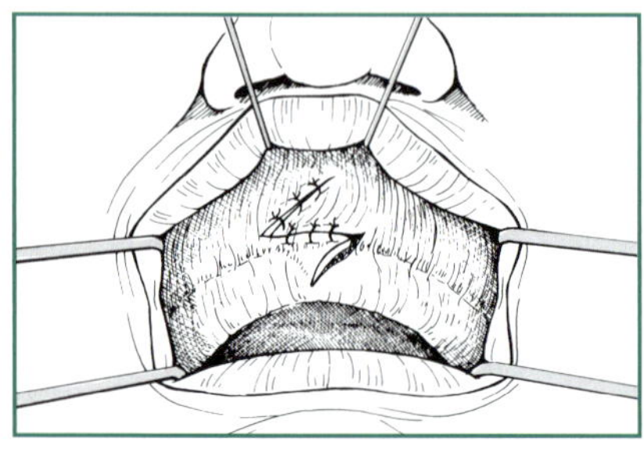

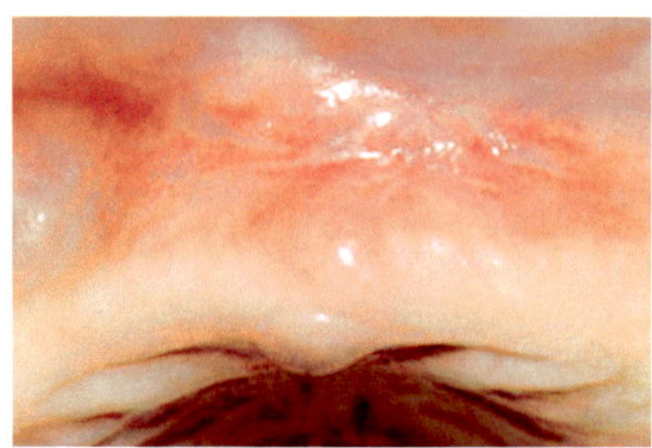

Fig 9-3 Suturing.

Fig 9-4 Result.

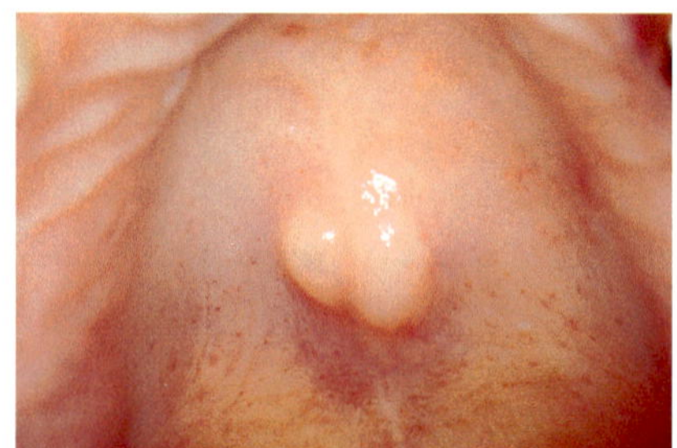

Fig 9-5 Palatal torus.

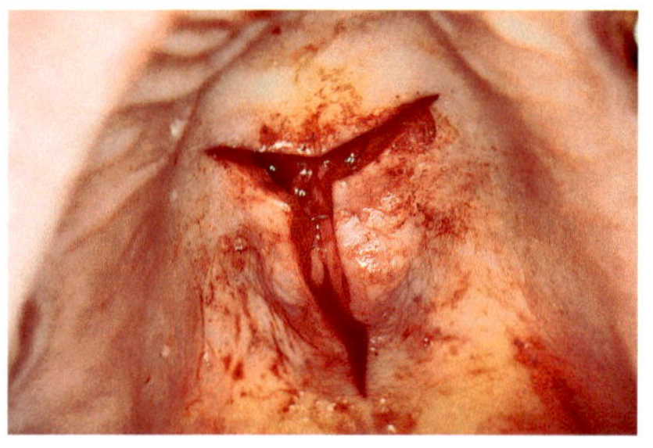

Fig 9-6 Incision to full depth.

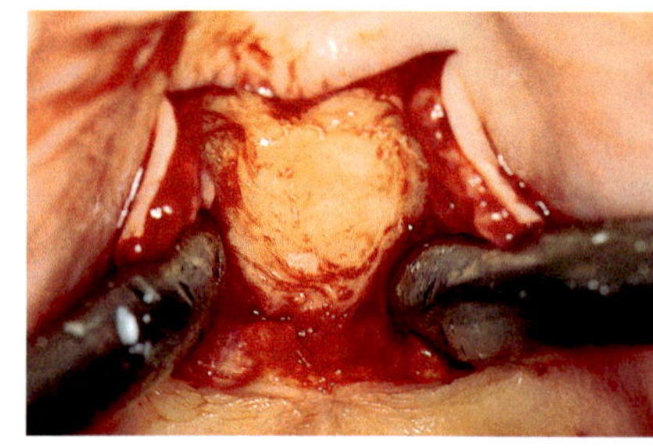

Fig 9-7 Exposure to show torus.

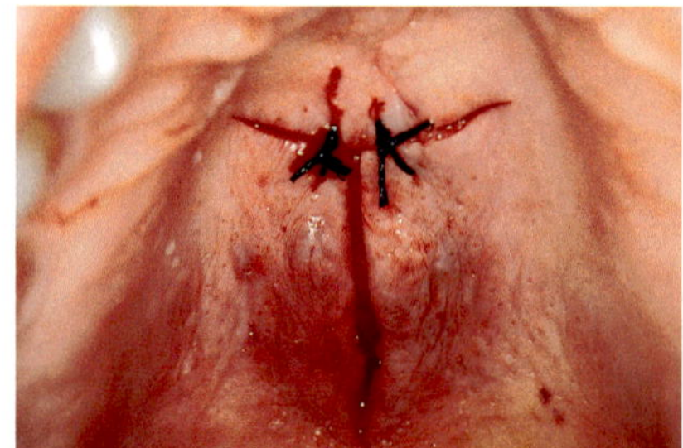

Fig 9-8 Suturing.

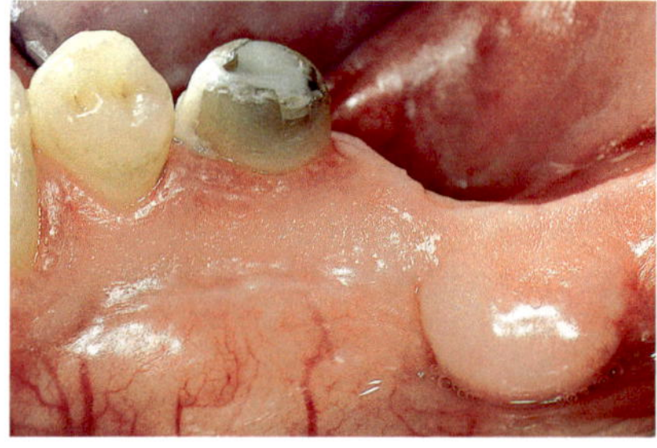

Fig 9-9 Mandibular tora.

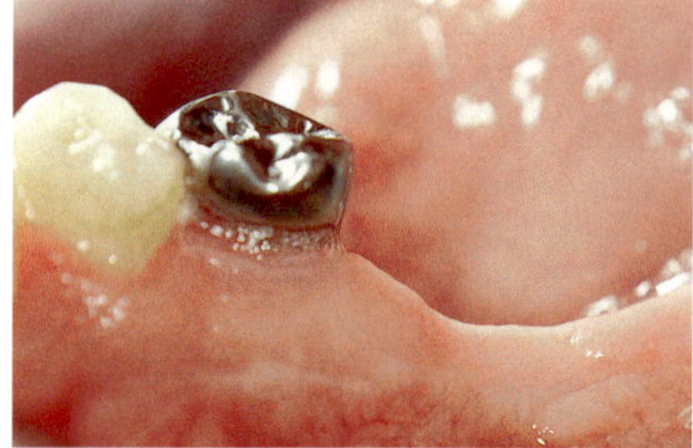

Fig 9-10 Result 15 days after surgery.

underlying alveolar bone. Laskin[3] reported that the surgical reduction of fluctuating ridges leads to a low and flat ridge or to a cutting ridge covered with thin mucosa and scar tissue, which do not support a complete denture.

When the fibrotic hypertrophy of the crestal mucosa impedes the renewal of a denture, surgical removal is necessary (Figs 9-11 to 9-23). Correcting flabby ridges can also be useful in cases where, after implant treatment, the thickness of the

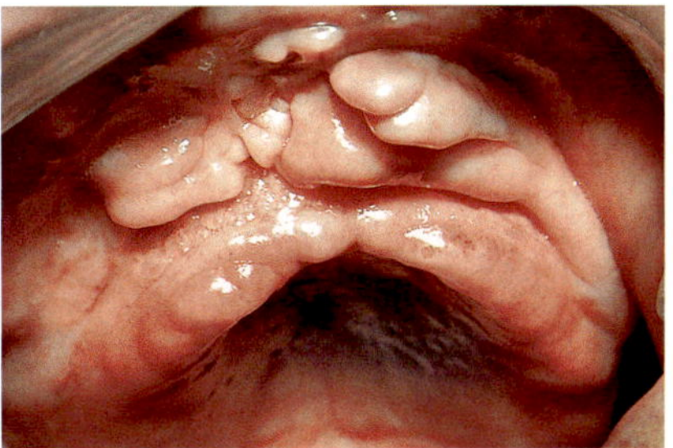

Fig 9-11 Maxillary fibroma.

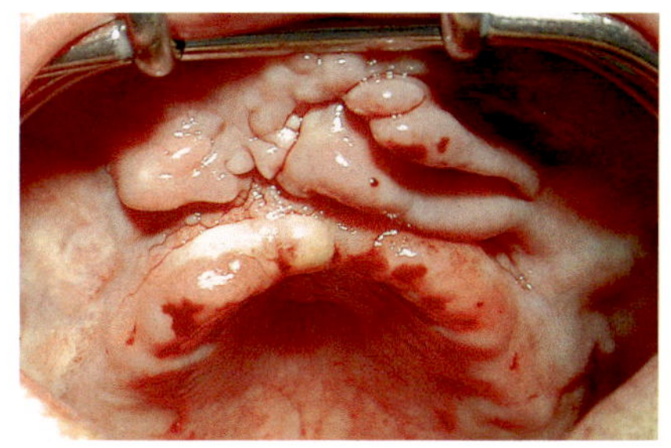

Fig 9-12 Maxillary fibroma divided into several sections.

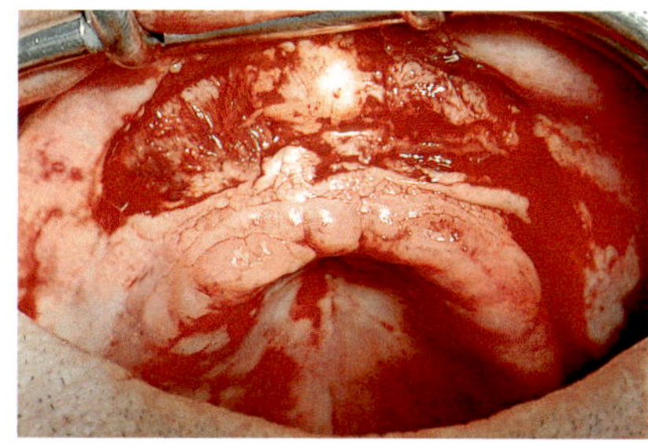

Fig 9-13 Surgical removal of half the thickness of the fibroma.

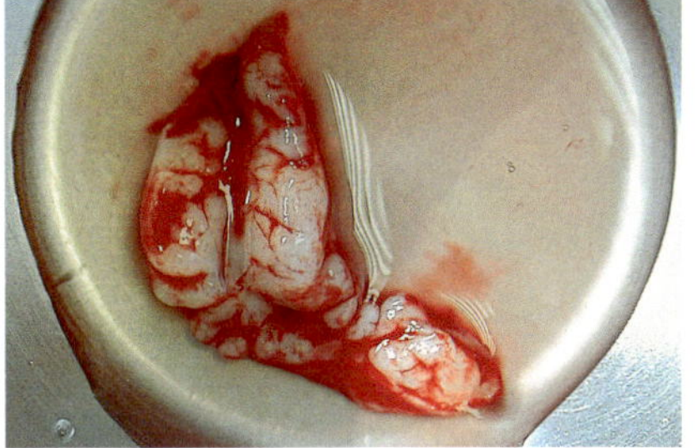

Fig 9-14 The removed fibroma.

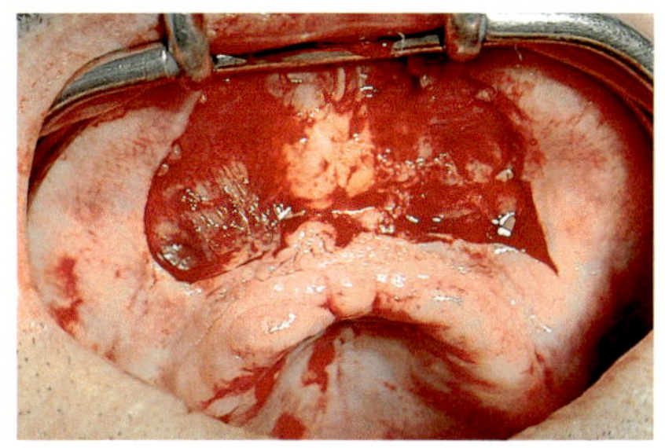

Fig 9-15 Only the periosteal tissue remains.

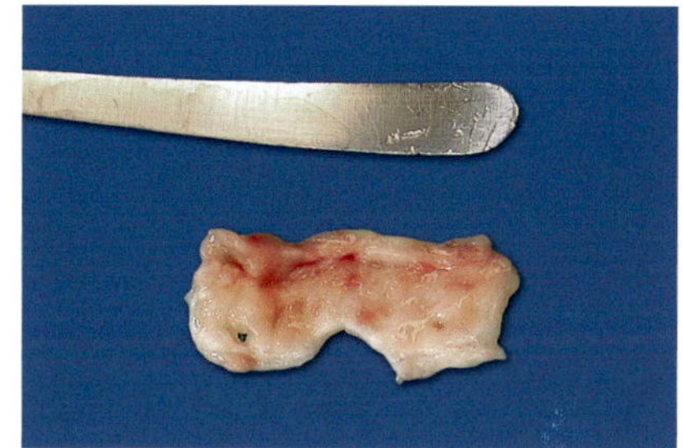

Fig 9-16 The fibroma is then sliced and modeled to be used as a mucosal graft.

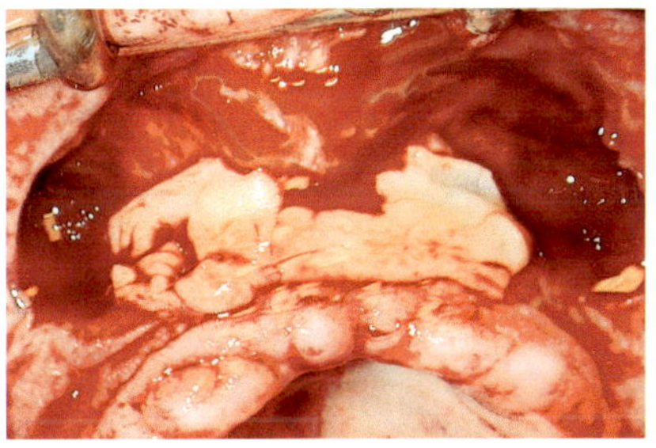

Fig 9-17 The graft placed in situ.

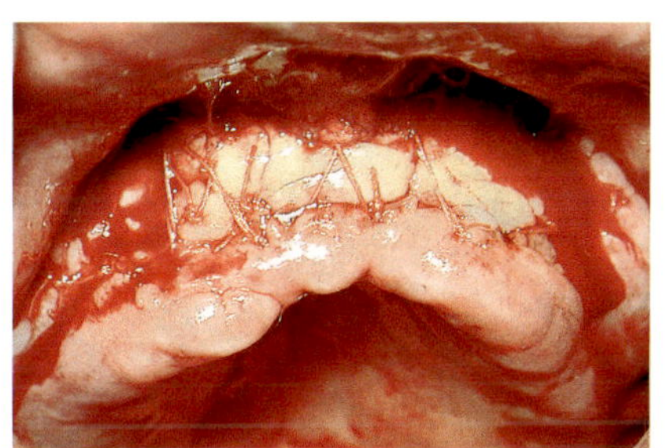

Fig 9-18 Suturing.

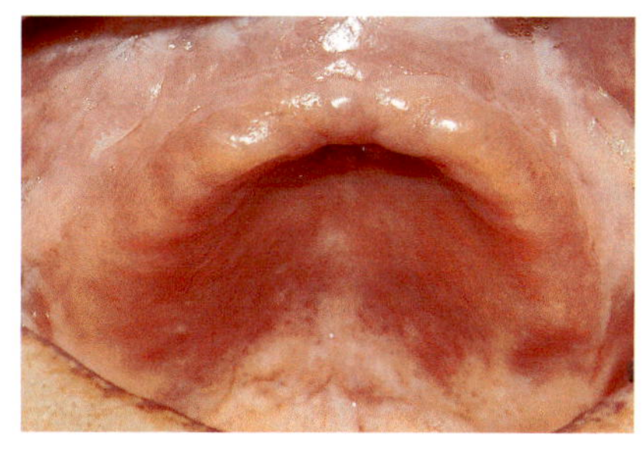

Fig 9-19 Healing after 15 days.

Fig 9-20 Incongruous denture. The body of the mandibular denture is not wide enough and causes pain.

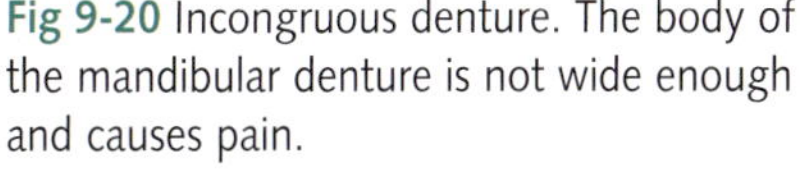

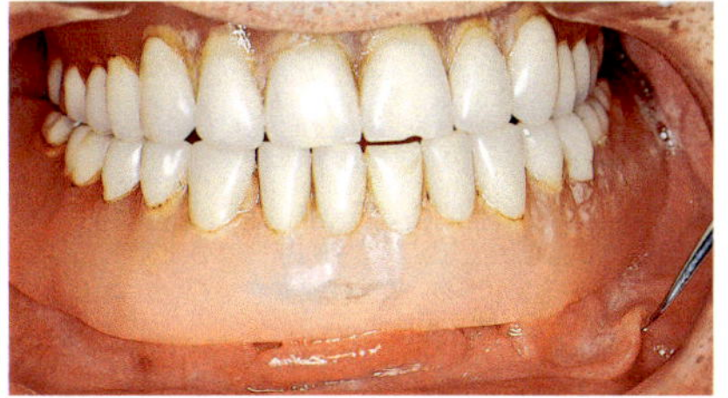

Fig 9-21 Fibroma of an incongruous prosthesis.

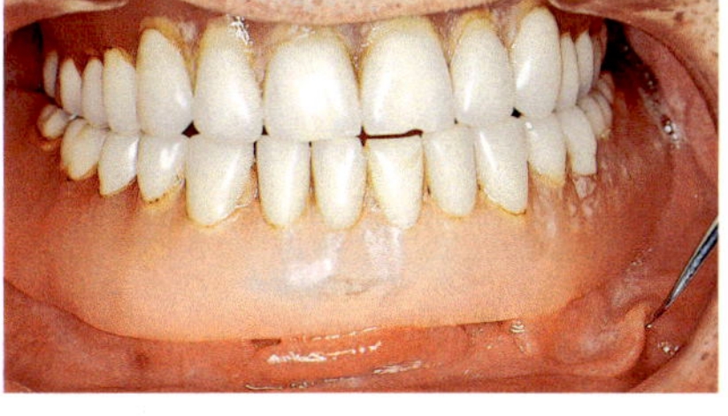

Fig 9-22 Detail of the fibroma.

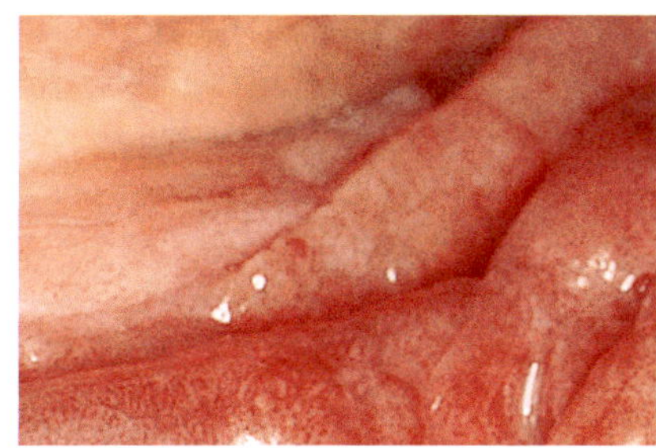

Fig 9-23 Healing of the mandibular fibroma.

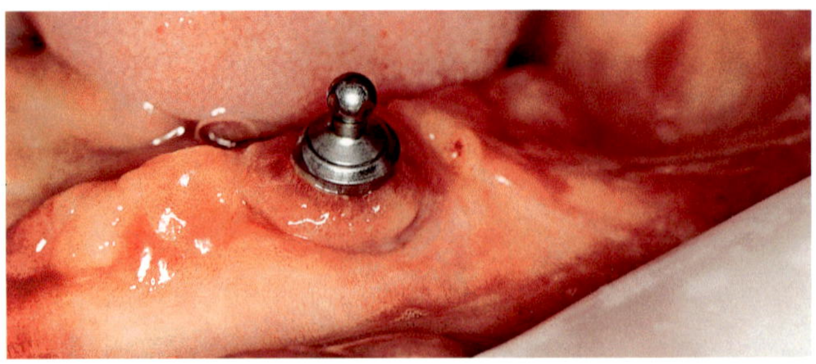

Fig 9-24 Peri-implantitis of the hypertrophic ntramucosal tunnel.

mucosa is such that a very long abutment is needed. An abutment that is too long presents a double disadvantage, however. From the biomechanical point of view it constitutes an unfavorable lever (arm). Furthermore, it encourages the development of anaerobic bacteria and spirochetes in the intramucosal tunnel, which can lead to peri-implantitis[4] (Fig 9-24).

Deepening the fornix

In cases in which there is a particularly reduced fornix with a frena very close to the ridge along with modest osseous atrophy, it is possible to deepen the fornix with a tissue graft, which can be taken from the palate or from the cheek.[5,6] The fornix assumes a more natural shape, and the grafted tissue has the same characteristics as the crestal mucosa. The only problem is the lack of available tissue that can be taken from the donor sites.

Tissue graft during implant placement

The objective of this procedure is to increase depth and create a band of keratinized tissue around the prosthetic abutment. In the immediate postoperative period, the stability of the graft is guaranteed by the prosthetic body, which is anchored to the implant and encourages success of the surgery. The success rate of implants does not depend on the presence or absence of the keratinized tissues around the implants; nevertheless, the presence of a well-shaped fornix and of (sufficient) peri-implant mucosa reduces the formation of pseudopockets and makes oral hygiene easier to maintain (Figs 9-25 to 9-33).

Reduction of a hypertrophic tuberosity

Bilateral hypertrophic tuberosities have a hard consistency, as they are mainly made up of dense fibrous connective tissue. When they are of significant dimensions and make positioning of the denture difficult, they must be surgically reduced (Figs 9-34 and 9-35).

Prosthetic Alternatives to Surgery

When the patient is not able to undergo surgery (for example, because of old age and/or systemic illnesses), it is necessary to use techniques in keeping with the construction principles.

Flabby ridge

When taking an impression, it is necessary to add a step to the conventional technique of molding borders with thermoplastic paste and relining with a mucostatic material to displace the flabby ridge. At the end of the normal procedure, the part of the tray that covers the flabby ridge is removed completely. The modified tray, repositioned in the mouth, must leave the entire flabby hypermobile area exposed. Keeping the tray in place, some fluid impression plaster is applied to the flabby ridge. Once the plaster is hardened, the tray is delicately removed to ensure that the impression obtained is of a mixed type.

Painful mylohyoid ridge

The removal or remodeling of a mylohyoid ridge that is painful on palpation (Figs 9-36 and 9-37) is a demanding procedure that can be avoided by placing implants. In the case of a fixed partial denture, there is no problem with interference. In the case of an implant-retained overdenture, interference can be avoided by reducing the prosthetic body. If it is not possible to use implants and the patient must be rehabilitated with a complete denture, the problem can be resolved in the following manner:

1. The prosthetic body is thickened over the mylohyoid ridge (Fig 9-38).
2. The thickening of the prosthetic body allows creation of a hollow that corresponds to the mylohyoid ridge (Figs 9-39 and 9-40).
3. The hollow is filled with a long-lasting soft resin material (Figs 9-41 to 9-44).
4. The procedure must be repeated at least once a year.

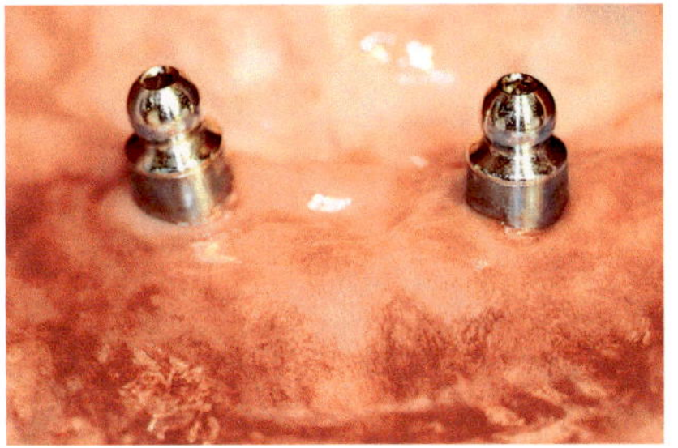

Fig 9-25 Absence of free mucosa around the edge of the two ball attachments.

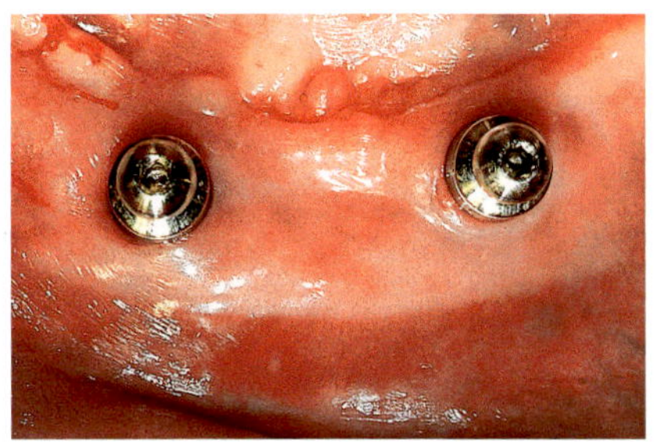

Fig 9-26 Occlusal view showing the mucosa around the circumferences of the patrices.

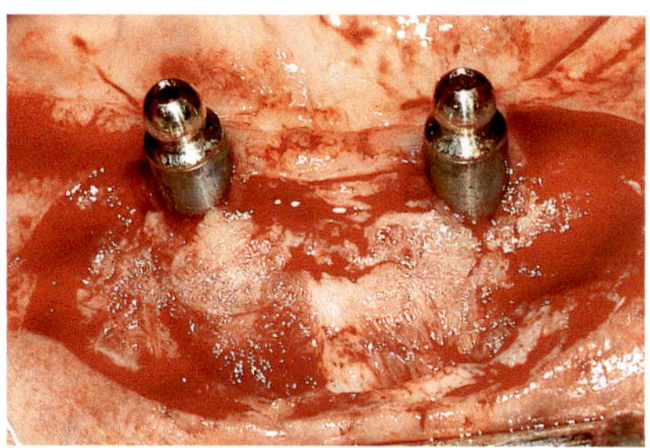

Fig 9-27 An incision of half the thickness to remove all of the alveolar mucosa around the ball attachment.

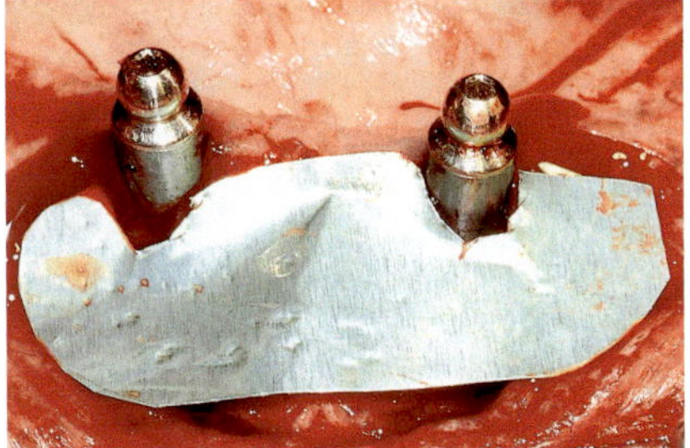

Fig 9-28 Site covered with tin foil pattern.

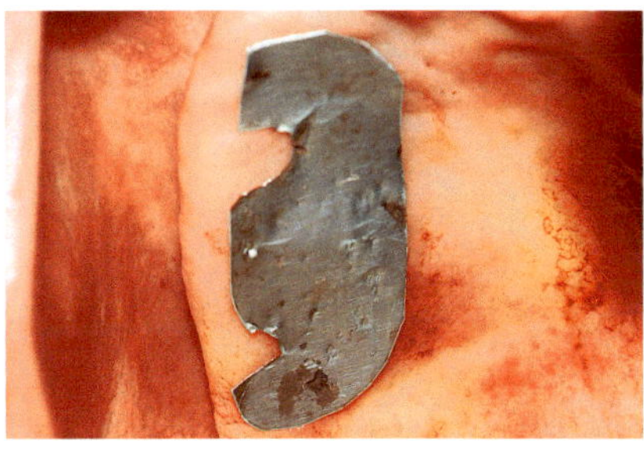

Fig 9-29 Tinfoil pattern is used to take a mucosal graft.

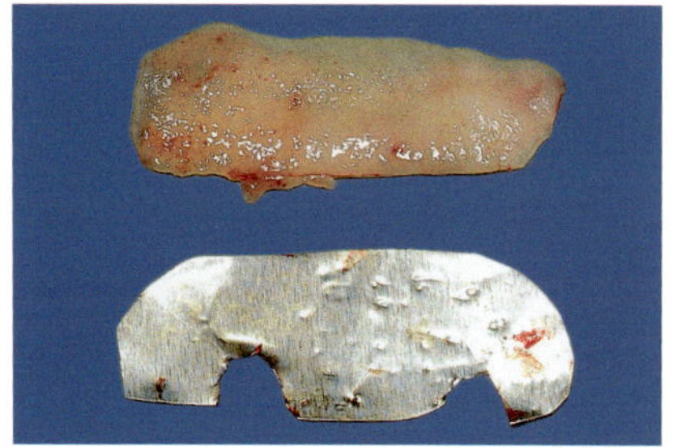

Fig 9-30 Remodeling the keratinized palatal graft.

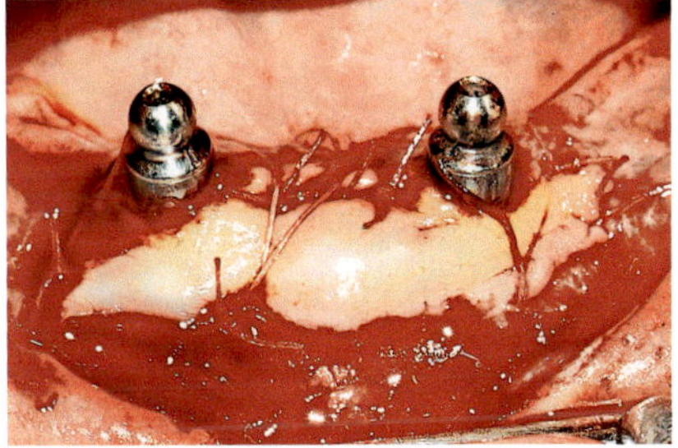

Fig 9-31 Sutured graft.

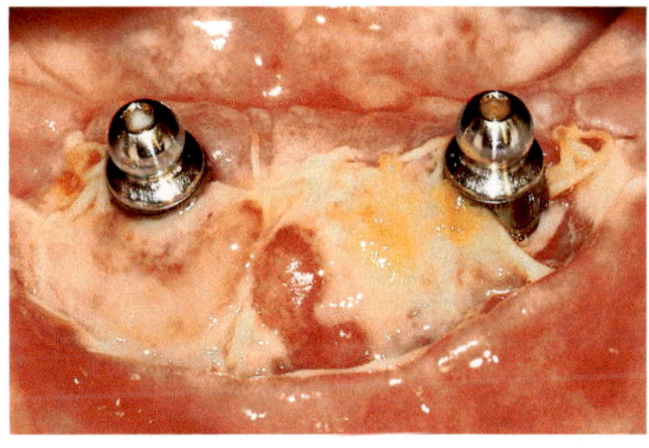

Fig 9-32 Healing after 7 days.

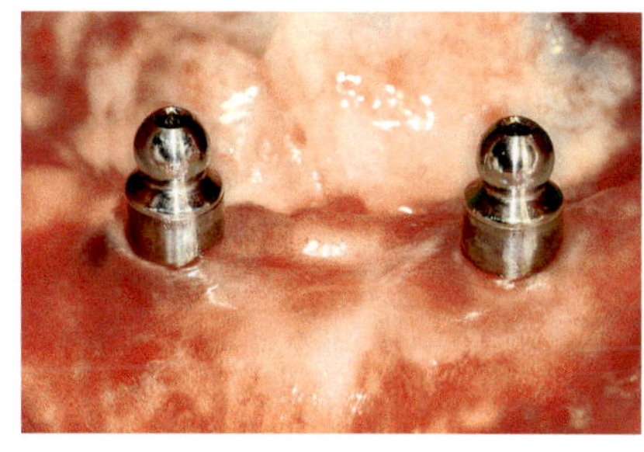

Fig 9-33 Healing after 15 days.

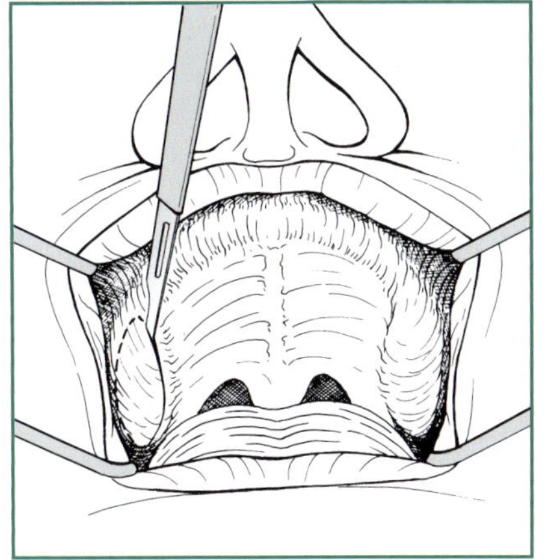

Fig 9-34 Diagram of incision.

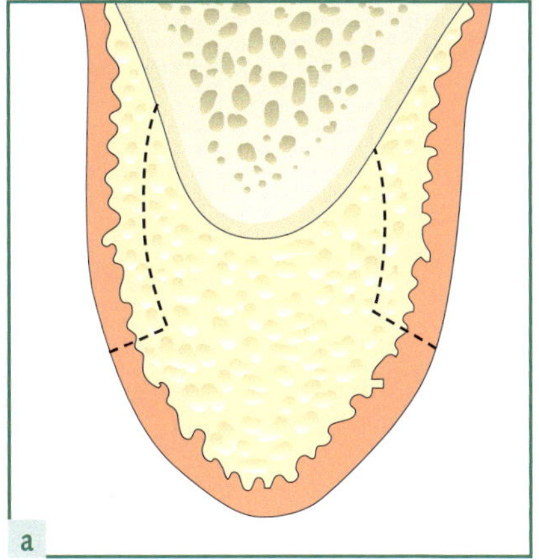
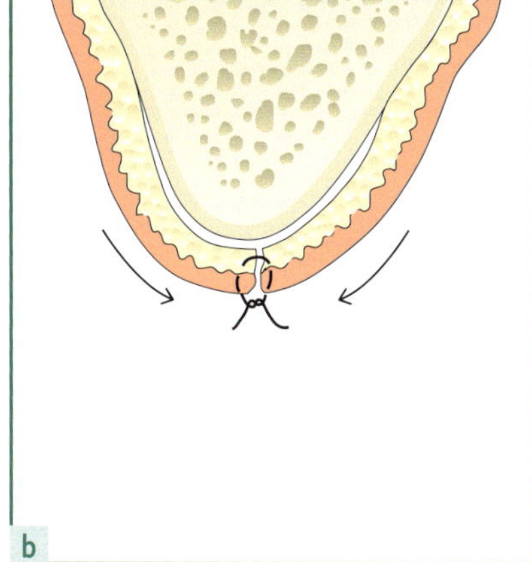

Fig 9-35 (a) Profile of the tuberosity. The excess fibromucosal tissue is removed. (b) Suture of the flap.

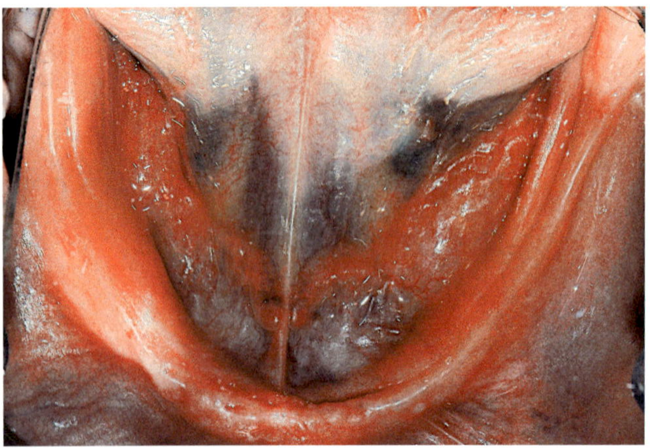

Fig 9-36 Mucosa showing an unfavorable mylohyoid ridge.

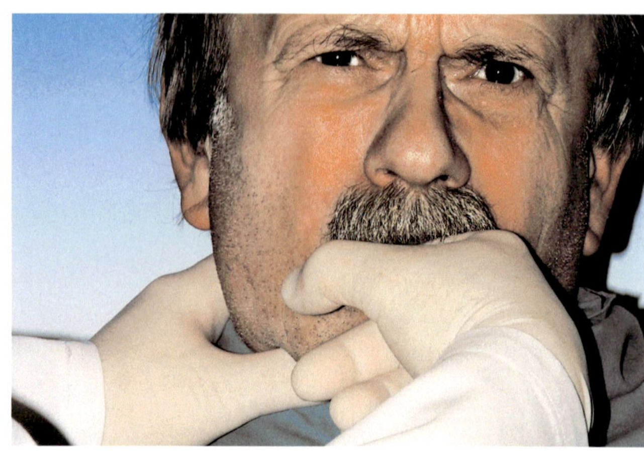

Fig 9-37 Palpation of the knife-edge mylohyoid ridge is painful.

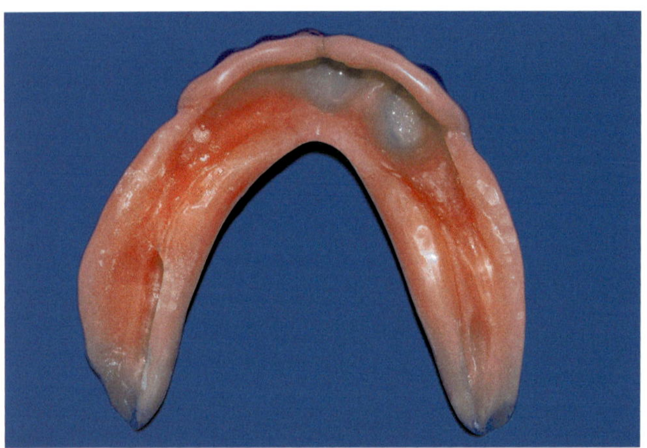

Fig 9-38 View of prosthetic flange in the area of the mylohyoid ridge.

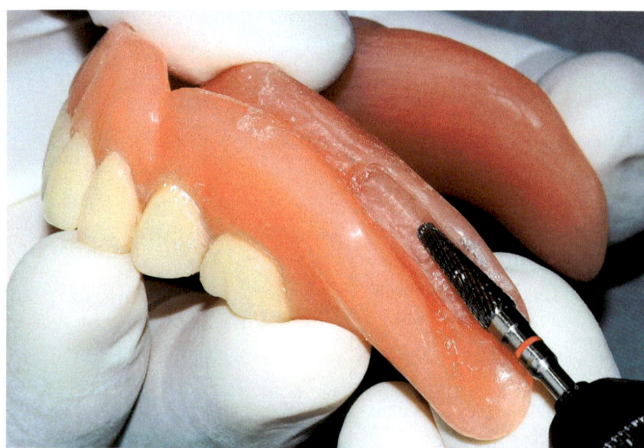

Fig 9-39 With a bur, a gutter is prepared in the body of the prosthesis.

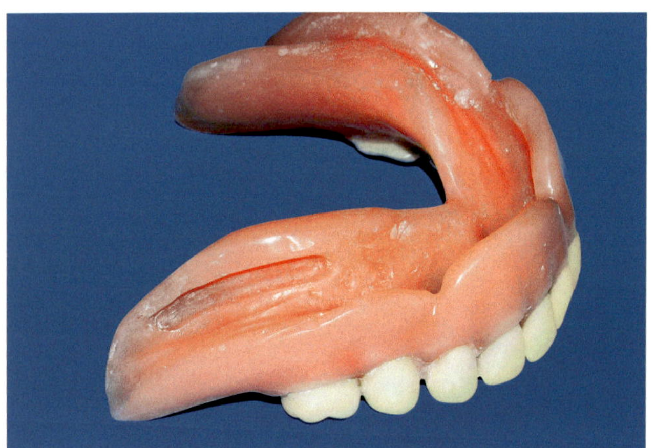

Fig 9-40 Placement of the gutter corresponds to the mylohyoid ridge.

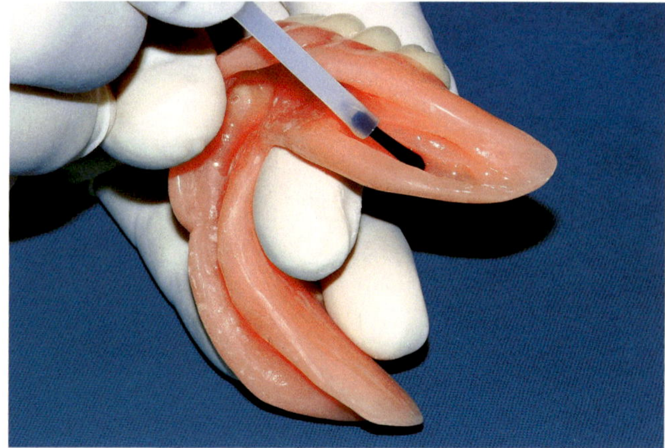

Fig 9-41 An adhesive liquid is applied to the gutter.

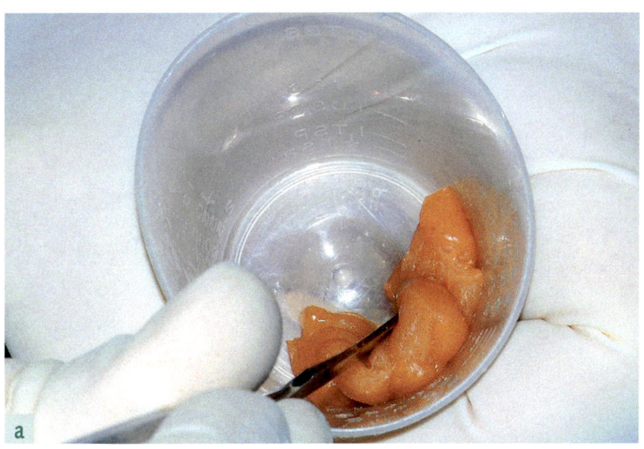
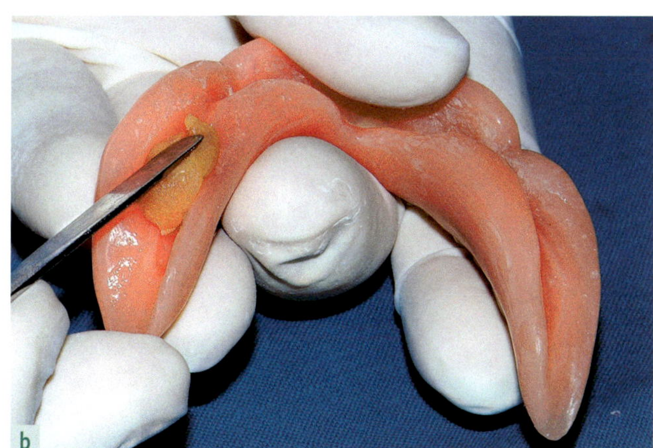

Fig 9-42 (*a and b*) Preparation and positioning the relining material.

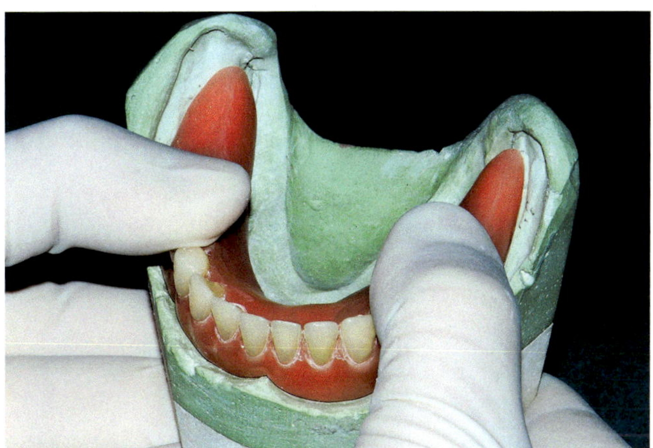
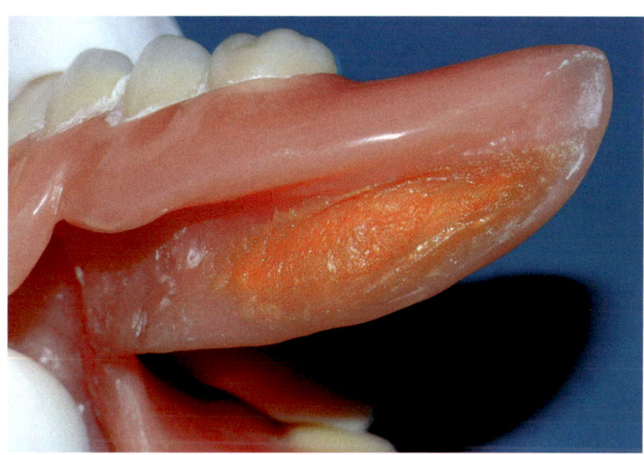

Fig 9-43 The prothesis is repositioned on the master cast. The soft resin material is then polymerized.

Fig 9-44 Prosthetic flange following polymerization.

References

1. Palla S. Problems of prosthetic treatment following preprosthetic measures in the maxilla. SSO Schweiz Monatsschr Zahnheilkd 1976;86:41–63. Cat. 7
2. Archer WH. Chirurgia Orale. Padova: Piccin, 1983. Cat. 7
3. Laskin DM. A sclerosing procedure for hypermobile edentulous ridges. J Prosthet Dent 1970;23:274–278. Cat. 8
4. Papaioannou W, Quirynen M, Nys M, van Steenberghe D. The effect of periodontal parameters on the subgingival microbiota around implants. Clin Oral Implants Res 1995;6:197–204. Cat. 4
5. de Koomen HA, Tideman H, Stoelinga PJW, Hubers AJ, Hendriks FHJ. Indikation, Technik und Ergebnisse der Unterkiefervestibulumplastik und Mundbodensenkung. Dtsch Zahnarztl Z 1982;37:509–512. Cat. 4
6. Hillerup S. Preprosthetic mandibular vestibuloplasty with buccal mucosal graft. A 2-year follow-up study. Int J Oral Surg 1982;11:81–88. Cat. 3

10

Burning Mouth Syndrome

Burning mouth syndrome (BMS)[1,2] is a clinical condition well known to dentists and specialists in oral medicine. It is characterized by a spontaneous burning sensation of the oral mucosa of the mouth, especially the tongue and palate and also the lips, which appear to be normal when examined. BMS is a relatively common phenomenon and affects mainly women during and after menopause. Many synonyms can be found in the literature, including stomatodynia, stomatopyrosis, glossodynia, glossopyrosis, oral dysesthesia, and "sore mouth of prosthetic origin" in removable denture wearers. These synonyms are frequently used in the literature and in clinical jargon to indicate illnesses of the mucosa other than BMS, such as geographic tongue, lichen planus, and oral candidiasis. Oral burning associated with a mucosal disease is not BMS, however. BMS is diagnosed when the clinical status is represented only by the symptom of oral burning or pain or one of the terms listed later on in the chapter, in the absence of evident signs of mucosal disease.

Epidemiology

There are few epidemiologic data concerning BMS in the general population and in different parts of the world. Most of the information reported in the literature comes from selected groups: dental patients, women in menopause, and diabetic patients.[3,4] All authors agree that BMS is much more common in women, with a ratio of 3:1 to 7:1.[5–8] In some cases, such as in patients with burning lips, the ratio is even more evident. (12:1).[9] Age groups older than 50 years are particularly vulnerable. The average age is about 62 years with a range of 36 through 84 years. BMS is rarely found in patients younger than 30 years, and it has never been found in children.[10] It has been estimated that the prevalence in the general population varies between 2.5% to 5.1%,[11] whereas it increases to 10% and 20% in patients in menopausal care centers.[12] The incidence varies in European and North American studies, from 5 to 10 cases per 100,000 per year.[3] Little or nothing is known about possible racial or geographic differences.

Symptoms

Patients describe a variety of symptoms that can be summarized in the following order of frequency: burning, scalding, tingling, stinging, prickling, and itching.[3,13] Sometimes they complain of "terrible pains," "unendurable torment," "enormous swelling,"[8] and "intolerable pain," although rarely does the illness cause physical disability.[14]

The symptoms are typically located in the following areas[15,16]: the anterior two-thirds of the mobile tongue is the most common site, and when this organ is involved, burning occurs at the tip, on the sides, and on the dorsum. The next most affected area is the hard palate, then the lips, the edentulous alveolar ridges (particularly in denture wearers), the gums, and the genial mucosa. The oral floor and the oropharynx are involved less frequently.[5,17] It is possible that only one of the above-mentioned sites is affected. The tongue is the most commonly affected area, but it is normal that patients report symptoms in different areas. It is possible that the symptoms are spread around the entire oral cavity. The symptoms are nearly always bilateral and, unlike neurologic illnesses, they do not have an anatomic-topographic distribution.

Oral burning can be associated with other symptoms, the most frequent being reduced salivary flow[18,19] (40% to 50% of cases) and saliva that is "viscous" or "glue like."[8] Other symptoms include taste disturbance (acidic, metallic, or bitter taste in about 30% of cases), reduction of olfaction, and dysphagia (although this symptom is rare).

The relationship between symptoms and daily activities is not clearly defined, although the study by Grushka[18] is important. It has been pointed out that psychologic tension, fatigue, talking, and chewing food worsen BMS in less that half of patients, whereas chewing food, eating cold foods, working, and various distractions improve BMS in the other half of the patients interviewed.

Patients with BMS have other symptoms and illnesses as well, such as headache, migraine, cervical pain and back pain, dermatitis or generalized cutaneous itching, spastic colitis or irritable bowel syndrome (IBS), alterations in the menstrual cycle with dysfunctional (uterine) bleeding, and sleep disturbances.[20] In most patients the symptoms are constant and persist for many years with diminishing intensity[3]; partial or total remission of symptoms after 6 to 7 years is reported in the literature.[20,21] It has been shown that, over time, the chronic nature of orofacial pain can bring about profound changes in patients. The depressive component is progressively associated with hypochondriac characteristics, and the patient gradually assumes unhealthy behavior in which lack of trust and incapacity to respond become predominant. Social relationships also become more sporadic.

Histologic Characteristics

There exists no histologic evidence of BMS. Thus, histologic examination should not be included in the routine study of these patients. Sometimes biopsies are necessary to exclude concomitant pathologies,[3,21] to be used for other examinations, and to be studied for research purposes.[22] This solid conviction has probably influenced the lack of study on the subject. It should be noted that there is only one study specifically dedicated to this topic.[23]

No author therefore proposes a biopsy as one of the examinations in the diagnostic protocol of this pathologic state.

Classification

Lamey and Lamb[9] have proposed that BMS should be classified into three subtypes (Table 10-1). These same authors have confirmed the validity of this classification, both from the epidemiologic point of view, noting that the distribution of the patients in the three subtypes is coincident in two different populations (English and North American),[24] and from the clinical and prognostic point of view, underlining the potential for improvement in treatment and in the approach to patients using a rational diagnostic and therapeutic protocol.[10]

Possible Causes

The cause or causes of BMS are unknown even today. A long series of possible triggering factors has been hypothesized, however. Some of these hypotheses are more convincing, since they are supported by significant research; others are less probable, because the experimental evidence is weak or has not been investigated sufficiently. No hypothesis properly answers all queries, and none can be considered valid in any or almost any of the cases. It is probable that BMS is a multifactorial illness, that there are one or more triggering factors, and that as the illness progresses, it involves or provokes other factors.

Oral candidiasis

Most investigators do not believe that candidiasis can cause a burning sensation in the oral cavity in the absence of clinical evidence. However, subclinical candidiasis has been indicated as a possible cause of BMS.[21,25]

This hypothesis has found possible confirmation in a study using the rinsing technique, in which BMS patients without apparent oral lesions showed a significant increase in some species of *Candida* and coliforms compared with healthy control subjects.[26] Given that previous studies did not obtain these results, the authors affirm that the sampling and culture techniques were very important. Successively, it has been affirmed that some species of *Candida* have been hosted in pathogenic quantities in these patients while the mucosa has maintained a healthy appearance.[15]

One way of investigating the role of *Candida* is through antimycotic therapy. In a study of BMS patients who showed *Candida*-positive results of the rinsing test, only 5% of patients benefited from antimycotic therapy, with evident elimination of the fungus.[16] The studies did not show a primary role of *Candida* in the pathogenesis of BMS, and it is possible that the presence of *Candida* species in patients with BMS could have been correlated with other factors implicated in this syndrome, such as reduced salivary flow, anemia, and the presence of a removable denture.

Table 10-1 BMS subtypes

Subtype	Patients (%)	Symptoms
1	35	Burning is present every day but not on waking up; onset is during the day, worsening until it reaches its peak in the evening
2	55	Burning is present every day on waking and maintains the same intensity until evening
3	10	Burning is not present every day and occurs in unusual places, such as the genial mucosa, the oral floor, and the throat

Removable dentures

Inadequate removable dentures can increase the level of functional stress of the whole stomatognatic system and therefore can cause BMS. It is necessary to specify that not all oral burning sensations in denture wearers can be ascribed to BMS. The principal differential diagnoses are prosthetic stomatitis and pain of prosthetic origin. Prosthetic stomatitis is a type of candidiasis characterized by erythema below the prosthetic base. This pathology can sometimes cause symptoms (burning, itching) but without the intensity and everyday occurrence of BMS. Furthermore, it can be resolved with adequate antimycotic therapy.[27,28] It is hence a pathologic state clearly distinguishable from BMS.

Much more uncertain is the differential diagnosis of pain of prosthetic origin, which some authors believe to coincide with prosthetic stomatitis, while others describe it as a distinct entity.[3,16] It is precisely this clinical entity that could be a confusing factor in these studies.

Some authors have attributed the problems of incongruous dentures to the cause of BMS in 50% of their patients with oral burning.[29] In these cases the most common cause was occlusion errors. In a study on 33 patients with BMS, an error that could be connected with the referred symptoms was pointed out in 50% of cases.[30] In subsequent controlled studies,[31–34] the role of removable dentures did not appear relevant. No significant difference was noted between BMS subjects and the control group, who all wore removable dentures. The authors therefore concluded that there is no direct correlation between the use of a denture and the symptom.

To the contrary, however, in a much wider study on 150 patients, of whom 120 were totally edentulous and 60% of these had incongruent dentures, the reconstruction of the dentures themselves improved the symptoms in 25% of cases.[16] This fact would imply that the role of the denture in the onset of BMS is very important. The same authors point out, however, that only a quarter of patients responded to the substitution of the dentures and that even in these cases, the denture can be just one of the possible causes in a multifactorial pathogenesis.

It has been observed that parafunction accompanies an excessive occlusal load, which was once attributed to the burning sensation because of the compression on the mucosa, but this fact has not been confirmed in recent literature. Patients with bruxism, however, push and rub the tongue between the teeth, which could provoke the onset of BMS. Also, patients who are anxious may unconsciously engage in this behavior.

A recent controlled study showed a significant increase in the frequency of pain on palpation of the masticatory muscles in patients with BMS who wore removable dentures. The examination of the prosthesis also showed significant differences: In the BMS group, errors of occlusion, reduced space for the tongue, and increase in vertical dimension were more frequent. Furthermore, these patients wore the denture for less time during the day.[35] These findings seem to support the hypothesis that dentures are correlated with other factors in the genesis of BMS.

Thus, dentures by themselves are not the cause of BMS, and BMS does not occur only in denture wearers. The current opinion is that, in patients with BMS, there is a complex interaction among general health factors, psychogenic factors, and inadequate dentures. If necessary, the denture must be reconstructed, paying particular attention to the vertical dimension, the space for the tongue to move, and the prosthetic base, which must be adequate and must ensure the best possible distribution of the masticatory loads. This intervention may not resolve BMS by itself; reconstruction must be combined with the support of other specialists.

Allergies

It is generally accepted that contact stomatitis is a rare event.[36] This condition is attributed to the rapid absorption and dispersion of the allergen throughout the mucosa and its subsequent removal and dilution through saliva. A survey of patients with oral burning found that dental materials such as metals or foods or preservatives can provoke an allergic reaction in these patients. Nevertheless, in many of these patients, there is evidence of stomatitis (erythematous and/or hyperplastic), and this finding excludes the diagnosis of BMS.[31]

Some authors have reported cases of oral burning in patients with healthy mucosa who had positive patch tests for sorbic acid (a preservative in food, ointment, and cream)[37] and cinnamic aldehyde (an aromatic agent in food and toothpastes).[34]

Allergic reactions to acrylic resins are somewhat rare[38] but not impossible. Rare cases of allergies to polymethylmethacrylate have been reported in patients with BMS and have responded positively to prosthetic reconstruction with alternative materials, such as nylon.[39]

Other authors have reported allergic reactions to dental materials, such as acrylics, mercury, and metals in patients with oral burning. However, in all of these cases, alterations to the mucosa were also present, such as erythema, edema, and in some, lichen planus. The removal of the allergen often brought about remission of the symptoms and the lesions, but in some patients only the lesions were resolved, leaving the oral burning unaltered.[40] Another study found positive patch tests for numerous metals currently used in dentistry, such as gold, palladium, zinc, molybdenum, gallium, indium, cobalt, chromium, nickel, iron, and selenium. These findings were significantly superior in patients with BMS compared with healthy patients, especially for palladium and nickel.[41]

117

A case of allergy to cadmium in a denture was reported, in which the burning sensation resolved 3 days after the denture was removed.[42] On the other hand, a recent controlled study did not find significant differences between patients with BMS and healthy volunteers in a comparison of the results of a series of epicutaneous patch tests for standard allergens and dental materials.[43] Although allergy to dental materials and to chemical compounds in foods or dentifrice is expressed by oral burning, the associated lesions exclude BMS as a diagnosis.

The allergic pathogenesis of BMS is strongly doubted. There are only a few controlled studies and surveys, with information gathered from too few subjects and mainly based on anecdotal evidence. It is not always clear whether a relationship exists between the elimination of the incriminating allergen and the resolution of the symptoms; further studies are necessary.

Saliva variations

Given that a relevant percentage of those affected by BMS also complain of xerostomia, it has been hypothesized that a reduced flow of saliva can be the cause or a contributing cause of the condition. Nevertheless, in these patients, a true reduction of the saliva flow is noticeable only in a modest percentage. A survey of BMS patients found that only 12% had a true reduction in parotid saliva flow after stimulation compared with 40%, who reported a subjective sensation of xerostomia.[16] Furthermore, there is no evidence of histologic alterations of the minor salivary glands in patients with BMS.

Because most patients with BMS are women in menopause or postmenopause, the reduced saliva flow has been attributed to hormonal changes. One study reported a reduction in parotid saliva flow during postmenopause, but a successive experiment did not show any difference in the saliva flow between postmenopausal women with BMS and a control group without BMS.[44]

It is necessary to observe that xerostomia and saliva flow are symptoms and signs caused by illnesses and multifactorial diseases, and it is possible that some of these factors, for example, the psychologic state of the patient, are also present in BMS patients. Also, xerostomia is a common adverse effect of various classes of drugs, such as tricyclic antidepressants, benzodiazepines, and antihistamines, all of which are commonly used by this category of patients.[45]

Other authors have proposed that it is the qualitative variations in the saliva that are responsible for oral burning, and they have documented an increase in the levels of proteins, phosphates, and potassium in menopausal patients with BMS.[46] This correlation between biochemical composition of saliva and BMS was not confirmed in a successive controlled study in which significant differences were found in the salival protein content of patients.[47] In an even more recent study, a new protein was identified in the parotid saliva of patients with BMS,[48] but the interpretation of the information and the role of the protein in the genesis of oral burning is not known.

Reduction in saliva flow or modifications in the biochemical composition of saliva cannot be considered a cause of BMS, even if they play a contributing role in some cases.

Hormonal state of menopause

The epidemiologic and clinical aspects of BMS indicate a possible correlation with the hormonal modifications of menopause. It has been observed, for example, that patients with BMS show a significant increase in menopausal symptoms with respect to control patients.[49]

An Australian study carried out on 149 women, both in menopause and not, showed that oral burning was significantly different between women in menopause (43%) and those who were not (6%).[12] Twenty-six percent of 114 English patients who attended a menopause treatment center had oral symptoms, such as burning and taste alteration.[29] In another study, a questionnaire administered to a group of 145 oophorectomized patients found that 17.9% of them experienced burning of the tongue and lips.[50] An important demonstration of the role that hormonal levels play in the genesis of oral burning would be the results obtained following hormone replacement therapy. Three studies reported conflicting results, with two finding an improvement[12,29] and the other[50] showing no improvement after therapy.

The fact that women in menopause have an increased risk for oral burning is indisputable, but whether this condition is due to estrogenic reduction is doubtful. The literature has yet to show whether hormone replacement therapy has an effect on the symptom of oral burning. Some authors think that such a symptom is more easily explainable as it relates to the neurotic and depressive features of menopause.

Poor nutrition

It has been documented that nutritional deficiency, such as iron deficiency anemia, megaloblastic anemia, and iron and folic acid deficiency can cause oral burning. However, the clinically evident mucosal lesions usually associated with these conditions (glossitis is typical) would exclude BMS as a diagnosis. Some hypothesize, however, that poor nutritional states can generate burning in the absence of clinical manifestations.[10]

Many years ago, a relationship between B vitamins and estrogen was hypothesized. One study documented that B complex therapy brought about the remission of oral symptoms in one-third of 86 patients with BMS in menopause.[10]

More recently, a study of 21 patients with BMS found that 6 patients (30%) were deficient in folic acid, and 1 patient (0.5%) was deficient in vitamin B_{12}.[29] In another study, 53% of 55 patients were sideropenic and 4% were lacking in folic acid. In this study, the substitutive therapy resolved the oral burning in about half of the deficient patients.[30]

A study of 70 English patients with BMS[51] reported that 28 patients were deficient in one or more B vitamins (B_1, B_2, and B_6). Supplemental vitamin therapy was administered to these patients and to 27 of the nondeficient control patients. In 3 months, BMS had resolved in 80% of the deficient patients and 7% of the controls. These findings were not confirmed in a subsequent study carried out with similar criteria.[52]

Deficient nutritional states merit careful consideration and must be evaluated; nevertheless, the published information is conflicting, and the data have not been confirmed. No single deficiency has been clearly correlated with oral burning; furthermore, studies have documented different and sometimes multiple deficiencies, but these deficiencies have not been found in a notable portion of subjects in a given study. The supplemental therapy administered in these studies seems to resolve the burning only in a portion of the patients, thus showing the importance but not the exclusivity of the cause. Furthermore, it is not clear whether these cases were true BMS or deficiency diseases without a subclinical manifestation.

Diabetes and severe hyperglycemia

For many years, it has been recognized that diabetes can be correlated to symptoms of oral burning. In one study, is was revealed that 39% of respondents to a BMS survey had abnormal oral glucose tolerance test (OGTT) results.[53] A survey of diabetic patients revealed symptoms similar to those of BMS in 10% of respondents, and another survey of diabetic patients reported that burning was the second most common oral symptom after xerostomia.[29]

Studies have found that patients with oral burning had positive OGTT results. One of 20[30] and 4 of 150[16] BMS patients were thus diagnosed as non–insulin-dependent diabetics. Other clinical studies[15,31] documented hyperglycemia in more than 3% of patients with BMS. In 43 cases of recently diagnosed non–insulin-dependent diabetics, 16 patients with BMS experienced a relief of their BMS at the onset of therapy.[54]

In conclusion, fasting glucose level and OGTT must always be used in patients with oral burning, because it is reasonable to think that a small percentage of these patients (1% to 5%) have oral symptoms associated with non–insulin-dependent diabetes and not BMS.

Polyneuropathy

Recently a group of Italian researchers proposed that peripheral polyneuropathy could be a cause of BMS.[22] The authors studied variations in touch, temperature, and taste sensitivity of the surface of the tongue and found anomalies of perception and lowering of the pain threshold associated with the loss of taste and a reduction in sensitivity to thermal stimuli. They also observed that the lower extremities of these patients were affected as well. If BMS were a clinical expression of a polyneuropathy, it is not, however, clear why it only affects the oral cavity. Further studies are necessary.

Psychogenic factors

In accordance with the current criteria of the *Diagnostic and Statistical Manual of Mental Disorders, Fourth Edition (DSM-IV)*,[33] BMS should be included among the somatoform disorders together with other painful and nonpainful disorders. In particular, it has been suggested that the onset of BMS is correlated with chronically stressful events or with negative triggering events,[55,56] but recent controlled studies have not confirmed this hypothesis.[57,58]

A good deal of literature, including case reports, psychoanalytic analysis, questionnaires, and controlled studies,[59] documents the relationship between BMS and associated psychiatric illnesses. There is a high prevalence of psychiatric illnesses and mental disorders in these patients. An investigation of this literature confirmed that at least 50% of BMS cases are associated with common psychiatric disturbances,[5,32,60,61] such as depression,[32,59,61–64] chronic anxiety,[16,65] hypochondria, and cancerphobia.[16,30,32,66] A recent controlled Italian study[58] showed psychiatric disturbance in 61 of 102 patients with BMS (71.6%, a significantly higher percentage than the control group). The authors used the diagnostic criteria of the *DSM-IV* to assess the subjects.

Psychogenic factors seem to be correlated with BMS, but the results of numerous studies do not agree on a possible association between adverse life events and the onset of BMS. It has been better documented that in more than 50% of patients with BMS, there are one or more associated psychiatric pathologies. It is therefore difficult to determine whether the association of these factors is proof of the psychiatric pathogenesis of BMS or whether, to the contrary, the syndrome itself can determine the onset of a psychiatric pathology by way of the chronic pain. Psychiatric pathology was proved to be preexistent in only some cases.

Therapy

Given that the causes of BMS remain fundamentally unknown, therapy should be established on a case-by-case basis. Inadequate dentures should be corrected and inappropriate materials substituted. Deficiency states (such as vitamins, iron, folate, estrogens, saliva substitutes) should be treated with replacement therapy. Apart form these remedies, the following suggested therapies are to be considered empiric and often are not supported by evidence-based studies.

Antidepressants

Although they are frequently prescribed for BMS patients, few controlled studies confirm the validity of antidepressants. Two studies are worth noting, however. A comparison between dothiepin and placebo[65] found a significant reduction in burning in patients receiving the experimental drug compared with control patients. In a study of trazodone versus placebo the effect of the drug was not significant.[67]

Clonazepam

In a study without control subjects, low doses of clonazepam were shown to be useful in reducing symptoms in 70% of patients with BMS.[68] Good results were also obtained with topical clonazepam.[69]

Psychotherapy

There is a lack of good studies supporting psychotherapy for BMS, although it is frequently advised[70] for these patients. A controlled study showed the validity of cognitive therapy for treatment-resistant BMS.[71]

Sucralfate

Commonly used to treat duodenal ulcers, sucralfate has shown to be a possible therapeutic option for BMS patients but is in need of further confirmation.[72]

Capsaicin

This alkaloid acts on nociceptive C-type (sensorial) neurons and has been reported to ease the pain in some neuropathies. Its use for BMS has also been proposed,[22,73] but further studies are necessary to determine its efficacy.

Diagnostic-Therapeutic Protocol

Patients with BMS should be investigated immediately and thoroughly to avoid a chronic condition. The following diagnostic-therapeutic protocol can be useful for these patients (Fig 10-1):

1. Assess the patient's medical and dental status.
2. Evaluate the health of the mucosa and, in case of lesions, refer the patient to the appropriate specialist. A biopsy is not useful in the diagnosis of BMS but may be useful in the differential diagnosis of some borderline cases.
3. Investigate possible parafunctional behavior including rubbing of the tongue on the teeth. If the patient wears a removable denture, evaluate the correct execution of the following parameters: space for the tongue, vertical dimensions, and insufficient extension of the support bases. If necessary, make a new denture.
4. Check hemoglobin, erythrocyte, ferritin, folate, and B_{12} values. In case of deficiency, prescribe replacement therapy and investigate the source of deficiency.
5. Check the values of vitamin B_1 and B_6; if this is not possible, administer vitamin B_1 (300 mg per day) and B_6 (50 mg three times per day) for 4 weeks, which can be repeated for another 4 weeks.
6. Check fasting glucose levels and carry out an OGTT). If the test is positive, refer the patient to a specialist.
7. In type 3 BMS, psychologically normal patients must be given patch tests for dental materials; for positive test results, removing the allergen should eliminate the symptoms.
8. If xerostomia is present, eliminate the possible causes (eg, medications) and recommend therapy with saliva substitutes.
9. Oral rinsing will determine the mycotic charge of the various types of *Candida*. When there are no evident clinical lesions, the borderline between colonization and infection is uncertain; nevertheless, if the mycotic charge is moderately elevated, it is advisable to start a 4-week course of antimycotic therapy (fluconazole 100 mg per day and miconazole oral gel). The patient must also be advised to restrict carbohydrates, and to maintain proper oral health.
10. If the patient is in menopause, evaluate with the gynecologist the possibility and limits of estrogen replacement therapy.
11. Investigate for the presence of cancerphobia and reassure the patient (remembering to reassure the patient again in the course of the follow-up visits).
12. Evaluate the patient's psychologic state. For screening purposes, questionnaires can be used. If indicated, psychiatric consultation should be recommended. Antidepressive therapy may then be advised.

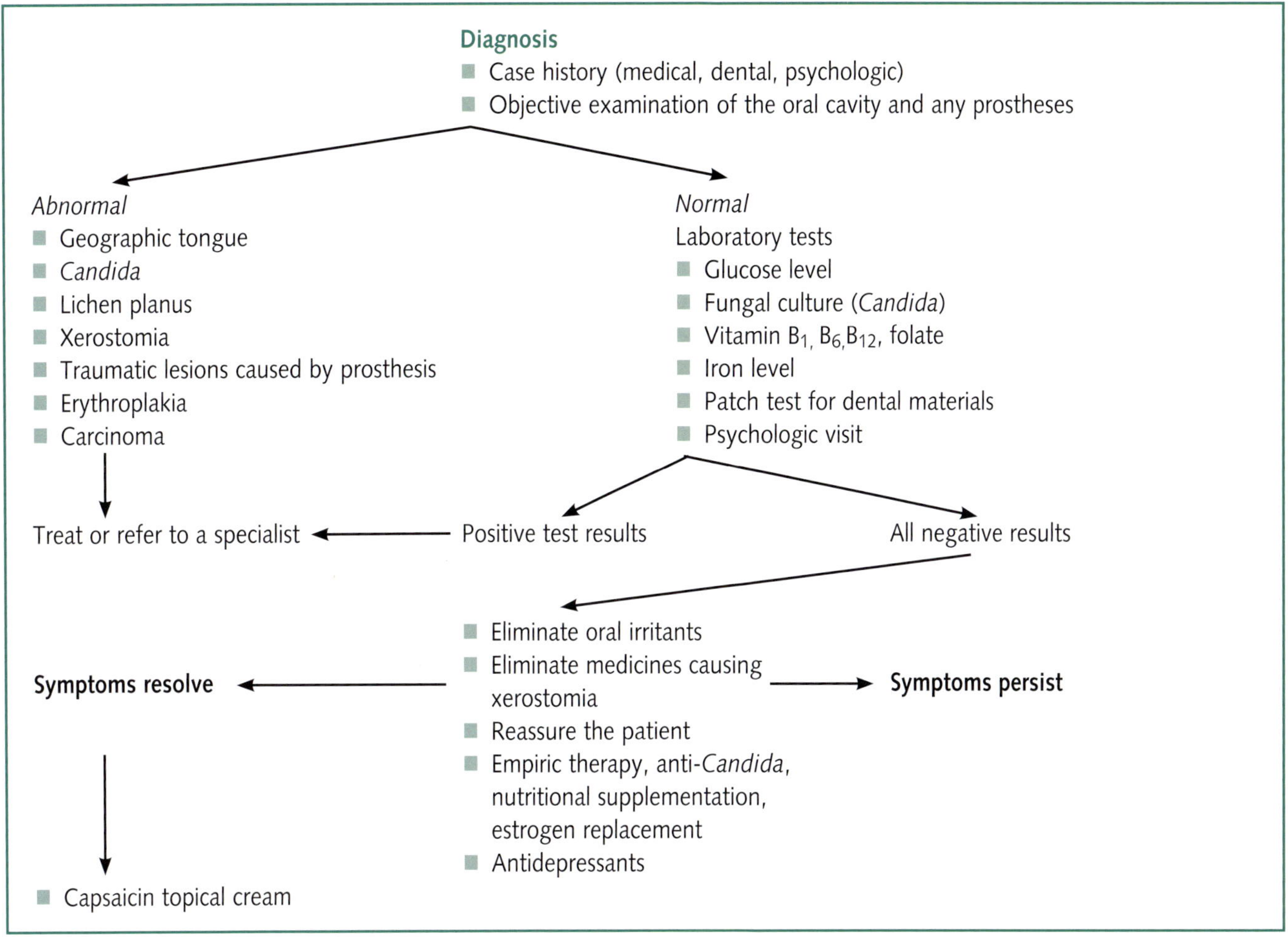

Fig 10-1 Algorithm for the treatment of BMS. (From Gandolfo et al.[74])

13. In case of treatment failure, evaluate new therapies, such as psychotherapy, sucralfate, topical capsaicin.

Whatever the chosen therapeutic approach, the psychologic needs of the patient are extremely important, because it is evident that these subjects need a great deal of attention and understanding.[8,54]

- It is necessary to be ready to listen at length to the clinical history of the patient, and to be interested even when it is complicated by particularities of no relevance.
- It is necessary to understand the patient's description of the condition as he or she interprets it. Avoid hurried judgments such as "there's nothing wrong with you."
- Investigate the possible presence of cancerphobia and reassure the patient (remembering to reassure him or her again in the course of the following visits).
- It is important that the patient be made aware that he or she is not the only one who suffers from this illness; hence, it is useful to show the patient a book or an article about the condition.

This approach comforts the patient and positively influences therapy, increasing its potential with a powerful placebo effect.

References

1. Muzyka BC, De Rossi SS. A review of burning mouth syndrome. Cutis 1999;64:29–35. Cat. 7

2. van der Waal I. The Burning Mouth Syndrome. Copenhagen: Munksgaard, 1990. Cat. 8

3. Engelbert A, Schulten JM, van der Waal I. Burning mouth syndrome. Innovations and developments in non-invasive orofacial health care. Northwood: Science Rev, 1996:27–38. Cat. 7

4. Lipton JA, Ship JA, Larach-Robinson D. Estimated prevalence and distribution of reported orofacial pain in the United States. J Am Dent Assoc 1993;124:115–121. Cat, 4

5. Van der Ploeg HM, van der Wal N, Eijkman MA, et al. Psychological aspects of patients with burning mouth syndrome. Oral Surg Oral Med Oral Pathol 1987;63:664–668. Cat. 4

6. Lamey PJ, Lewis MAO. Oral medicine in practice: Burning mouth syndrome. Br Dent J 1989;167:197–200. Cat. 7

7. Tammiala-Salonen T, Hiidenkari T, Parvinen T. Burning mouth in a Finnish adult population. Community Dent Oral Epidemiol 1993;21:67–71. Cat. 4

8. Vescovi P, Manfredi M, Savi A, et al. Burning mouth syndrome: Clinical experience on 75 patients. Minerva Stomatol 2000;49:169–177. Cat. 9

9. Lamey PJ, Lamb AB. Lip component of burning mouth syndrome. Oral Surg Oral Med Oral Pathol 1994;78:590–593. Cat. 4

10. Lamey PJ. Burning mouth syndrome. Dermatologic Clinics 1996;14:339–353. Cat. 7

11. Locker D, Grushka M. Prevalence of oral and facial pain and discomfort: Preliminary result of a mail survey. Community Dent Oral Epidemiol 1987;15:169–172. Cat. 4

12. Wardrop RW, Hailes J, Reade PC. Oral discomfort at menopause. Oral Surg Oral Med Oral Pathol 1989;67:535–540. Cat. 4

13. Huang W, Rothe MJ, Grant-Kels J. The burning mouth syndrome. J Am Acad Dermatol 1996;34:91–98. Cat. 7

14. Hughes AM, Hunter S, Still D, et al. Psychiatric disorders in a dental clinic. Br Dent J 1989;166:16–19. Cat. 4

15. Gorsky M, Silverman Jr S, Chinn H. Clinical characteristics and management outcome in the burning mouth syndrome: An open study of 130 patients. Oral Surg Oral Med Oral Pathol 1991;72:192–195. Cat. 4

16. Lamey PJ, Lamb AB. Prospective study of etiological factors in burning mouth syndrome. Br Med J 1988;296:1243–1246. Cat. 4

17. Forman RL, Settle RG, Brighatman V, et al. The prevalence by history of burning mouth syndrome among veterans [abstract]. J Dent Res 1989;68:278. Cat. 4

18. Grushka M. Clinical features in burning mouth syndrome. Oral Surg Oral Med Oral Pathol 1987;63:30–36. Cat. 2

19. Maresky LS, Van der Bijl P, Gird I. Burning mouth syndrome: Evaluation of multiple variables among 85 patients. Oral Surg Oral Med Oral Pathol 1993;75:303–307. Cat. 4

20. Feinmann C, Harris M. Psychogenic facial pain. Part 1. The clinical presentation. Br Dent J 1984;156:165–168. Cat. 4

21. Zegarelli DG. Burning mouth: Analysis of 57 patients. Oral Surg Oral Med Oral Pathol 1984;58:34–38. Cat. 4.

22. Lauritano D, Spadari F, Formaglio F, et al. Etiopathogenetic, clinical-diagnostic and therapeutic aspects of the burning mouth syndrome. Research and treatment protocols in a patient group. Minerva Stomatol 1998;47:239–251. Cat. 3

23. Vidas I. A histological basis of stomatopyrosis in the postmenopausal period. Acta Stomatologica Croatica 1988;22:31–37. Cat. 3

24. Killough S, Rees T, Lamey PJ. Demographic study of sub-type of burning mouth syndrome in an UK and USA population. J Dent Res 1995;74:892. Cat. 4

25. Gorsky M, Silverman S, Chinn H. The burning mouth syndrome: A review of 98 cases. J Oral Medicine 1987;42:7–9. Cat. 4

26. Samaranayake LP, Lamb AB, Laney PJ, MacFarlane TW. Oral carriage of candida species and coliforms in patients with burning mouth syndrome. J Oral Pathol Med 1989;18:233–235. Cat. 2

27. MacEntee MI, Scully C. Oral disorders and treatment implications in people over 75 years. Community Dent Oral Epidemiol 1988;16:271–273. Cat. 4

28. Lombardi T, Budtz-Jorgensen E. Treatment of denture-induced stomatitis: A review. Eur J Prosthodont Restor Dent 1993;2:17–22. Cat. 7

29. Basker RM, Sturdee DW, Davenport JC. Patients with burning mouth: A clinical investigation of causative factors, including the climateric and diabetes. Br Dent J 1978;145:9–16. Cat. 4

30. Main DMG, Basker RM. Patients complaining of burning mouth. Br Dent J 1983;154:206–211. Cat. 4

31. Ali A, Bates JF, Reynolds AJ, et al. The burning mouth sensation related to the wearing of acrylic dentures: An investigation. Br Dent J 1986;161:444–447. Cat. 4

32. Browning S, Hislop S, Scully C, et al. The association between burning mouh syndrome and psychosocial disorders. Oral Surg Oral Med Oral Pathol 1987;64:171–174. Cat. 1

33. American Psychiatric Association, Diagnostic and Statistical Manual of Mental Disorders, 4th Edition (DSM-IV). Washington, DC: American Psychiatric Association, 1994. Cat. 8

34. Brown RS, Hays GL, Flaitz C, et al. Burning mouth syndrome due to xerostomia and/or a tartar control dentifrice: Report of a case. J Greater Houston Dent Soc 1991;62:3–4. Cat. 8

35. Svensson P, Kaaber S. General health factors and denture function in patients with burning mouth syndrome and matched control subjects. J Oral Rehabil 1995,22:887–895. Cat. 2

36. Helton J, Storrs F. The burning mouth syndrome: Lack of a role for contact urticaria and contact dermatitis. J Am Acad Dermatol 1994;31(2pt1):201–205. Cat. 3

37. Lamey PJ, Lamb AB, Forsyth A. Atypical burning mouth syndrome. Contact Dermatitis 1987;17:242–243. Cat. 8

38. Devlin H. Watts DC. Acrylic allergy? Br Dent J 1984;157:272–275. Cat. 7

39. Dutree-Meulenberg RO, Kozel MM, van Joost T. Burning mouth syndrome. A possibile etiologic role for local contact hypersensitivity. J Am Acad Dermatol 1991;26:935–940. Cat. 3

40. Skoglund A, Egelrud T. Hypersensitivity reactions to dental materials in patients with lichenoid oral mucosal lesions and in patients with burning mouth syndrome. Scand J Dent Res 1991;99:320–328. Cat. 3

41. Van Loon LA, van Elsas PW, van Joost T, et al. Test battery for metal allergy in dentistry. Contact Dermatitis 1986,14:158–161. Cat. 1

42. Purello-D'Ambrosio F, Gangemi S, Minciullo P, et al. Burning mouth syndrome due to cadmium in a denture wearer. J Investig Allergol Clin Immunol 2000;10:105–106. Cat. 8

43. Virgili A, Corazza M, Trombelli L, et al. Burning mouth syndrome: The role of contact hypersensitivity. Acta Derm Venereol 1996;76:488–490. Cat. 1

44. Glick D, Ben-Aryeh H, Gutman D, et al. Relation between idiopathic glossodynia and salivary flow rate and content. Int J Oral Surg 1976;5:161–165. Cat. 2

45. Cibirka RM, Nelson SK, Lefebre CA. BMS : A review of etiologies. J Prosthet Dent 1997;78:93–97. Cat. 7

46. Ben-Aryeh H, Filmar S, Gutman D, et al. Salivary phosphate as an indicator of ovulation. Am J Obstet Gynaecol 1976;15:871–874. Cat. 0

47. Tammiala-Salonen T, Soderling E. Protein composition, adhesion, and agglutination properties of saliva in burning mouth syndrome. Scand J Dent Res 1993;101:215–218. Cat. 2

48. Sarna L, Beeley JA, Lamb AB, et al. Sialochemical changes in burning mouth syndrome [abstract.]. J Dent Res 1995;74:892. Cat. 2

49. Grushka M. Sessle BJ. Burning mouth syndrome. Dent Clin North Am 1991;35:1717–184. Cat. 7

50. Ferguson MM, Carter J, Boyle P, et al. Oral complaints related to climateric symptoms in oophorectomized women. J R Soc Med 1981;74:492–498. Cat. 1

51. Lamey PJ, Hammond A, Allam BF, et al. Vitamin status of patients with burning mouth syndrome and the response to replacement therapy. Br Dent J 1986;160:81–84. Cat. 3

52. Hugoson A, Thorstensson B. Vitamin B status and response to replacement therapy in patients with burning mouth syndrome. Acta Odontol Scand 1991;49:367–375. Cat. 3

53. Brody HA, Pendergast JJ, Silverman S. The relationship between oral symptoms, insulin release, and glucose intolerance. Oral Surg Oral Med Oral Pathol 1971;31:777–782. Cat. 4

54. Gibson J, Lamey PJ, Lewis M, et al. Oral manifestations of previously undiagnosed non-insulin dependent diabetes mellitus. J Oral Pathol Med 1990;19:284–287. Cat. 4

55. Hammaren M, Hugoson A. Clinical psychiatric assessment of patients with burning mouth syndrome resisting oral treatment. Swed Dent J 1989;13:77–88. Cat. 4

56. Jontell M, Haraldson T, Persson LO, et al. An oral and psycosocial examination of patients with presumed oral galvanism. Swed Dent J 1985;9:175–185. Cat. 2

57. Eli I, Kleinhauz M, Baht R, et al. Antecedents of burning mouth syndrome (glossodynia)—Recent life events vs. psychopathologic aspects. J Dent Res 1994;73:567–572. Cat. 4

58. Bogetto F, Maina G, Ferro G, et al. Psychiatric comorbidity in patients with burning mouth syndrome. Psychosomatic Medicine 1998;60:378–385. Cat. 2

59. Zilli C, Brooke RI, Lau CL, et al. Screening for psychiatric illness in patients with oral dysesthesia by means of the General Health Questionnaire—twenty-eight items version (GHQ-28) and the Irritabilty, Depression and Anxiety Scale (IDA). Oral Surg Oral Med Oral Pathol 1989;67:384–389. Cat. 4

60. Rojo I, Silvestre FJ, Bagan JV, De Vicente I. Prevalence of psychopathology in burning mouth syndrome. A comparative study among patients with and without psychiatric disorders and controls. Oral Surg Oral Med Oral Pathol 1994;77:312–316. Cat. 2

61. Rojo L, Silvestre FJ, Bagan JV, De Vicente I. Psychiatric morbidity in burning mouth syndrome. Psychiatric interview versus depression and anxiety scales. Oral Surg Oral Med Oral Pathol 1993;75(3):308-311. Cat. 4

62. Schoenberg B, Carr AC, Kutscher AH, et al. Chronic idiopathic orolingual pain: Psychogenesis of burning mouth. NY State J Med 1971;71:1832–1837. Cat. 8

63. Lamey PJ, Lamb AB. The usefulness of the HAD scale in assessing anxiety and depression in patients with burning mouth syndrome. Oral Surg Oral Med Oral Pathol 1989;67:390–392. Cat. 4

64. Brooke RI, Seganski DP. Aetiology and investigation of the sore mouth. Can Dent Assoc J 1977;43:504–506. Cat. 4

65. Feinmann C, Harris M. Psychogenic facial pain. Part 2. Management and prognosis. Br Dent J 1984;156:205–208. Cat. 1

66. Lowental U, Pisanti S. The syndrome of oral complaints. Etiology and therapy. Oral Surg 1978;46:2–6. Cat. 4

67. Tammiala-Salonen T, Forssel H. Trazodone in burning mouth pain. A placebo controlled, double-blind study. J Orofac Pain 1999;13: 83–88. Cat. 1

68. Grushka M, Epstein J, Mott A. An open-label, dose escalation pilot study of the effect of clonazepam in burning mouth syndrome. Oral Surg Oral Med Oral Pathol 1998;86:557–561. Cat. 3

69. Woda A, Navez ML, Picard P, et al. A possible therapeutic solution for stomatodynia (burning mouth syndrome). J Oralfac Pain 1998; 12:272–278. Cat. 3

70. Demange C, Husson C, Poi-Vet D, et al. Burning mouth syndrome and depression: A psychoanalytic approach. Rev Stomatol Chir Maxillofac 1996;97:244-252. Cat. 9

71. Bergdahl J, Anneroth G, Perris H. Cognitive therapy in the treatment of patients with resistant burning mouth syndrome: A controlled study. J Oral Pathol Med 1995;4:213–215. Cat. 1

72. Campisi G, Spadari F, Salvato A. Sucralfate in odontostomatology. Clinical experience. Minerva Stomatol 1997;46:297–305. Cat. 3

73. Epstein JB, Marcoe JH. Topical application of capsaicin for treatment of oral neuropathic pain and trigeminal neuralgia. Oral Surg Oral Med Oral Pathol 1994;77:135–140. Cat. 3

74. Gandolfo S, Scully C, Carrozzo M. Patologia e Medicina del Cavo Orale. Torino: UTET, 2001. Cat. 7

Mandibular Implant-Retained Overdenture

The first prosthetic implant rehabilitation of the edentulous mandible[1] was a fixed prosthesis sustained by five or six implants positioned in the region between the two mental foramina. The wide-scale clinical application of this protocol, preceded by basic research on animals, has been perfected over time.[2] When the correct techniques and principles of biomechanics are applied, it has proved to be effective, lasting, and reliable.

In the 1980s, the idea of combining the rehabilitation protocol of edentulism with a complete denture and the latest in implantology was introduced to reduce costs and operating times and to make implants more accessible.[3] In a short time, mandibular implant-retained overdentures (MIR-OVDs) received widespread attention in the international literature. In a recent analysis, Brunski[4] underlined how many clinics hurried to adopt new implant rehabilitation protocols without waiting for the basic clinical research results because they were under pressure to rehabilitate patients. He pointed out that "...the criteria for the planning and the use of dental implants has often been dictated by a commercial environment which is extremely aggressive in terms of productivity, rather than by results acquired by scientific means in the field of biomaterials, biomechanics and bone biology."

The procedure followed by the international scientific community to confirm the rehabilitation protocol for implant-retained fixed prostheses (ie, observation of the osteointegration process, realization of the prosthetic design, experimentation, clinical application, results, definitions, and publishing of the protocol) has been completely disregarded for MIR-OVDs, since this technique, as Taylor[5] recently reported, has been revealed as being effective, relatively simple, and economically accessible.

Even in 1988 the lack of basic research was pointed out by Naert,[6] when the clinical and operative protocol of MIR-OVDs had already been defined and widely adopted. A couple of years later, Brånemark[7] re-emphasized the difficulty and dangers of this method. The scientific community has only recently begun to investigate questions about the nature and quality of the support tissues (bone, implants, and mucosa of the distal edentulous regions). What are the modalities of load transmission to implants in the anterior region and to the distal alveolar ridges? How does the mucosa and bone in the distal regions change over the long term? Is it possible to influence, in the long term, the extent of osseous resorption of the distal ridges using different methods of retention? Is the evaluation of the tissue response and oral function a key factor in predicting long-term success?

Only since 1990 has basic and clinical research provided a scientific foundation for the MIR-OVD rehabilitation protocol and analyzed its biomechanical, biologic, and functional aspects. In the field of biomechanics, research has focused on examining the modalities of distribution of the masticatory load to the supporting structures. As described by Taylor,[5] the reference design for MIR-OVDs is constituted by two implants placed in the canine region (or slightly more mesial) to provide anchorage for the denture[3,8–11] and can be either joined through a bar or independent. The most common forms of retention—the bar method[12] and the ball method—allow a rotation of the prosthetic body under masticatory load and thus the load transmission to the supporting structures differs in a substantial way from that studied in implant-retained fixed rehabilitation.[13] Until the second half of the 1990s, the theory that masticatory load is distributed on implants and on the mucosa of the edentulous distal ridges had only been proved indirectly.[14,15]

In an in vivo study published in 1991, Jemt and colleagues[15] hypothesized that a reduction in tension and compression loads transmitted through the implants to the peri-implant bone in the MIR-OVD could depend on the resilience of the mucosa of the distal edentulous ridges compared with that observed in fixed dentures,[6–17] Jemt and colleagues also pointed out that despite the reduction in masticatory load, implants that anchor

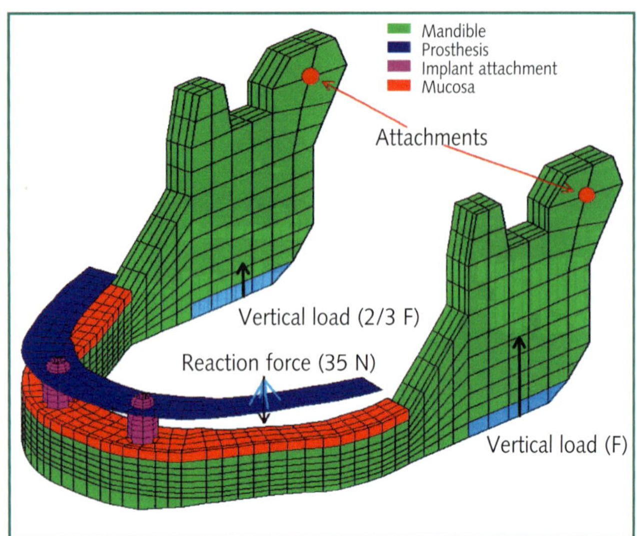

Fig 11-1 Mathematic model of the MIR-OVD with the ball anchor method. The model includes the mandible, mucosa, implant, ball attachments, and overdenture.

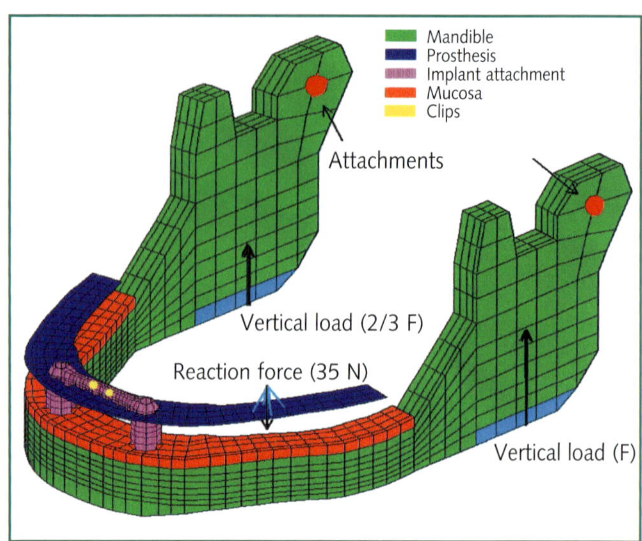

Fig 11-2 Mathematic model of the MIR-OVD with the bar anchor method. The model includes the mandible, mucosa, implant, bar, and overdenture.

the MIR-OVD are subjected to both axial and transverse forces[15,16]; transverse forces are less intense but potentially more damaging.[18]

In 1998, the Turin University dental school published two studies[19,20] in which retention of the MIR-OVD was evaluated in terms of load transmission to the supporting structures: implants, peri-implant bone, mucosa, and distal ridges. The first of the two studies[19] was based on the analysis of a finite element mathematical model (FEM), a method that is widely used and described in the international literature.[21,22] The mathematical model reproduces an edentulous mandible, the mucosa, two titanium implants positioned in the area of the canines, and one MIR-OVD anchored by two ball attachments (Fig 11-1) or a bar with two clips (Fig 11-2). All of the components represented by FEM, including the mucosa,[23–26] are considered to be isotropic, homogeneous, and linearly elastic.[22–23,26] The elastic properties are listed in Box 11-1 and have been chosen

on the basis of the information reported in the literature.[27] The prosthetic design was adopted in accordance with the protocol proposed by Naert[6] in 1988. In order to simulate the action of the elevator muscles, two vertical forces directed upward (Fig 11-1 and Fig 11-2) were applied bilaterally in correspondence with the lower posterior margins of the horizontal ramus of the mandible.[22,27–29] The intensity of these two forces resulted in a reaction force equivalent to a vertical masticatory load of 35 N at the area of the first molar of the denture.[30] A clinical study was then carried out using the strain gauge technique on three patients wearing MIR-OVDs for 3 years, and a conventional complete maxillary denture.[20] The load transmitted to the mucosa and to the distal edentulous ridges was recorded via a load cell interposed between the prosthetic body and the mucosa, while stresses were generated in the working-side implant by means of a prosthetic abutment equipped with four strain gauges[31–43] (Fig 11-3).

Box 11-1 Elastic properties of the materials indicated in FEM

	E	Poisson ratio
Titanium	103.400 N/mm^2	0.35
Cortical bone	13.700 N/ mm^2	0.30
Spongiform bone	1.370 N/mm^2	0.30
Resin	3.000 N/mm^2	0.35
Mucosa	1 N/mm^2	0.37
Gold alloy	100.000 N/mm^2	0.30

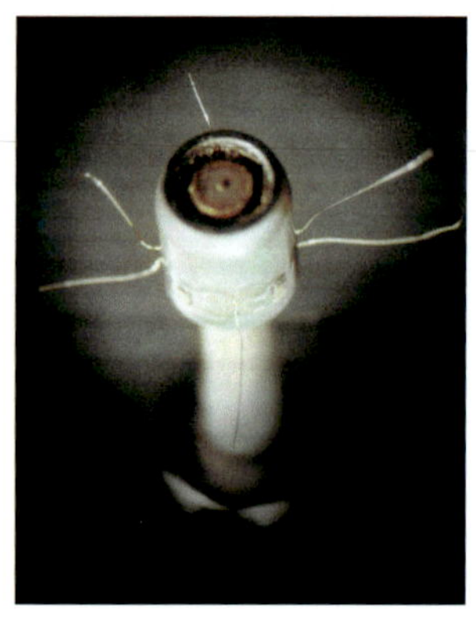

Fig 11-3 Prosthetic abutment equipped with four sensor gauges.

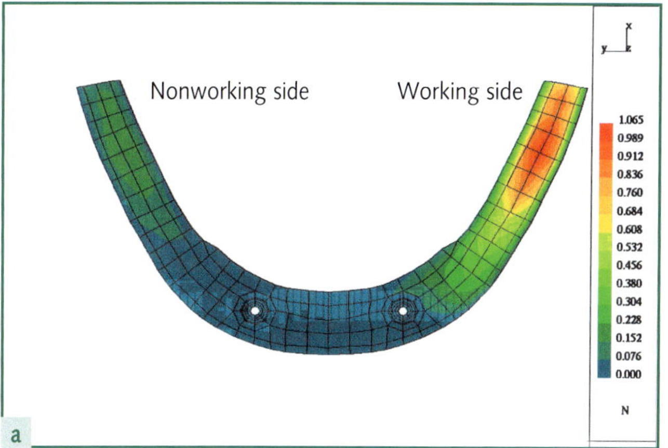
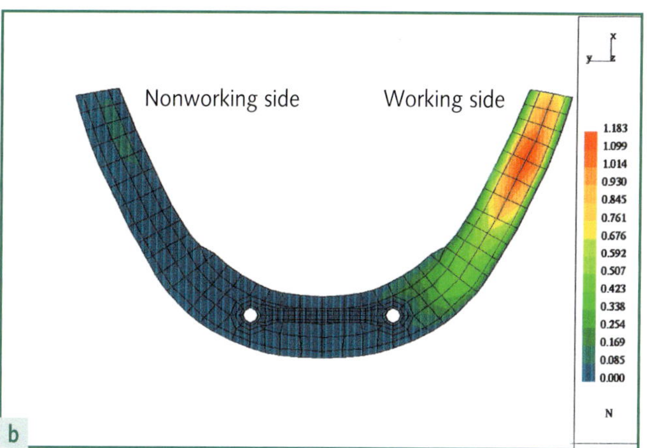

Fig 11-4 Mathematic model of the MIR-OVD with the *(a)* ball and the *(b)* bar methods: reaction force on the edentulous distal mucosa on both working and nonworking sides. The edentulous crest on the nonworking side undergoes more stress with the ball attachment compared with the bar attachment. When the prosthesis is anchored by a ball attachment, the reaction force on the distal edentulous mucosa of the nonworking side results in distribution on a more extensive area *(green)*.

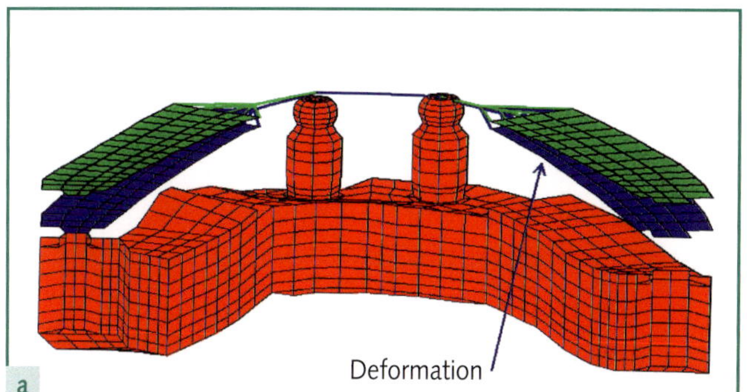
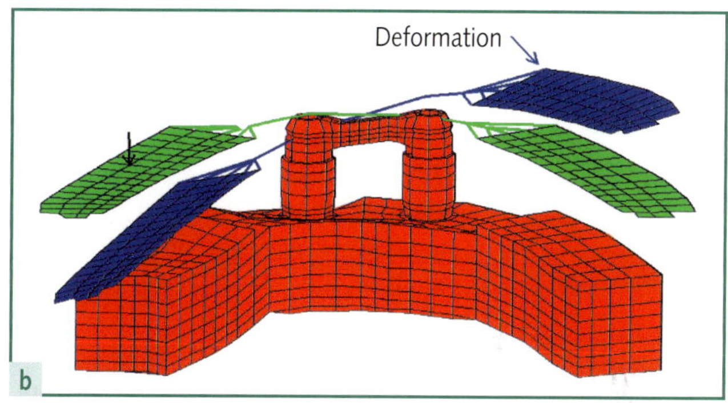

Fig 11-5 When the MIR-OVD is anchored by a bar, *(a)* the prosthesis moves more easily. *(b)* The hinges of the two clips are closer with respect to the ball attachments.

The patients had to undergo a masticatory cycle lasting 10 seconds while wearing the MIR-OVD anchored with the two different retention systems. The FEM analysis and the clinical evidence did not show substantial differences in the stresses recorded in the prosthetic abutment and the working-side implant. In the FEM, the particular distribution of stress around the implants seems to have been influenced by torsion of the mandibular body.[44–49]

With the ball attachments, the central area of the mandibular body deformed without interference from the implants, whereas if a bar was present, the stresses preferably transmit through this structure to the area around the implants. This observation seems to confirm the results obtained by Hobkirk and Schwab[44] in an in vivo study on mandibular prosthesis deformation in patients with implants joined by a rigid super-

structure, as well as by Meijer.[21–24] Nevertheless, these differences in stress are modest, and it is difficult to believe that they can influence the success rate of the bar versus the ball retention systems.

The FEM analysis and the clinical investigation have provided important indications concerning the distribution of the masticatory load to the distal edentulous regions: The ball retention system appears to encourage a more uniform load distribution to both distal edentulous ridges (Fig 11-4). This effect depends on the greater stability that the ball attachments provide the prosthetic body because of their greater distance with respect to the clip (Fig 11-5).

Only a careful evaluation of the tissue reactions and the functional alterations of the stomatognatic apparatus can provide indications on how the denture-implant retention system

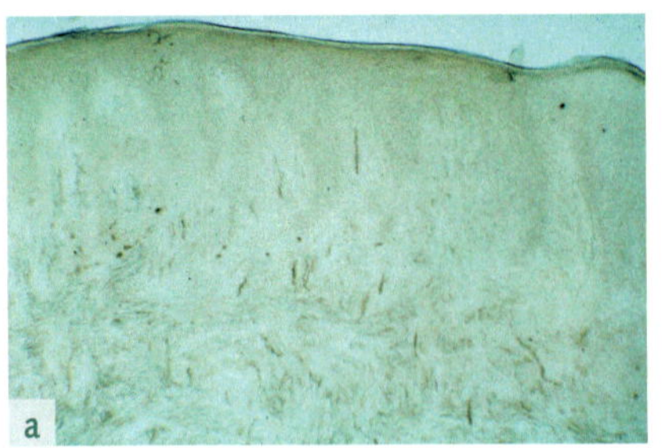 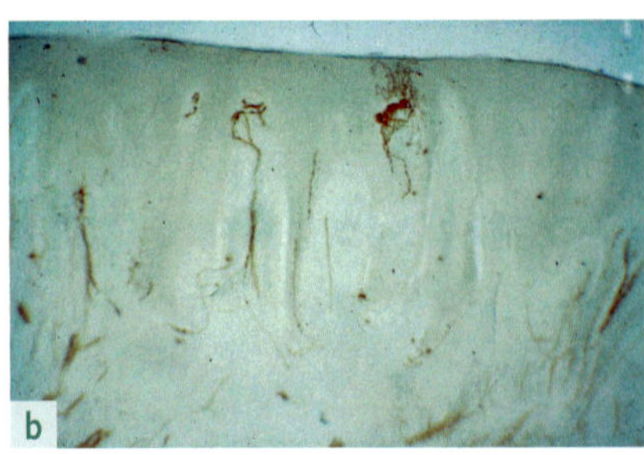

Fig 11-6 *(a)* The mucosa that covers the edentulous crest near the molars. Very few nerve fibers can be seen (in brown). *(b)* Mucosa sampled in the same site a year after anchorage of the complete mandibular denture showing numerous nerve fibers.

influences the structural prophylaxis. From the immunohistochemical, functional, and histologic points of view, research is substantially orientated in two directions: *(1)* to determine the variations in peri-implant tissues and the distal edentulous ridges that occur as a consequence of adopting this type of denture and *(2)* to evaluate the presence of an effective functional advantage that the patient can obtain from MIR-OVDs.

At the University of Turin, a study was carried out[50] to analyze the histologic changes induced in the edentulous mucosa at the area of the first mandibular molar following attachment of a complete pre-existent denture to implants. Mucosa samples were taken from this area when two implants were placed in the interforamina area, when the denture was attached to the implants, and 1 year after loading. The following were histologically analyzed: epithelial thickness, morphology of the corneal layer and stromal papillae, the presence of inflammatory infiltrate in the (submucosal) stroma, and the distribution of the cytokeratins in the epithelium as revealed by immunoperoxidase analysis.[51,52] The results suggest how anchorage of a complete mandibular denture encourages an increase in the tropism of the edentulous mucosa as a result of a more uniform load distribution.

Various authors[53–56] have noted how the loss of periodontal neural innervation due to the extraction of all teeth contributes to a reduction in masticatory efficiency and tactile discrimination. In edentulous patients, this loss of innervation is partially substituted by receptors in the mucosa covering the edentulous ridges despite the reduction in mucosal innervation.[57]

To establish how MIR-OVDs can influence the level of tactile innervations of the mucosa of edentulous ridges, a study was undertaken[58] on a control group with a natural opposing dentition. At the moment of surgical intervention, the number of receptors in the mucosa of complete denture wearers was lower than that of the control subjects; following implant placement and denture attachment, a marked increase in receptors was observed (Fig 11-6). One year after denture attachment, the total number of sensory receptors in the peri-implant soft tissues and in the mucosa covering the edentulous ridges was higher than that evaluated before the surgical implant, but lower than in the control group. The number of receptors in

the distal areas was comparable to that of the control subjects, however. These results support the hypothesis that the use of implants for complete denture retention impedes overload of the mucosa, which causes degeneration of the mucosal nervous fibers in patients wearing conventional complete dentures.

Another study[59] analyzed the changes in mucosal sensory innervation in patients with complete dentures, in those with MIR-OVDs, and in a group of dentate control subjects, by means of growth-associated protein 43 (GAP-43) expression in the nerve fibers of the mucosa covering the distal ridges. GAP-43 is a neuropeptide produced by peripheral nerve fibers during embryonic neurogenesis and only during regeneration of nerve fibers in the adult.[60–62] In the tissue samples taken from patients rehabilitated with a complete denture, a considerable quantity of GAP-43 was found, whereas in patients with MIR-OVDs, the quantity of GAP-43 was minimal. In control subjects, the presence of GAP-43 was not detectable. The presence of this neuropeptide in the mucosa of patients with complete nonanchored dentures confirms data suggesting a poorly innervated alveolar mucosa in these conditions.

From the biomolecular point of view, the production of cytokines in the soft peri-implant tissues and in the distal edentulous ridges has been studied.[63] Cytokines are involved in the modulation of tissue generation by mechanical stimuli and have been shown to cause osseous remodeling.[64–69] Their action on oral tissues, however, is not yet very clear. An attempt has been made to analyze the modulating action of cytokines on the mandibular bone in totally edentulous patients rehabilitated with MIR-OVDs. The samples consisted of soft tissues taken from the distal edentulous ridge and from the mucosa adjacent to the implants in the interforamina area, taken at the stage-one and stage-two surgical phases and at 4, 8, and 12 months after denture anchorage. The results showed how the occlusal load distribution obtained by anchoring the total denture to the implants can encourage the expression of cytokines, which can in turn encourage osseous deposition in the peri-implant area and in the distal edentulous ridge.

Studies investigating oral function in patients with MIR-OVDs have looked at patient satisfaction,[70–72] masticatory efficiency,[73–76] maximum occlusal force,[77,78] discrimination threshold of interocclusal thickness,[79,80] quality and length of masticatory cycles,[81] and level of stereognostic ability.[82] The data for each parameter show a greater degree of function in the MIR-OVD groups compared with the control subjects.

The University of Turin[79] evaluated the interocclusal thickness discrimination threshold using shimstock in groups of patients with either conventional complete dentures or MIR-OVDs. The day after placement of the conventional dentures, it was possible to record a definite reduction in the thickness discrimination threshold, which could be evaluated even after 4 days. After about 3 months the threshold increased notably. The patients with MIR-OVDs had reduced threshold values in discriminating interocclusal thicknesses both immediately and over time.

In a recent study,[80] the influence of selective grinding on the thickness discrimination threshold in two groups of patients rehabilitated with either a conventional complete denture or MIR-OVD was evaluated. The capacity to discriminate interocclusal thickness was quantified with shimstock . The patients then underwent extraoral and intraoral recording of the maxillomandibular relationships. The patients' dentures were subjected to selective grinding when necessary. Afterward, the patients again underwent tests to determine the threshold perception of interocclusal thicknesses. The results indicated that patients with an MIR-OVD had a lower interocclusal thickness discrimination threshold than those with a conventional complete denture, confirming the efficiency of implant anchorage for structural prophylaxis.

To quantify the variations in width of the masticatory cycles and masticatory efficiency in the same group of patients, the values recorded before and after anchorage of the mandibular complete denture to the implants were compared.[81] The masticatory cycles were evaluated by a sirognatograph, and masticatory efficiency was evaluated using the Olthoff protocol,[83] which consists of preparing cubes of condensation-cured silicon of 5.6 mm^2 per side, which the patient subjects to a given number of masticatory cycles. The resulting fragments are separated by size through sieves. After denture-implant anchorage, it was possible to record a significant increase in the width of the masticatory cycles and in masticatory efficiency. Furthermore, a direct correlation between the area of the masticatory cycles and masticatory efficiency was verified: The greater the area, the greater the efficiency. This information agrees with that obtained in the past by other authors,[84] according to whom wide masticatory cycles constitute an index of elevated masticatory efficiency.

Summary of MIR-OVD

The ball retention method has the following advantages:

- Functional load distribution on the mucosa, and therefore on the bone, is wider than that obtained by the bar retention method.
- Separated implants do not interfere with the physiologic deformation of the mandible during function. Interference occurs when uniting the implants with a bar. The deformation of the mandible during function could be important in relation to osseous remodeling.
- Residual oral structures are maintained in good health over time.
- Oral function is improved. Tissue reaction to functional loads demonstrates improved tropism of the mucosa covering the distal edentulous ridges.
- Sensory receptors in the mucosa increase in number.
- Physiologic behavior of innervation is more similar to that in dentate patients.
- Increased expression of cytokines stimulates the osteogenic activity of fibroblasts of the mucosa covering the edentulous ridges.

In a global population living significantly longer, the MIR-OVD offers the advantages of osseointegration at an acceptable cost for those who are most in need. The International Symposium "Towards Optimized Management of the Edentulous Predicament"[85] established that MIR-OVDs could be the optimum standard of treatment for the edentulous mandible.

MIR-OVD: Clinical Procedures

Rehabilitation of the edentulous mandible by anchoring a complete denture to two osseointegrated implants positioned between the mental foramina has a high success rate in terms of both the implant and prosthetic components.[2,5,6,8–11,14,86–114] Such a procedure improves oral function,[71,73,76,80,81,115–121] is efficient for the prophylaxis of the residual oral structures,[63,122,123] and therefore is recommended for all edentulous patients, independent of age,[124–133] even when the residual alveolar process is still well maintained (Fig 11-7).

An important part of the rehabilitation of a totally edentulous patient, regardless of the type of retention, is preparation of a definitive prosthesis prior to positioning of the implants. The complete denture, even if it will be anchored to implants, must respect the construction principles of conventional rehabilitation.

After a period of adaptation (2 months), implants can be placed in the canine areas of the edentulous mandible; these

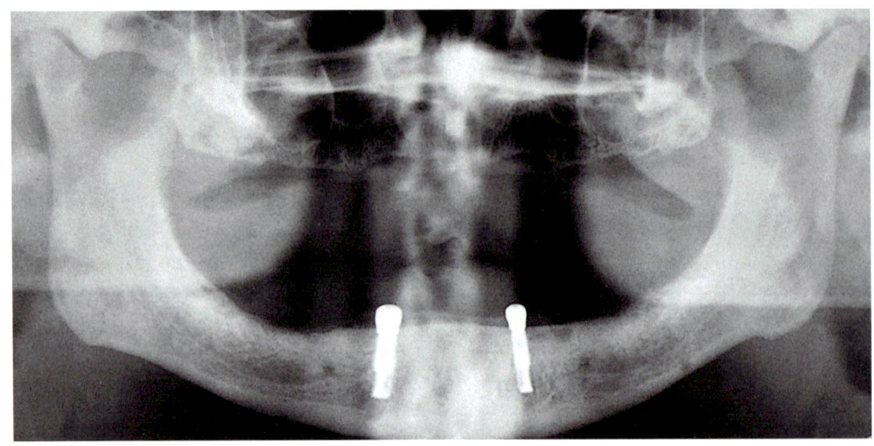

Fig 11-7 Orthopantomograph of edentulous jaws with two Brånemark implants (Nobel Biocare). The resdiual bone structures are well represented.

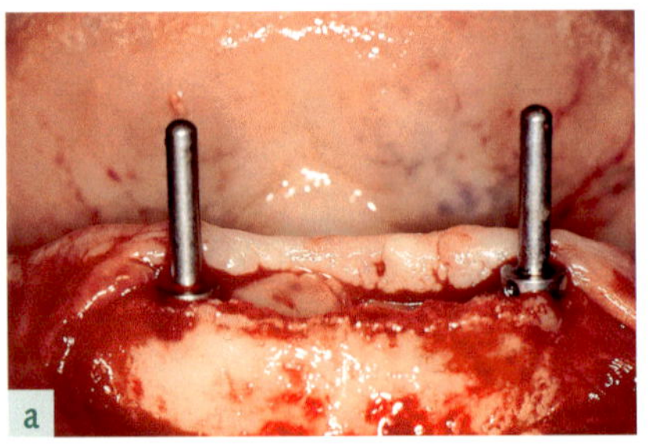

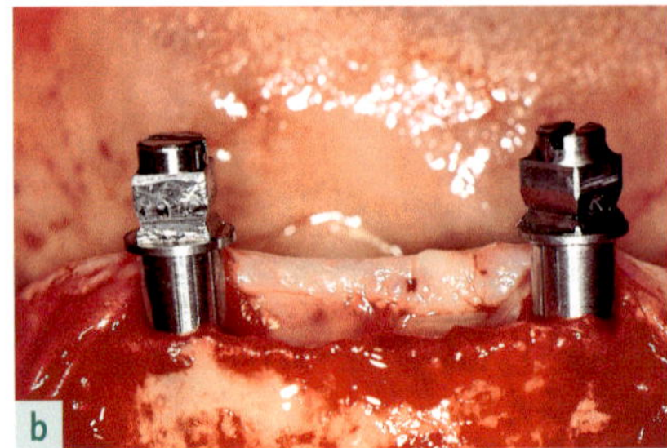

Fig 11-8 First surgical intervention involves positioning the implants according to the Brånemark protocol. *(a)* The implants are positioned as parallel as possible in the canine area. *(b)* The implants are placed in the bone with the disposition indicators still in position.

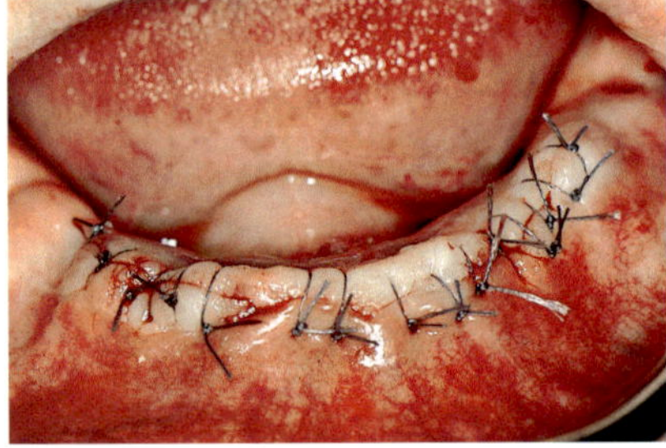

Fig 11-9 Sutures at the end of stage-one surgery. Because postoperative edema increases over time, it is not advisable to use the mandibular prosthesis immediately.

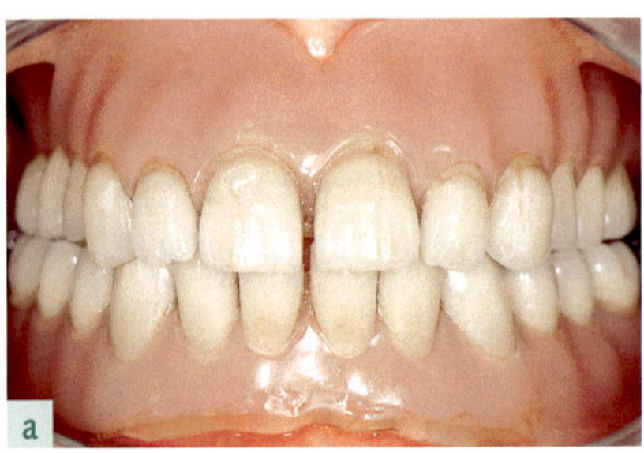

Fig 11-10 *(a)* The prosthetic body was relined with a soft conditioner (Functional Impression Tissue Toner; or Visco gel). *(b)* The mandibular prosthesis can then be inserted after healing and suture removal, about 10 to 15 days. Postsurgical edema has nearly resolved.

must be as parallel to each other as possible in accordance with the surgical protocol proposed by Brånemark[6] (Fig 11-8). In the period immediately after the operation until 10 to 15 days postoperatively, the patient must not wear the mandibular denture to allow the mucosa to heal (Fig 11-9). The denture is then relined with soft conditioning materials (Functional Impression Tissue Toner, Kerr; or ViscoGel, Dentsply DeTrey) (Fig 11-10). This procedure is repeated once every 15 days during the period necessary to obtain osseointegration (about 3 months).

During the second surgical phase, after having placed healing abutments (Fig 11-11), the denture is again relined with the conditioning material. Once the peri-implant tissues have healed, after about 3 or 4 weeks (Fig 11-12), it is possible to proceed with anchorage of the denture[13,134–147] (Fig 11-13).

Bar retention

It is necessary to evaluate certain parameters before placing implants when planning bar retention. Bar retention often presents space problems. Three factors influence the feasibility of this method: *(1)* the position of the implants, *(2)* the morphology of the bar, and *(3)* the position of the bar clips in the denture. The implants must be positioned at a distance that allows the bar to run straight and parallel to the

Fig 11-11 Stage-two surgery involves positioning the healing abutments. Because the space around the healing abutments is extremely reduced in this phase, it is possible to insert the relined prosthesis as soon as the incision has been made around the head of the implants.

Fig 11-12 Peri-implant mucosa 4 weeks after stage-two surgery.

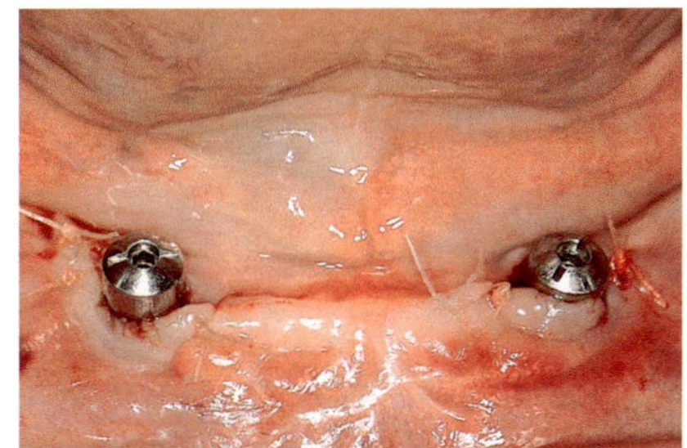
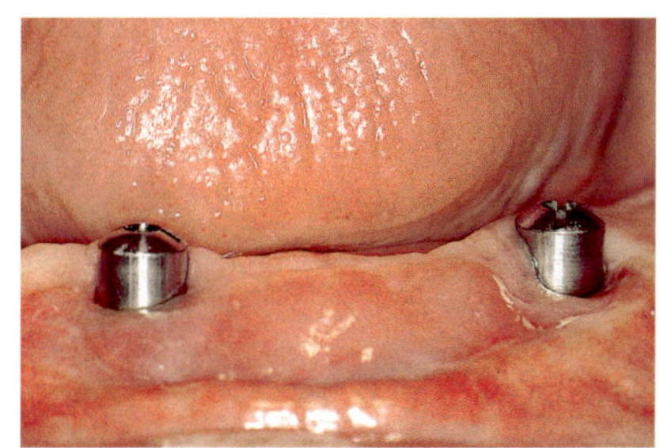

Fig 11-13 Anchorage systems for the mandibular prosthesis supported by implants: *(a)* bar attachments; *(b)* ball attachments.

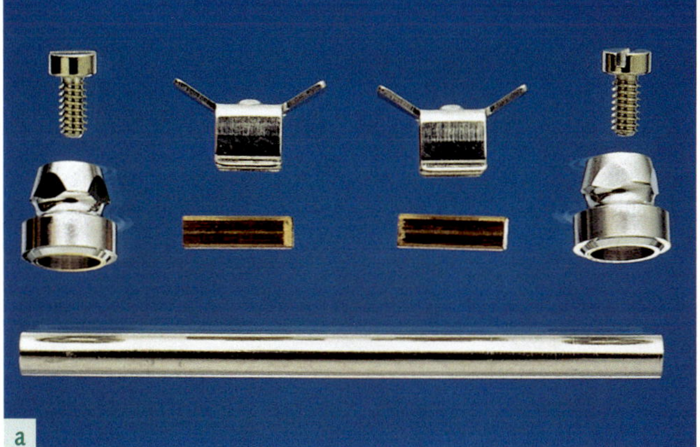
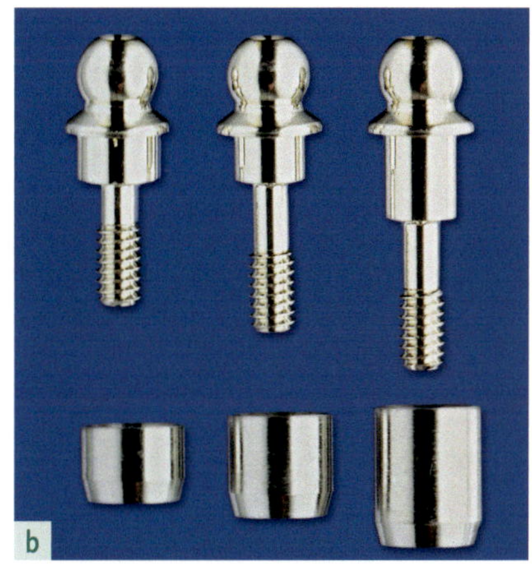

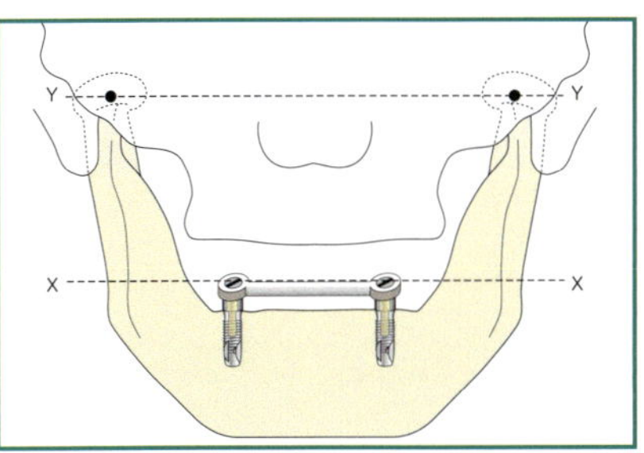

Fig 11-14 Note that the bar (x) should parrallel a line connecting the rotational axes of the condyles (y).

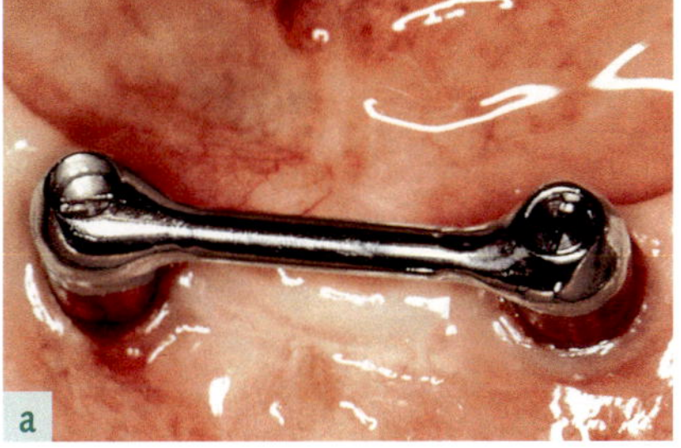

Fig 11-15 *(a)* Clinical view of the bar attachment.. *(b)* Radiograph of the same case.

intercondylar rotation axis[148] and perpendicular to the sagittal plane[149] (Fig 11-14), avoiding the space occupied by the tongue. The bar must be straight[150] without extensions distal to the implants[151,152] and must respect a distance of 4 to 5 mm from the mucosa to allow for oral hygiene procedures (Fig 11-15).[153,154] The two prosthetic bar clips must be positioned as far as possible from each other (Fig 11-16).

At times it is difficult to position the mandibular incisors and canines in the neutral zone, and the consequences are often negative to the function and esthetics. It is therefore necessary to evaluate the available space.[155] If it is not sufficient, the following problems can occur:

■ The space for the tongue will be reduced.
■ The lower lip will be pushed forward, and the labial sulcus will be reduced or eliminated.
■ Underneath the bar, tissue hyperplasia can occur, more frequently in the absence of adequate adherent mucosa[156,157] (Fig 11-17).

Furthermore, bar retention requires more and longer clinical sittings as compared with the ball retention method.[12,158]

131

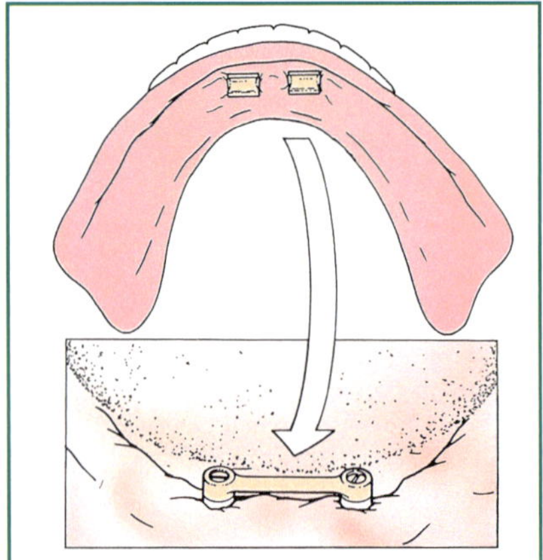

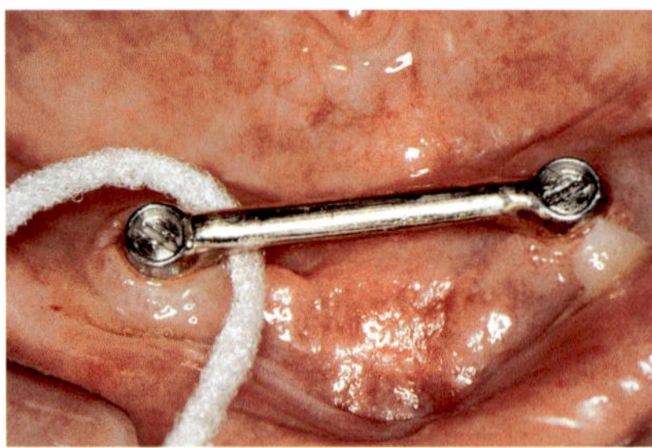

Fig 11-16 Position of the clip attachments in the prosthetic body.

Fig 11-17 Hyperplastic tissue under the bar may be due to the absence of adherent mucosa or to insufficient space for hygiene practices.

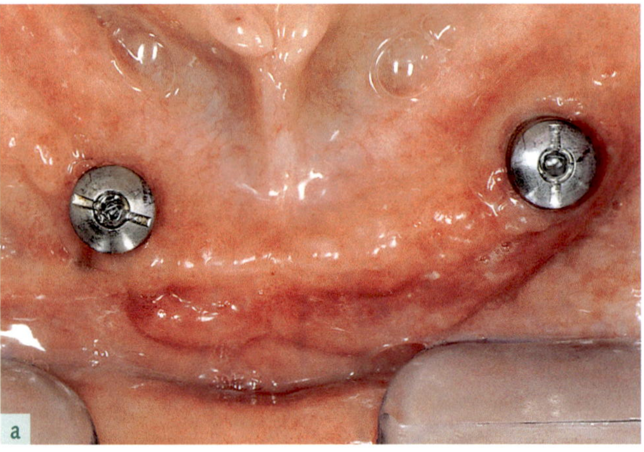
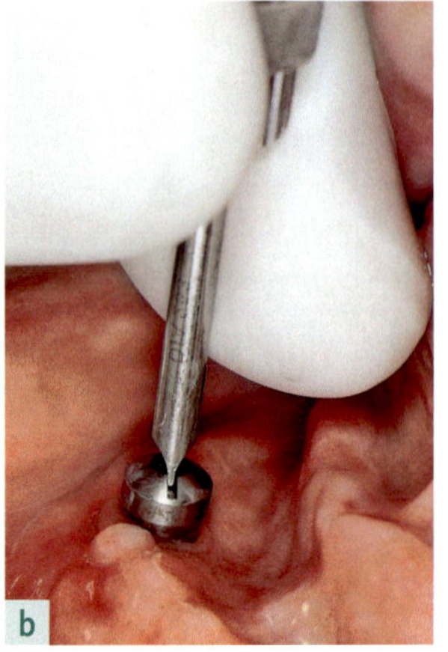
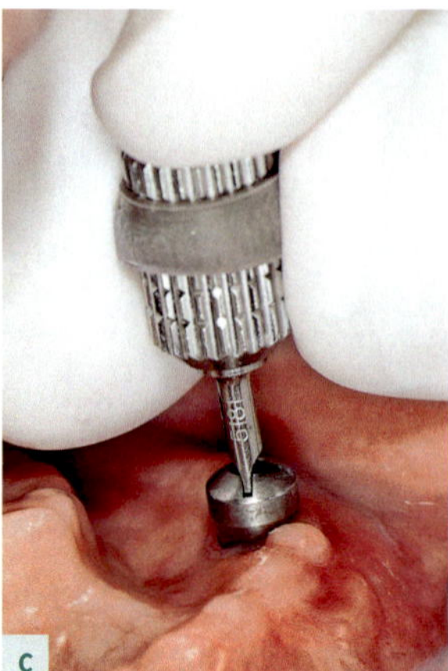

Fig 11-18 (a) Healing abutments in situ. (b and c) Removal with the appropriate screwdriver (Nobel Biocare).

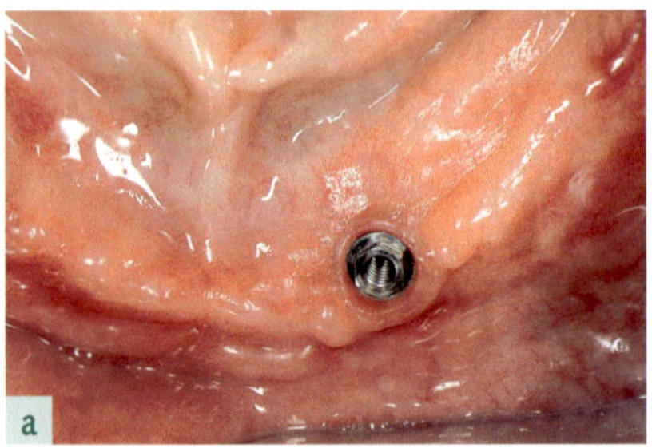
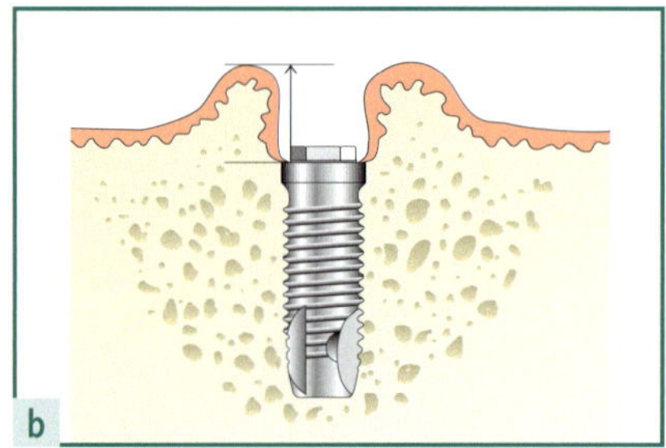

Fig 11-19 (a) Implant head after removal of healing abutment . (b) Transmucosal pathway from the head of the implant to the margin of the peri-implant mucosa.

Ball retention

For the aforementioned clinical and biomechanical aspects,[19,20,23,31] ball retention is the option most chosen by the University of Turin, even if bar retention is the method most quoted in the literature.

About 3 or 4 weeks after stage-two surgery, the healing abutments are removed and the ball retention system is placed (Fig 11-18). Proper execution of this procedure requires the following:

- The choice of height of the prosthetic abutment is determined by the transmucosal pathway between the head of the implant and the free margin of the peri-implant mucosa (Fig 11-19). A millimeter gauge (Figs 11-20 and 11-21) should be used for measurement.
- The upper part of the abutment must emerge from the mucosa by 1.5 to 2.0 mm to make hygiene practices easier (Figs 11-22 and 11-23).
- The upper profiles of the ball attachments must be at the same height, and the line that joins them must be parallel to

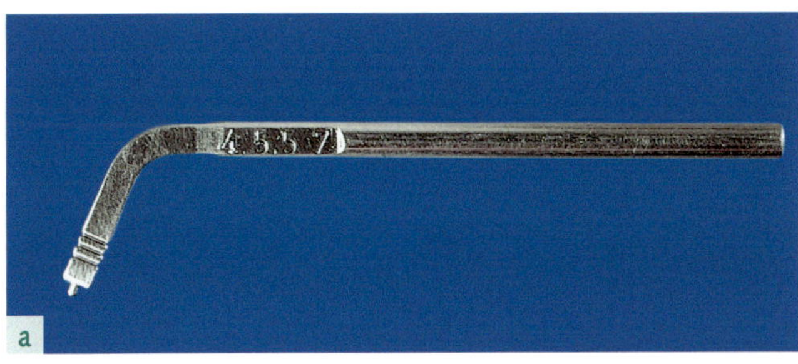
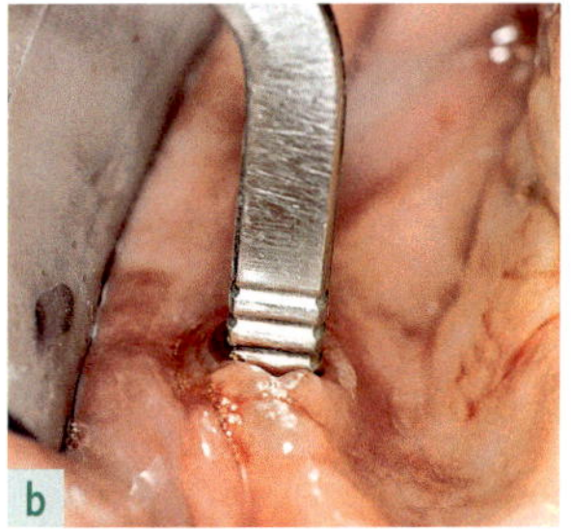
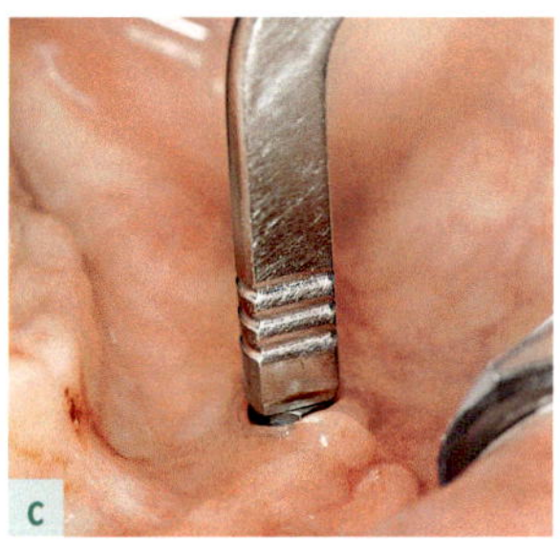

Fig 11-20 *(a)* Stainless steel gauge with millimeters indicated (Nobel Biocare). It is necessary to measure the transmucosal pathway in order to select the appropriate prosthetic abutment. *(b and c)* In this patient the height is different in the two sites (4 to 5 mm and 5 to 7 mm).

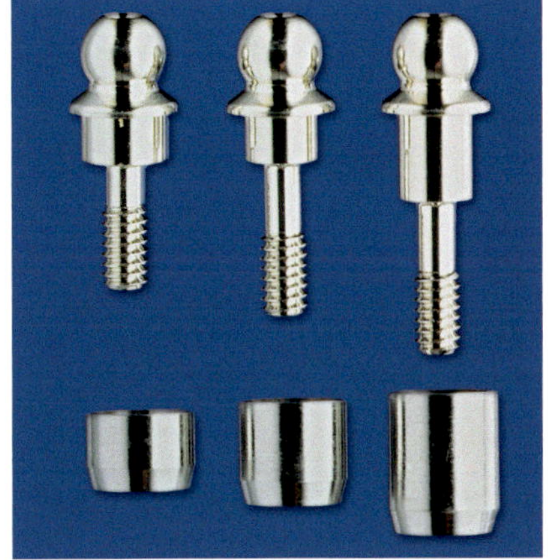
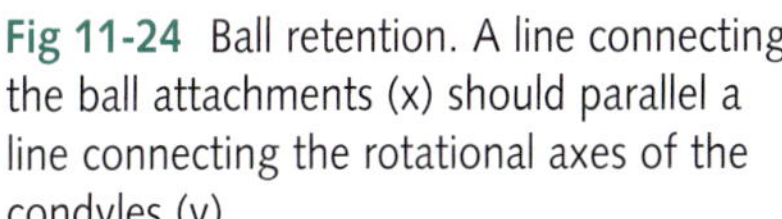
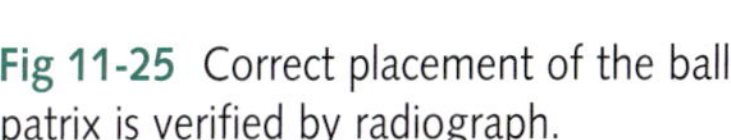

Fig 11-21 Prosthetic ball attachments with pillars of various dimensions (3 to 5.5 mm). The diameter of the ball patrix is about 4 mm.

Fig 11-24 Ball retention. A line connecting the ball attachments (x) should parallel a line connecting the rotational axes of the condyles (y).

Fig 11-25 Correct placement of the ball patrix is verified by radiograph.

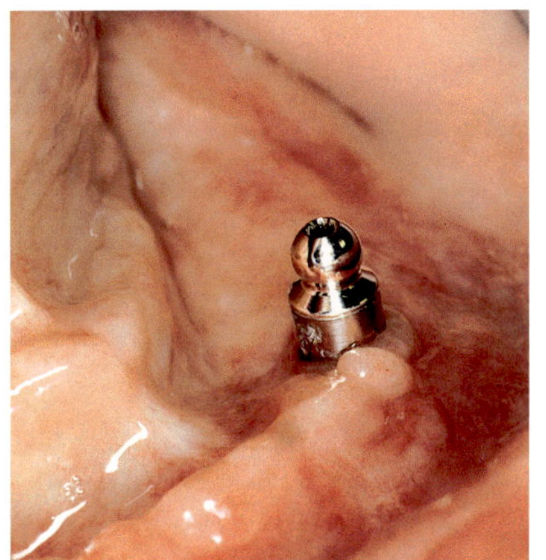

Fig 11-22 Ball attachment screwed onto the implant.

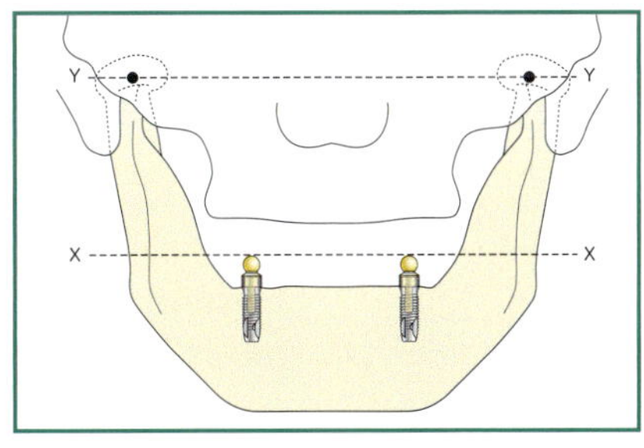

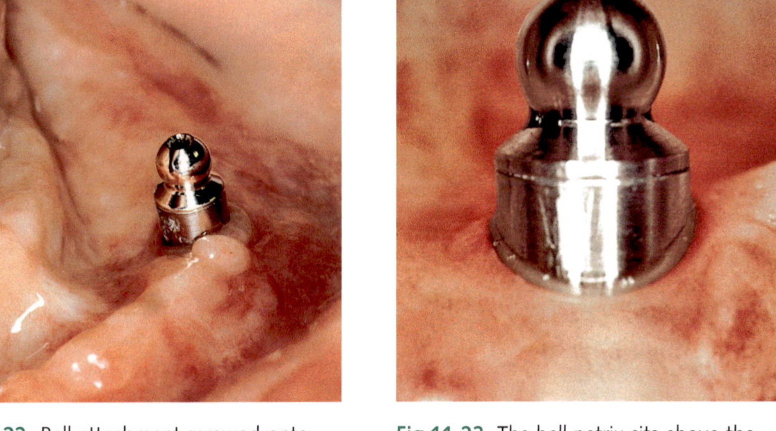

Fig 11-23 The ball patrix sits above the mucosa, which facilitates hygiene care.

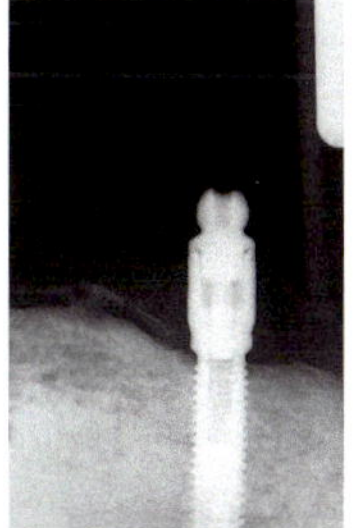

the intercondylar rotation axis (Fig 11-24). It is often necessary to use prosthetic abutments of different heights.

■ Perfect adaptation between the attachment components is indispensable to avoid the interposition of mucosa. Screwdrivers and pliers suitable for prosthetic abutments should be used.

Initially, the ball attachment is screwed manually onto the head of the implant, but not tightened. Intraoral radiographs with a centering device are useful to verify the correct adaptation between components (Fig 11-25). If there are no errors of positioning, tightening is continued to 20 Ncm using a screwdriver mounted on a contra-angle handpiece at low speed (Torque Controller, Nobel Biocare).

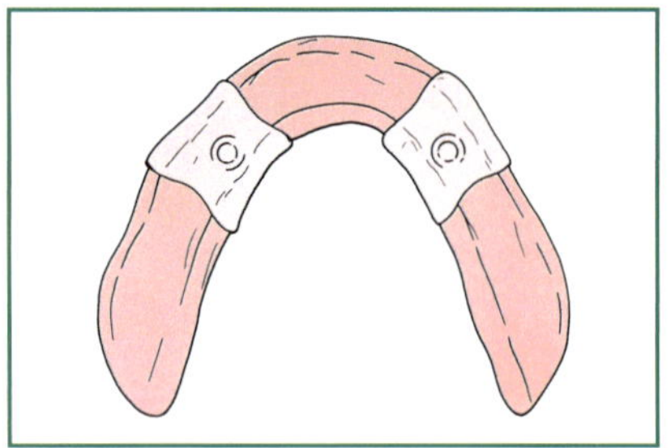

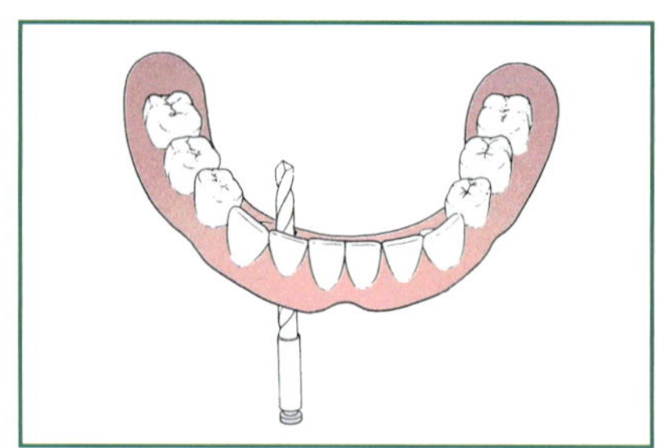

Fig 11-26 Wax positioned on the interior surface of the prosthetic body indicates the position of the ball attachments. (From Bassi F et al.[142])

Fig 11-27 The prosthetic body is drilled to correspond with the wax markings. (From Bassi F et al.[142])

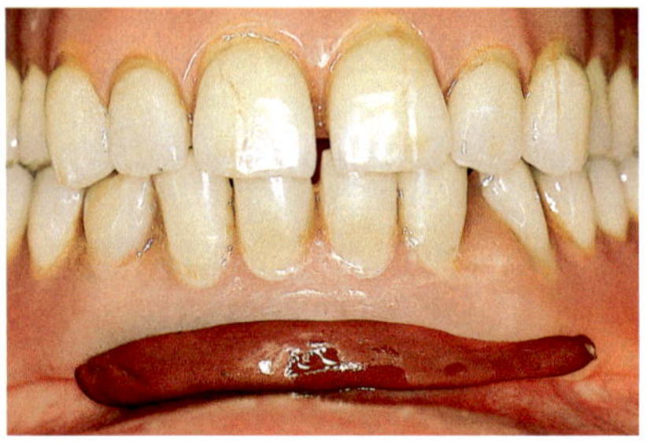

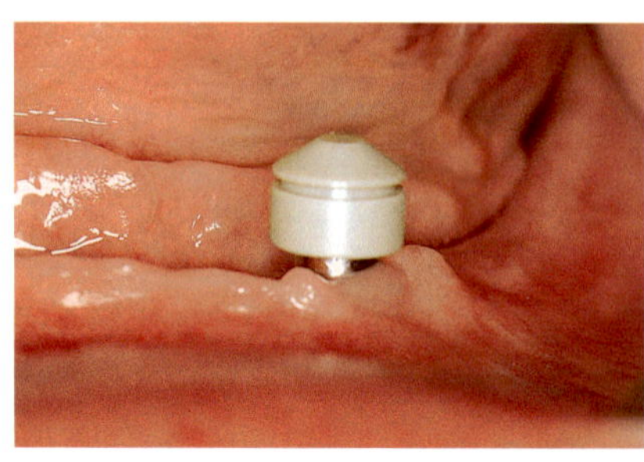

Fig 11-8 Edging with thermoplastic paste.

Fig 11-29 Retention matrix on the ball patrix.

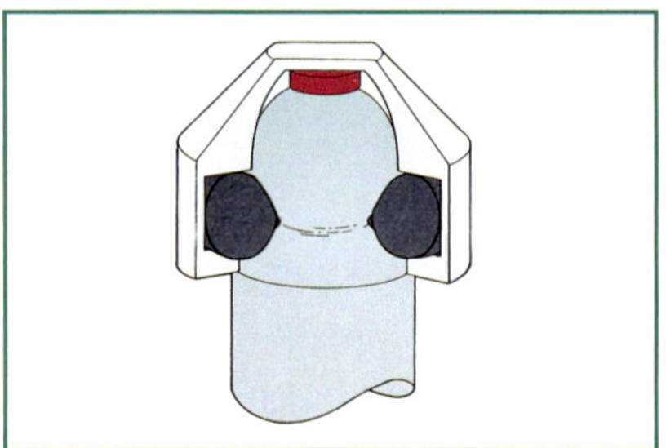

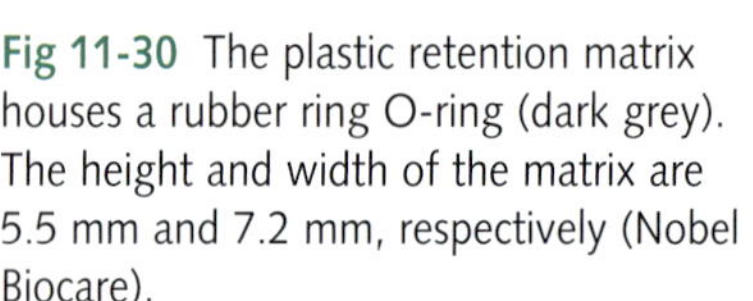

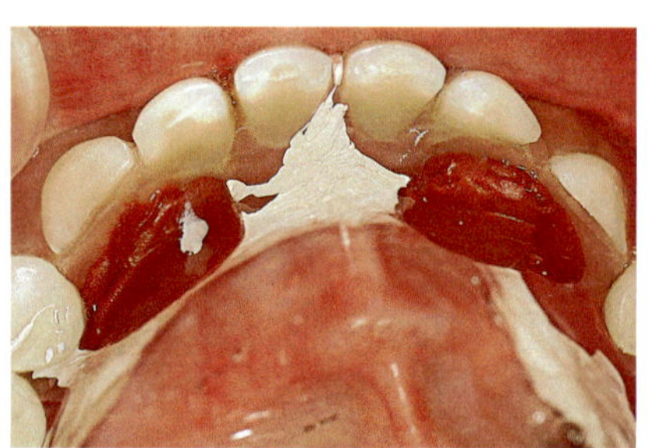

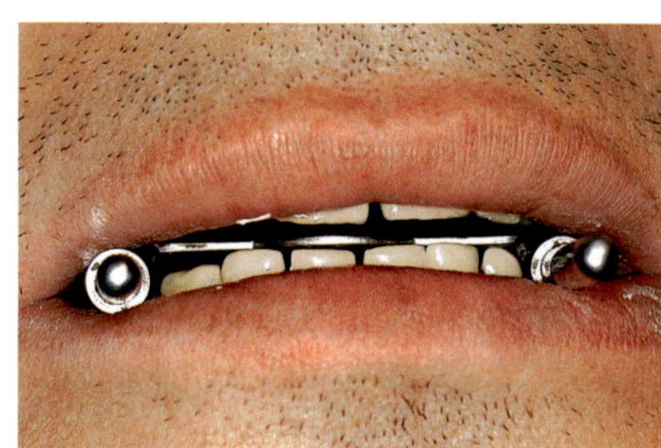

Fig 11-30 The plastic retention matrix houses a rubber ring O-ring (dark grey). The height and width of the matrix are 5.5 mm and 7.2 mm, respectively (Nobel Biocare).

Fig 11-31 Occusal view of the impression. Note the positioning of the thermoplastic paste in the perforations made in the prosthetic body to block the plastic retention matrix.

Fig 11-32 Registration of the maxillomandibular relationship using a gothic arch.

Indirect retention technique

The conditioning material is removed, and a thin layer of wax (Tenatex, KemDent) is placed inside the prosthetic body to identify the position of the ball attachments (Fig 11-26). Holes are drilled through the entire thickness of the denture in keeping with the marks left on the wax to allow for adequate lodging of the retention system (Fig 11-27). Where necessary, it can be molded with thermoplastic paste (red impression compound, Kerr) (Fig 11-28). The two matrices are positioned on the ball attachments with an inner ring of plastic (Nobel Biocare) (Figs 11-29 and 11-30).

Before taking the impression, it is necessary to confirm that the retention system is secure. Sometimes it is necessary to remove the artificial teeth from the prosthetic body to avoid interferences. A silicone index, taken before their removal, allows the teeth to be remounted in the identical position.

At the same time a zinc-eugenol impression is taken, the two plastic matrices are placed in the drilled holes and covered with red impression compound (Fig 11-31). When the impression material has hardened, the denture is removed. It is important to verify that the matrices are stable. Finally, the maxillomandibular relationships are recorded (Fig 11-32).

Laboratory phases

The analogs of the ball attachments are positioned in the matrices, blocked in the prosthetic body (Figs 11-33 and 11-34). Plaster casts are then made, and the master cast is mounted on the articulator. The analogs have small plastic spacers of

Fig 11-33 Laboratory analog of the ball matrix and patrix.

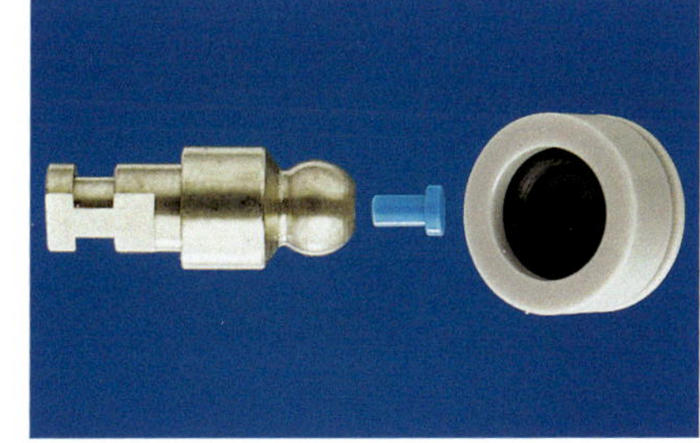

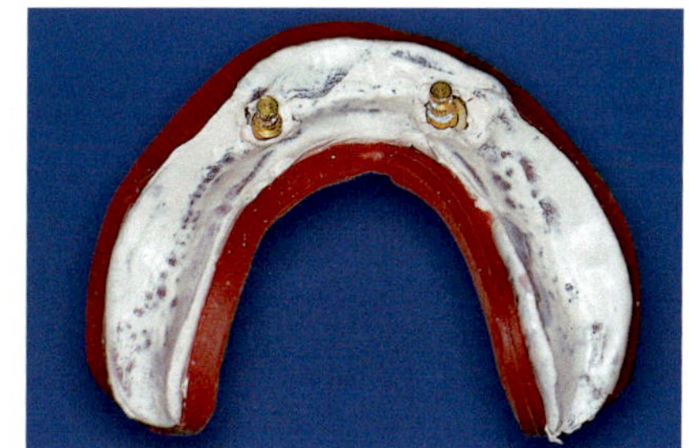

Fig 11-34 Positioning of the analog retention matrix.

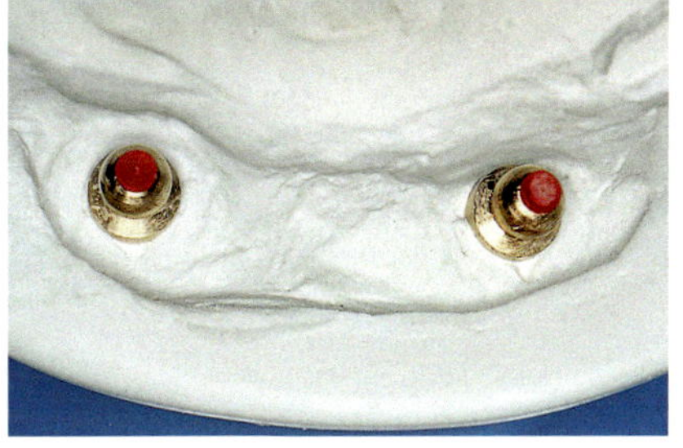

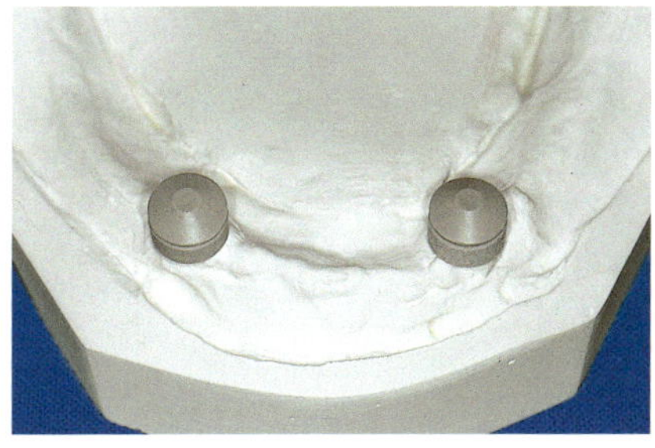

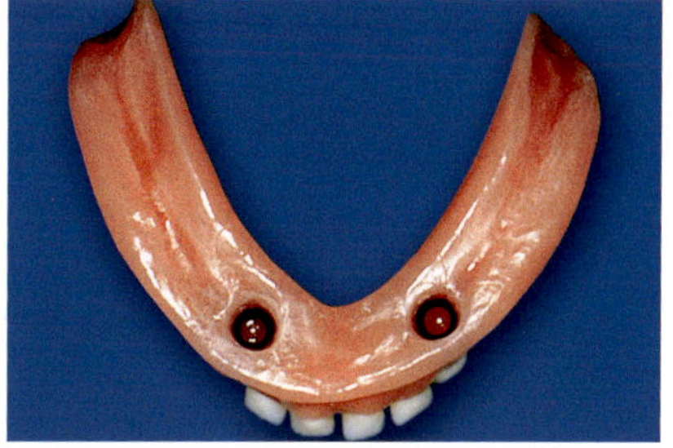

Fig 11-35 The master cast with the analog to reproduce the position of the ball attachment. Note the spacing blocks (red) that simulate the resilience of the mucosa. Spacing blocks of different colors indicate various grades of resilience.

Fig 11-36 Matrix inserted in the analog of the master cast.

Fig 11-37 Definitive prosthetic body with the retention matrix in position.

Fig 11-38 Ball attachments of smaller dimensions. Pillar heights of attachments are 3, 4, and 5.5 mm; ball diameters are 2.25 mm with a height of 2.60 mm.

Fig 11-39 Titanium retention matrix (Nobel Biocare). These matrices are removable to allow substitution with a steel ring. The external plastic spacer does not adhere to the prosthetic resin and is placed in preparation for substitution with the steel ring. In this way, a substitution can be made without removing the entire matrix from the prosthetic body.

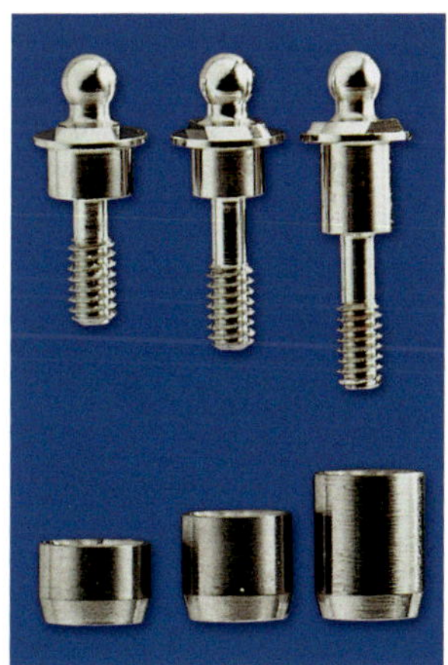

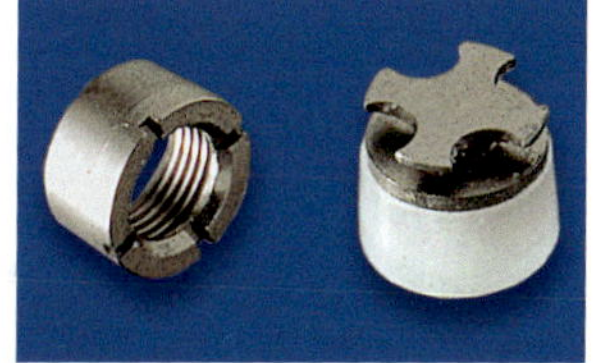

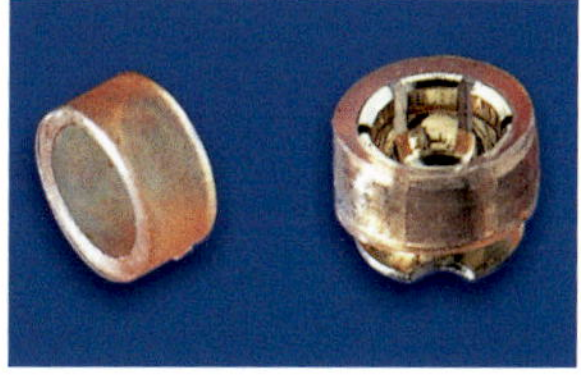

Fig 11-40 Gold retention matrix (Nobel Biocare).

different heights, which simulate the resilience of the patient's mucosa; therefore the degree of resilience dictates the proper spacer to use (Fig 11-35).

The plastic matrices are removed from the denture and inserted on the analogs (Fig 11-36). The prosthetic body is again inserted on the cast, fixing it at three points with sticky wax. The master cast, with the denture in place, is removed from the articulator for preparation and polymerization of the resin.

Once the polymerization has finished, the plastic matrices are incorporated definitively, and the prosthetic body is refined and polished. It is again placed on the articulator, the occlusion is checked, and selective grinding is carried out (Fig 11-37).

The method just described is that used most at the University of Turin. When the amount of space is reduced, a ball attachment with a diameter of 2.25 mm (Nobel Biocare) is used. The height of the prosthetic abutments remains unvaried (Fig 11-38). In this case, the retention matrices can be of two types: titanium or gold alloy (Figs 11-39 and 11-40). The clinical procedure for positioning the abutment remains the same (Figs 11-41 and 11-42). The laboratory phases are the same if the indirect method is used (Figs 11-43 and 11-44); nevertheless,

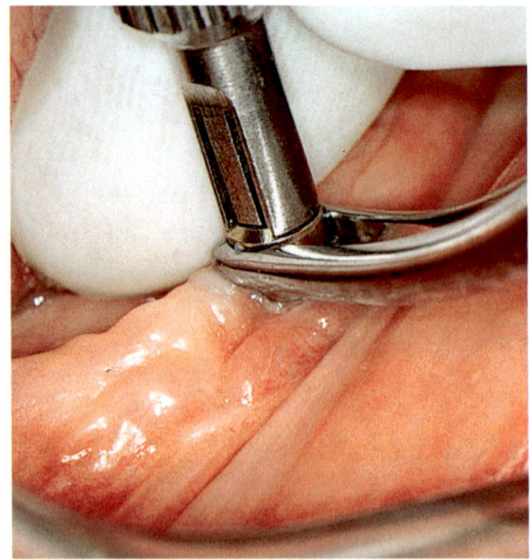

Fig 11-41 Placement of a ball attachment on the implant (Nobel Biocare).

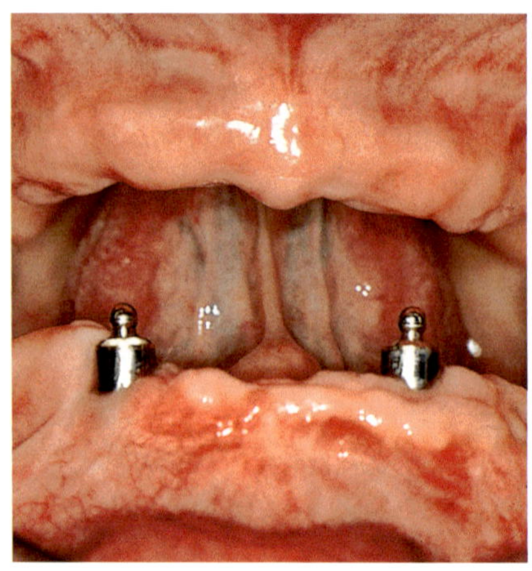

Fig 11-42 Ball attachment of 2.25 mm in situ.

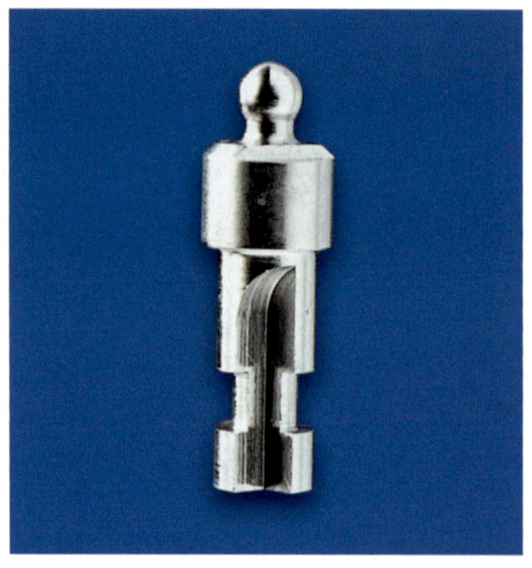

Fig 11-43 Laboratory analog of the ball attachment with a diameter of 2.25 mm.

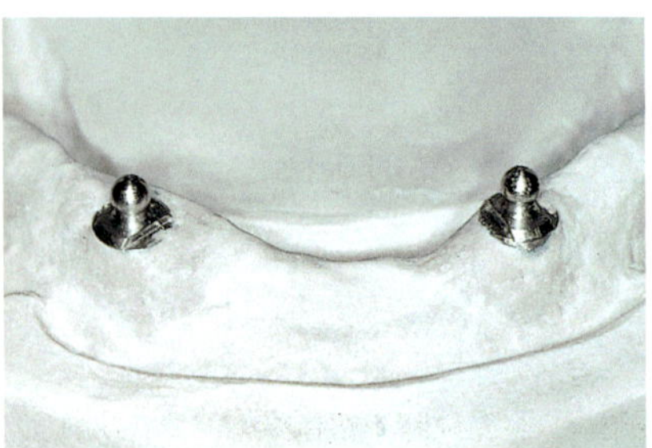

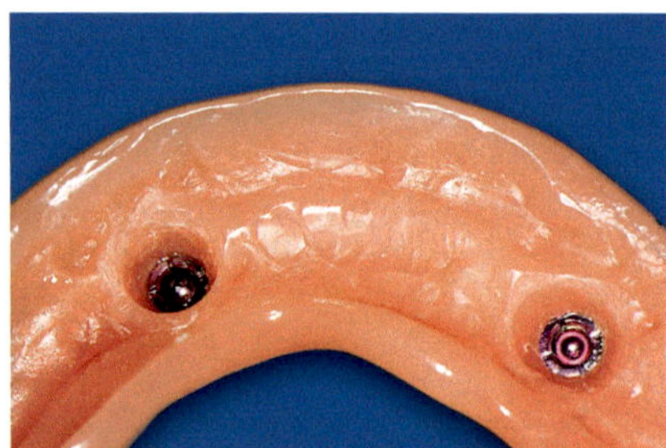

Fig 11-44 Master cast with a laboratory analog.

Fig 11-45 Prosthetic body with a titanium retention system.

the reduced dimensions of these attachments allow the retention matrices to be blocked directly in the mouth (Fig 11-45).

Peri-overdenture

The Perio-overdenture (POVD) is a variant of the overdenture, developed by Koller and Palla in 1988.[159] In this technique, a metal substructure is anchored to two osseointegrated implants that are positioned in the interforamina region using two precision ball attachments 2.25 mm in diameter.

This method is used for prosthetic rehabilitation of the edentulous mandible when: *(1)* the lingual caruncles are very close to the alveolar ridge (Fig 11-46); or *(2)* one or more implants have been placed too close to the lingual caruncles (Fig 11-47). In both cases, the flange of the conventional denture would block the ducts of the salivary glands (Fig 11-48), resulting in a stagnant pool of saliva and tumefaction in the submandibular cavity.

Clinical and laboratory phases

Figures 11-49 to 11-54 illustrate the preparation phases for impression taking. Using suitable transfers and an individual tray, the impression is made with a polyether material (Figs 11-55 to 11-57). It must cover the entire edentulous mandible and at the same time record the position of the implants (Fig 11-58).

In the laboratory the analogs are positioned, the plaster (type IV) is cast, and the master cast is obtained (Figs 11-59 and 11-60).

The correct positioning of the components is visually evaluated (Fig 11-61), and the prosthetic abutments are then screwed into the implant analogs (Fig 11-62).

The impression-taking technique and the master cast preparation described above achieve greater precision in transferring the position of the head of the implants, direct control of the positioning of the various components during the laboratory phases, the possibility of preparing in conditions identical to those of the mouth, and locking of the retention matrices in the metal substructure in the laboratory.

It is, however, possible to take the impression of the ball attachments directly in the mouth of the patient, using a plastic

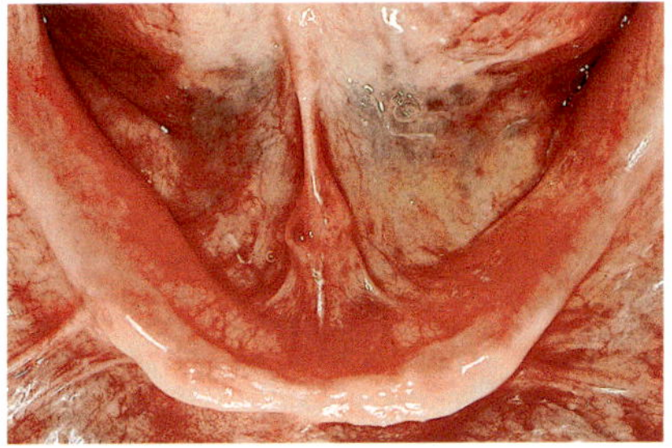

Fig 11-46 In this edentulous patient, the distance that separates the lingual caruncle from the mandibular bone is minimal.

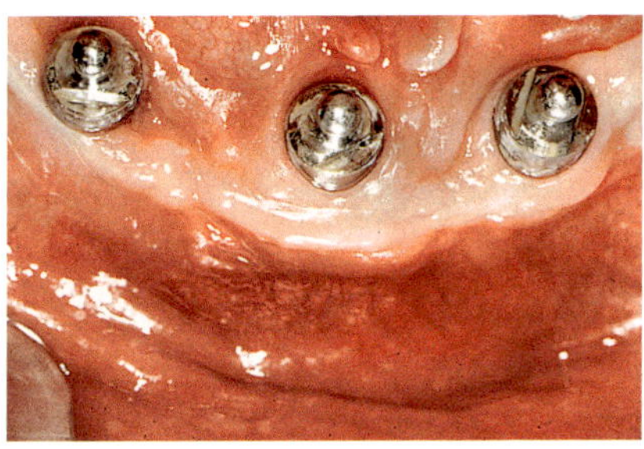

Fig 11-47 Implant positioned behind the lingual caruncle.

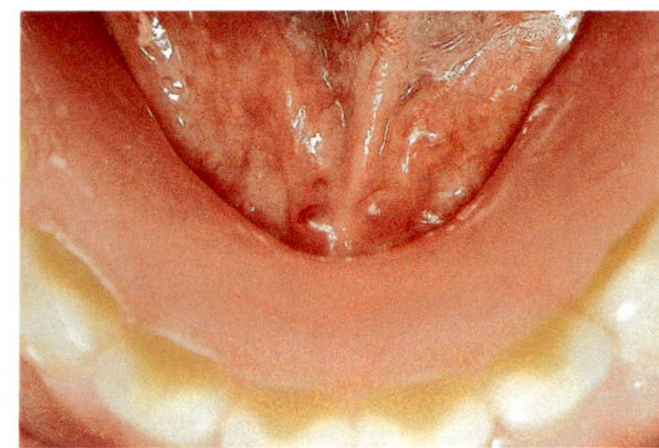

Fig 11-48 Complete mandibular prosthesis in situ. Note that the lingual area of the prosthetic flange compresses the outlet of the submandibular and sublingual secretory ducts of the salivary glands. To avoid this interference, the anterior portion of the lingual flange must be removed.

Fig 11-49 Clinical view of the edentulous mandible before the stage-two surgery.

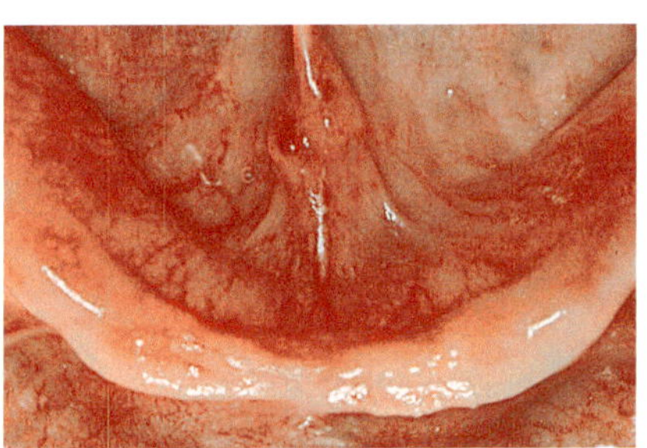

Fig 11-50 Healing abutments 4 weeks after the stage-two surgery.

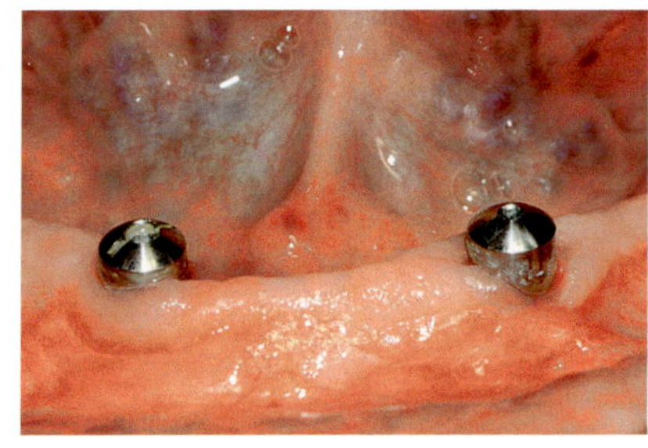

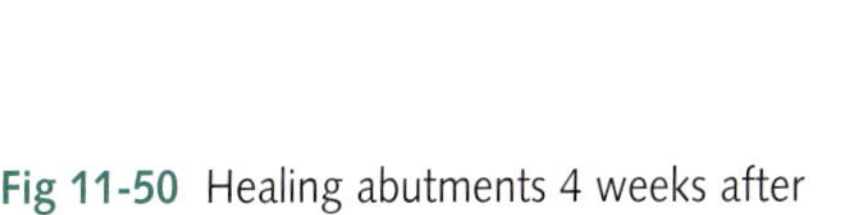

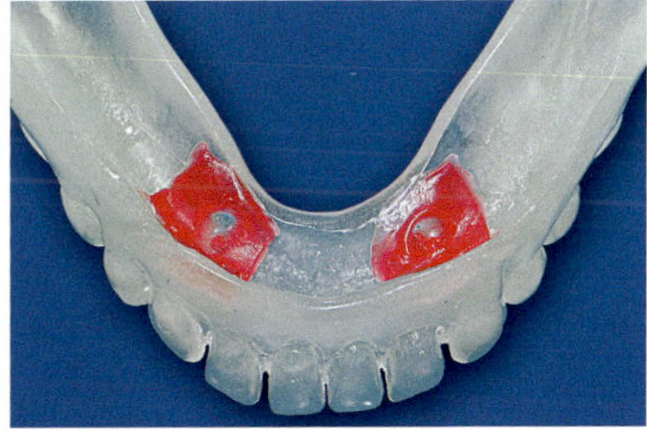

Fig 11-51 Duplicate of the complete denture in transparent resin. This will be used as a preimplant radiologic guide, a surgical guide for positioning the implants, a custom impression tray, and for registation of the maxillomandibular relationships for the mounting into the articulator.

Fig 11-52 Wax is placed on the duplicate to register the positions of the healing abutments.

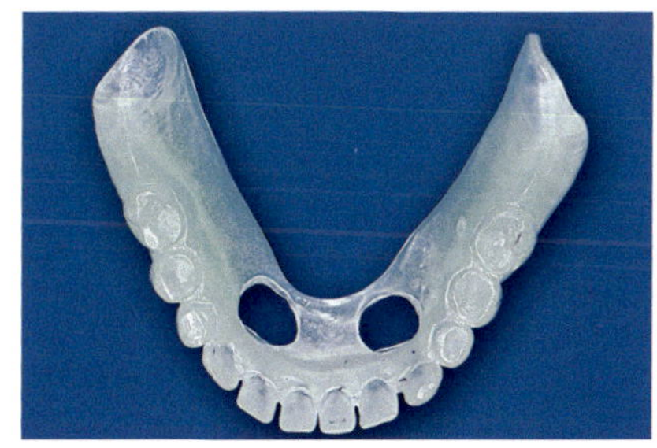

Fig 11-53 Holes are drilled to correspond to the wax positions.

Fig 11-54 (*a and b*) Measuring the transmucosal path to help select the appropriate height of the prosthetic abutments.

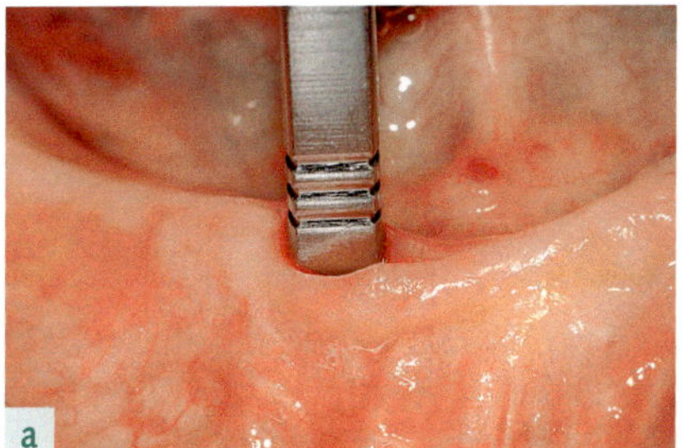

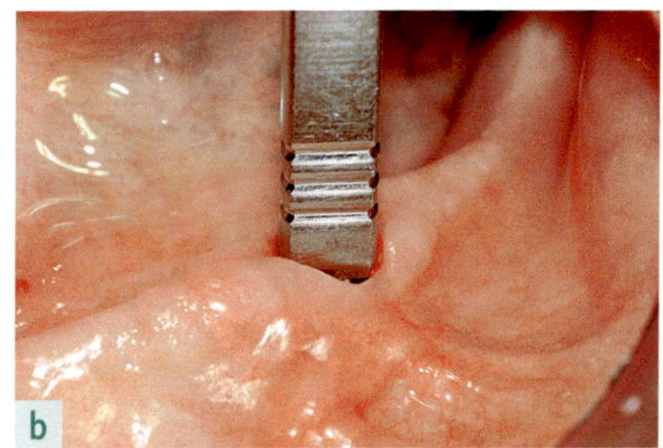

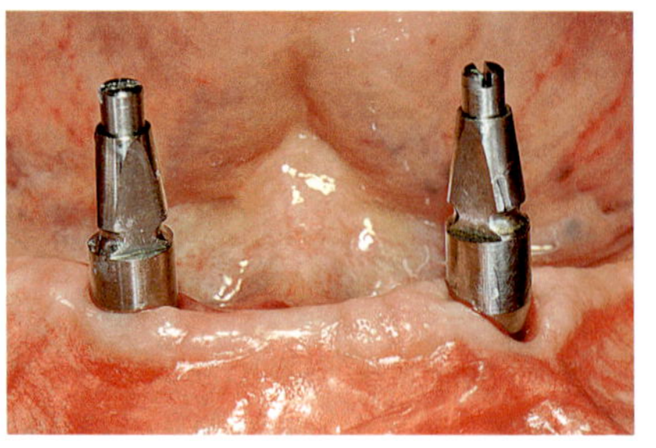

Fig 11-55 Transfer abutment (Nobel Biocare) in place to register on the impression.

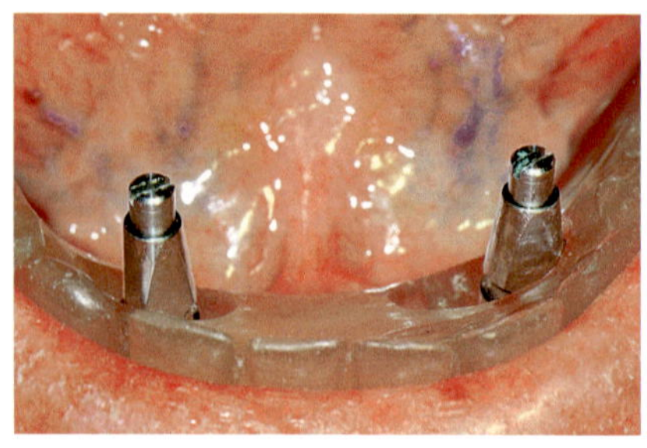

Fig 11-56 The position in the oral cavity is evaluated for interference with the transfer abutment.

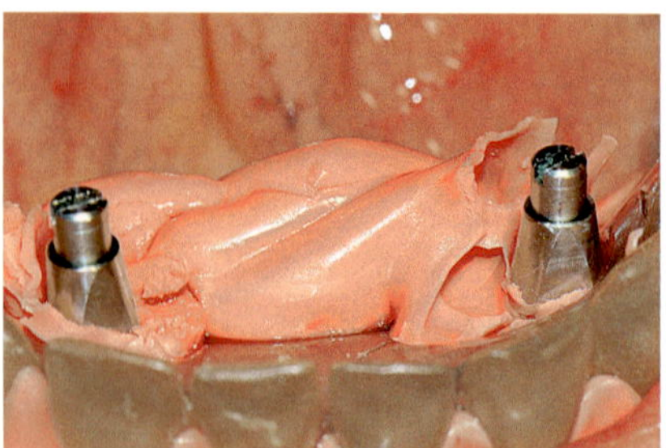

Fig 11-57 Taking an impression using polyether of medium consistency. The trophic properties and precision and degree of rigidity of this material helps to guarantee correct positioning. After hardening, the impression material is unscrewed and then moved to the duplicate.

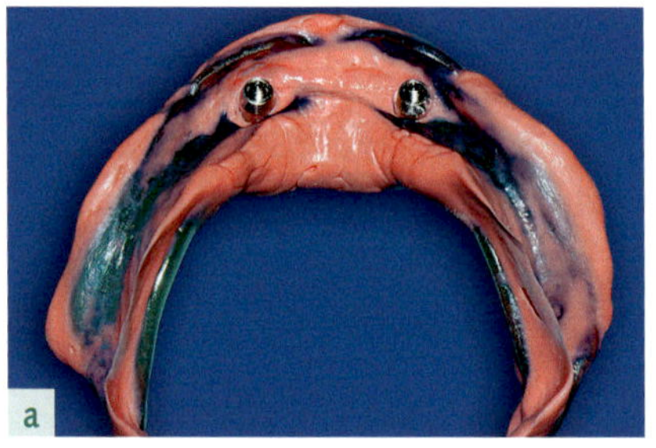

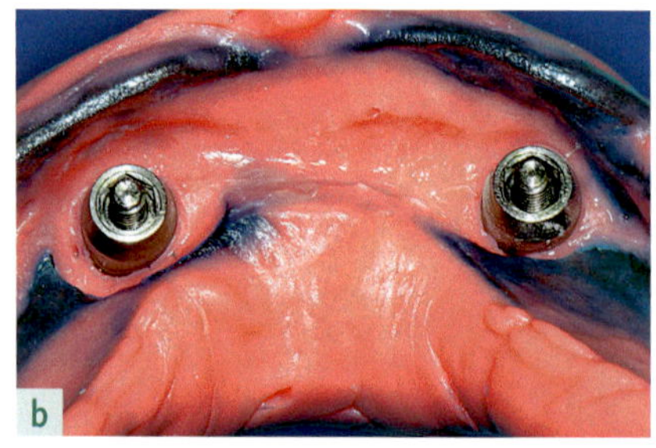

Fig 11-58 *(a)* The impression. *(b)* Details of the transfer position. The impression material moves mostly to the anterior area where stage-one and stage-two surgeries were done.

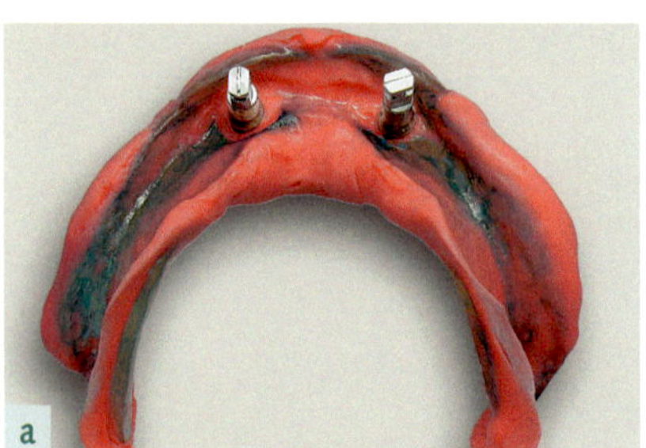

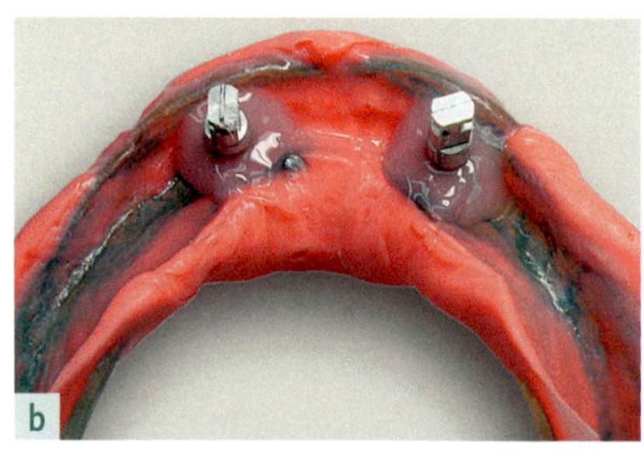

Fig 11-59 *(a)* Laboratory analog of the implants positioned in the impression. *(b)* Soft pliable silicone resembles the soft tissues of the peri-implant.

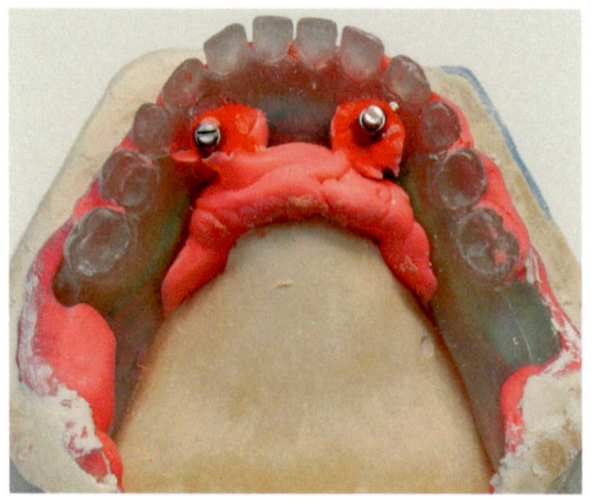

Fig 11-60 Master cast with type IV plaster.

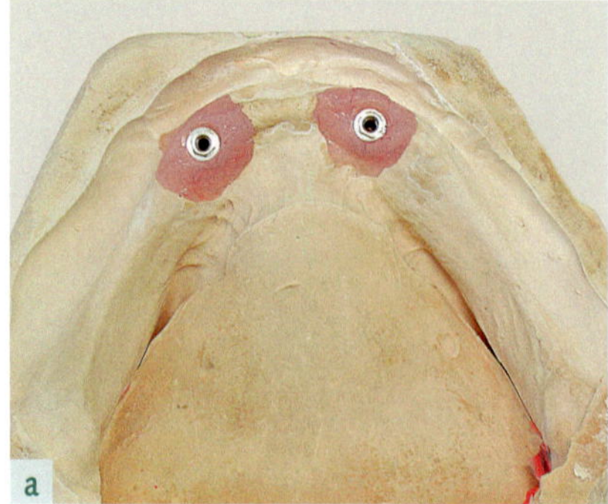

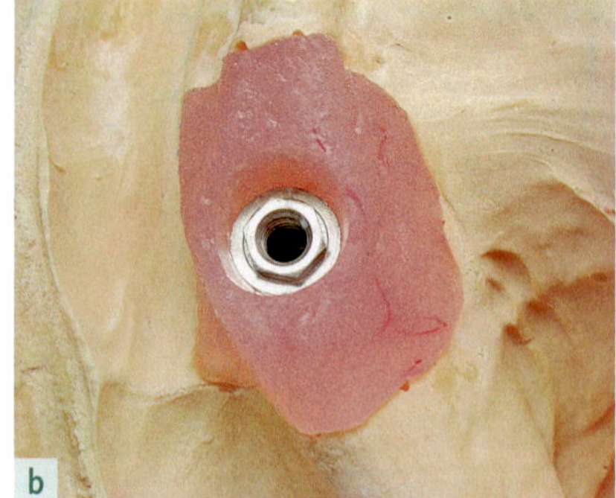

Fig 11-61 *(a)* Master cast after the removal of the impression. *(b)* Detail of the implant head with artificial mucosa in pliable silicone. By removing the artificial mucosa during the last phase of the work, it is possible to evaluate the correct positioning of the components.

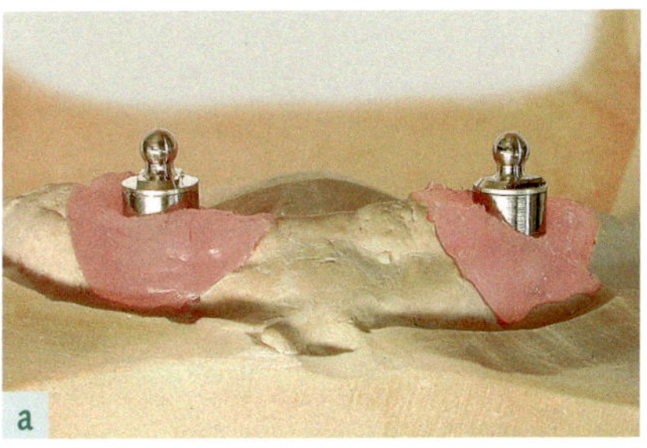 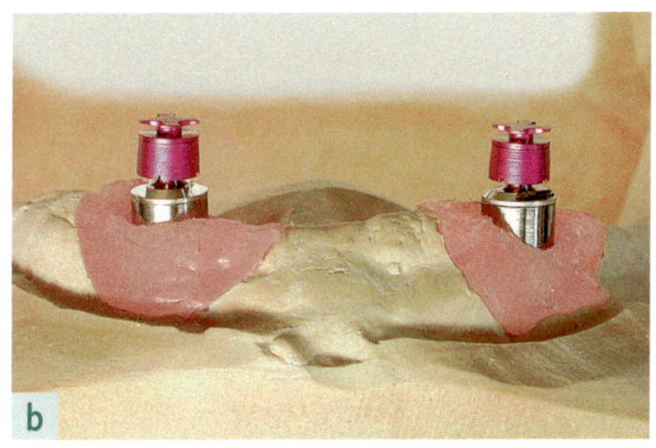 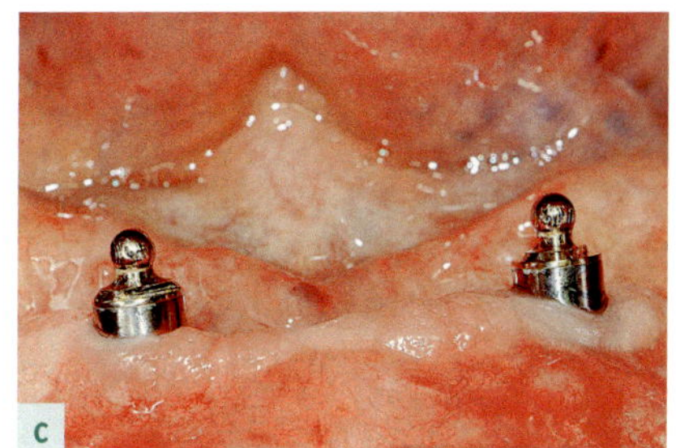

Fig 11-62 Ball attachments with a diameter of 2.25 mm *(a)* on the cast and *(b)* with the retention matrix. *(c)* The ball attachments must be positioned at the same height in the oral cavity.

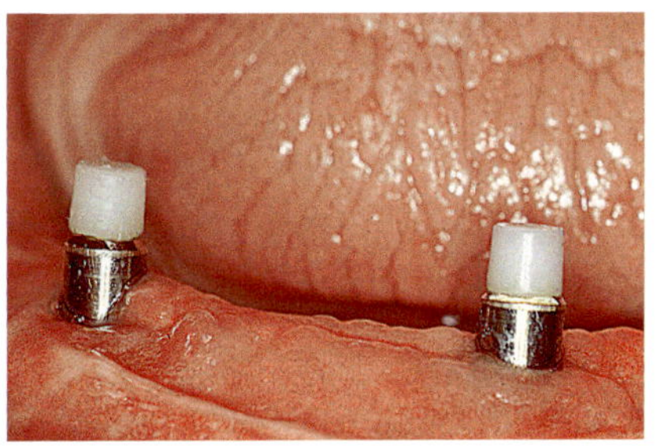 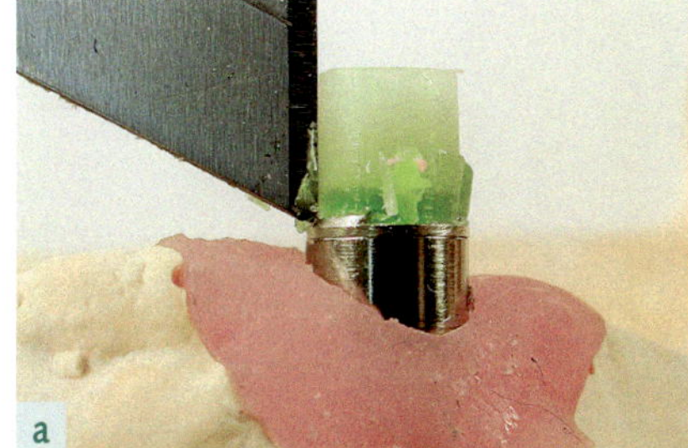 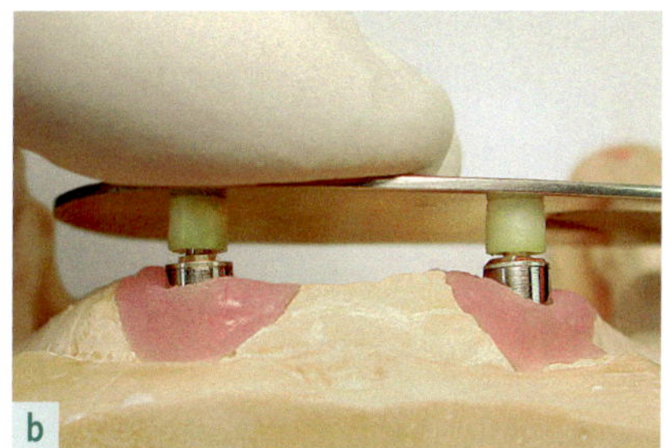

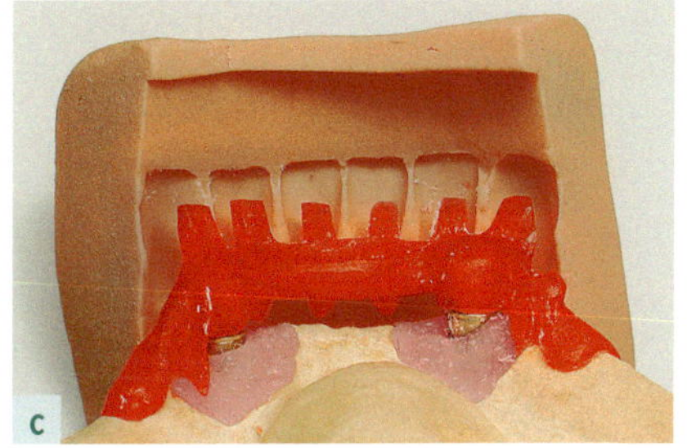 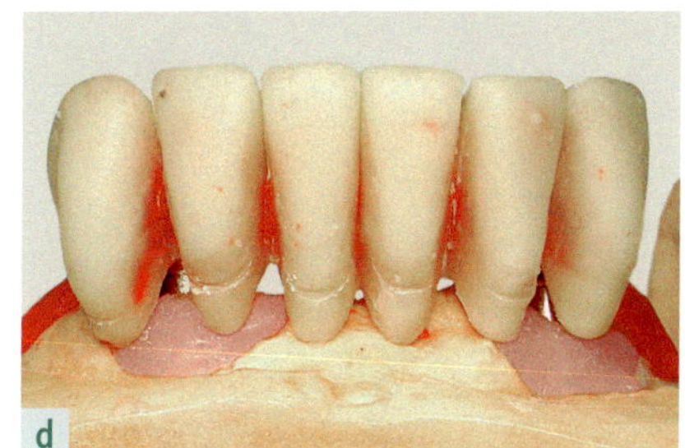

Fig 11-63 Plastic retention matrix used for recording the position of the ball patrix in an impression.

Fig 11-64 *(a and b)* Waxing the attachment patrix. *(c)* Modeling the incisive and canine teeth. their position is dictated by the silicone guide made on the transparent resin guide. *(d)* The cast is made comprising the implant abutments.

transfer, an individual impression tray, and polyether material (Fig 11-63). This technique allows for the maintenance of the ball attachments in the oral cavity once positioned.

When the master cast has been obtained, the following steps are taken:

- Modeling of the teeth in wax from one abutment to the other (Fig 11-64)
- Elimination of the undercuts from the cast (Fig 11-65)
- Duplication of the master cast in refractory material (Fig 11-66)

The previously prepared waxup of the teeth can be adapted to the refractory cast and finished by waxing up the secondary connectors for the resin (Fig 11-67).

The waxup of the incisors and canines is not carried out on the refractory cast but on the plaster master cast mounted on the articulator, to evaluate the available space and the maxillomandibular relationships.

The substructure of the POVD is then cast (Fig 11-68), removed from the refractory cast, finished, polished, and adapted to the master cast. Finally, the matrices are positioned and locked with resin or composite cement (Fig 11-69).

The substructure is tried in the mouth, the anterior, esthetic portion is created, and the posterior teeth are mounted (Figs 11-70 and 11-71). If there is sufficient anterior space, the waxup of the teeth can be avoided and commercial teeth can be used (Fig 11-72).

Rehabilitation by means of a POVD offers greater comfort for the patients, makes hygiene easier, and offers esthetic advantages. Nevertheless, compared with the overdenture, the costs are greater, and the time needed is longer (Figs 11-73 and 11-74).

139

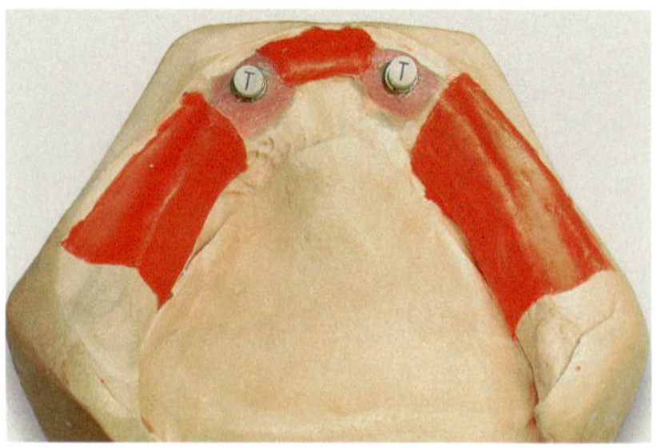

Fig 11-65 Wax calibrator for eliminating the undercuts on the master cast.

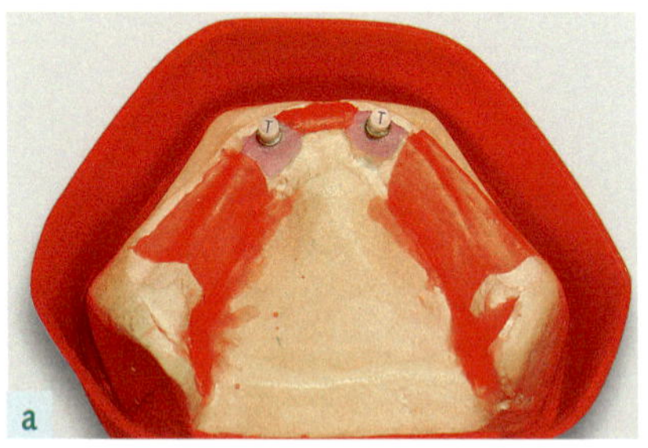
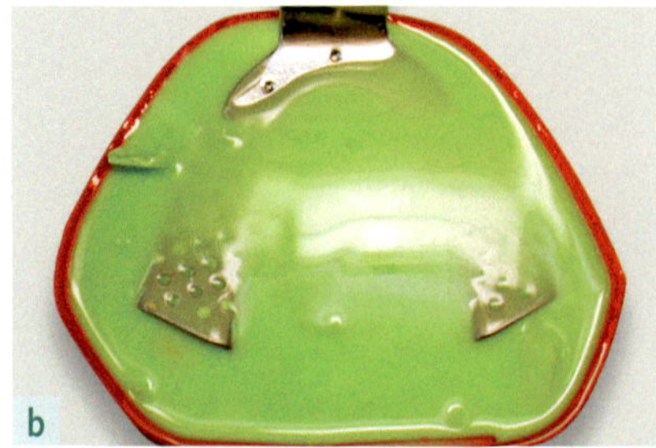
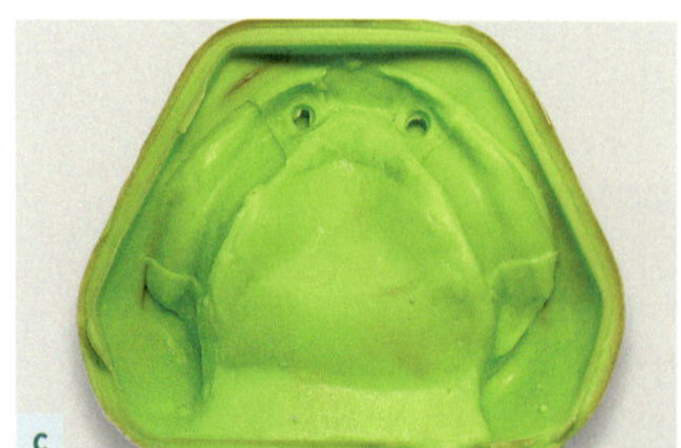

Fig 11-66 *(a to c)* Phases of the duplication of the master cast in refractory material.

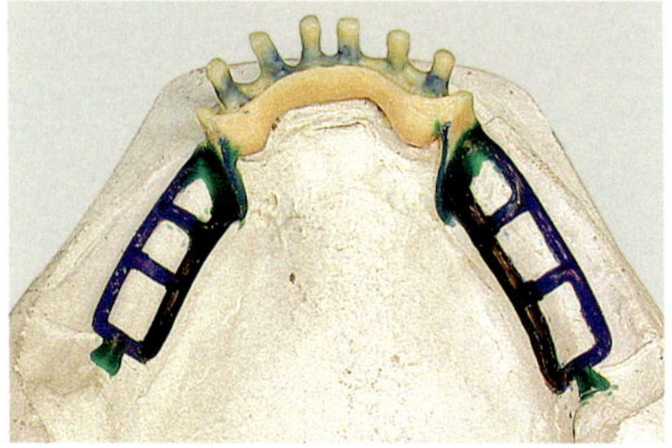
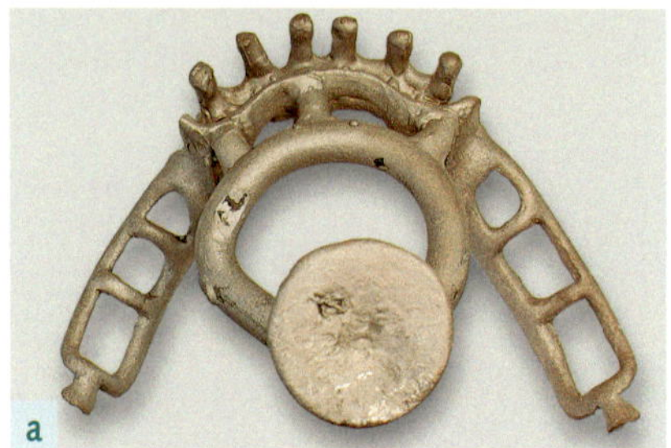

Fig 11-67 Refractory cast with the adjusted waxup of the incisors and canines and the secondary connectors.

Fig 11-68 The metal substructure. *(a)* Occlusal view; *(b)* interior view.

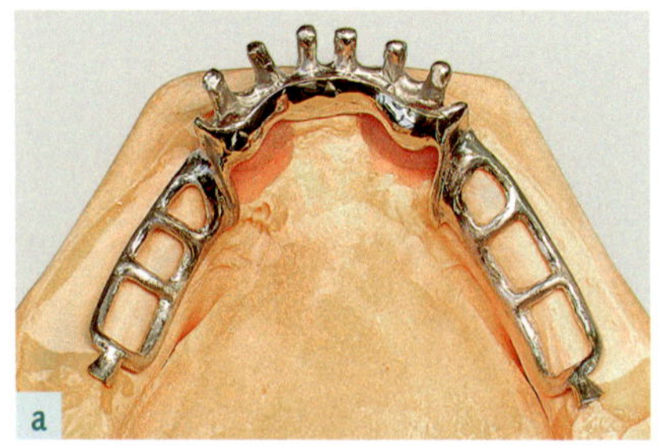
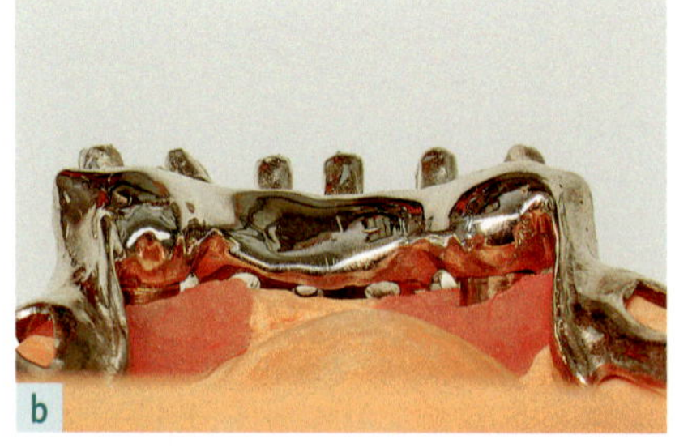
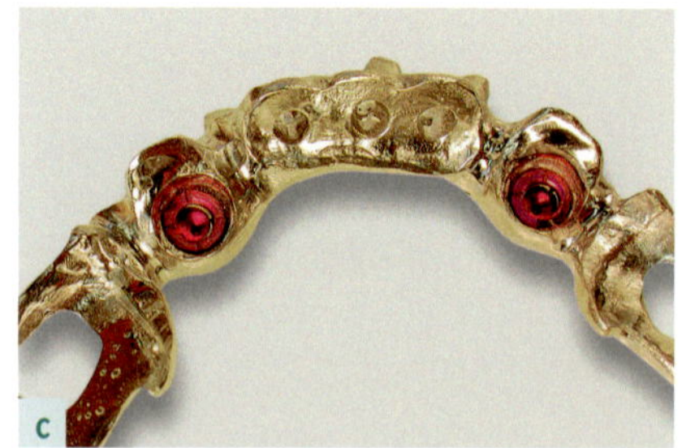

Fig 11-69 *(a)* Completed POVD in chromium-cobalt. *(b)* Details of anterior section. *(c)* Definitive position of the matrix in the frame.

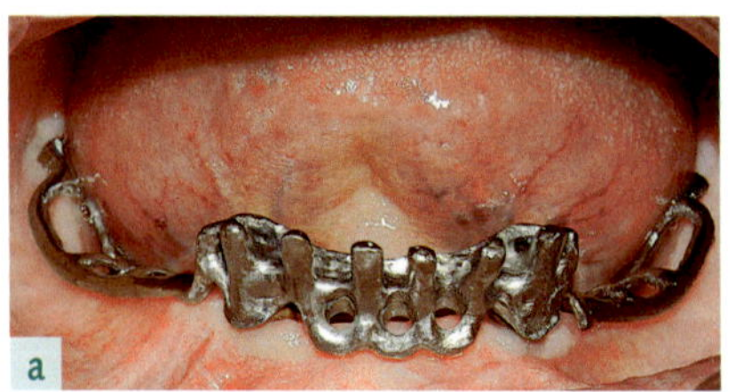
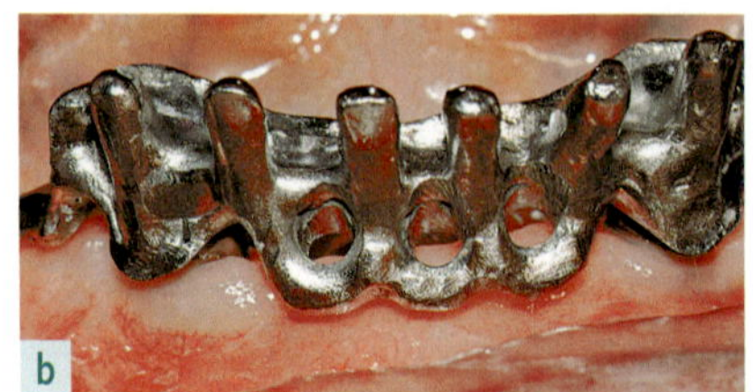
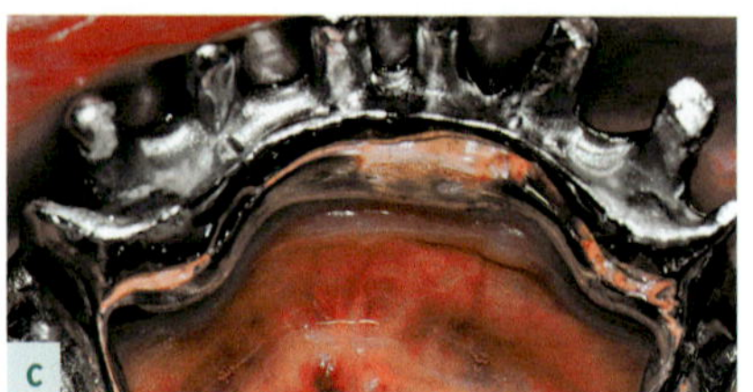

Fig 11-70 *(a)* Clinical try-in. The framework is about 1 mm from the abutment. *(b)* Detail of anterior section; *(c)* lingual view.

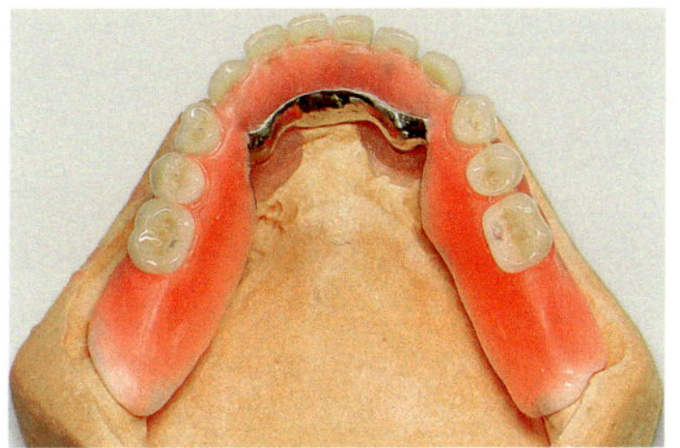
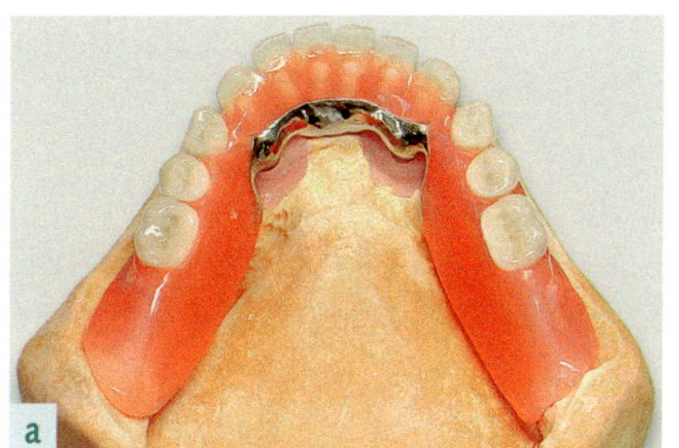
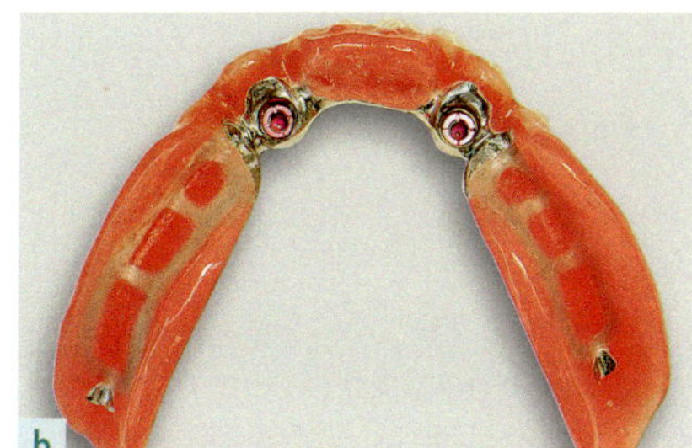

Fig 11-71 Master cast with the prosthetic body.

Fig 11-72 POVD *(a)* covered in resin; *(b)* view of interior surface; *(c)* palatal view of anterior section; *(d)* labial view of anterior section. The resin flange is only in the buccal region for anchorage of the incisors and canines.

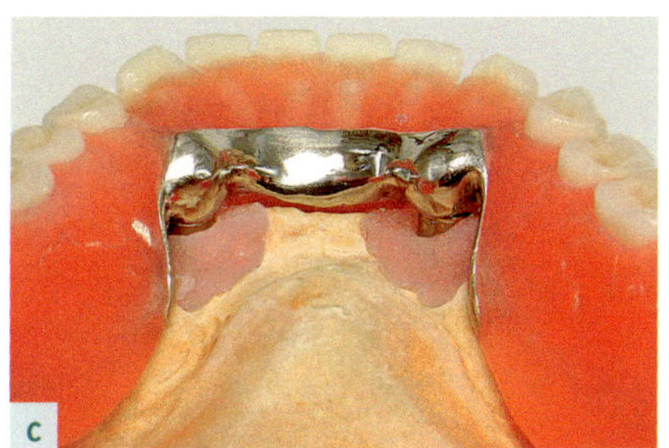
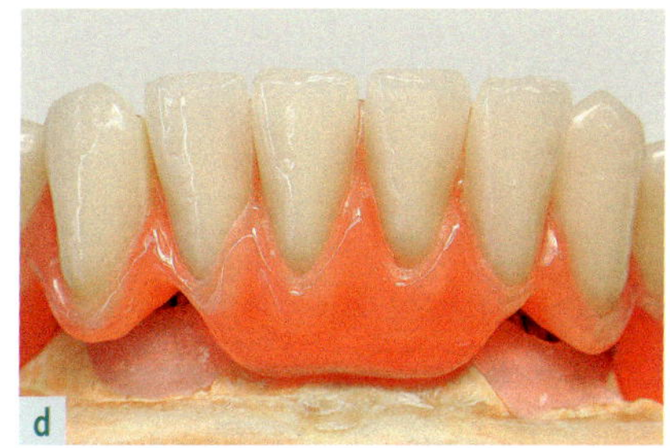

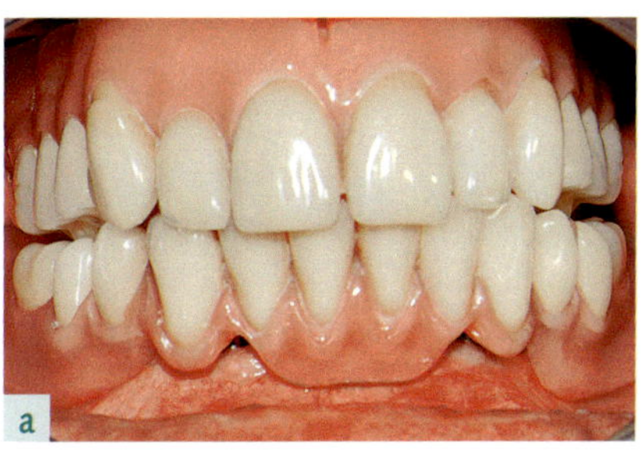
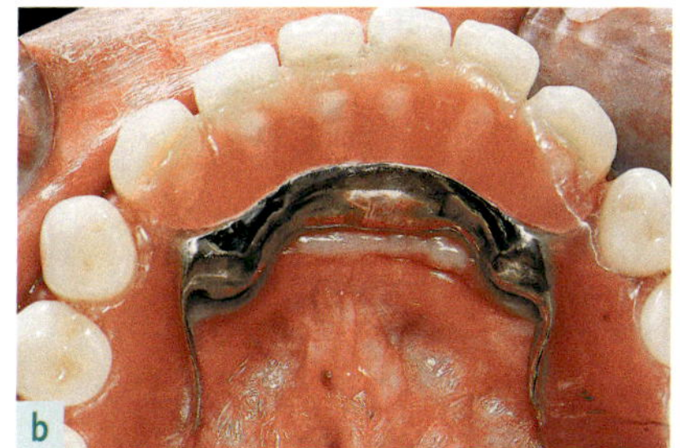

Fig 11-73 Completed POVD in situ: *(a)* frontal view; *(b)* lingual view. View of the same case with an overdenture: *(c)* frontal view; *(d)* lingual view.

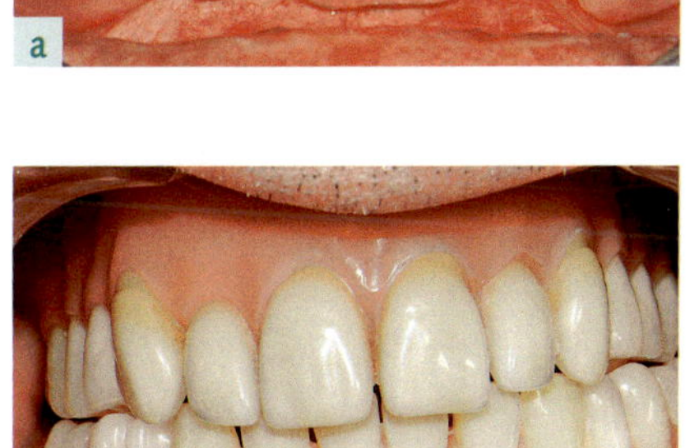
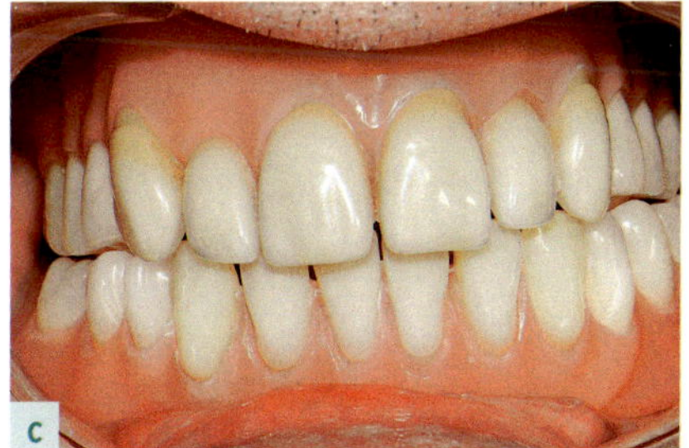
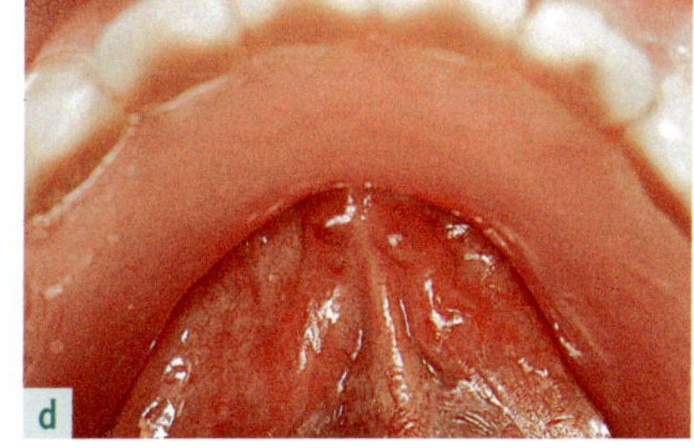

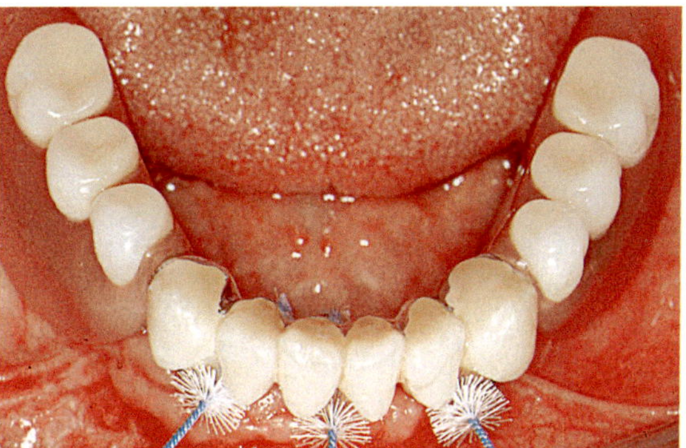

Fig 11-74 POVD. The morphology of the anterior part of the prosthesis permits optimal cleaning of the implant abutment.

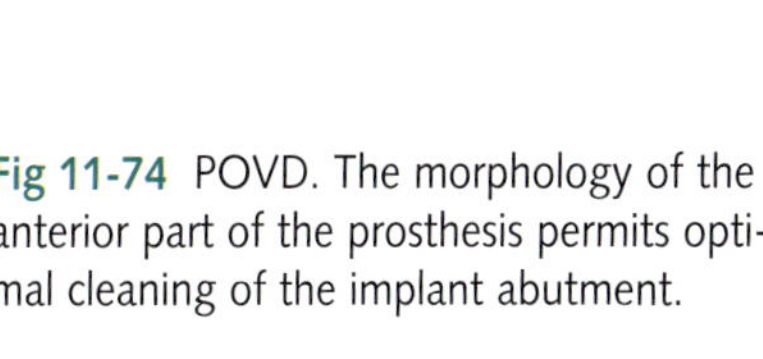

Maxillary Implant-Retained Overdenture

Implant-supported prosthetic rehabilitation of the edentulous maxilla requires a more complex surgical and prosthetic procedure than the edentulous mandible. The indications for a maxillary implant-retained overdenture are the impossibility of stabilizing the denture, an irrepressible gag reflex, and prevention of the Kelly syndrome.

Instability of the denture

Instability of the maxillary denture can be due to biologic, functional, and anatomic causes.

Biologic causes

Decrease or absence of the salival flow can be caused by pharmacologic[160] or radiation[161] therapy.

Functional causes

Reduction of neuromuscular control is characteristic of older patients.[162]

Anatomic causes

Greatly resorbed alveolar ridges, exostoses, or voluminous lingual tori may cause instability. In the latter case, anchoring the denture to implants allows reduction of the prosthetic body to avoid interference caused by these osseous formations.[163,164]

Irrepressible gag reflex

Anchoring the complete denture to implants allows elimination of the lingual portion of the prosthetic body, which induces the gag reflex.[165]

Prevention of the Kelly syndrome

In 1972, having observed complete maxillary denture wearers with natural opposing teeth in the anterior region, Kelly[166] described a syndrome characterized by resorption of the anterior maxilla, hypertrophy of the maxillary tuberosities, and marked resorption of the mandibular edentulous ridges. Generally the patient is unaware of any anterior maxillary pain because of compression of the vascular-nervous bundle. Other authors observed the same syndrome in patients who had a complete maxillary denture with an opposing implant-retained denture.[167–169] Anchoring the complete maxillary denture to implants can prevent this phenomenon.[168,169]

Rehabilitation protocol

For the maxilla, the integration of implant techniques with the protocol for complete conventional dentures has given life to different rehabilitation methods.[100,111] Because the osseous quality of the maxilla is inferior to that of the mandible, the denture should be anchored to more than two implants rigidly splinted to each other by means of a bar.[170] The operative protocol is more complex in cases in which there is marked resorption of the maxilla.

Misch and Judy[171] identified four classes of osseous morphology on which a surgical and prosthetic treatment plan can be based[172] (Box 11-2). Based on this system, classes A and B can be rehabilitated by means of a bar-retained overdenture supported by four implants.[126] Figures 11-75 to 11-97 show the rehabilitation stages of an edentulous maxilla with class A resorption, with an implant-supported overdenture.

In cases of serious atrophy of the posterior maxilla, Brånemark[1] proposed, as an alternative to bone grafts, fixed rehabilitation using zygomatic implants assisted by at least two implants positioned in the anterior maxilla. Zygomatic implants are threaded and vary from 30 to 55 mm in length. The implants are inserted in the zygomatic bone, passing through the maxillary sinus and emerging in the oral cavity at about the level of the first molar. The follow-up after 10 years shows a success rate of 97% (164 implants in 81 patients).

The zygomatic implant tends to bow easily under transverse loads. This behavior is due to the length and the reduced surface in contact with bone (the implant is inserted only at the two extremities in the alveolar ridge and in the zygomatic bone, crossing the maxillary sinus). For this reason the zygomatic implants must be joined to at least two standard implants in the anterior region.

It is important to remember that the zygomatic implants emerge in the first molar area in a more palatal position compared with traditional implants. These are indicated in Misch class C, characterized by a posterior atrophic alveolar ridge and a volume of anterior bone adequate for placing traditional

Box 11-2 Classification of osseous morphology according to the height and thickness of the edentulous crest

	Thickness	Height
Class A	> 5 mm	> 10 to 13 mm
Class B	2.5 – 5 mm	> 10 to 13 mm
Class C	< 2.5 mm	< 10 mm
Class D	Severe atrophy	

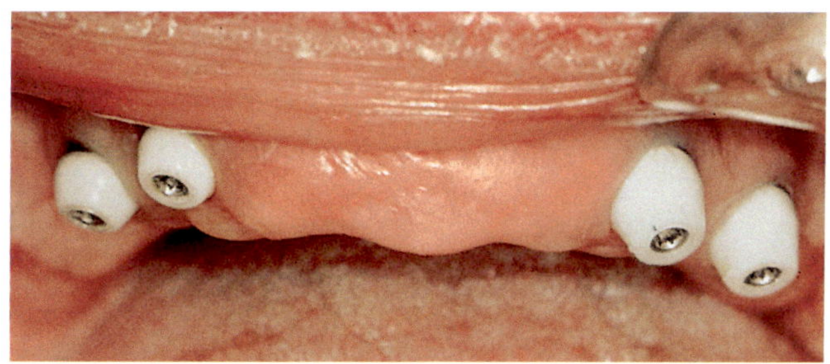

Fig 11-75 Maxilla after placement of implants in the maxillary left and right canine and first premolar sites. The plastic caps protect the implant abutments and will be removed for the taking the impression.

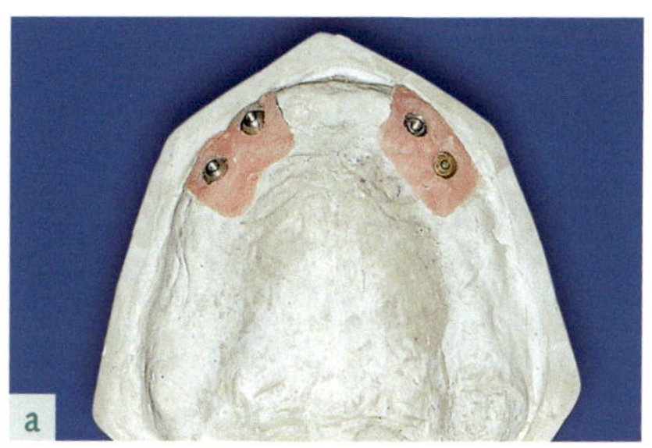

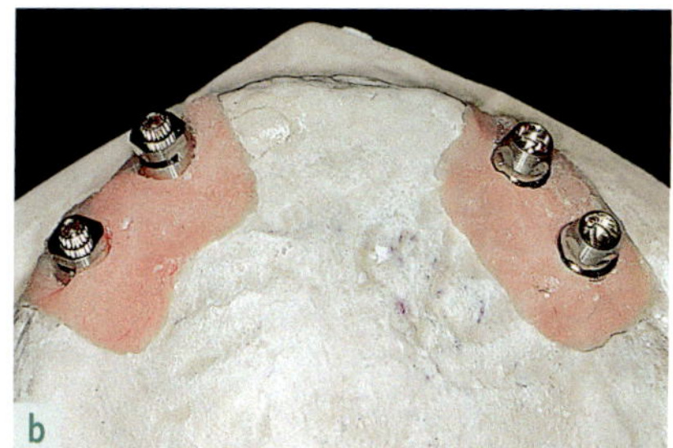

Fig 11-76 Master cast with analog of the prosthetic abutments. *(a)* The guide in pliable silicone simulates the peri-implant soft tissues. *(b)* Details of the gold cylinders positioned on the prosthetic abutment analogs.

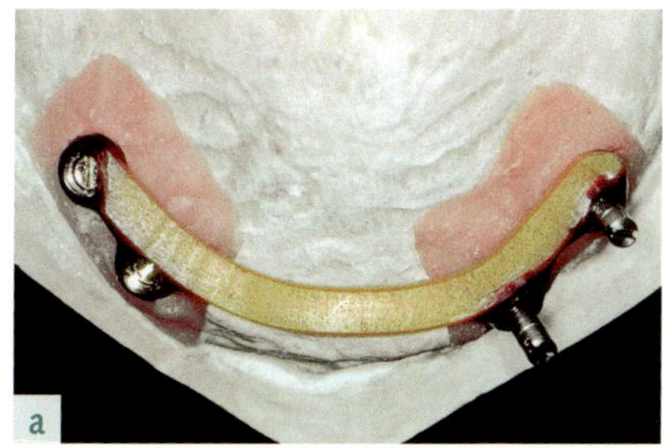

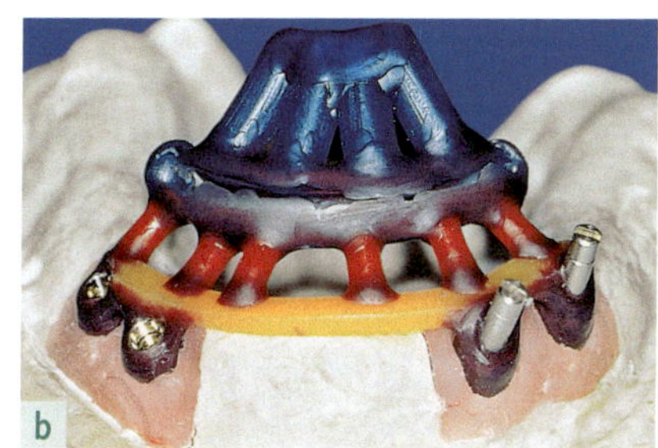

Fig 11-77 *(a)* Waxup of the bar on the master cast. *(b)* Details of the casting pins.

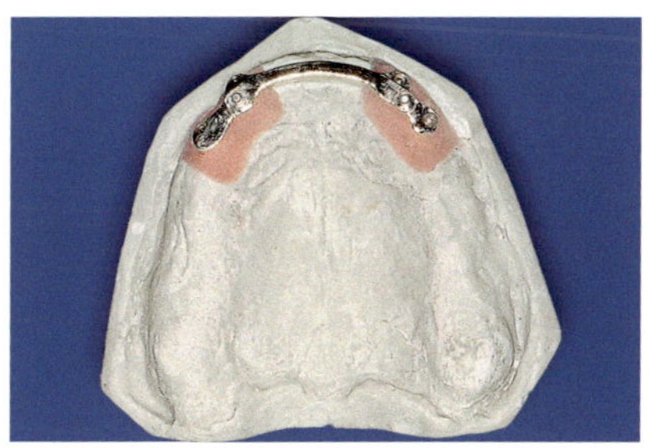

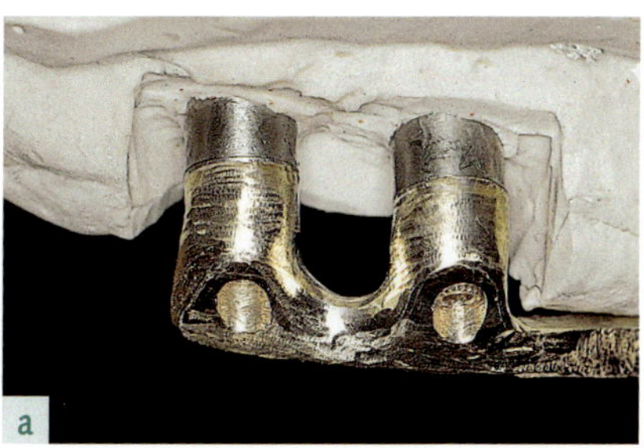

Fig 11-78 Master cast with the completed bar.

Fig 11-79 *(a and b)* Detail of the the bar attachment.

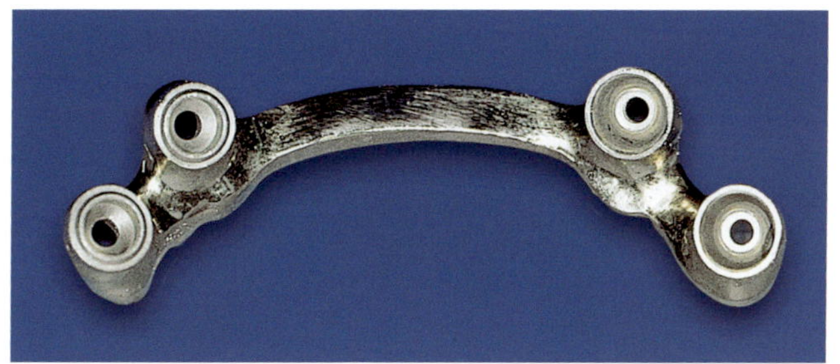

Fig 11-80 Bar before polishing; the gold cylinders have been included in the cast structure.

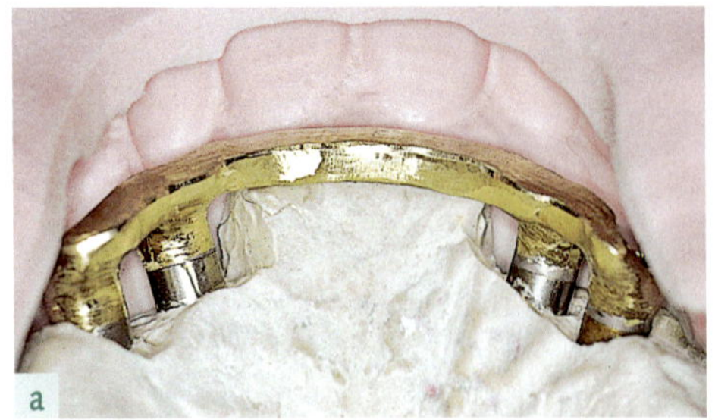
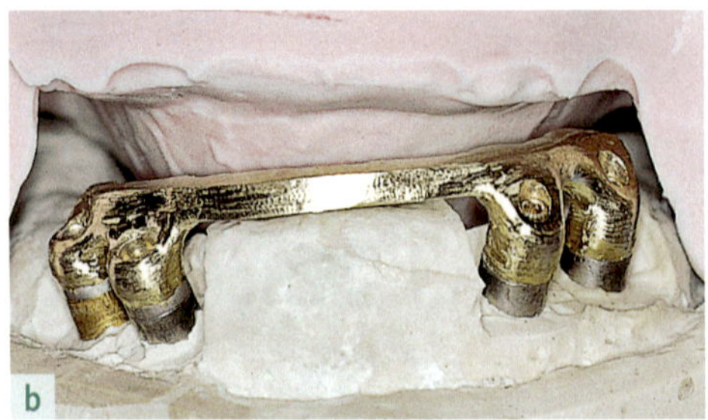

Fig 11-81 Evaluation of the (a) horizontal plane and the (b) vertical plane using the silicone guide constructed on the prosthesis.

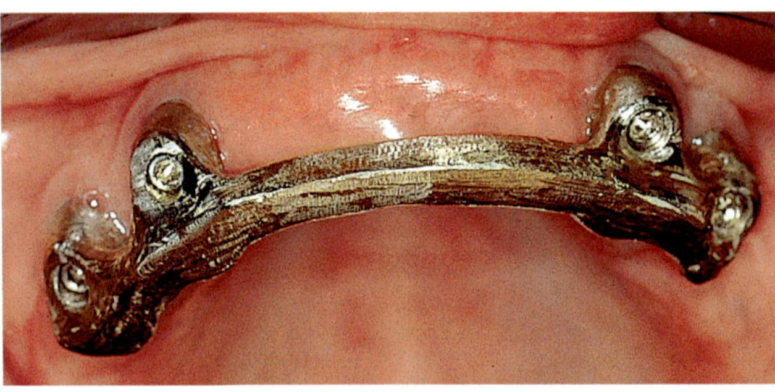

Fig 11-82 Clinical try-in of the bar.

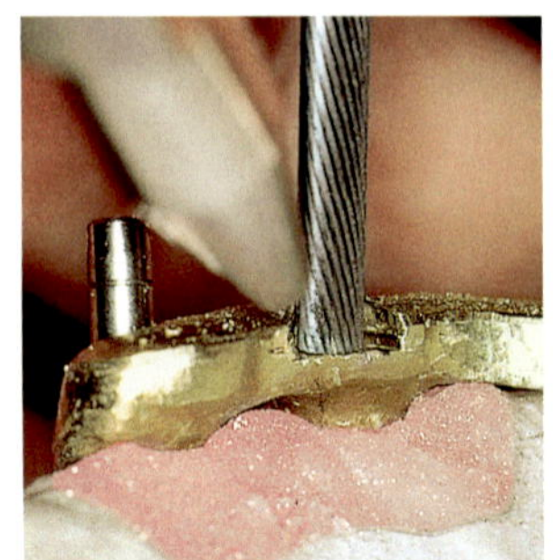

Fig 11-83 Milling the base of the cylindrical attachment.

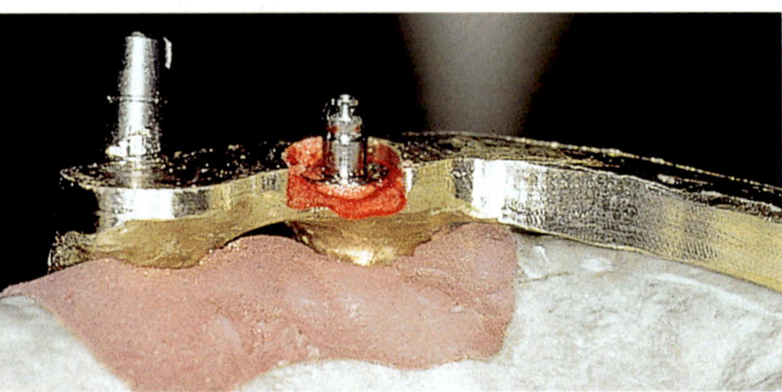
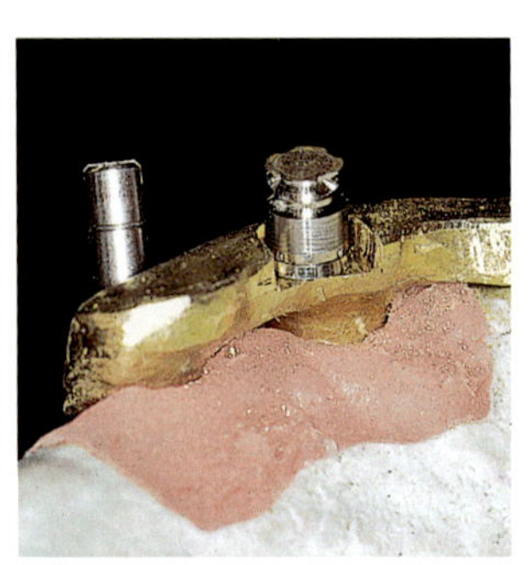
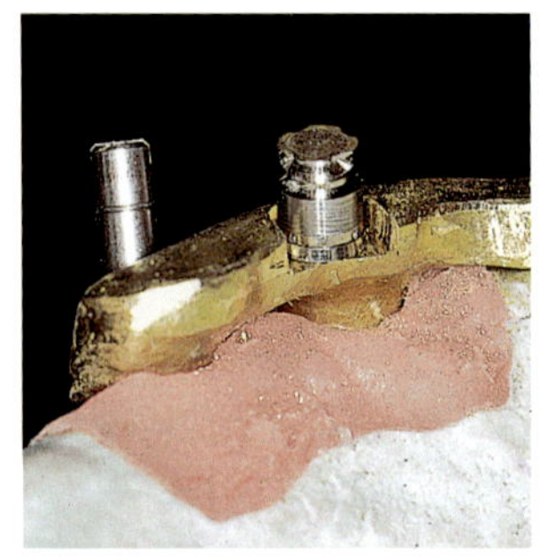

Fig 11-84 Cylindrical attachment blocked with self-polymerizing resin before soldering.

Fig 11-85 Retention matrix positioned on the cylindrical connection.

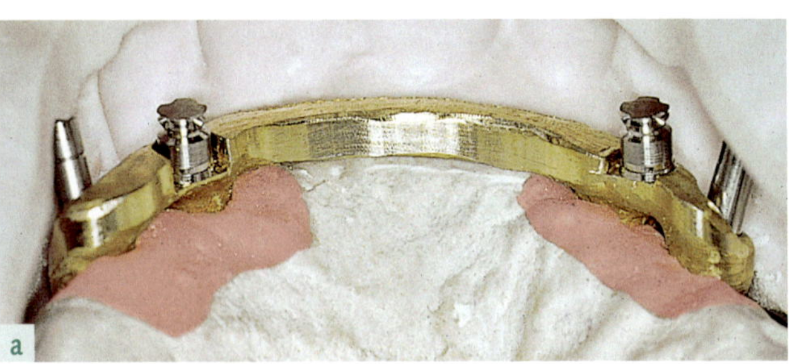
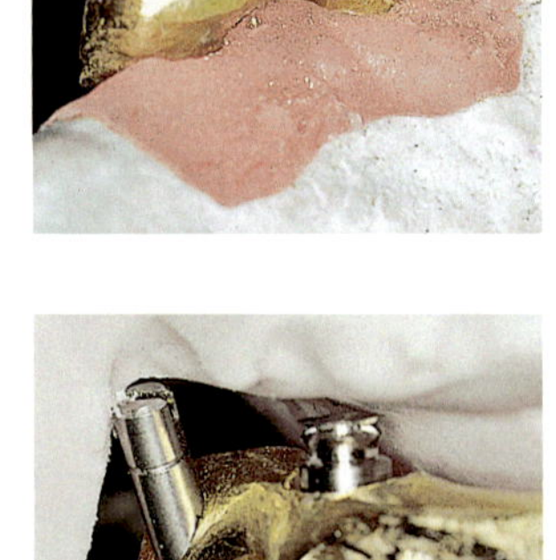

Fig 11-86 (a) Evaluation of the space occupied by the bar and the attachments through the silicone guide. (b) Close-up view.

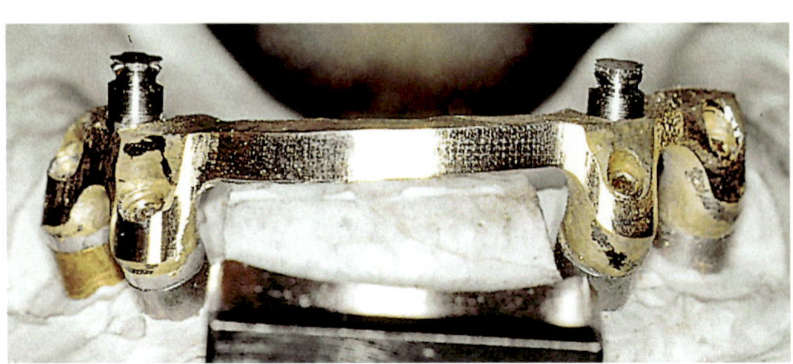

Fig 11-87 Retention matrix positioned on the cylindrical attachment.

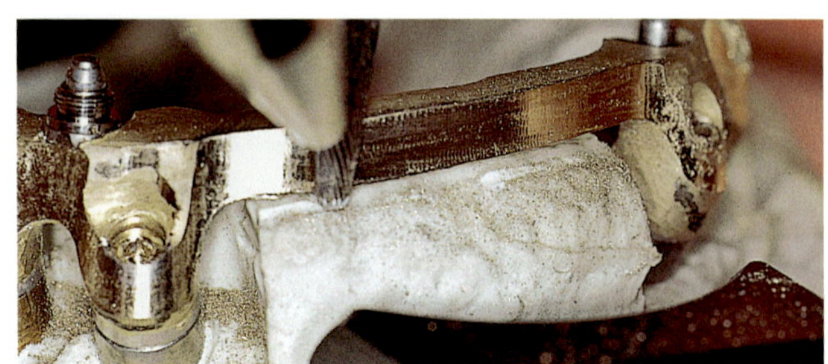

Fig 11-88 Finishing the bar to an angle of 6 degrees

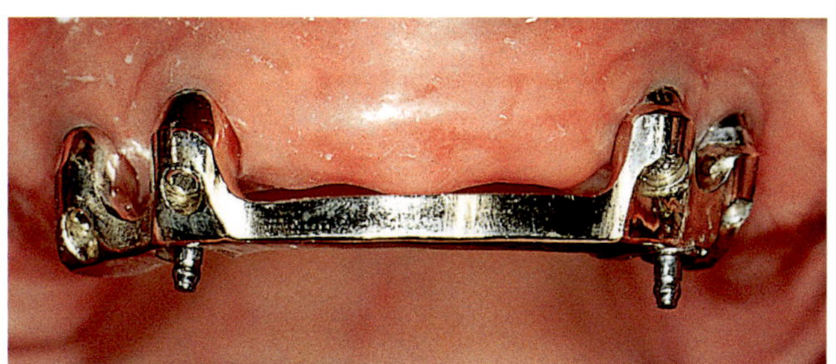

Fig 11-89 Clinical try-in of the definitive bar.

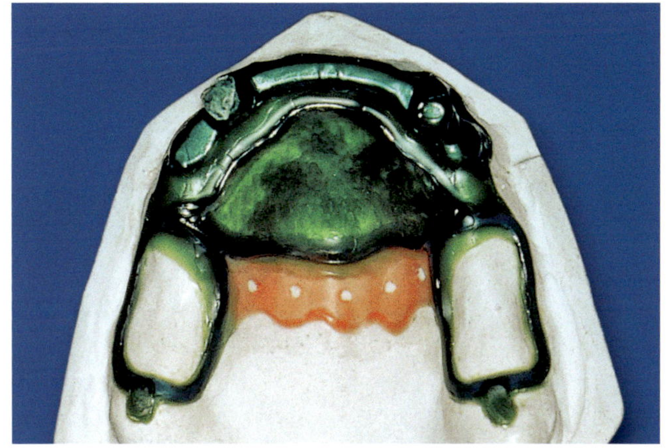

Fig 11-90 Refracted cast on which the framework of the prosthesis is modeled in wax.

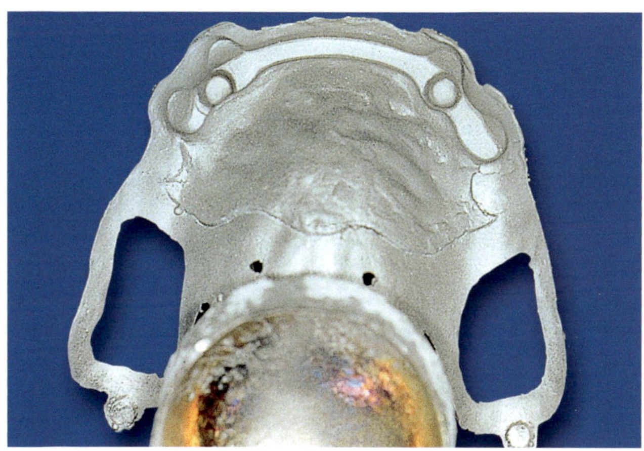

Fig 11-91 Completed cast of the titanium metal structure.

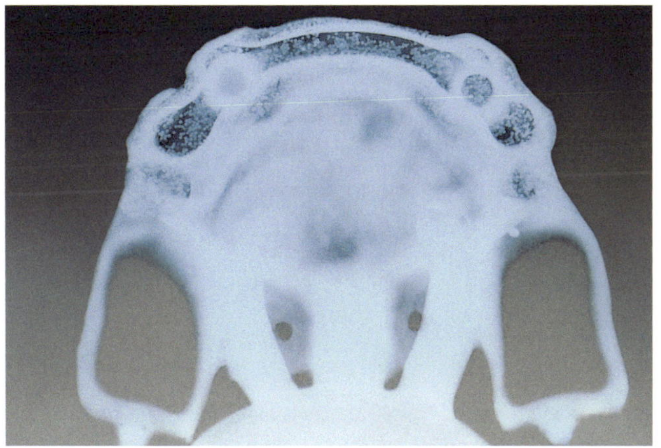

Fig 11-92 Radiograph verifying that there are no porosities.

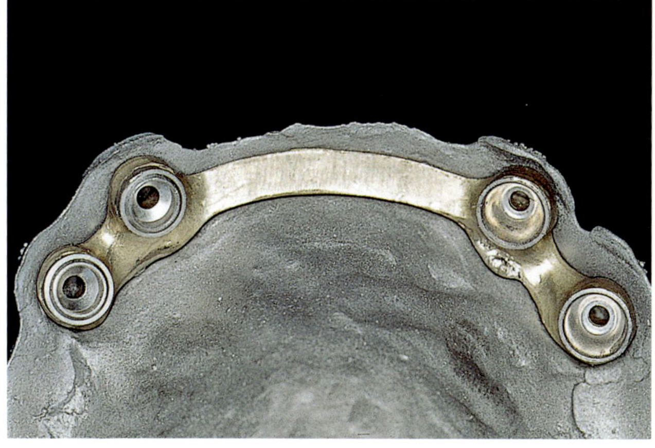

Fig 11-93 Adaptation of the bar to the titanium substructure.

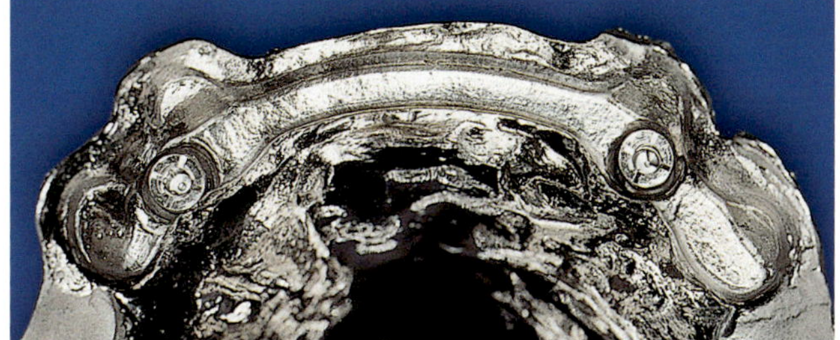

Fig 11-94 Blockage of the retention matrix with resin or composite cement on the titanium framework.

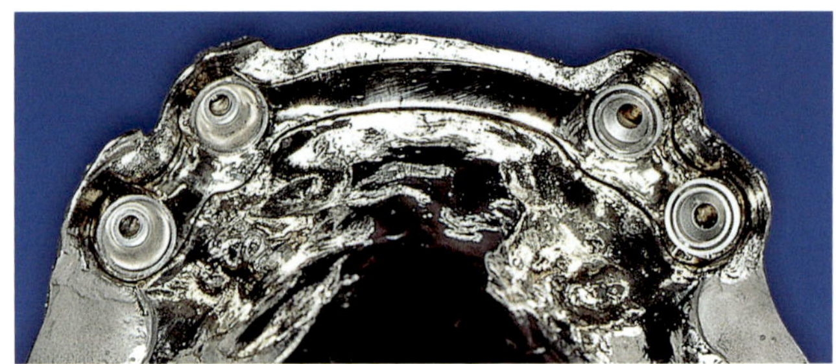

Fig 11-95 Checking the retention system.

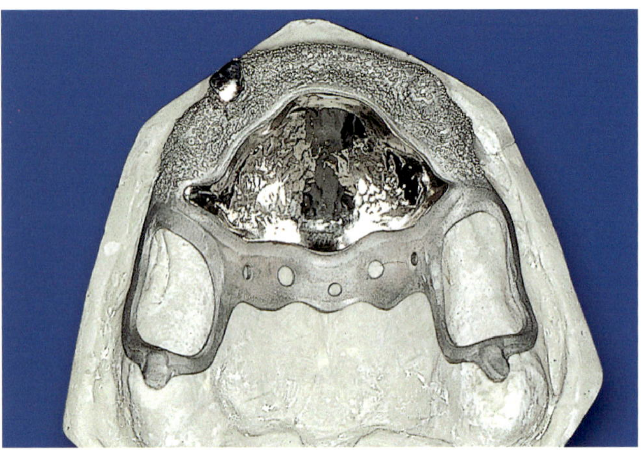

Fig 11-96 Cast with metal framework in position.

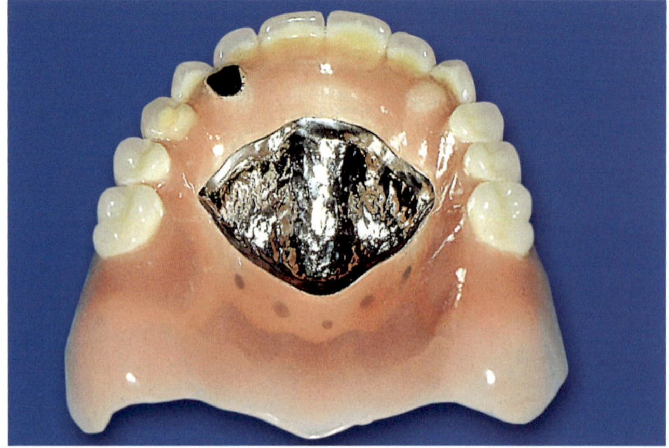

Fig 11-97 Completed prosthetics body.

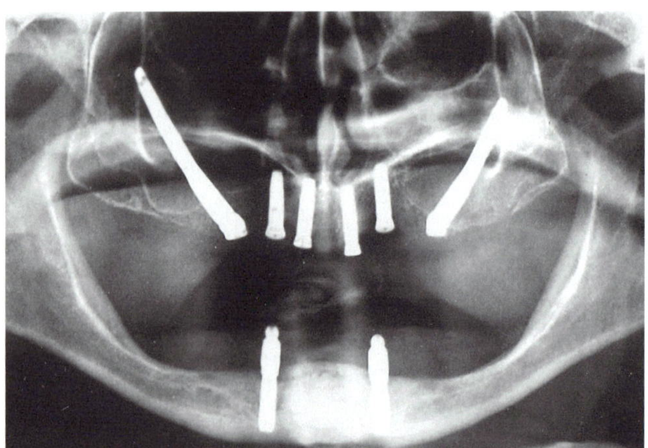

Fig 11-98 Radiograph of the edentulous maxilla after placement of implants. Note the two zygomatic implants in the posterior region.

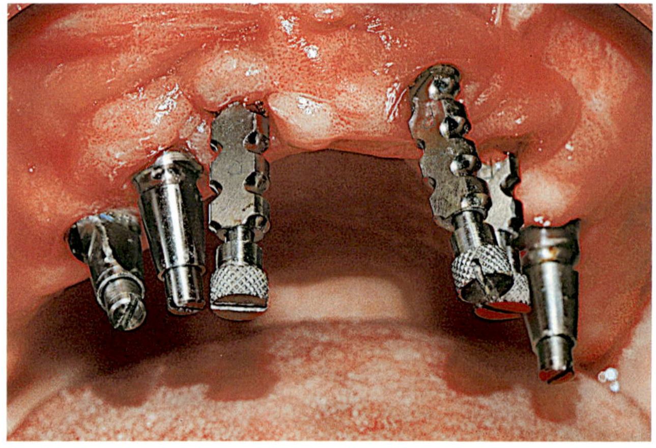

Fig 11-99 Positional transfer abutments for surveying the impression.

implants; in Misch class D, a bone graft in the anterior region is needed as well as the zygomatic implants.

Due to marked resorption of the maxilla in classes C and D, the best cheek and lip support is obtained more easily with an overdenture than with a fixed partial denture. For this reason it is preferable to rigidly splint the implants (as demanded by the protocol) with a bar on which an overdenture is anchored. Figures 11-98 to 11-107 describe the rehabilitative protocol of this technique.

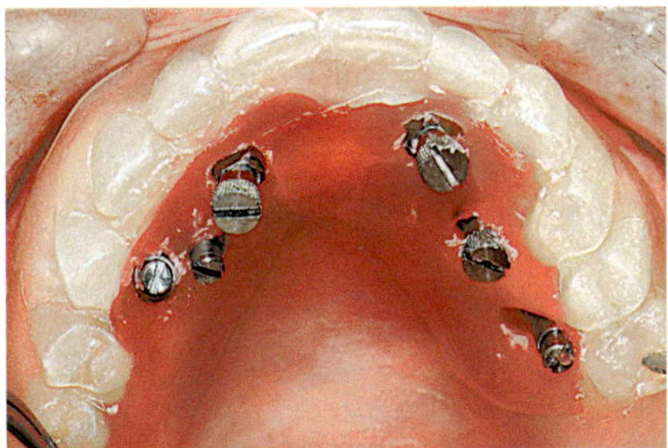

Fig 11-100 The resin duplicate is used as a custom impression tray. The tray is in situ; note the holes in the wax to allow the transfer position to be identified.

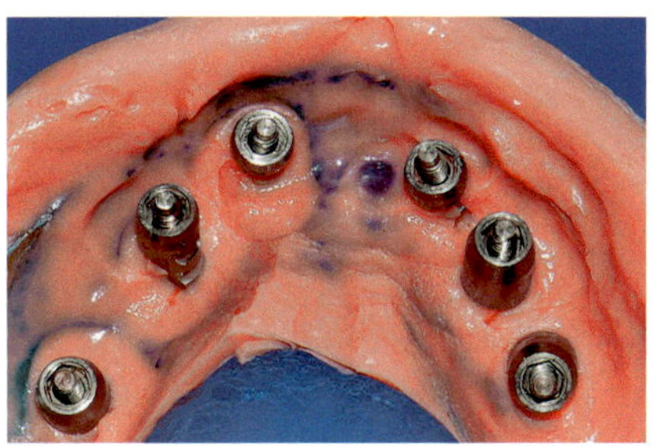

Fig 11-101 Detail of the impression in polyether with the transfter position on the implant heads.

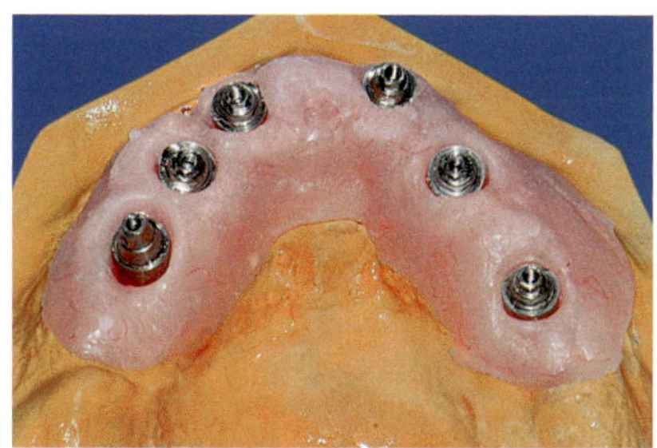

Fig 11-102 Master cast with the prosthetic abutments unscrewed.

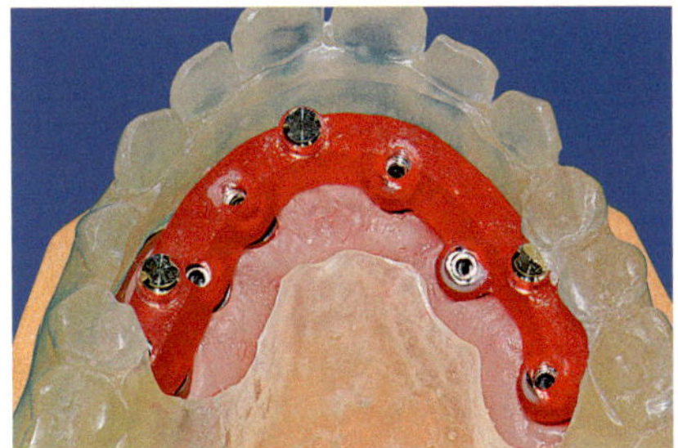

Fig 11-103 Waxup of the bar and duplicate of the complete denture to check for spaces. Note the matrix positioned on the wax to determine the position of the ball attachments.

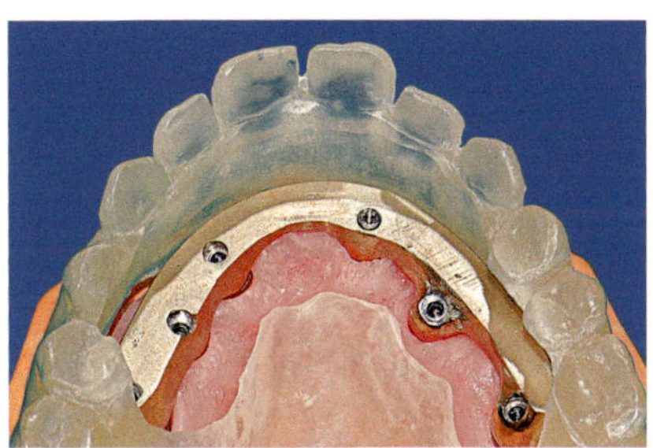

Fig 11-104 The complete bar before soldering the ball attachment. The spacing is rechecked on the resin duplicate. Due to the marked resorption, there is a difference between the positioning of the implants and the correct position of the teeth. Use of a removable prosthetic body provides adequate support for the lips and cheeks.

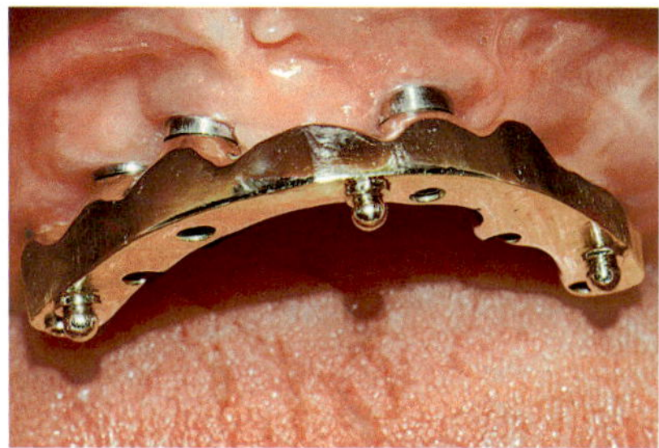

Fig 11-105 Clinical try-in of the bar with soldered abutments.

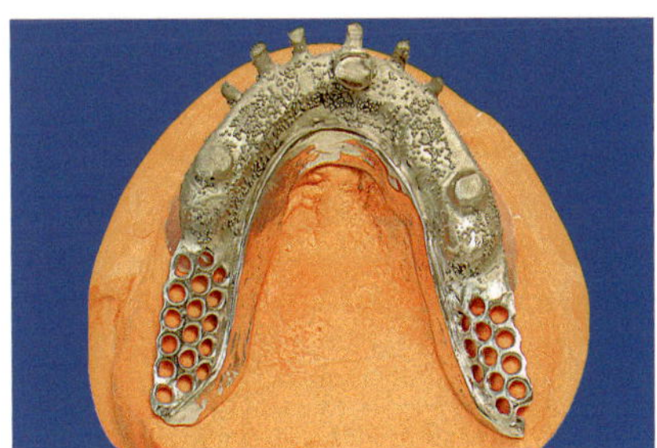

Fig 11-106 Metal structure that will be incorporated into the prosthesis.

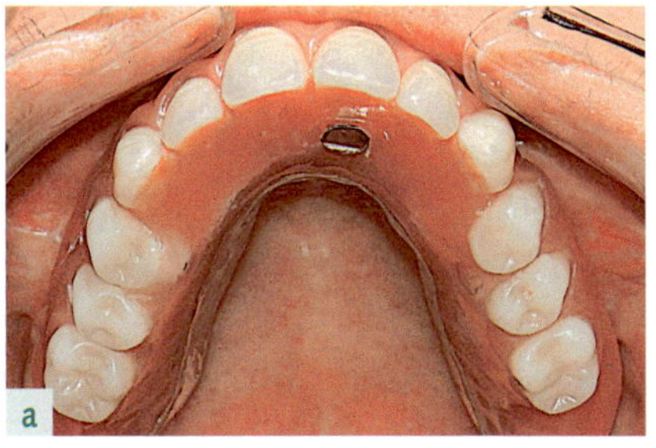

Fig 11-107 *(a and b)* Definitive prosthesis. Note that the distal support by the zygomatic implant has allowed the removal of the lingual resin portion.

References

1. Brånemark PI, Zarb GA, Albrektsson T. Tissue-integrated prostheses: Osseointegration in clinical dentistry 3rd ed. Chicago: Quintessence, 1985. Cat. 7

2. Adell R, Lekholm U, Rockler B, Brånemark PI. A 15-year study of osseointegrated implants in the treatment of the edentulous jaw. Int J Oral Surg 1981;10:387–416. Cat. 3

3. Jemt T, Book K, Linden B, Urde G. Failures and complications in 92 consecutively inserted overdentures supported by Brånemark implants in severely resorbed edentulous maxillae: A study from prosthetic treatment to first annual check-up. Int J Oral Maxillofac Implant 1992;7:162–167. Cat. 4

4. Brunski JB, Puleo DA, Nanci A. Biomaterials and biomechanics of oral and maxillofacial implants: Current status and future developments. Int J Oral Maxillofac Implants 2000;15:15–46. Cat. 7

5. Taylor TD, Agar JR, Vogiatzi T. Implant prosthodontics: Current perspective and future directions. Int J Oral Maxillofac Implants 2000;15:66–75. Cat. 7

6. Naert I, De Clercq M, Theuniers G, Schepers E. Overdentures supported by osseointegrated fixtures for the edentulous mandible: A 2.5 year report. Int J Oral Maxillofac Implants 1988;3:191–196. Cat. 3

7. Brånemark PI. Possibilities and limitations in the clinical application of osseointegration. Leuven, Belgium: Leuven University Press, 1998. Cat. 7

8. Naert I, Quirynen M, Theuniers G, van Steenberghe D. Prosthetic aspects of osseointegrated fixtures supporting overdentures. A 4-year report. J Prosthet Dent 1991;65:671–680. Cat. 3

9. Johns RB, Jemt T, Heath MR, et al. A multicenter study of overdentures supported by Brånemark implants. Int J Oral Maxillofac Implants 1992;7:513–522. Cat. 3

10. Engquist B, Bergendal T, Kallus T, Linden U. A retrospective multicenter evaluation of osseointegrated implants supporting overdentures. Int J Oral Maxillofac Implants 1988;3:129–134. Cat. 4

11. Smith DE, Zarb GA. Criteria for success of osseointegrated endosseous implants. J Prosthet Dent 1989;62:567–572. Cat. 7

12. Jennings KJ, Lilly P. Bar-retained overdentures for implants—technical aspects. J Prosthet Dent 1992;68:380–384. Cat. 8

13. Donatsky O. Osseointegrated dental implants with ball attachments supporting overdentures in patients with mandibular alveolar ridge atrophy. Int J Oral Maxillofac Implants 1993;8:162–166. Cat. 3

14. Hutton JE, Heath MR, Chai JY, et al. Factors related to success and failure rates at 3-year follow-up in a multicenter study of overdentures supported by Brånemark Implants. Int J Oral Maxillofac Implants 1995;10:33–42. Cat. 3

15. Jemt T, Carlsson L, Boss A, Jöurnéus L, In vivo load measurements on osseointegrated implants supporting fixed or removable prostheses: A comparative pilot study. Int J Oral Maxillofac Implants 1991;6:413–417. Cat. 8

16. Mericske-Stern R, Geering AH, Bürgin WB, Graf H. Three-dimensional force measurements on mandibular implants supporting overdentures. Int J Oral Maxillofac Implants 1992;7:185–194. Cat. 6

17. Setz J, Krämer A, Benzing U, Weber H. Complete dentures fixed on dental implants: Chewing patterns and implant stress. Int J Oral Maxillofac Implants 1989;4:107–111. Cat. 4

18. Rangert B, Jemt T, Jorneus L. Forces and moments on Brånemark implants. Int J Oral Maxillofac Implants 1989;4:241–247. Cat. 7

19. Menicucci G, Lorenzetti M, Pera P, Preti G. Mandibular implant-retained overdenture: Finite element analysis of two anchorage systems. Int J Oral Maxillofac Implants 1998;13:369–376. Cat. 6

20. Menicucci G, Lorenzetti M, Pera P, Preti G. Mandibular implant retained overdenture: A clinical trial of two anchorage systems. Int J Oral Maxillofac Implants 1998;13:851–856. Cat. 2

21. Meijer HJ, Kuiper JH, Starmans FJ, Bosman F. Stress distribution around dental implants: Influence of superstructure, length of implants and height of mandible. J Prosthet Dent 1992;68:96–102. Cat. 6

22. Meijer HJ, Starmans FJ, Bosman F, Steen WH. A comparison of three finite element models of an edentulous mandible provided with implants. J Oral Rehabil 1993;20:147–157. Cat. 6

23. Meijer HJ, Starmans FJ, Steen WH, Bosman F. Location of implants in the interforaminal region of the mandible and the consequences for the design of the superstructure. J Oral Rehabil 1994;21:47–56. Cat. 6

24. Meijer HJ, Starmans FJ, Steen WH, Bosman F. A three-dimensional, finite-element analysis of bone around dental implants in an edentulous human mandible. Arch Oral Biol 1993;38:491–496. Cat. 6

25. Besimo C, Kempf B. In vitro investigation of various attachments for overdenture on osseointegrated implants. J Oral Rehabil 1995;22:691–698. Cat. 6

26. Kydd WL, Daly CH, Wheeler JB III. The thickness measurements of masticatory mucosa in vivo. Int Dent J 1971;21:430–441. Cat. 4

27. van Zyl PP, Grundling NL, Jooste CH, Terblanche E. Three-dimensional finite element model of a human mandible incorporating six osseointegrated implants for stress analysis of mandibular cantilever prostheses. Int J Oral Maxillofac Implants 1995;10:51–57. Cat. 6

28. Picton DC, Wills DJ. Viscoelastic properties of the periodontal ligament and mucous membrane. J Prosthet Dent 1978;40:263–272. Cat. 5

29. Moller E. The chewing apparatus. An electromyographic study of the action of the muscles of mastication and its correlation to facial morphology. Acta Physiol Scand Suppl 1966;280:1–229. Cat. 4

30. Haraldson T, Jemt T, Stalblad PA, Lekholm U. Oral function in subjects with overdentures supported by osseointegrated implants. Scand J Dent Res 1988;96:235–242. Cat. 4

31. Kenney R, Richards MW. Photoelastic stress patterns produced by implant-retained overdentures. J Prosthet Dent 1998;80:559–564. Cat. 6

32. Carr AB, Brunsky JB, Hurley E. Effects of fabrication, finishing and polishing procedures on preload in prostheses using conventional "gold" and plastic cylinders. Int J Oral Maxillofac Implants 1996;11:589–598. Cat. 6

33. Benzing UR, Gall H, Weber H. Biomechanical aspects of two different implant-prosthetic concepts for edentulous maxillae. Int J Oral Maxillofac Implants 1995;10:188–198. Cat. 8

34. Richter EJ. In vivo vertical forces on implants. Int J Oral Maxillofac Implants 1995;10:99–108. Cat. 4

35. Glantz PO. Strandman E, Svensson SA, Randow K. On functional strain in fixed mandibular reconstructions. I. An in-vitro study. Acta Odontol Scand 1984;42:241–249. Cat. 6

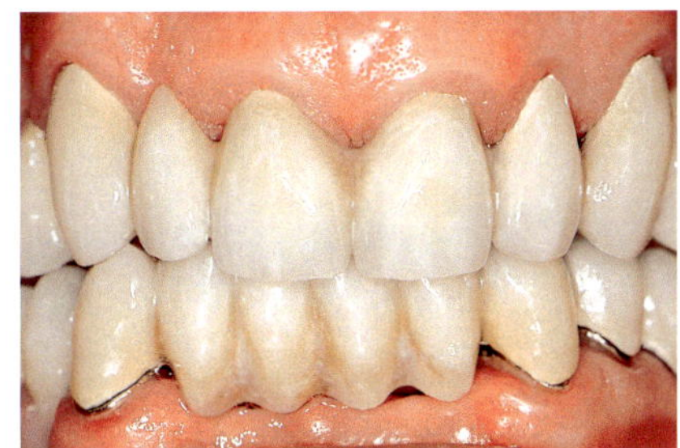

Fig 12-9   Mandibular OVD: The buccal flange is absent.

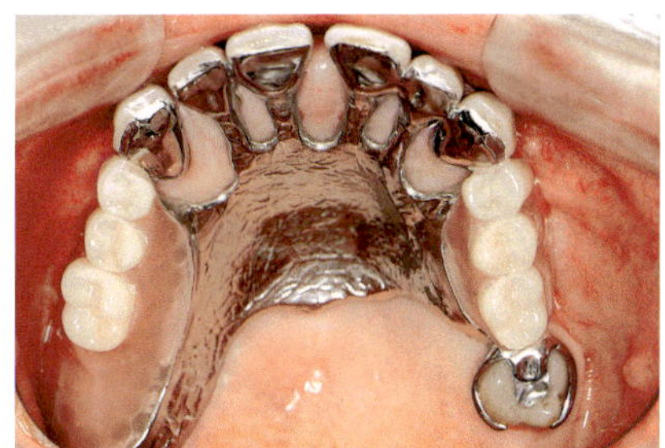

Fig 12-10   Metal structure of a maxillary OVD.

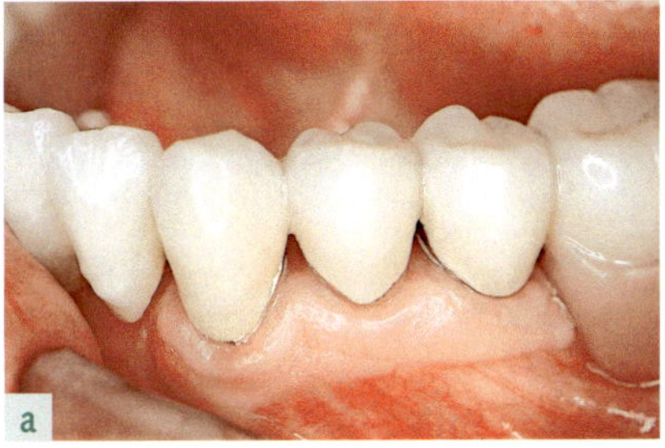

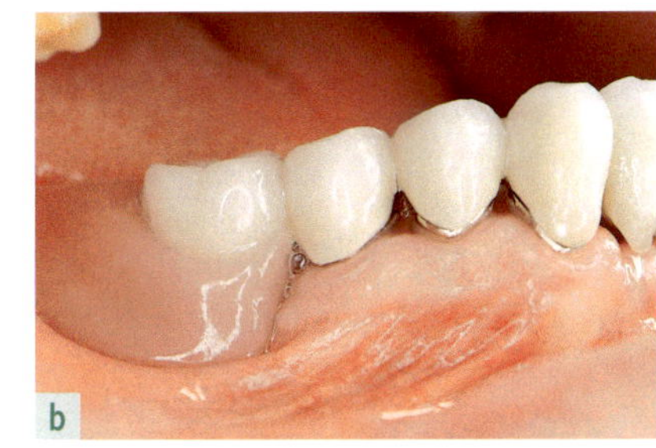

Fig 12-11   (*a and b*) Anatomic reconstruction of the abutment teeth without the gingival margin and an open interdental space.

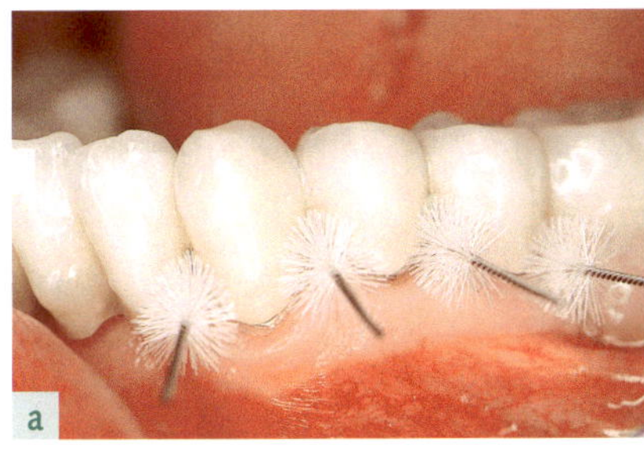

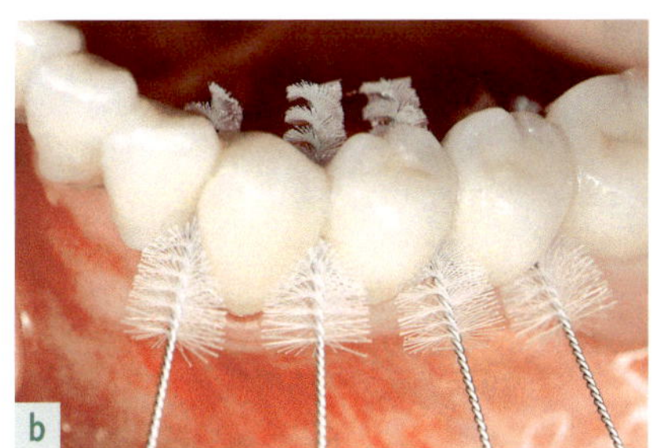

Fig 12-12   (*a and b*) The guide is applied to the interdental surfaces, facilitating the insertion of a special toothbrush to maintain proper hygiene.

ferent. The POVD has a metal superstructure that is therefore very rigid, similar to the removable partial denture from which it is derived (Fig 12-10). The superstructure is less bulky and allows for the anatomic reconstruction of the supporting teeth while respecting the correct emergence profile and maintaining open interdental spaces (Fig 12-11).

This prosthetic design is well tolerated by the periodontal tissues because it does not traumatize them, and the accumulation of plaque is reduced. Furthermore, the patient is able to clean the supporting teeth without removing the denture by means of an interproximal toothbrush inserted between the interdental surfaces of the superstructure. The interproximal surfaces guide and facilitate the hygiene procedures, particularly for patients with reduced dexterity (Fig 12-12).

The classic OVD has relatively minimal costs. To the contrary, the POVD involves complex procedures, including planning and construction phases, which incur higher costs.

Indications and Contraindications

OVD with simple root coverage (overlay) is used for a significantly reduced, severely compromised residual teeth. Therefore, it should be considered as a transition to a traditional, mucosa-supported complete denture.

The root-anchored OVD with bar or ball attachment is used when there is a very reduced residual complement of teeth that have good periodontal support. Because of its complexity and higher costs, POVD is recommended for those patients who require a more refined prosthetic rehabilitation. This prosthesis is preferable when the conditions of the residual teeth do not ensure a favorable long-term prognosis for the rehabilitation or when the eventual extraction of a single tooth could compromise the result of the entire restoration.

The POVD is a modular prosthetic system that allows for the eventual extraction of teeth without substantial modifications of the prosthetic superstructure. This type of prosthesis is also recommended for patients with major osseous undercuts in which the flange of the conventional OVD would distress the

155

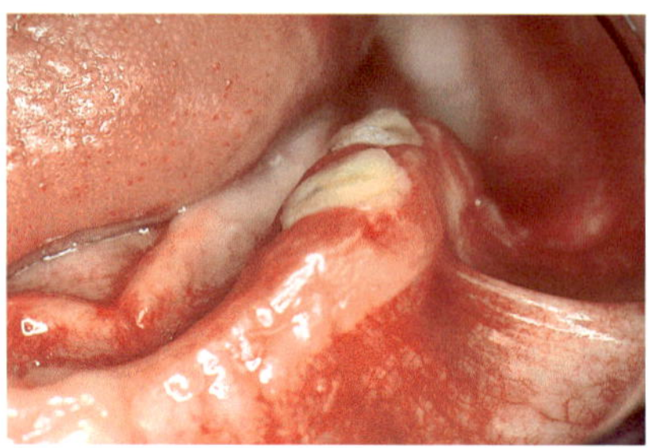

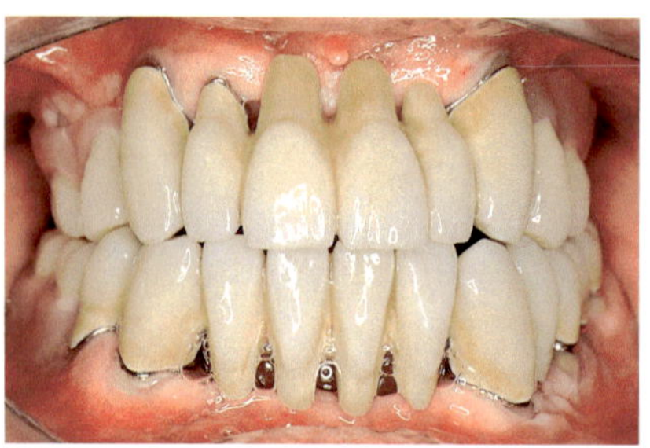

Fig 12-13 Residual roots on a crest with a substantial overhang. An OVD flange would traumatize the tissue and provide undesirable esthetics.

Fig 12-14 Exaggerated tooth length and excessive open interdental spaces due to substantial bone loss.

supporting tissues and would have poor esthetic results (Fig 12-13). POVD is further recommended in cases where a chairside setup is required for esthetic reasons or when the lingual space is reduced.

The POVD is not recommended when the health of the patient does not allow difficult and frequent sittings, when the residual teeth have unfavorable prognoses, or in cases of insufficient motivation on behalf of the patient. The use of a POVD restoration is also limited if there is significant bone loss in the anterior sector. In this case, a POVD would require very long teeth with very open interdental spaces, resulting in possible esthetic and phonetic problems (Fig 12-14).

The type of prosthesis needed is based on the analysis of the indications described. Patient health and economic conditions permitting, POVD is preferable because it preserves the periodontal tissues by virtue of the anatomic reconstruction of the supporting teeth without covering the marginal gingiva.

Implant or Denture Rehabilitation: Choice Criteria

Keeping residual teeth or extracting them for implant placement depends on the careful evaluation of general, local, and economic factors. Age and health status are of primary consideration. In elderly patients who are not able to cope with excessively long therapeutic procedures such as the placement of implants, it is preferable to preserve the residual teeth. Likewise, implants are not advised for patients with serious hematologic diseases, untreated or uncontrolled diabetes, osteoporosis, or who are undergoing prolonged corticosteroid therapy.

Another factor that affects the therapeutic choice is the endodontic and periodontal status of the residual teeth. In the presence of lesions or in cases of uncertain prognosis, tooth extraction and placement of osseointegrated implants is indicated.

A third consideration regards the jaw to be rehabilitated. According to the literature, the best results in implant therapy can be obtained in the mandible. The interforamina area has

the greatest success rate (98%). The long-term cost-benefit relationship supports implant treatment, which avoids the costs associated with caries and endodontic pathology. On the other hand, in the posterior region of the mandible, the operative difficulties due to the position of the mandibular canal lowers the success rate and supports the decision to maintain the residual teeth and choose a conventional denture.

The maxilla is less favorable in terms of osseous quality and is therefore less often recommended for implant rehabilitation. Furthermore, in this region, the retention offered by the active factors (musculature) and passive factors (saliva film) is generally sufficient to maintain a conventional removable denture.

Implant placement in the maxilla is recommended in cases of serious generalized atrophy with a flat palate—a situation that does not guarantee valid retention and stability. In addition, it is recommended when the opposing arch has natural teeth in the anterior region, which can cause significant resorption of the anterior maxilla because of transmitted loads.

If a root-anchored denture is proposed, additional considerations should be made concerning the position of the residual teeth and their radicular morphology. In the maxilla, the canines and central incisors are the most important teeth, because their radicular anatomy contributes to conserving the structural integrity of the anterior maxilla. In the mandible, the main strategic teeth are the premolars and the canines for their important role in mechanical retention. Incisors are often maintained even though their radicular morphology is less favorable from both the endodontic and the periodontal perspective.

An interesting and relevant work by Kalk[29] subdivides the arches into four areas of relevance (1: canine; 2: premolar, 3: incisor; and 4: molar) (Fig 12-15) and underlines the importance of symmetric anchorage. Ideally, four supporting abutments should be placed in zones 1 and 2 to create a supporting polygon, as in traditional removable partial dentures, thus eliminating the rotation axes of the denture (Fig 12-16). An alternative solution is to place one abutment per demi-arch, in the canine or premolar and canine area. However, this situation creates a rotation axis, respectively frontal or transversal (Fig 12-17).

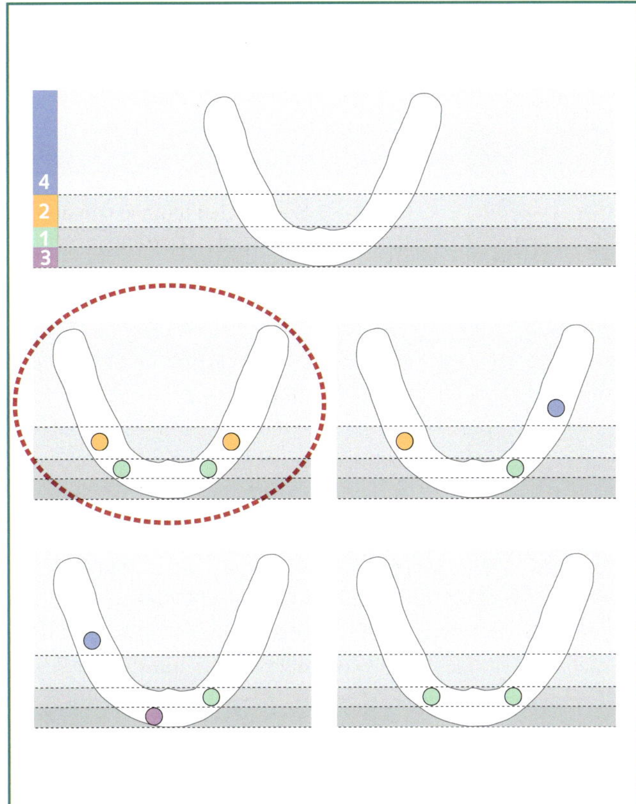

Fig 12-15 Ideal abutment placement (*circled*) highlighting the symmetic placement in zones 1 and 2. Asymmetric placement or placement in zones 3 and 4 would be less effective because of the unfavorable rotation axis.

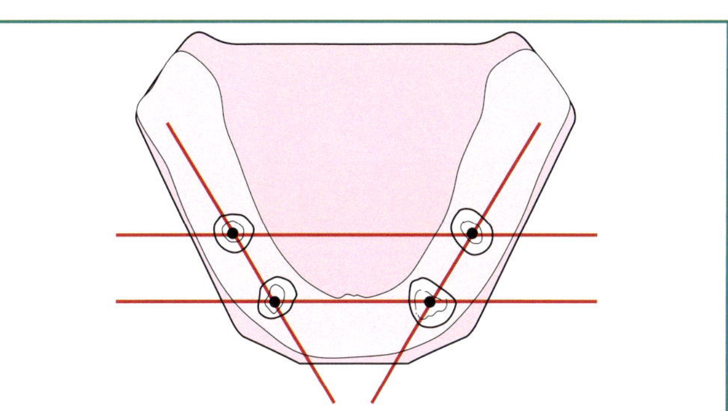

Fig 12-16 Polygon support on four residual teeth; there is no rotational axis.

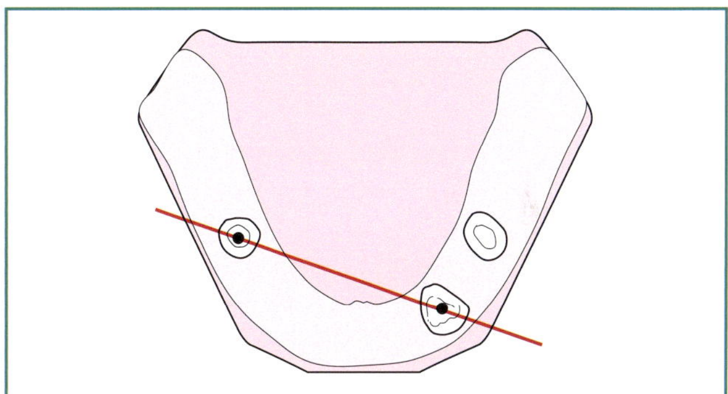

Fig 12-17 Transverse rotational axis with three residual roots.

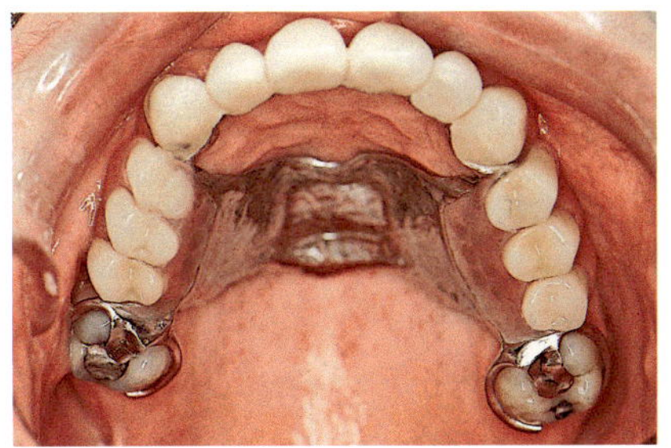

Fig 12-18 Maxillary POVD seated in resin with palatal structure.

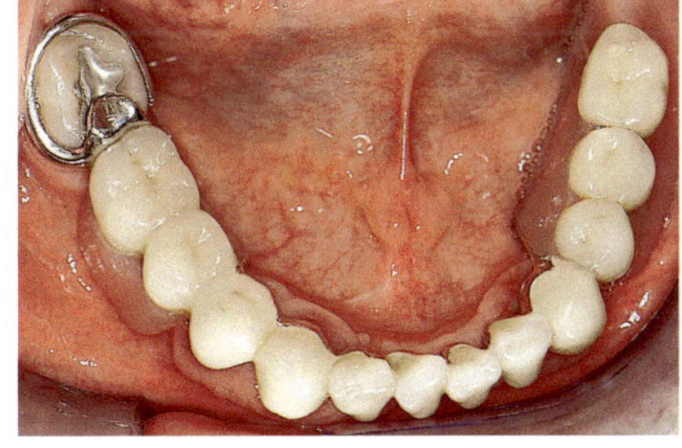

Fig 12-19 Mandibular POVD seated in resin. The major attachment is an integral part of the anterior support.

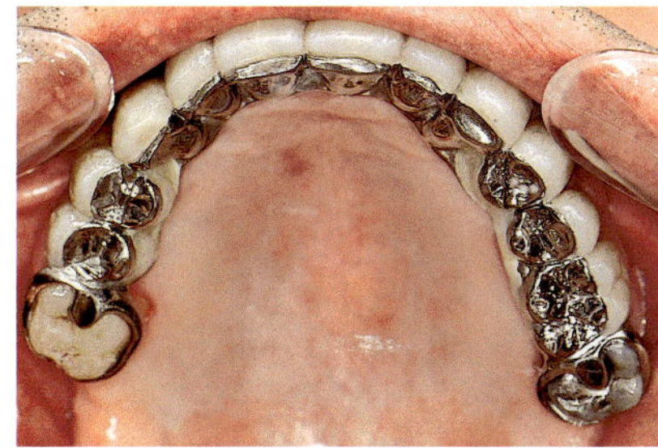

Fig 12-20 Maxillary POVD seated in resin and with only dental supports.

POVD Design

The information necessary for denture planning is obtained from clinical and radiologic evaluation and from the analysis of the patient's study casts, which are used to evaluate the position of the residual teeth and the shape of the alveolar ridges. The study casts are also used for analyzing the available space and creating a diagnostic waxup. All of these data are needed to decide which teeth will be used for retention, the design of the definitive denture, and the type of attachments. The morphologic characteristics of the POVD vary in relation to the number of residual teeth and the degree of preservation of the alveolar bone. In the presence of serious resorption of the ridges or a reduced number of residual teeth, a POVD similar to a removable partial denture with resin saddles and major connectors can be applied (Fig 12-18). On the contrary, if well-

157

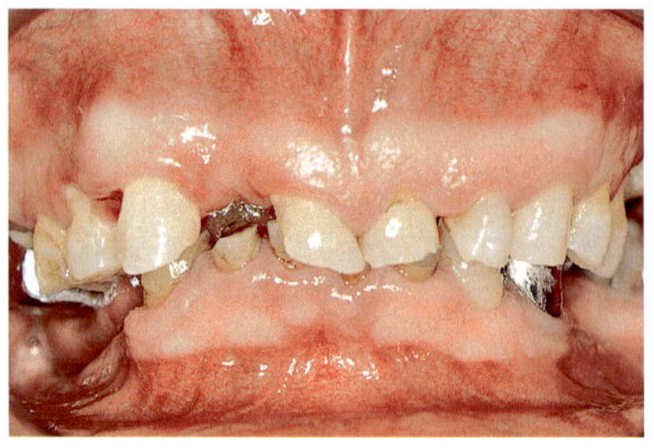

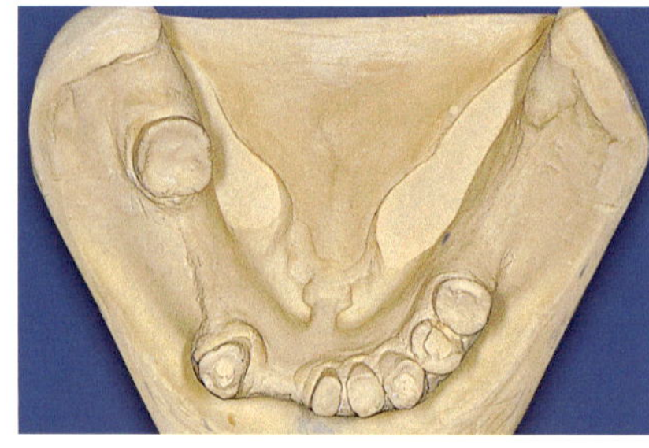

Fig 12-21 Initial clinical situation.

Fig 12-22 Cast of the mandibular arch.

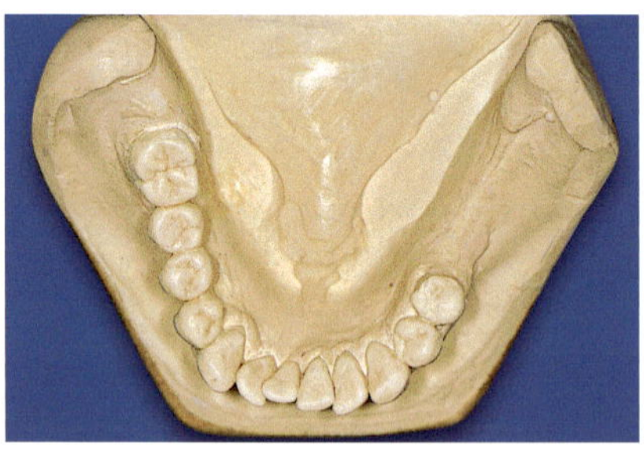

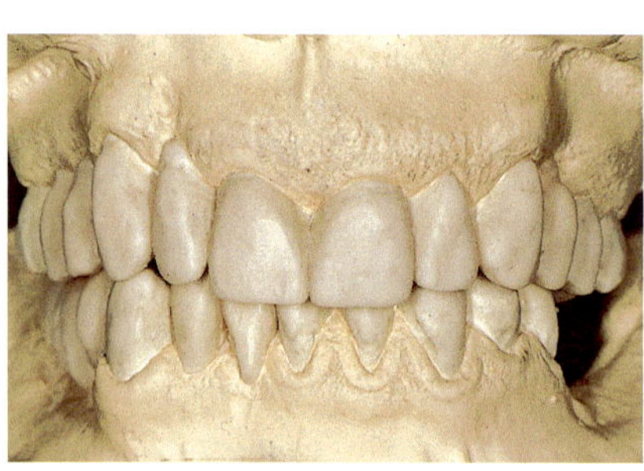

Fig 12-23 Diagnostic waxup of the mandibular arch.

Fig 12-24 Diagnostic waxup of the maxilla and the mandible in an articulator.

shaped ridges and a sufficient number of teeth are present, a POVD without major connectors but with resin saddles can be created (Fig 12-19) or with only dental support (Fig 12-20). A rigid metal structure would be needed in this case.

Final Considerations and Therapeutic Approach

- Keeping residual teeth, even just the roots, offers psychologic, functional, and biologic advantages.
- The periodontal receptors retain proprioception, and the roots stimulate alveolar bone, keeping it trophic.
- The therapeutic approach depends on the conditions of the roots and their strategic positions.
- The decision to maintain or extract the roots depends on whether implants will be used. It is advisable to keep the roots when:
  - The roots are in good condition, the patient is very old, or his or her health does not make implants advisable.
  - The roots are in a position in which, because of poor bone quality and quantity, implants cannot be placed or could have a poor prognosis (maxillary and posterior mandibular regions).
  - The roots are located in the anterior maxilla and prevent bone resorption in this area.

It is advisable to extract roots whose maintenance would need complex and expensive endodontic and periodontal treatment.

Clinical Planning and Construction of the POVD

The clinical procedure for a POVD supported by natural teeth is described in the following case (Fig 12-21).

Study casts and waxup

After diagnosis and initial preparation, study casts are taken (Fig 12-22) and mounted on an articulator, on which the diagnostic waxup is made (Fig 12-23). The waxup defines the morphology of the prosthetic structure and allows silicone keys to be constructed to guide the final esthetic modeling (Fig 12-24).

Preparation of the supporting abutments

Particular attention should be paid to the positioning of the restoration margin if a good esthetic result is to be obtained. In conventional preparation, the margin of the abutment cap is placed supragingivally, where it is visible, particularly in patients with a very high smile line. It is preferable to substitute the conventional beveled preparation with an unbeveled one, which allows placement of an abutment cap level with the marginal gingiva (Figs 12-25 to 12-30).

Adaptation of the provisional prosthesis

The esthetic result of the rehabilitation depends on the provisional prosthesis (Figs 12-31 to 12-33).

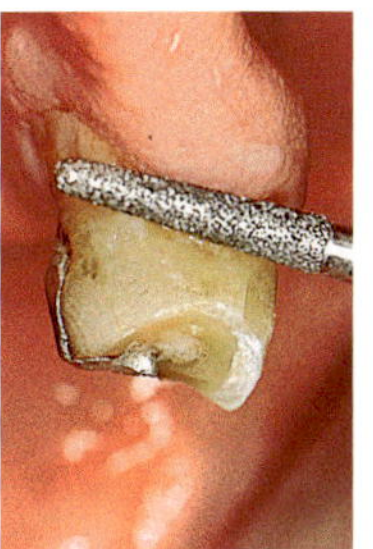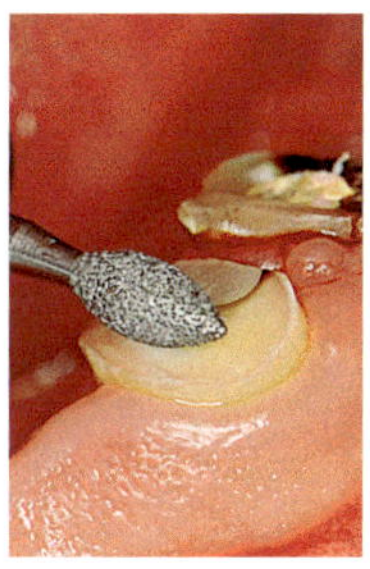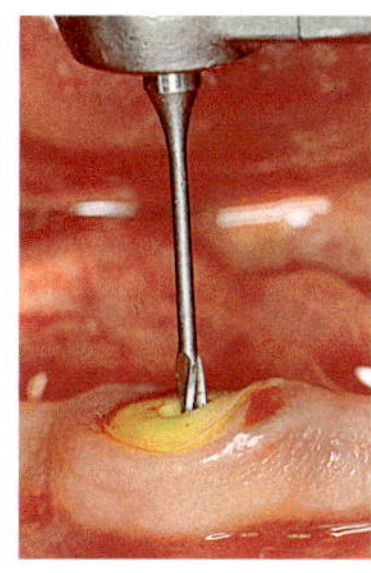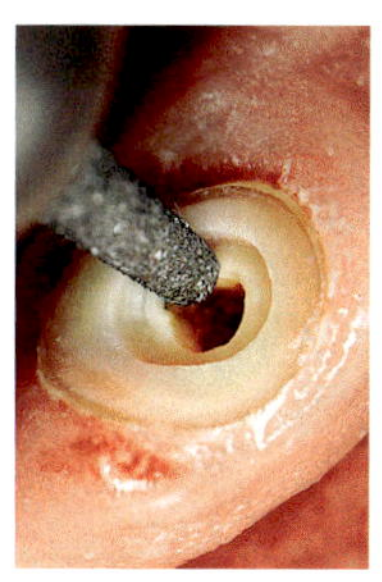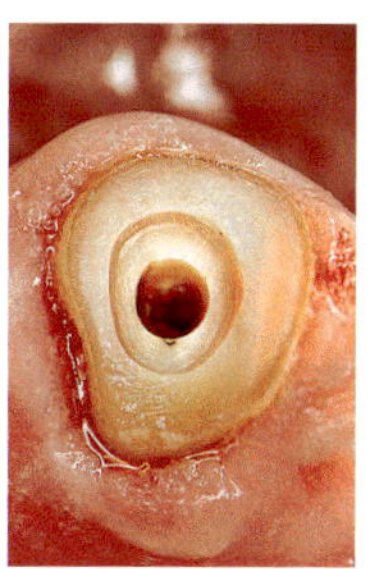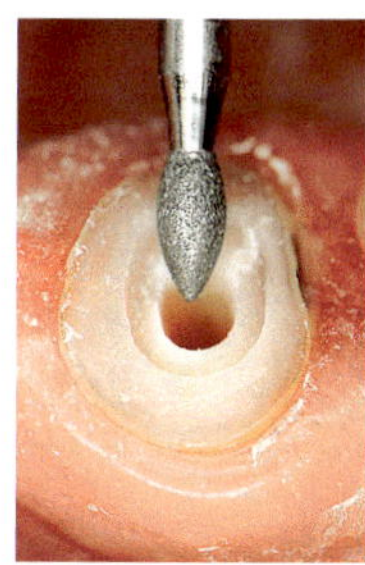

Figs 12-25 to 12-30 *(from left to right)*

Fig 12-25 The teeth are shortened to the gingival level with a cylindrical diamond bur (diameter, 0.12 mm) mounted on a handpiece.

Fig 12-26 An occlusal cavity made by a football-shaped bur (diameter, 0.23 mm).

Fig 12-27 Prepartion of a root canal with a large bur (no. 2–4) to seat a cylindrical or conical pin 7 to 8 mm in length (the length of the pin varies according to the root length from one-half to two-thirds of the root.

Fig 12-28 Prepartion of an occlusal drain with a depth of 2 mm, made with a conical diamond bur (diameter, 0.14 mm).

Fig 12-29 Occlusal view of preparation. The dentin must have a minimal thickness of 1 mm.

Fig 12-30 The margin of the canal drain and the occusal surface are chamfered, and the preparation is finished with a football-shaped diamond bur (diameter, 0.16 mm).

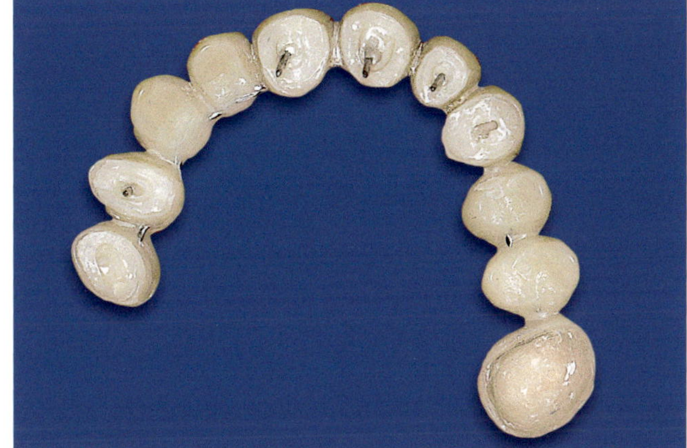
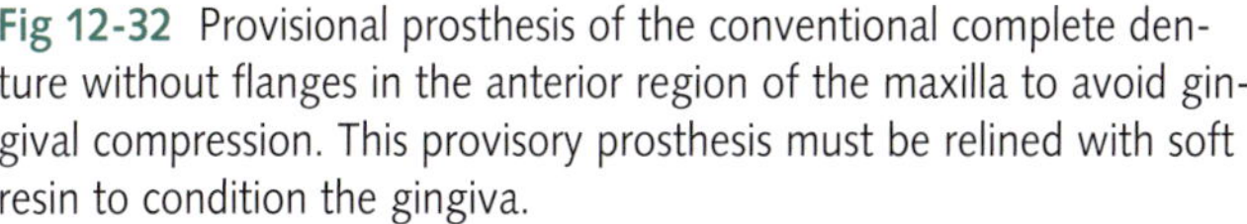

Fig 12-31 Provisionsl prosthesis with radicular anchorage in resin reinforced with metal threads.

Fig 12-32 Provisional prosthesis of the conventional complete denture without flanges in the anterior region of the maxilla to avoid gingival compression. This provisory prosthesis must be relined with soft resin to condition the gingiva.

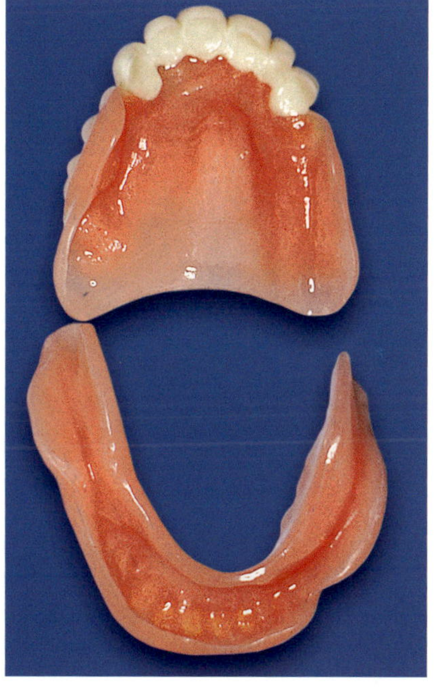
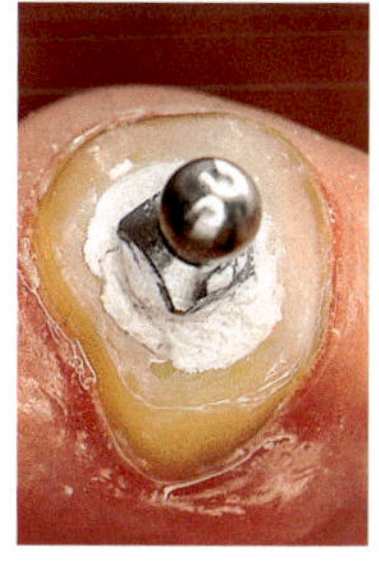

Fig 12-33 *(far right)* Provisional ball attachment (Dalbo-Rotex, Cendres et Metaux) cemented with zinc oxide, onto which the provisional prosthesis is anchored. This attachment is shortened to 3 to 4 mm to facilitate removal.

Impression for the root caps

The material used for the impression of the root preparation must guarantee resistance to lacerations, elastic behavior, and dimensional stability. Such characteristics are provided by silicones and polyethers. If silicone is used, the two-step technique must be followed. With the polyethers, a one-step, two-paste technique is made using a custom impression tray to guarantee greater precision, better support for the material, and a uniform thickness (Figs 12-34 and 12-35).

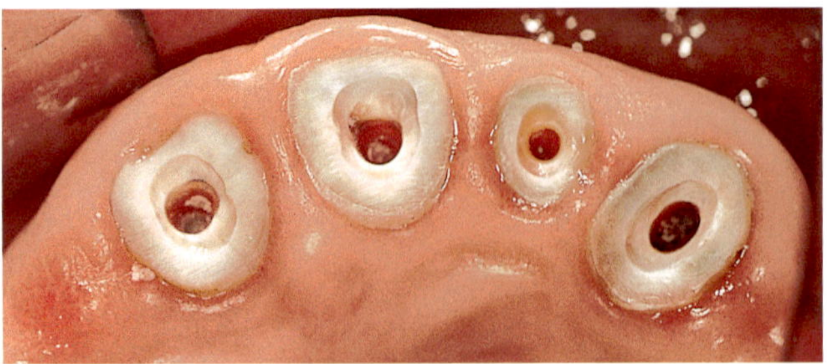

Fig 12-34 Retraction of gingival margin using a nonimpregnated cord and a pin adapted to prevent contact with the sides of the interradicular preparations.

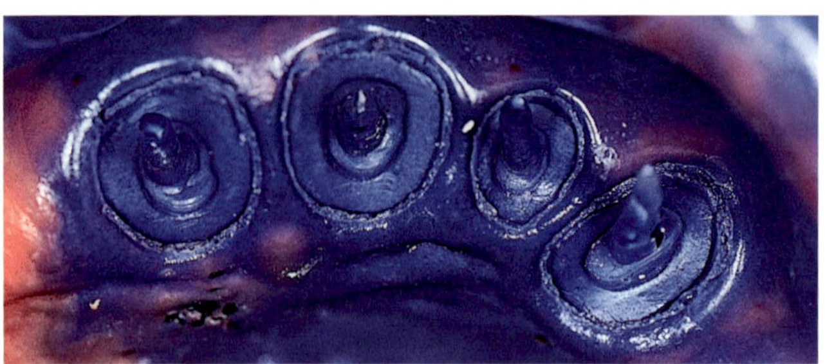

Fig 12-35 Impression showing the lighter lining material that is placed inside the first impression using a syringe and a handle-mounted lentulo.

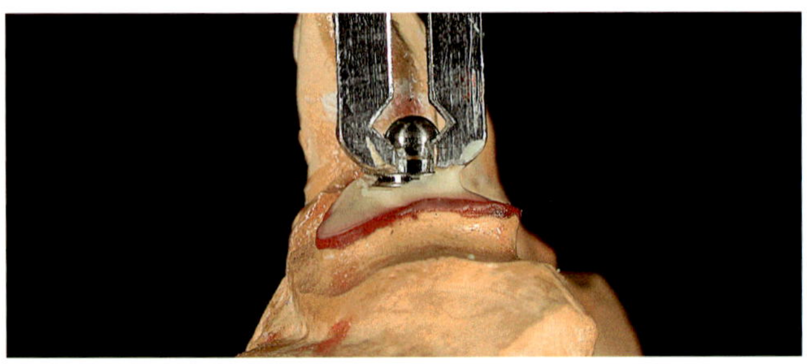

Fig 12-36 Preparation of radicular cap. The caps are waxed on a cast with the pin inserted into the canal. A thickness of at least 1 mm is needed for corrections of the occlusal surfaces when the retention device is positioned.

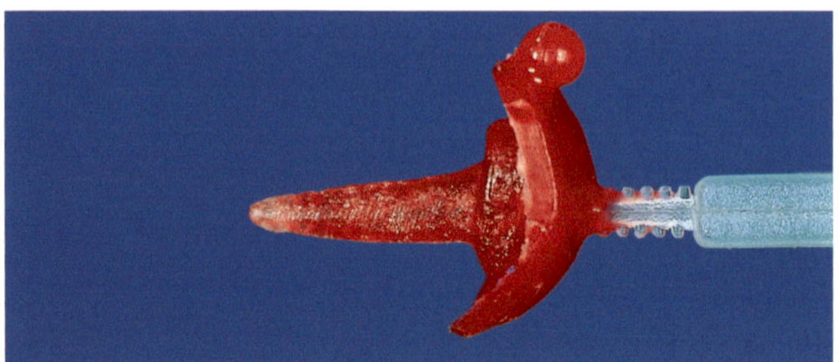

Fig 12-37 Occlusal shape of the gold cap is prepared perpendicularly to the axis of insertion, controlled by a parallel meter. The element is fixed depending on the space needed (between 1.3 and 1.5 mm).

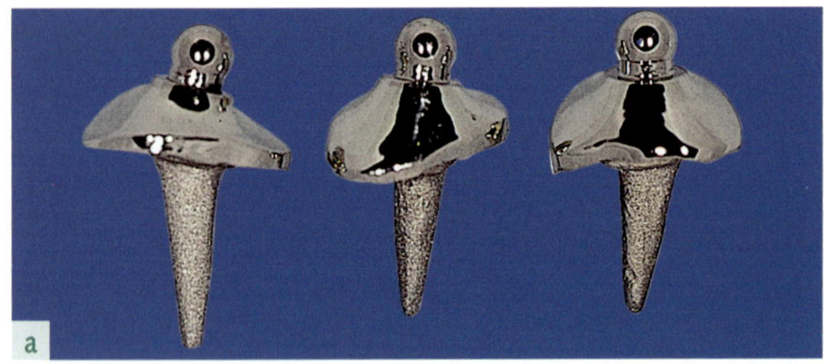

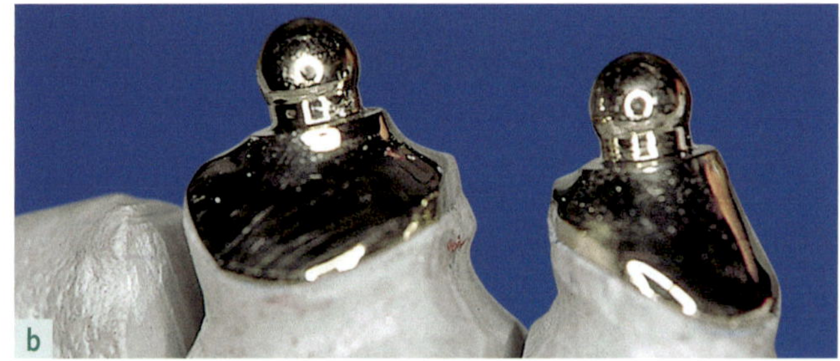

Fig 12-38 (a and b) Vestibular part of the cap is reduced to a thickness of 0.1 to 0.2 mm after treatment in a 400°C ceramic oven for 15 minutes to temper the metal; the metal prepared for the oral cavity remains thick for guaranteed stability.

Preparation of the root caps

Root caps try-in

The correct fitting of the root caps is carried out by means of contact indicators (Figs 12-36 to 12-38). The relationship of the gingival margin with the cap is then checked by a precision impression created using a one- or two-paste polyether material. The gingiva are reproduced in silicone to obtain an esthetic model of the cap margins, which will be clinically evaluated (Fig 12-39).

Cementation of the caps

Both the internal surface of each cap and the dentin must be conditioned to increase adhesion to the composite cement and impede contraction, which could provoke the formation of a marginal gap. The cap is cemented with composite cements

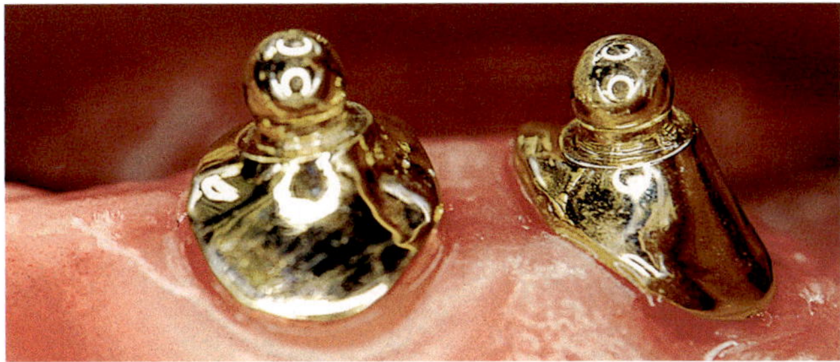

Fig 12-39 Checking the correct positioning of the gold cap.

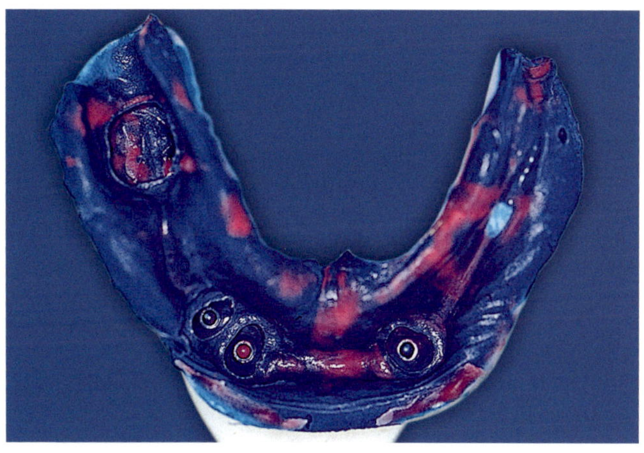

Fig 12-40 Polyether impression with a custom impression tray.

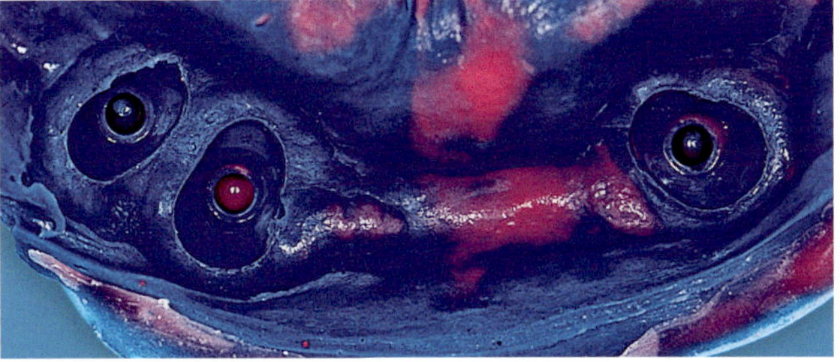

Fig 12-41 Detail of the impression of the cap shown in Fig 12-40.

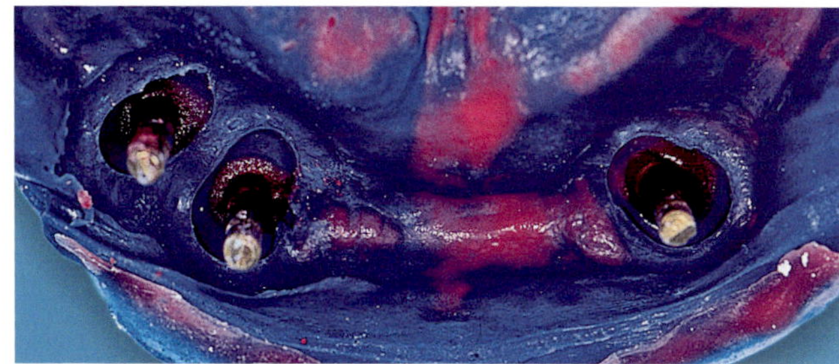

Fig 12-42 Replica of the attachment in the impression.

(Panavia 21, Kuraray America; Allbond, Bisco; or Superbond C&B, Morita) within 10 minutes of conditioning. The cement is applied on the internal surface of the cap and must not be introduced into the canals.

Impression for the metal structure

A custom impression tray that enables a uniform thickness of the material will result in good precision when taking the impression for the metal structure. The most common materials are polyethers because of their elasticity and dimensional stability. Based on the type of material, it is possible to use either two-paste (Permadyne, 3M ESPE) or a one-paste (Impregum, 3M ESPE) material with the one-stage technique (Figs 12-40 to 12-43).

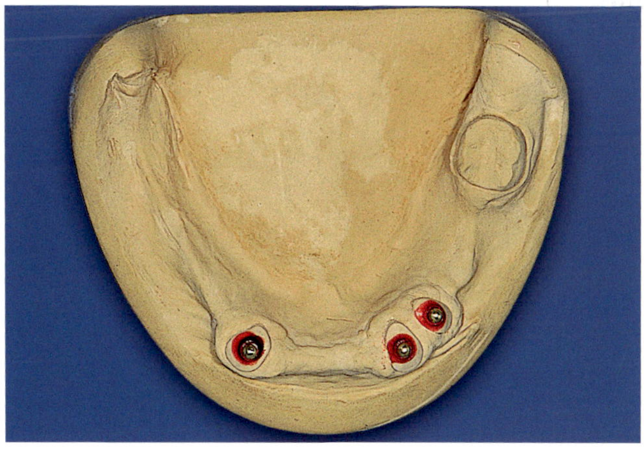

Fig 12-43 Master cast showing the same position as the cemented cap in the patient's mouth.

Esthetic and functional try-in

In this phase, teeth are waxed up on a resin support that includes the attachment matrices. This waxup, based on the initial diagnostic waxup, allows direct esthetic control and

161

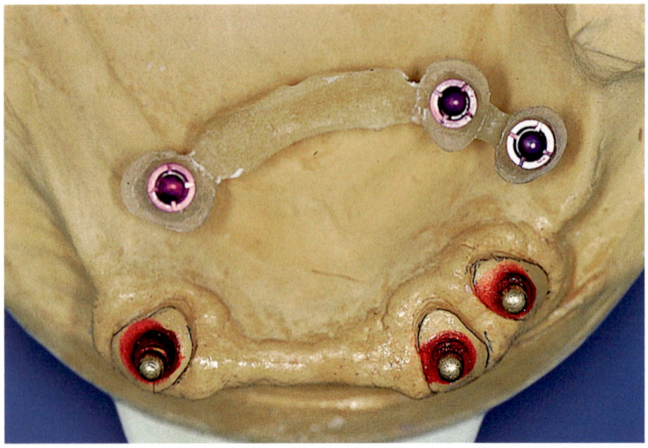

Fig 12-44 Strucure of the resin support prepared on the master cast in which the matrix attachments are incorporated.

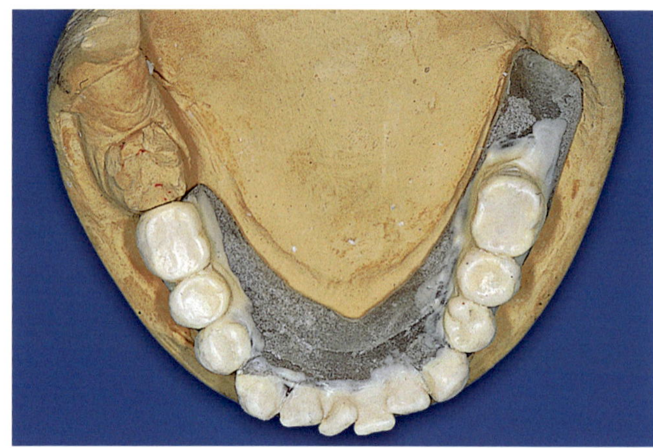

Fig 12-45 Definitive waxup based on the diagnostic waxup made in the planning phase.

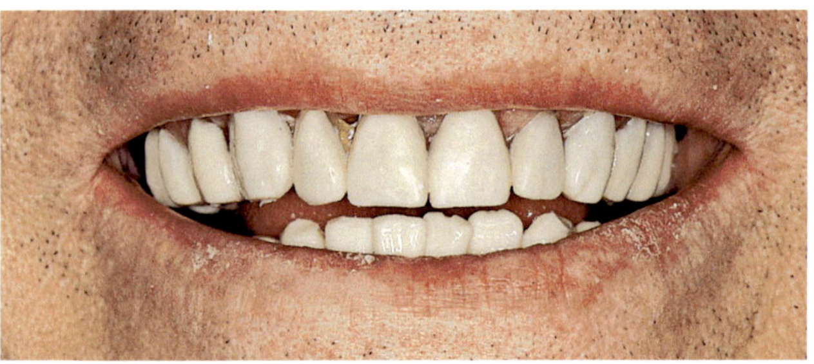

Fig 12-46 Try-in to check the esthetics and the maxillomandibular relationship.

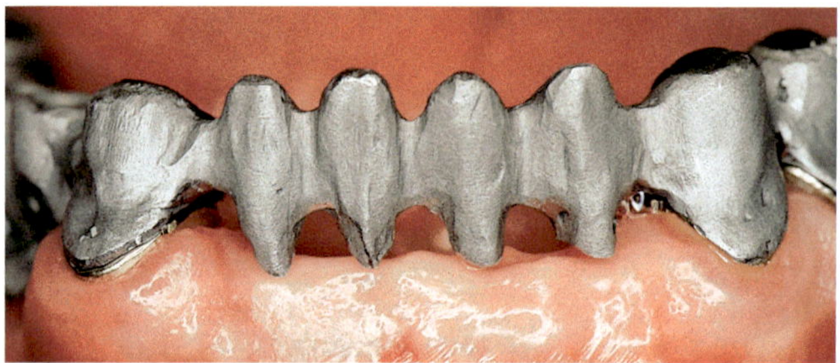

Fig 12-47 Correct positioning of the metal structure.

guides the technician in creating the metal superstructure. The attachments give stability to the product and allow confirmation of the correct positioning of the retentive elements (Figs 12-44 to 12-46).

Metal superstructure try-in

This step verifies the correct adaptation of the structure, which already includes the attachments blocked with resin. The correctly positioned metal superstructure must be stable. To verify the presence of precontact areas of the supporting elements and on the root caps, pressure spot indicators are used. If the position of the attachment matrices is not correct, they should be removed and blocked at the time of denture delivery. The emergence profiles and the correct closure of the crowns are also checked in this phase (Fig 12-47).

Altered cast

If the edentulous ridges are very wide or incorrectly registered (mucosa incorrectly placed on the underlying osseous ridge), it is necessary to proceed with the modified cast technique. This method consists of preparing resin saddles with a metal structure, which requires a custom tray for taking an impression with appropriate materials. The modified cast is created based on the new impression (Figs 12-48 and 12-49). (See also chapter 13.)

Mounted teeth try-in

The prosthetic teeth are made with composite materials and is based on the waxup used for the esthetic try-in. However, it is useful to remember that in the premolar and molar area, it is sometimes possible to use commercial ceramic teeth (Figs 12-50 and 12-51).

Fig 12-48 The seating is edged with thermoplastic paste to protect the mucosa on the underlying alveolar crest.

Fig 12-49 Taking an impression with zinc oxide–eugenol paste.

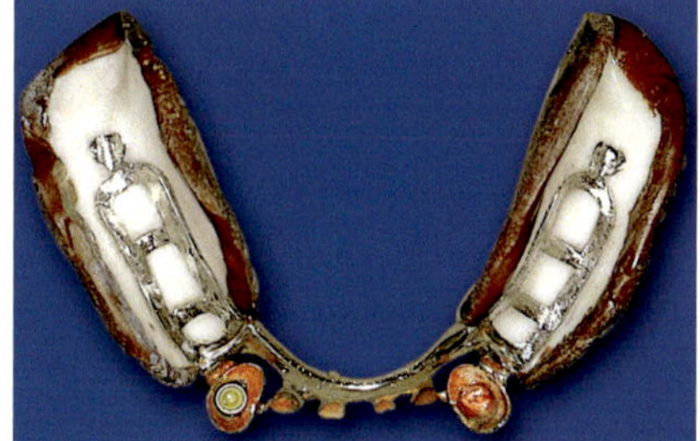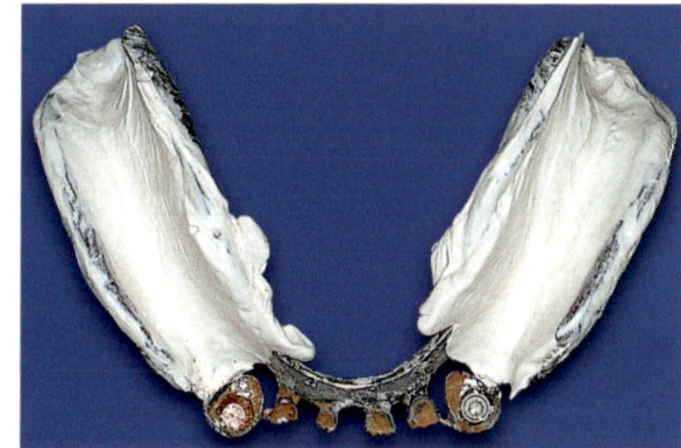

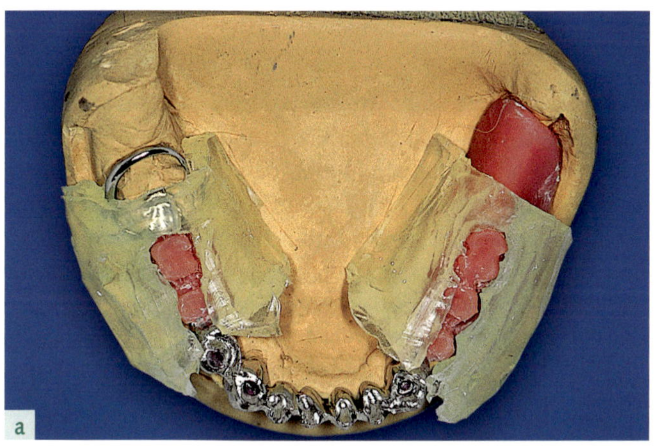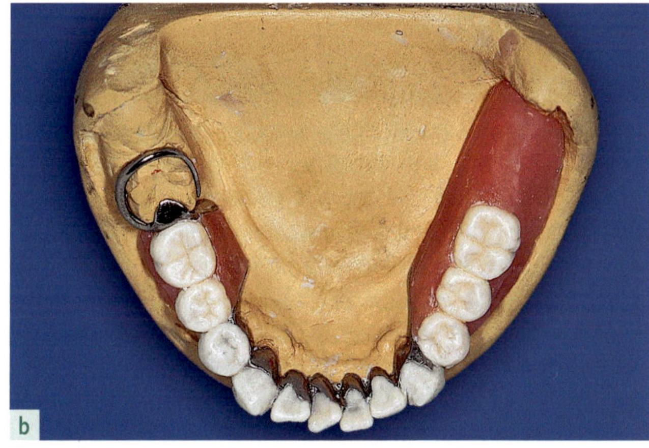

Fig 12-50 Preparing the prosthetic teeth in composite on the metal structure with the assistance of the silicone key prepared from the waxup.

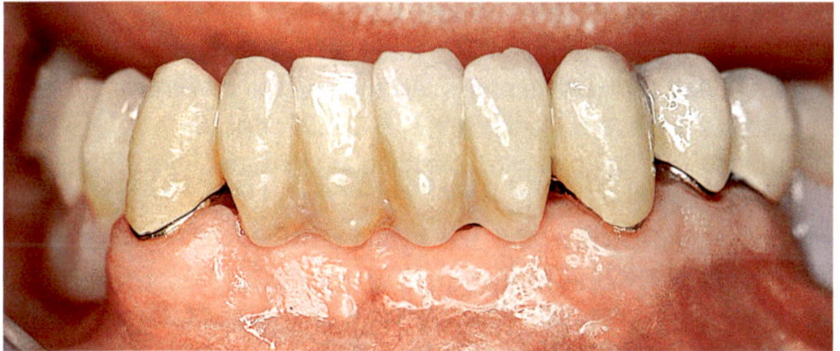

Fig 12-51 Checking the correct positioning of the margins.

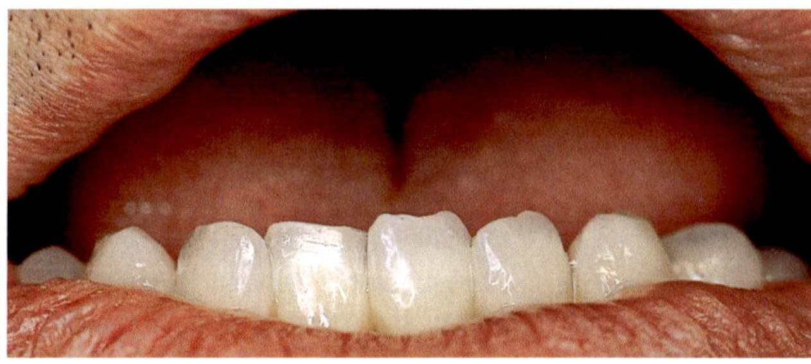

Fig 12-52 Checking the esthetics.

Delivery of denture

The last phase of rehabilitation is the delivery of the prosthesis. Particular attention must be given to the following aspects:

- Positioning of the margins of the esthetic components of the superstructure.
- Stability of the superstructure and eventual blocking of the attachment matrices with resin or composite cements.
- When resin saddles are used, the extension and fitting with frena.
- Occlusal stability.

On insertion of the denture, the patient must be instructed on how to maintain oral hygiene at home, and a follow-up hygiene consultation should be scheduled (Figs 12-52 to 12-55).

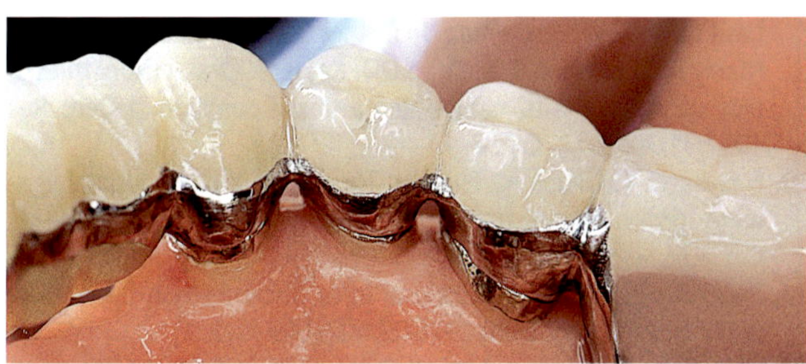

Fig 12-53 Checking the periodontal situation.

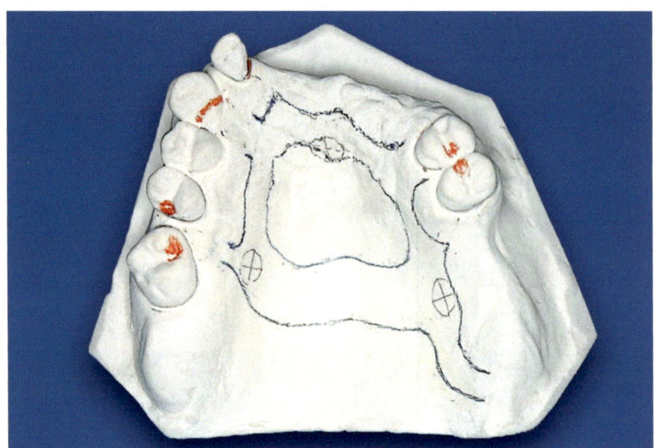

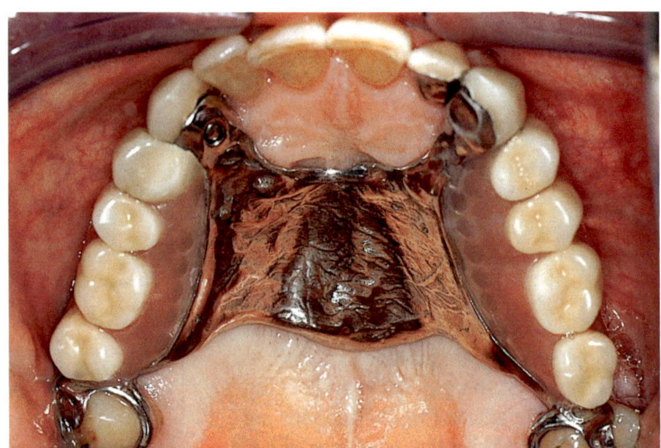

Fig 13-21 Design sequence proceeds with the selection of the principal connector. For anterior edentulism, a double bar is an alternative to a palatal plate, which needs ample space and is not well tolerated by patients.

Fig 13-22 Palatal plate as the principal connector in the maxilla. It provides good vertical support and sufficient rigidity and can be readily adapted by the patient.

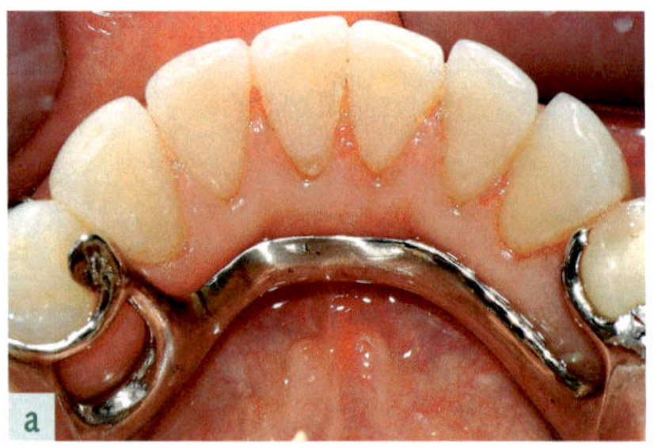

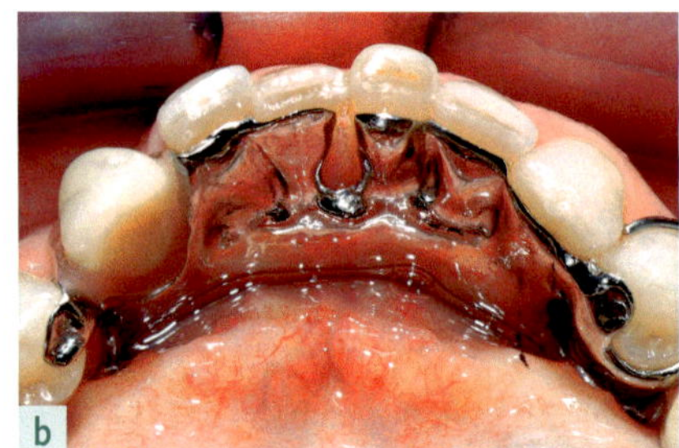

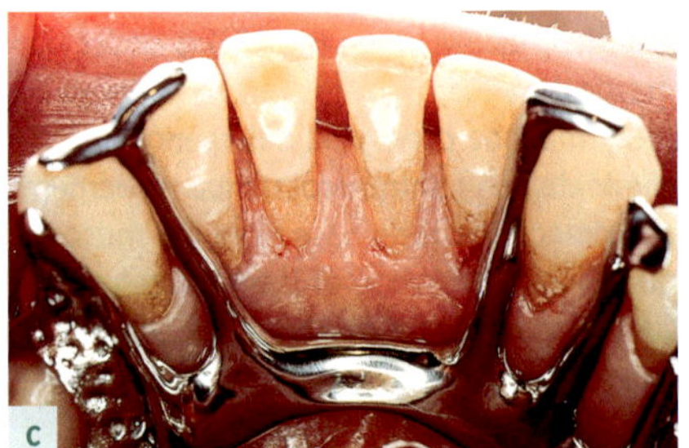

Fig 13-23 Principal mandibular connectors. *(a)* Lingual bar. *(b)* Lingual plate. *(c)* Sublingual bar.

prosthetic distal extensions (Fig 13-21). The maxilla and mandible have different characteristics and therefore need specific primary connectors. In the maxilla, the palate is an excellent area for the positioning of the primary connector because of the large fibromucosa-coated surface, which provides excellent vertical support for the RPD. The safe distance between the gingival margin and the edge of the primary connector is about 6 mm. Among the various types of maxillary primary connectors, the palatine band is the most versatile and most used (Fig 13-22). It is the connector to which the patient adapts most easily. The curved shape of the palate allows for construction of a thin layer with the necessary rigidity. Circumferential thickening provides sealing or "beading," increases rigidity, offers greater comfort for the patient, and does not have areas where food can accumulate.

In the mandible, the choice and the positioning of the primary connector depend on the morphology of the sublingual sulcus. The safety distance between the gingival margin and the edge of the primary connector is about 3 mm. If there is enough height, the first choice connector is the lingual bar (Fig 13-23a). The half-pear profile guarantees sufficient rigidity and access for hygiene.

In the presence of serious resorption of edentulous ridges and periodontally compromised residual teeth, the lingual plate is recommended (Fig 13-23b). The lingual plate is made up of two parts. The base has a half-pear–shaped profile and a thin coronal part that follows the lingual surfaces of the teeth. The upper margins of the lingual plate pass above the cingulum and must be in close contact with the dental surface and the adjacent soft tissues to prevent the creation of areas of plaque accumulation. The disadvantage of the lingual plate is the large contact surfaces, which encourage the accumulation of plaque if the patient's hygiene practices are substandard. In the case of periodontally compromised residual teeth with insufficient space for the lingual bar, a sublingual bar can be used (Fig 13-23c). Unlike mandibular connectors that use the lingual plate, the sublingual bar is positioned on the sublingual sulcus. The use of this area requires the construction of a custom

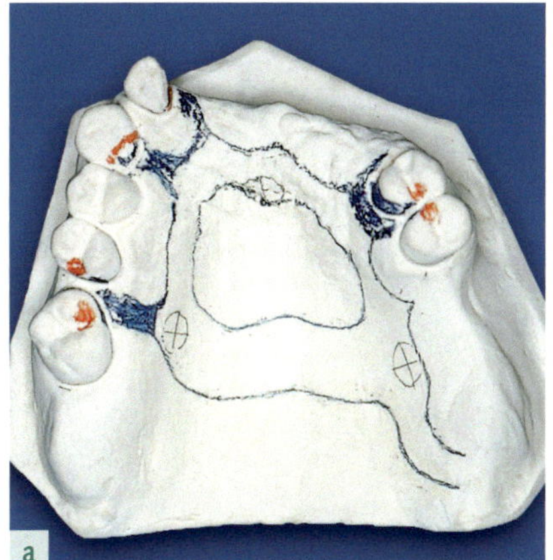
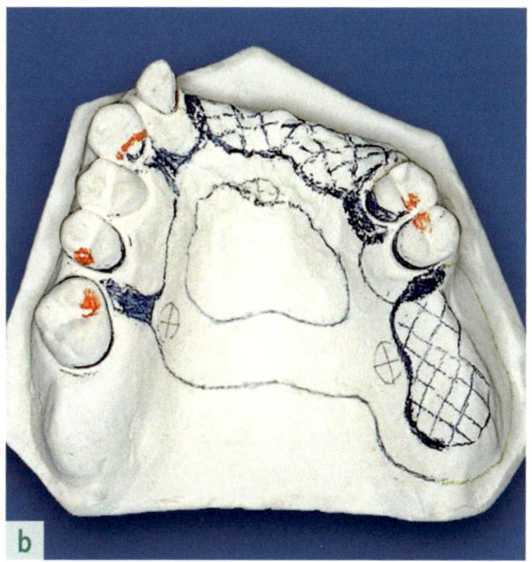
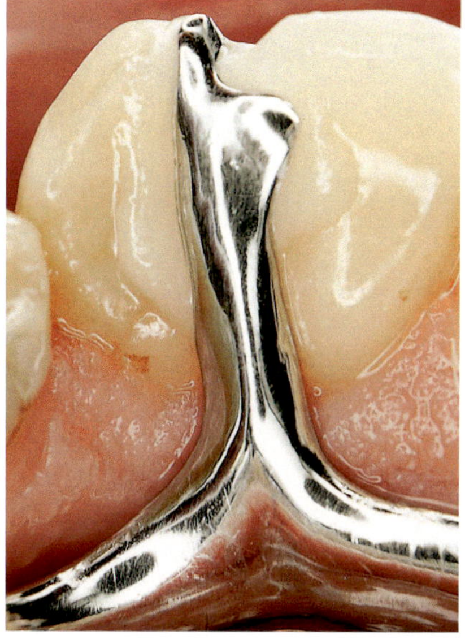

Fig 13-24 *(a)* Secondary connectors unite the clasps and the support areas to the principal connectors. *(b)* Then, the secondary connectors unite with the resin base.

Fig 13-25 This secondary connector unites the support with the principal connector at 90 degrees, with a rounded margin.

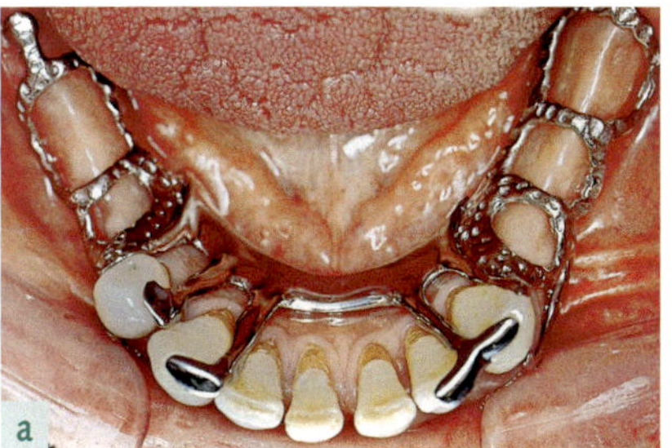
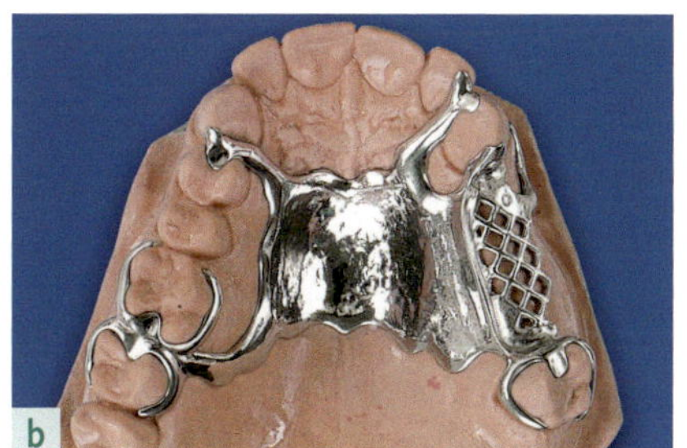
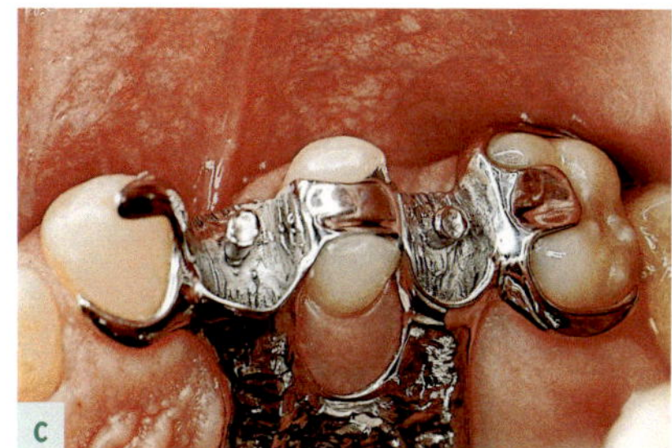

Fig 13-26 *(a)* Secondary connector with a large loop. *(b)* Secondary connector in a mesh grid. *(c)* Secondary connector with a pin connector.

impression tray to carefully plan the position of the connector so as to avoid interference with the movements of the tongue.

Secondary connectors join the primary connectors to all of the other components of the RPD. This group includes connectors that join the clasps and the rests to the primary connector (Fig 13-24a) and connectors that act as retention to the resin base (Fig 13-24b).

The secondary connectors of the first group are positioned in the interdental spaces in triangular forms or on the surfaces of the guide planes acting as proximal plates. Positioning of these connectors in the interdental spaces or on the guide planes of the most distal teeth assists insertion and removal of the denture and increases its stability. In addition, these connectors originate from the primary connector at a 90-degree angle with rounded margins and are placed perpendicular to the mucosa so that they pass over it without contact (Fig 13-25).

The secondary connectors that join the resin base to the primary connector must provide good anchorage without interfering with the positioning of artificial teeth. These connectors can be divided into large loops, a mesh grid, or a pin connector (Fig 13-26).

When in contact with the supporting teeth, the clasps keep the denture in place, both during function and rest (Fig 13-27). The retention of clasps is provided by a flexible and nondeformable arm that is lodged in an undercut of the tooth, creating resistance to the displacing forces.

There are many different types of claps for different clinical situations, including suprabulge and infrabulge clasps (Fig 13-28) and whether the retention arm originates above or below the height of contour of the tooth. The basic components of the clasp, which allow the fundamental functions of retention, stabilization, and support, are the retention arm, the reciprocal arm, and the rest. In the case of edentulous gaps, the choice depends on the position of the undercut, the position of the abutment tooth, and the esthetic considerations. For distal extension edentulism, the clasp must have a mesial rest, allowing the disengagement of the retention arm during rotational movement due to the difference in resilience

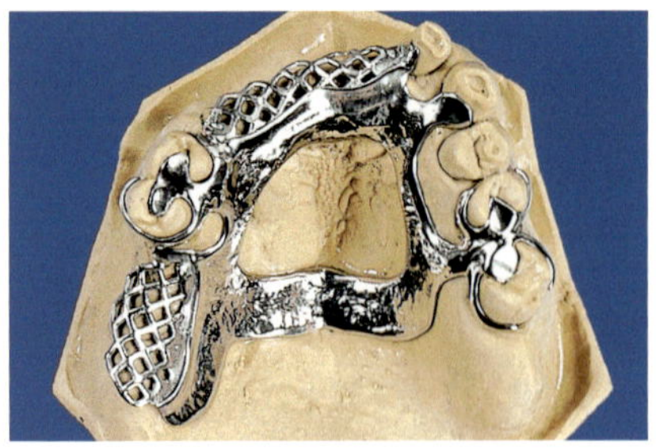

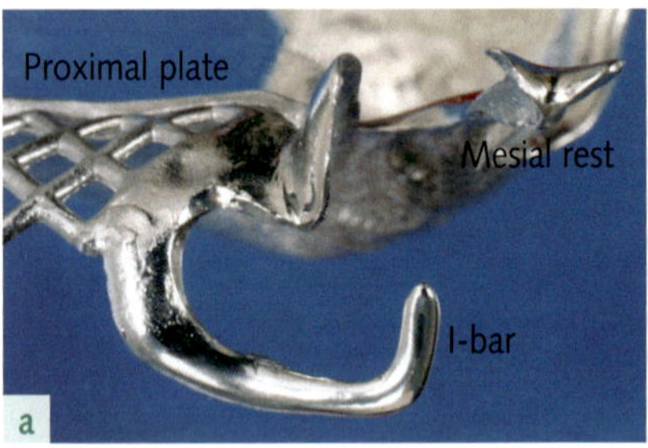

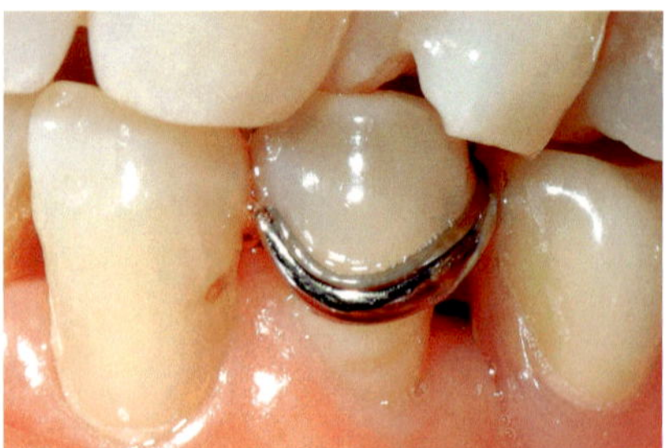

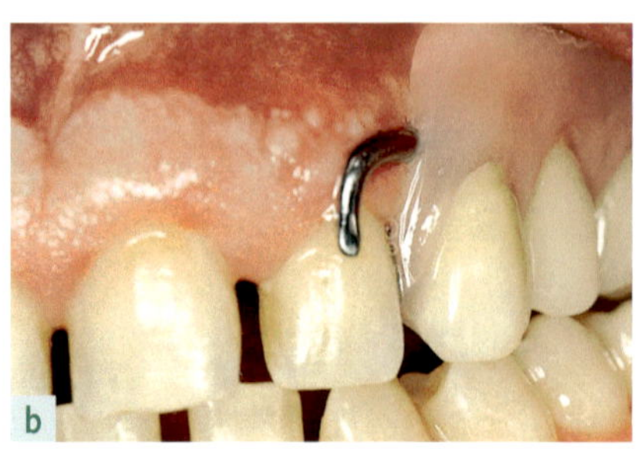

Fig 13-27 Design sequence is completed by the selection and placement of the clasps. On the left second premolar, a posterior clasp determines the positon of the mesial support at the retentive extremity. On the right first molar and second premolar, a double Bonwill clasp is used.

Fig 13-28 The origin of this clasp retention is suprabulge the tooth.

Fig 13-29 *(a)* I-bar clasp proposed by Kratochil with retention originating inferior to the height of contour of the tooth, a mesial rest, and a proximal plate that guides the insertion and removal of the prosthesis. *(b)* Clinical view in situ.

between the alveolar ligament and the mucosa. The clasp that satisfies the biomechanical requirements and the charcateristics of simplicity and hygiene is the mesial rest,[73] proximal plate, and I-bar (RPI) system proposed by Kratochvil (Fig 13-29). The I-bar is the retention arm, which must be positioned at the level of maximum curvature of the tooth, as close as possible to the center of the buccal surface. Its top is placed at the level of the height of contour, and the retentive portion is lodged in an undercut of 0.25 mm. The mesial rest is mesial to the retention arm of the I-bar. The proximal plate will be in contact with the guide plane, which must be prepared on the distal surface of the supporting tooth. The configuration of the I-bar has some advantages when compared with other types of clasps. These include the possibility of obtaining a better esthetic result, less contact between metal and tooth, less stress on the supporting tooth, better vertical distribution of the forces on the edentulous ridge, minimal alteration of the dental profile, and consequently, improved self-cleaning ability.

Preparation of the mouth

The parts of the supporting teeth that need the most preparation concern the guide planes for the minor connectors, the sites for the rests, and the height of contour for the retention arms or for the rigid parts that cannot engage in an undercut. Modifications of the supporting tooth can be accomplished through simple ameloplasty or a partial or total crown.

Enamel contouring. This procedure is used when modifications can be made in the enamel layer. Modifications are planned on the study cast based on the design of the metal structure and can be accurately transferred to the mouth. So as not to alter the circumferential margin of the rests, use the following steps: Preparation of the guide planes (Fig 13-30), determination of the height of contour (Fig 13-31), determination of the width of the undercut (Fig 13-32), and preparation of the sites for the rests (Fig 13-33).

Partial and total crowns. If preparation also includes dentin, and the abutment teeth are structurally compromised, these structures will need prosthetic reconstruction as well (Fig 13-34). Once the necessary modifications have been made to the residual teeth, an impression is taken for the master cast, and the correct preparation is verified with the parallelometer. Through duplication, the cast is obtained in refractory material on which the metal structure is constructed.

Try-in and clinical adaptation of the metal framework

The metal structure is positioned correctly when all of the rests are in contact with the relative sites (Fig 13-35). The checkup and adaptation of the other components of the RPD can then be undertaken.

Physiologic adjustment. In the case of distal extensions situations, it is necessary to check that the metal structure does not cause torsion stresses to the abutment teeth during function. If it is impossible to prevent rotational movement caused by the viscoelastic behavior of the alveolar ligament and the mucosa, then it is necessary to reduce the stress to a minimum both on the abutment tooth and the edentulous ridge. This result can also be obtained through physiologic adjustment and with the modified cast. Physiologic adjustment allows for identification

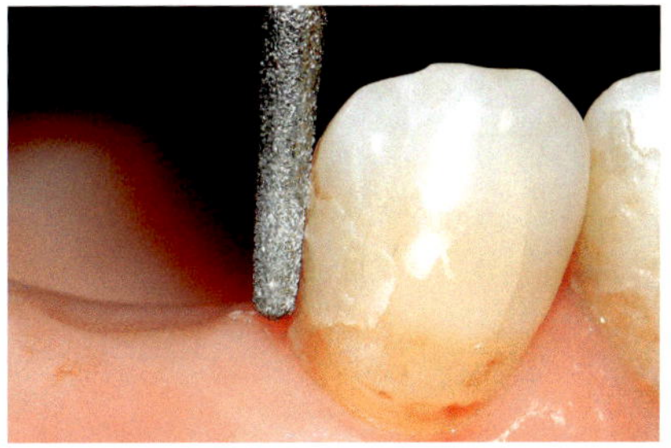

Fig 13-30 Preparation of the guide plane on the proximal surface of the abutment tooth. It is necessary to respect the curvature of the tooth on the horizontal plane in removing a minimal uniform thickness of enamel and to maintain the optimal retention of the clasp.

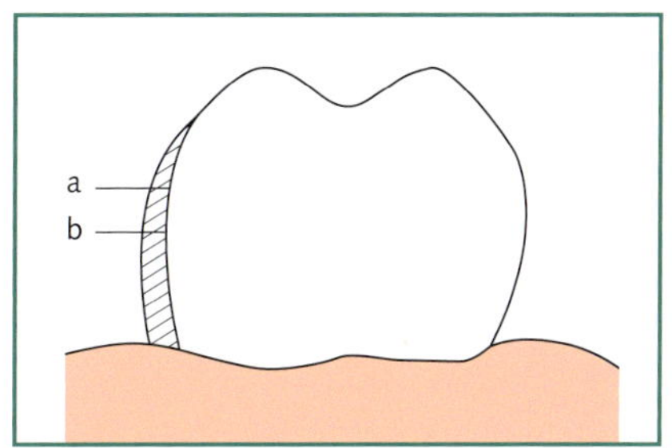

Fig 13-31 Enamel contouring makes it possible to vary the placement of the height of contour on the abutment tooth. *(a)* Initial height of contour. *(b)* After the correction.

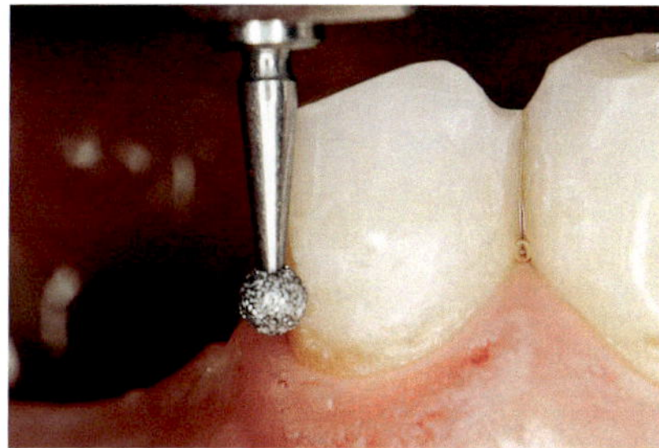

Fig 13-32 Enamel contour increases the undercut. The slight depression with rounder margins must have an extension of around 4 mm in the mesiodistal direction and about 2 mm in the occlusogingival direction.

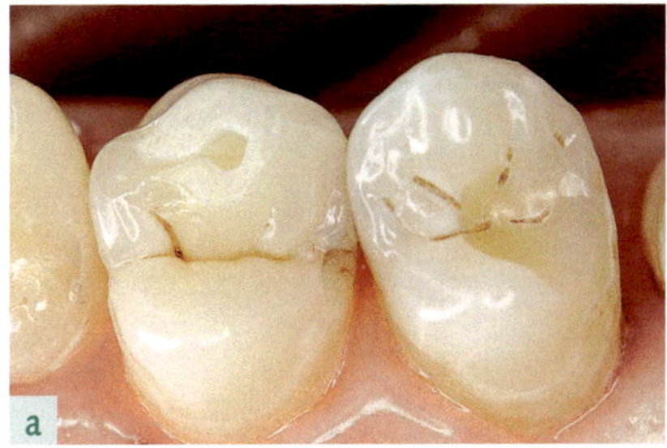

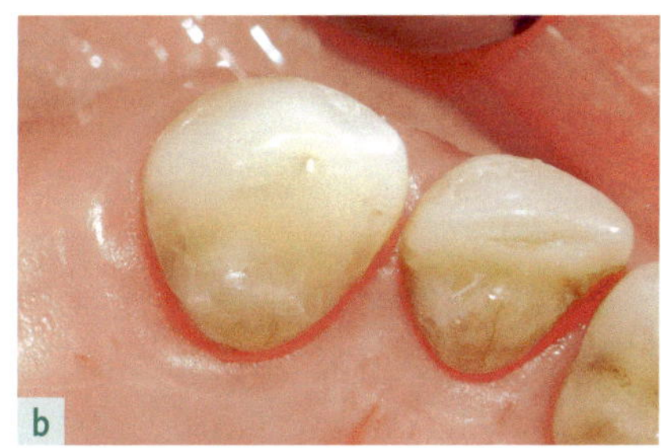

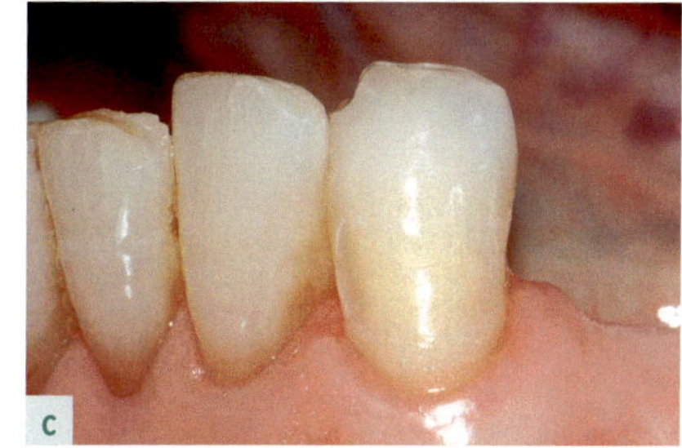

Fig 13-33 Types of preparation or support sites: *(a)* occlusal, *(b)* cingulum, *(c)* incisal.

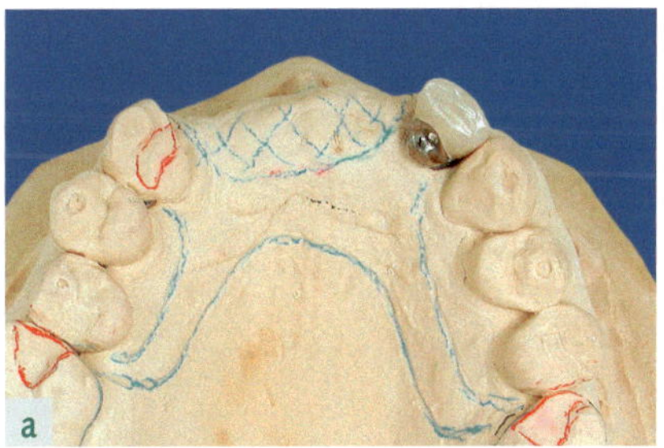

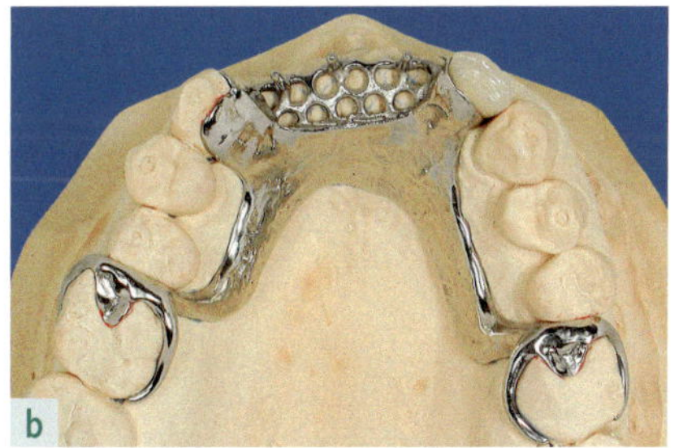

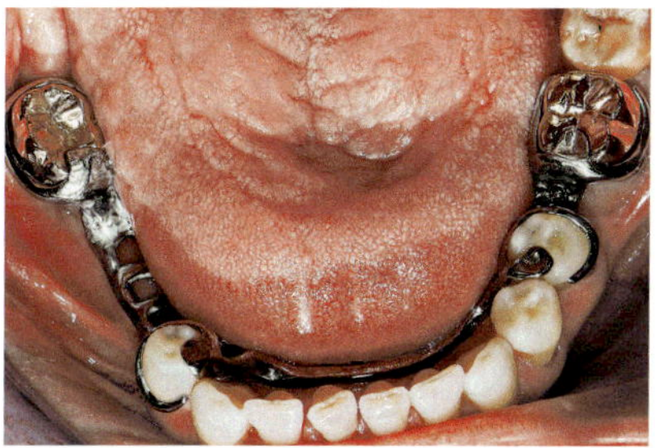

Fig 13-34 *(a)* Preparation for support on the left canine is completed during the waxup, prior to the analysis of the parallelism and the design of the metal armature. The fused crown will be, in effect, the guide plane, the site for support, and the ideal undercut. On the cingulum of the metal-ceramic crown, the site for support is clear. *(b)* The metal structure of the RPD is then prepared.

Fig 13-35 The positioning of the metal structure is considered correct when all supports are in contact with the related sites.

and elimination of the areas of greater friction between the rigid metal structures and the supporting teeth during function (Fig 13-36).

Constructive principles of the dental base

These principles are the same as the complete denture in terms of the morphologic characteristics and the installation of the artificial teeth.

The master cast on which the metal structure has been constructed does not reproduce the distal edentulous extension situation with the details necessary for constructing a prosthetic body (Fig 13-37).

Impression of the edentulous area. Altered cast. In this cast, the impression of the residual teeth is kept intact and the impression of the edentulous ridge is renewed. The alveolar ridges are

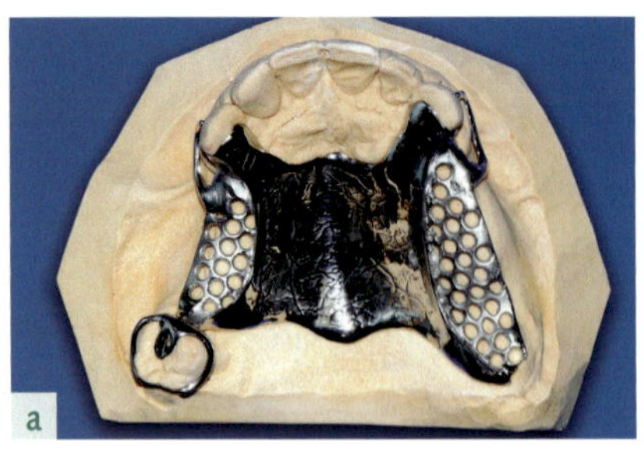
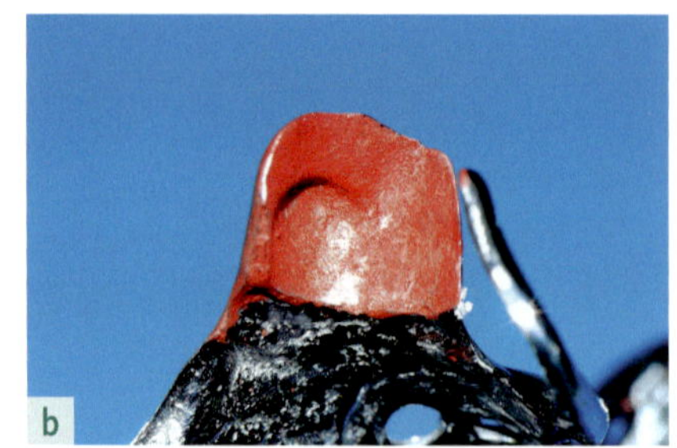

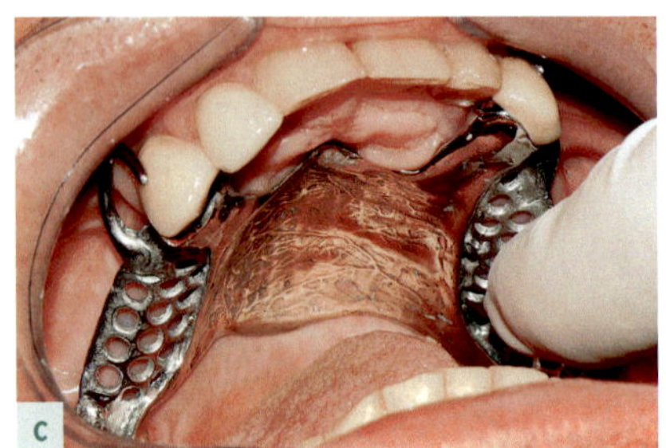
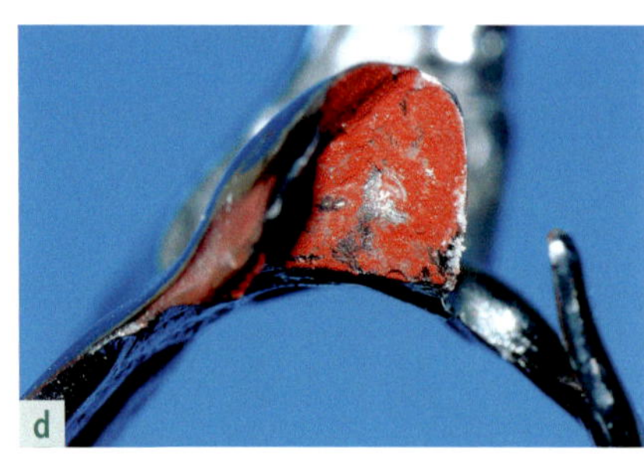

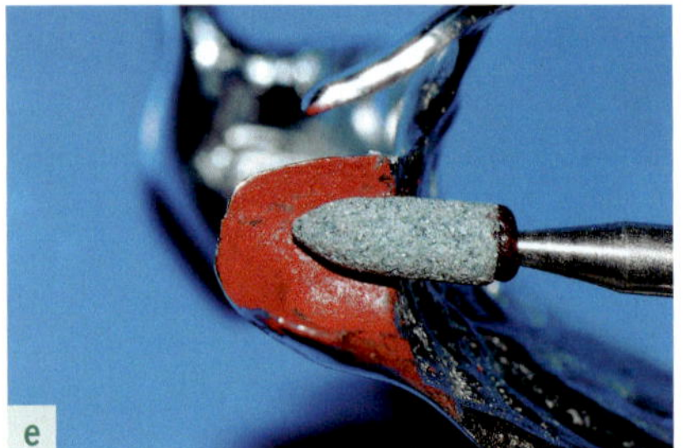
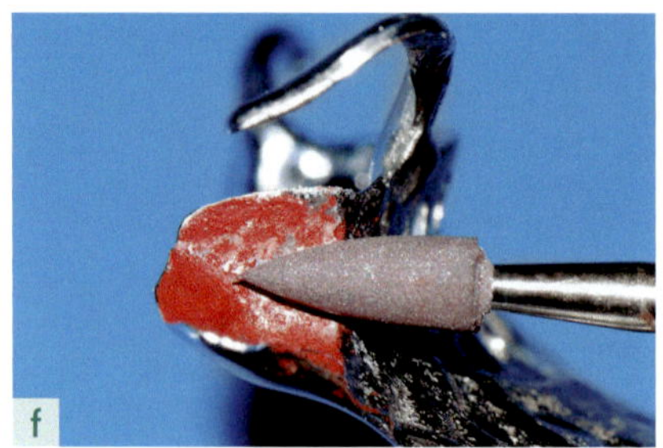

Fig 13-36 *(a)* The metal structure on the cast. Modified Kennedy Class II with a principal palatal plate connector, with an I-bar clasp on the maxillary left and right canines, and a circumferential clasp on the right second molar. *(b)* A fine layer of red plaster of Paris disolved in chloroform is applied to the clasps. *(c)* After seating and verifying the correct position by pressing on the distal extension, a rotational movement is provoked in the RPD, which detaches at the support on the right canine. *(d)* Removing the metal framework the area of friction corresponds to the areas with red plaster of Paris. *(e)* With a carborundum bur, remove and correct the contour and repeat until the area of friction disappears. *(f)* Polish the metal with a rubber tip.

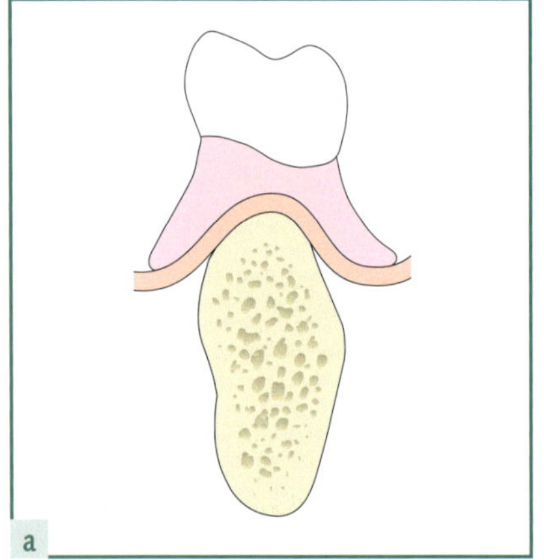
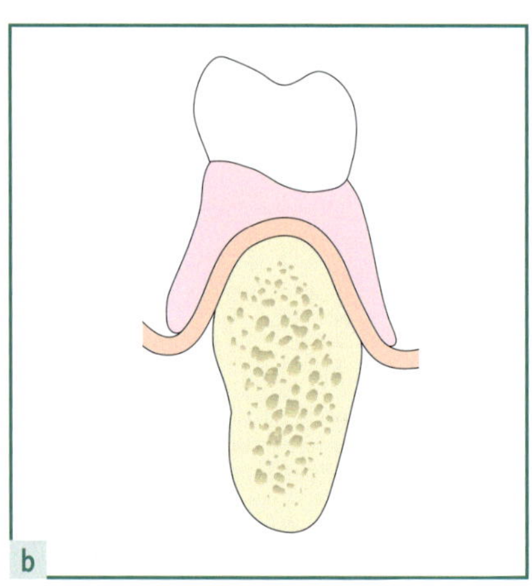

Fig 13-37 *(a)* The first resin impression has too wide a base, and the masticatory loads would be transmitted only at the center of the crest corresponding to the adhering mucosal tissue. *(b)* The altered cast allows a restoration with the mucosa adapted to the underlying bone structure in resin, which allows a wider and more uniform distribution of the functional load.

reproduced with the mucosa adapted on the underlying bone profile, resulting in an excellent distal extension (Fig 13-38).

Delivery and patient instruction

When the RPD is delivered, a control check must be carried out on the adaptation and extension of the prosthetic body and the occlusal relationship. The patient must also be instructed on how to maintain optimal oral hygiene, and a follow-up schedule should be designed to ensure a successful rehabilitation (see chapter 14).

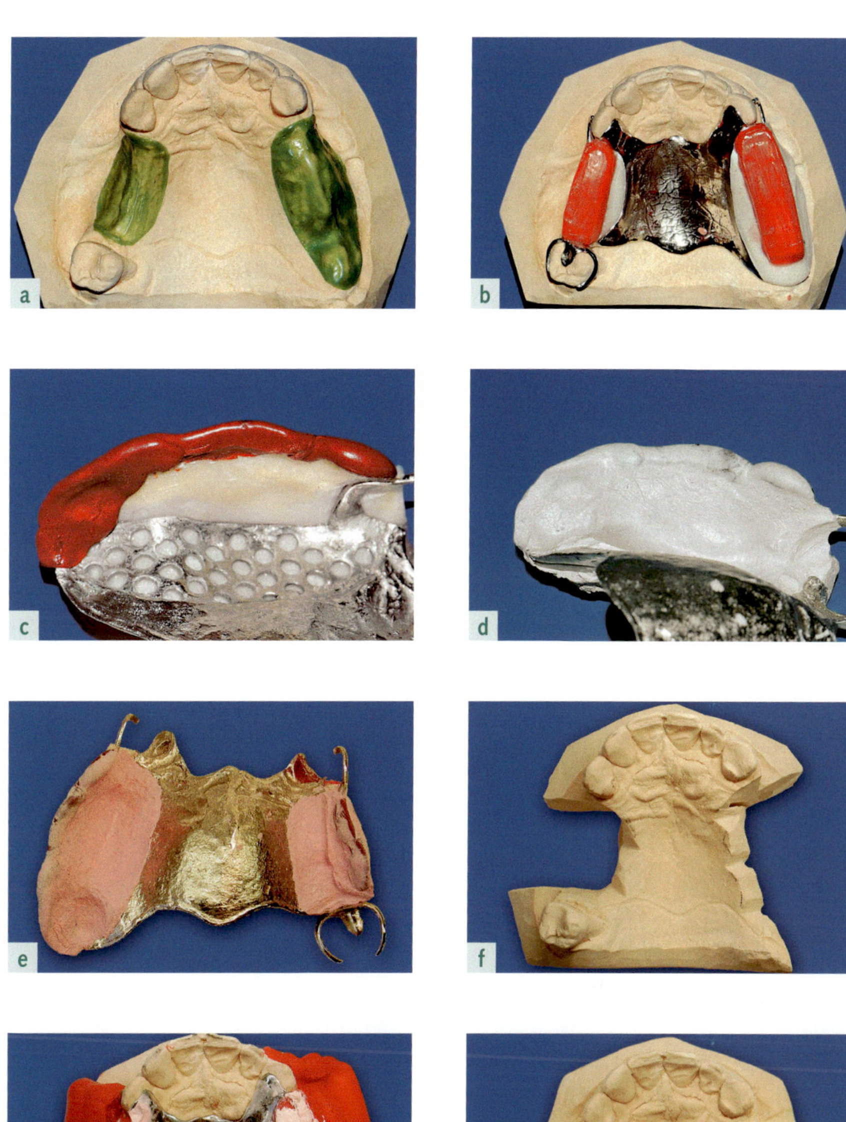

Fig 13-38 *(a)* Technique for a modified cast. With the use of autopolymerizing resin, the denture base can be used as custom tray to take the impression of the edentulous crest. On the cast the edentulous areas are then coated with a 0.4-mm layer of wax. *(b)* The heated framework is seated in position on the cast. The denture base is constructed with the same characteristics as a custom impression tray for the full prosthesis. It is possible to adapt the rims in wax. *(c)* After having checked the correct extension of the base with a border of thermoplastic paste, take an impression with zinc oxide–eugenol material. *(d)* Detail of the right distal extension. (e) Both edentulous areas. *(f)* The master cast is then adapted, eliminating the parts corresponding to the impressions of the edentulous crest. *(g)* Replace the framework by checking the position of the primary and secondary supports and mark for the base. *(h)* The resulting cast includes the dentition from the master cast on which the metal structure was constructed as well as the replica of the edentulous ridges obtained with the new impression.

Esthetics in RPDs

The metal parts of the RPD cannot always be masked; the retention arm and rests are visible when speaking.

A Dutch study[84] evaluated patients' needs (subjective) versus surgeons' needs (objective) for better esthetic results. It was considered necessary for 63% of surgeons and 40% of patients. The discrepancy between the objective and subjective needs increased with the patients' age and has been linked to the greater critical requirements of the surgeon. The patient's esthetic requirements are only evaluated during function.

During function, however, the lips are not open wide enough to reveal the metal parts of the RPD (Fig 13-39).

Older patients are less likely to be bothered enough by the esthetics to request a more complicated and expensive operation, as shown by Taylor and colleagues.[85] The authors compared subjects in two age groups, 55 through 64 years and 65 through 74 years, and found that esthetics were less important in the older group.

If a patient cannot tolerate the visible metal parts, it is possible to eliminate the anterior clasps using axes of rotational

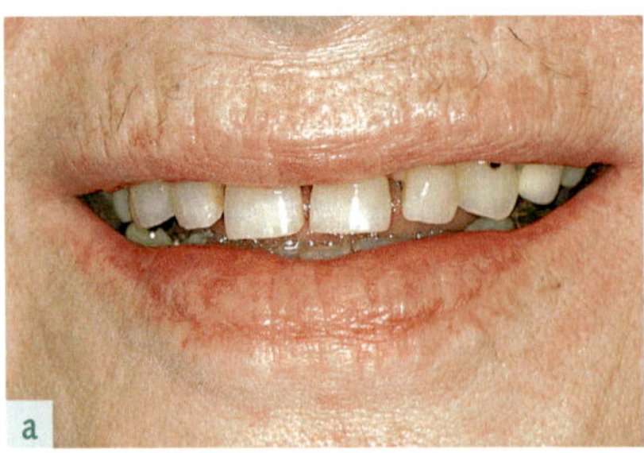 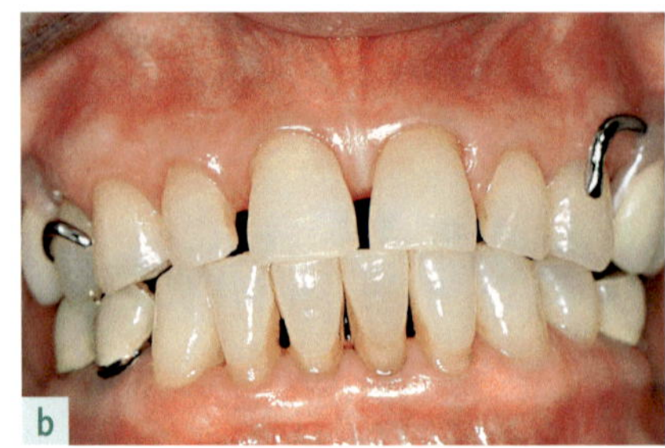

Fig 13-39 Esthetic considerations. The metal structure, clasps, and supports cannot be eliminated from the anterior region, but they can be positioned with care for a better esthetic impact. The retentive arms can be placed in the buccal cervical portion of the teeth. Supports at the cingulum must respect the incisal area. Esthetic interference must also be considered while the patient is talking or smiling *(a)* and without the distraction of the lips *(b)*.

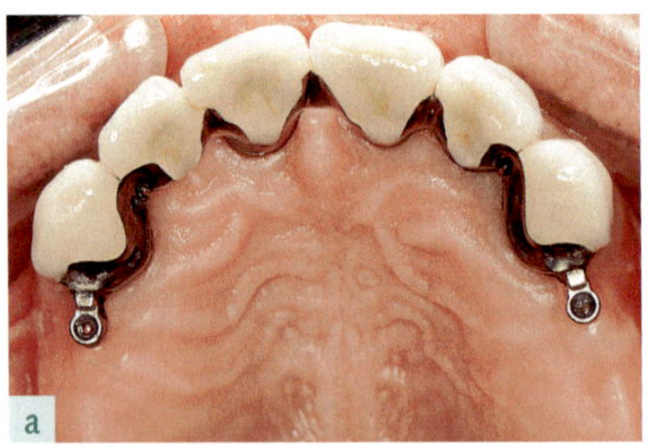 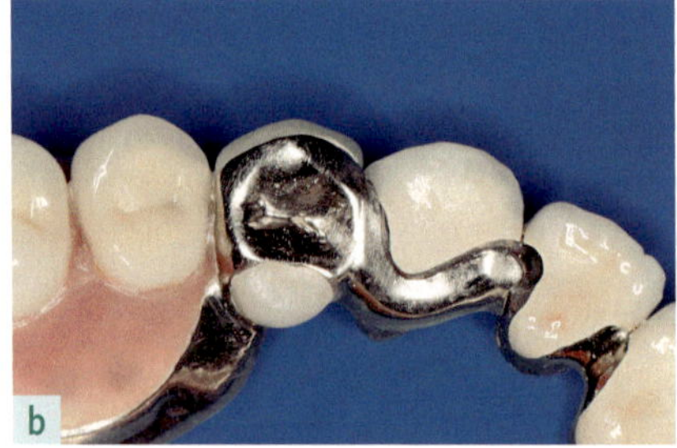

Fig 13-40 *(a)* Patients with high esthetic expectations need precison attachments. A clincal occlusal view of the metal-ceramic anterior teeth in with extracoronal precison attachments (Conex). *(b)* Removeable components (RPD) inserted into an FPD.

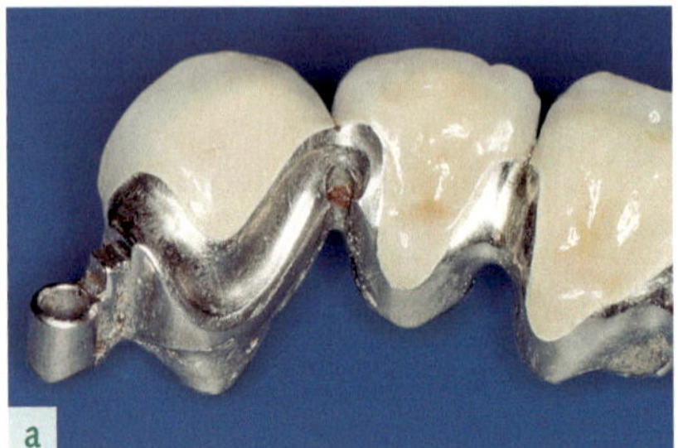 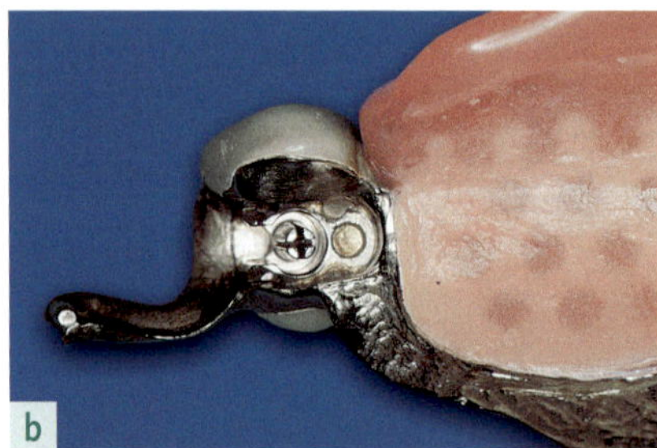

Fig 13-41 Attachment comprising two components: *(a)* ball attachment (or patrix) applied to a fixed crown and *(b)* matrix attached to the RPD.

insertion. These can be used almost exclusively in the presence of edentulous gaps adjacent to natural teeth. It is possible to use adhesive or soldered precision attachments on prosthetic crown, or with radicular clasps (see chapter 12) to satisfy the esthetic needs of these patients.

RPDs with precision attachments

This type of RPD is recommended only if the esthetic requirements are demanding and if the supporting teeth must be replaced by a prosthesis (Figs 13-40 and 13-41). A simple clasp gives similar functional results to those of a precision attachment.

There are many types of precision attachments. A simple classification separates the attachments into radicular (Figs 13-42c and 13-43), intracoronal (Figs 13-42a and 13-44), and extracoronal (Figs 13-42b and 13-45) in relation to the application area of the attachment.[86] In the rehabilitation of a distal extension situation, given the stresses caused by the masticatory loads and the different reactions of the support structures, the use of extracoronal attachments is recommended.[75] The extracoronal attachments are prefabricated units made up of two matching components: *(1)* the patrix, applied to the external walls of a crown, and *(2)* the matrix, usually fixed to the removable denture. The main advantages of the extracoronal attachments are prefabrication and good metallurgic quality; good adaptation; replaceable matrix; and vertical support, retention, reciprocity, and passivity. The disadvantages include its dimensions in the standard size, cost, and complexity. The attachment can be fused or soldered with the metal structure of a crown.

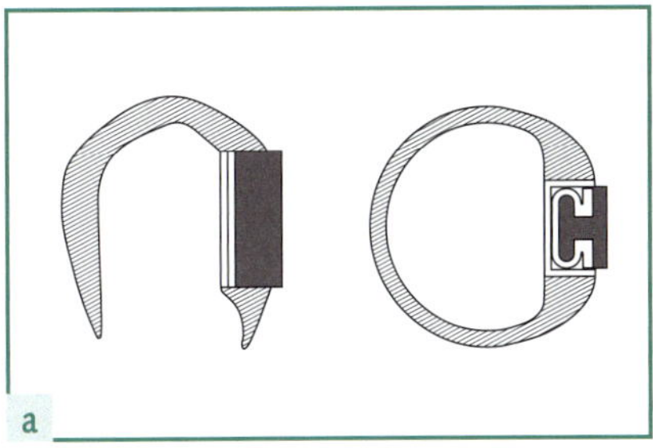 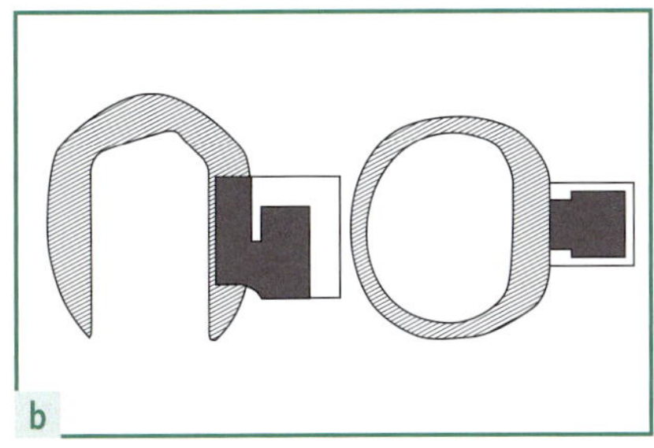 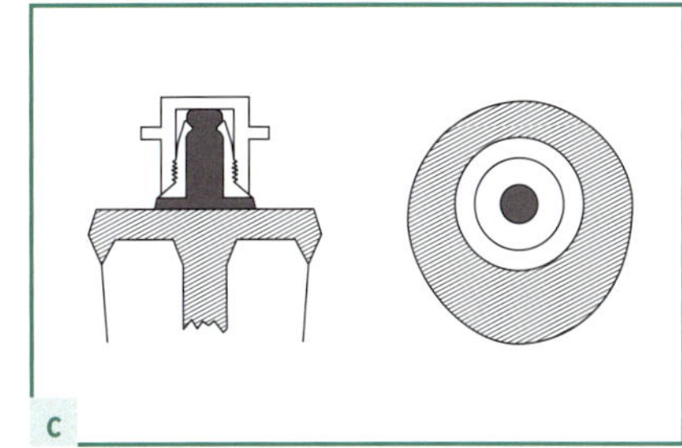

Fig 13-42 Classification of precision attachments according to the areas where they will be applied: *(a)* intracoronal; *(b)* extracoronal; *(c)* radicular.

Fig 13-43 Radicular attachment: *(a)* ball attachment (patrix) soldered to a Richmond base; *(b)* matrix fixed to the metal structure of an RPD.

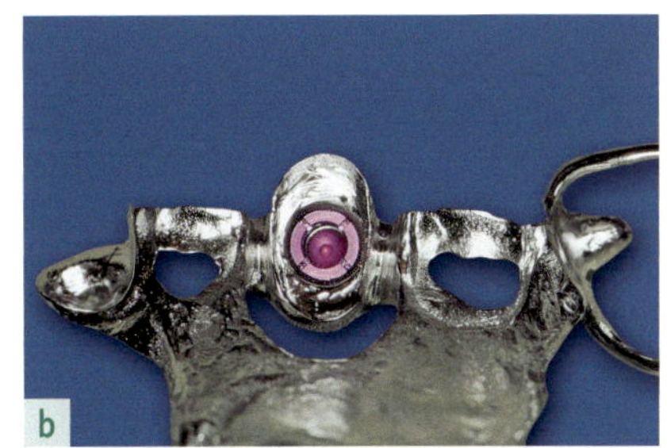

Fig 13-44 Intracoronal attachment: *(a)* patrix attachment used in the internal profile of the crown; *(b)* patrix attachment fixed to the RPD. Retention is obtained by friction with a spring-loaded ball attachment (Ipsoclip, Cendres et Metaux).

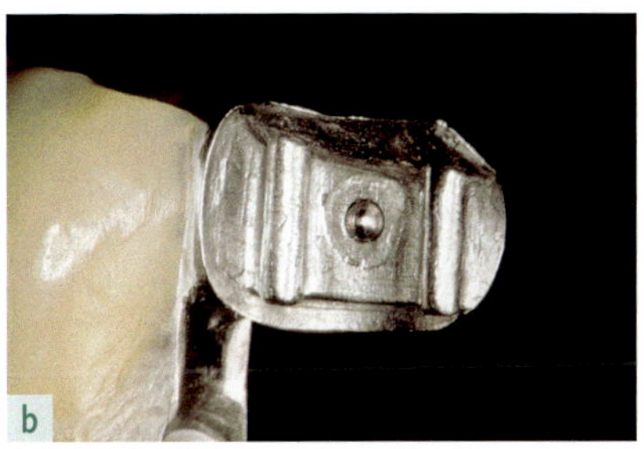

Fig 13-45 Extracoronal attachment SG (Cendres et Metaux): *(a)* patrix soldered to the external profile of the crown; *(b)* matrix fixed to the RPD; the retention is obtained with easily interchangeable plastic friction-grip sleeves located in matrix (center).

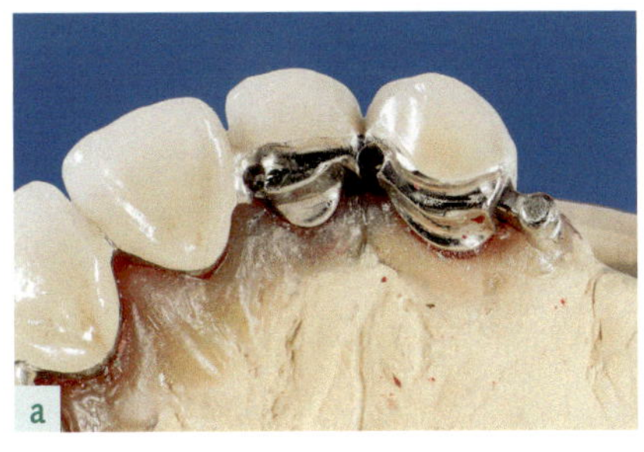 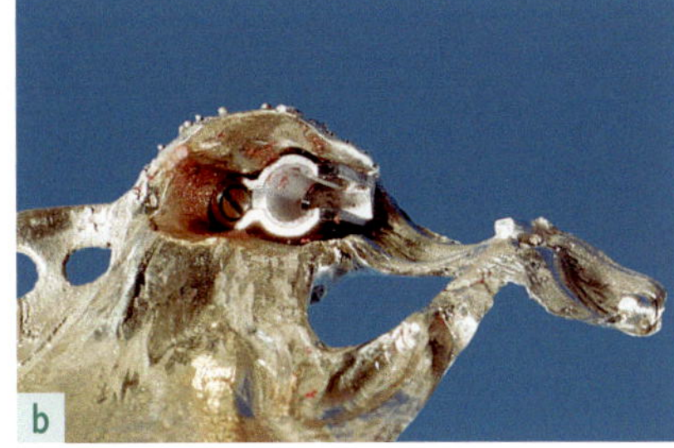

The available height of the distal wall of the supporting tooth as well as the vertical and buccolingual space must be clinically evaluated for the placement of extracoronal attachments (Figs 13-46 and 13-47). Adequate space must be available in order to position the attachment with respect to the abutment without interfering with function and esthetics. Particular attention must be given to the alignment of the attachments on both the sagittal and vertical planes.

This solution offers the best esthetic and functional results but requires a technical and clinical procedure that is costly in terms of maintenance. A retrospective study 2 years after the insertion of the RPD with precision attachments showed

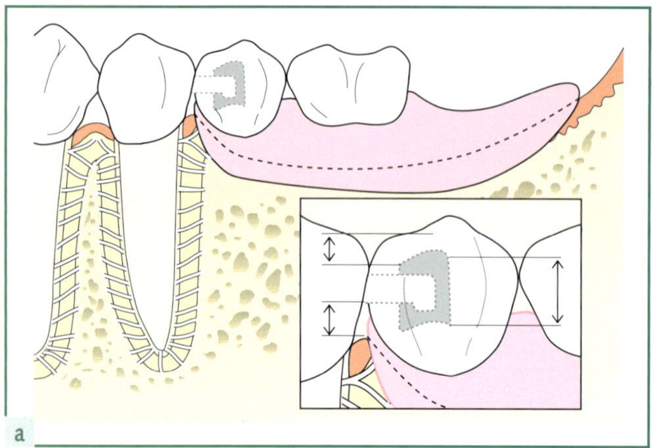

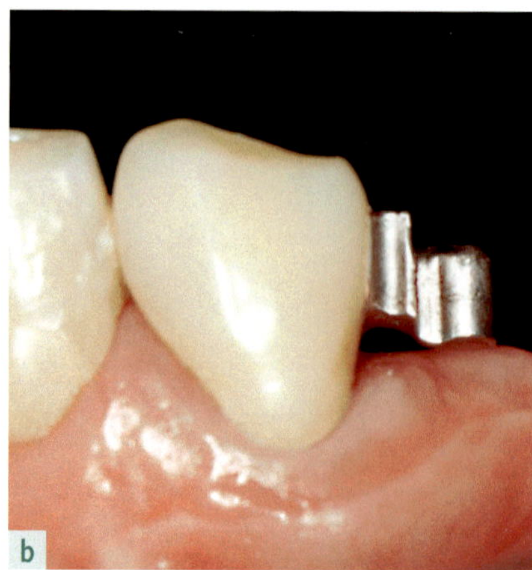

Fig 13-46 *(a)* Vertical space needed for an extracoronal attachment. With conventional attachments the space needed in the proximal area is 7 mm, of which 5 mm is for the standard measure of the attachment, 1 mm for the esthetic occlusal material, and 1 mm to respect the periodontal margins. *(b)* This lateral view shows the correct vertical positioning of an extracoronal attachment.

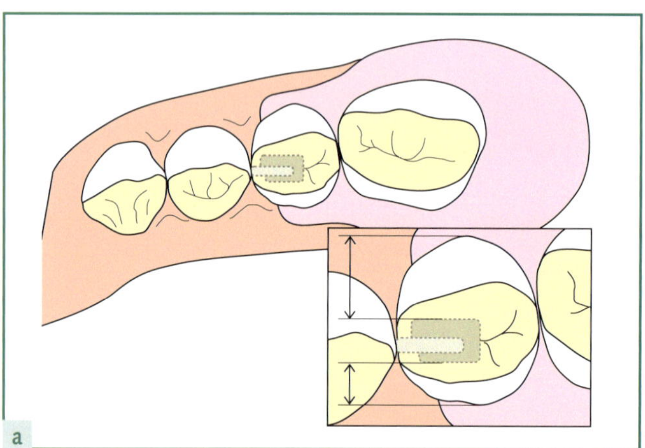

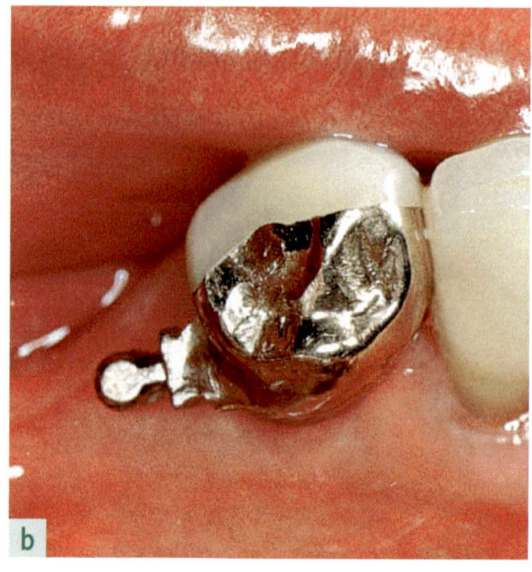

Fig 13-47 *(a)* Buccolingual space available on the distal surface of the crown that determines the position of the attachment. *(b)* Clinical view: The position of the attachment is slightly lingual to allow adequate thickness on the buccal aspect for esthetics. The alignment of the attachment on the sagittal plane is not always necessary, whereas perfect alignment on the vertical plane is essential.

how the initial satisfaction of the patient and surgeon tends to diminish because of the high incidence (63%) of complications.[87]

RPDs with adhesive attachments

With elderly patients, the age-related changes in the dental and periodontal tissues must be taken into consideration when choosing the type of anchorage. Dental abrasion and gingival retraction occurs frequently in this group. Morphologic changes in teeth, and crowns that are clinically longer than the anatomic ones, with excessive inclinations, often cause difficulty when

correctly positioning the clasps (Fig 13-48). In such cases, to position the retentive and reciprocal arms on the enamel and in the areas with an undercut less than 0.50 mm, the clinician must use areas that are too close to the occlusal surfaces, resulting in esthetic and functional problems (eg, unfavorable leverage arm) (Fig 13-49). A solution to such problems could be a fixed prosthesis, which is not always appropriate in elderly patients for economic and biologic reasons. Furthermore, it is almost always necessary to resort to endodontic treatment and a post reconstruction for the crown.

A more convenient solution can be found in adhesive attachments,[88–90] which are relatively simple to prepare and

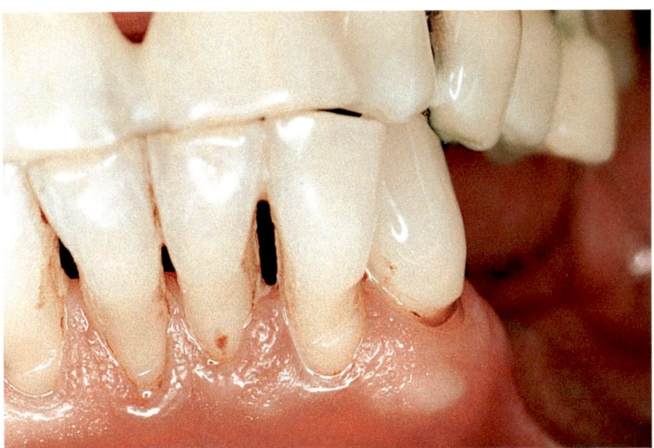

Fig 13-48 Altered morphology in an elderly patient. The crowns are lengthened in the mandibular incisors with exposed cementum and erosion around the neck of the teeth. The incisors are fanned out, and the left canine is destabilized with a lingual inclination. In such situations, the only support area in the undercut for positioning a retentive clasp is often too close to the roots.

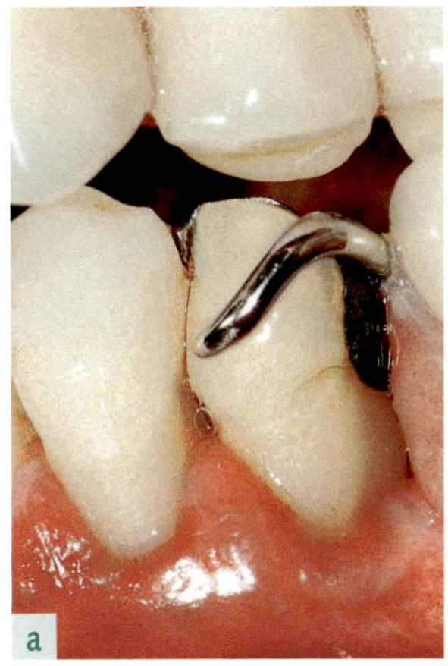
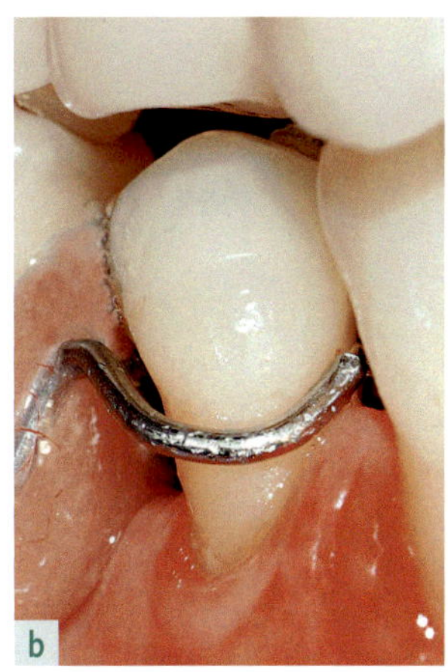

Fig 13-49 *(a)* In the presence of neck errosion, the retentive arm can be attached to an occlusal surface, but this is unfavorable for function and esthetics. *(b)* Use of mixed retention allows the use of a wire retentive arm that can be placed in a more favorable cervical position to suit the undercut.

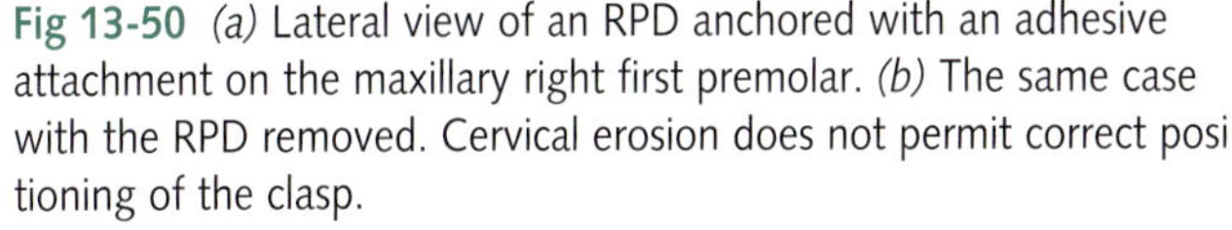

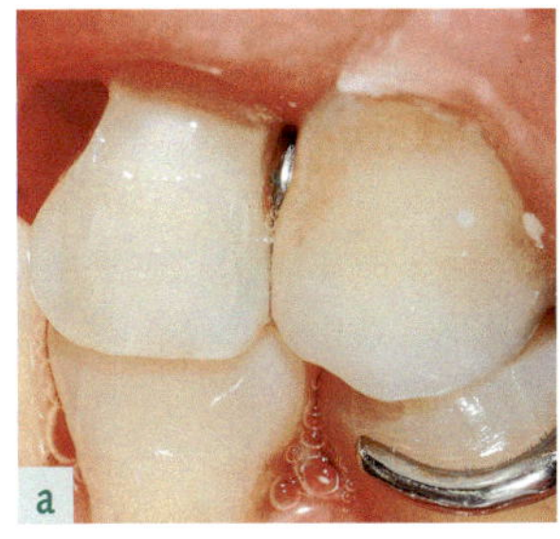
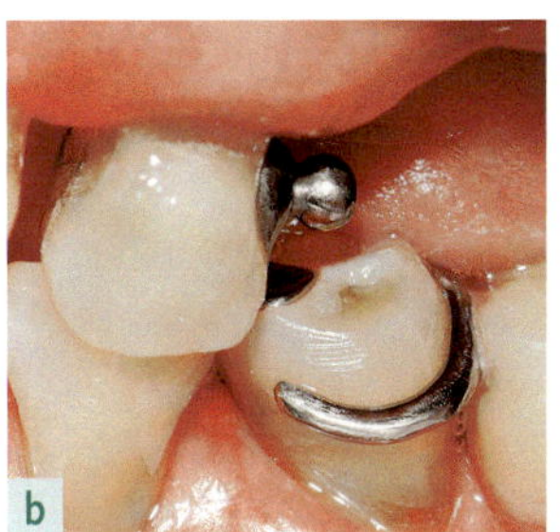

Fig 13-50 *(a)* Lateral view of an RPD anchored with an adhesive attachment on the maxillary right first premolar. *(b)* The same case with the RPD removed. Cervical erosion does not permit correct positioning of the clasp.

are priced reasonably (Fig 13-50). The preparation techniques, execution, and cementation of the adhesive prosthesis are described in part II of this chapter.

Until a few years ago, the contraindications for the use of this type of attachment were linked to the quantity of enamel, particularly on the occlusal surface.[90] Adhesives were not very effective on the dentin. Now, with dentin-enamel adhesives, it is possible to extend adhesion to the dentin without losing retention.[91] This method is advantageous in terms of esthetics, retention, simplicity, the speed with which it is accomplished, reversibility, and the ease of repair in cases of failure.

Implant-supported RPDs

If there is enough bone, one or two implants can be placed in a strategic position and can thus modify the RPD.[75,92] The implant-supported RPD is an affordable therapy that is moderately invasive and technically simple. The strategic placement of a reduced number of implants allows the clinician to optimize the rotation axes of the RPD with mixed support (Figs 13-51 to 13-53, *next page*), eliminate the rotation axes to re-establish a supporting polygon for the FPD (Figs 13-54 to 13-56), and to

avoid placement of clasps on teeth with low periodontal support or esthetic importance (Figs 13-57 and 13-58).

Conclusion and considerations

1. Whether or not to recommend prosthetic rehabilitation in the case of partial endentulism depends on:

- Patient's general health
- Condition of the residual teeth
- Periodontal situation
- Patient motivation and expectations
- Patient's ability to maintain oral hygiene and attend follow-up visits
- Occlusal relationships and dental function
- Advantages, disadvantages, and long-term prognosis of the reconstruction
- Complications that limit the probability of clinical success
- Cost

2. The morphologic restoration of all dental arches can, in some conditions, constitute overtreatment.

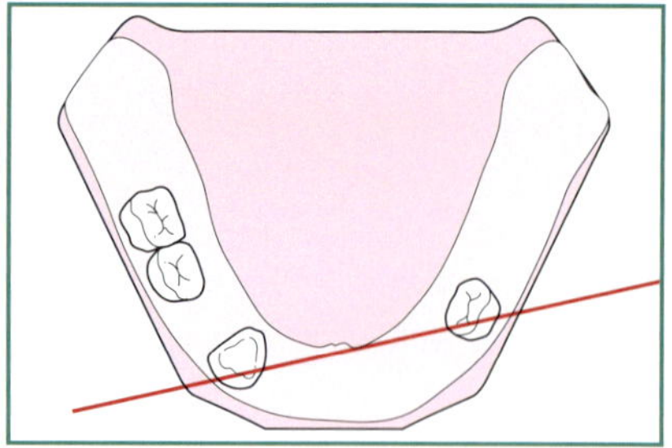

Fig 13-51 Optimization of a Kennedy Class II modified mandible with an unfavorable rotational axis. The axis of rotation from the left second premolar to the right canine is oblique with respect to the frontal plane. The interposed edentulous gaps accentuate the curve. Thus, the interposed occlusal load would be difficult to control and dangerous for abutment teeth.

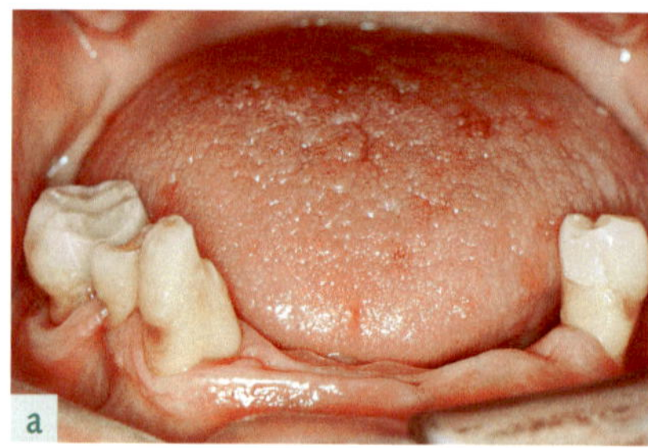

Fig 13-52 Mandible missing strategic abutments: the left canine and first molar. (a) Labial view; (b) occlusal view.

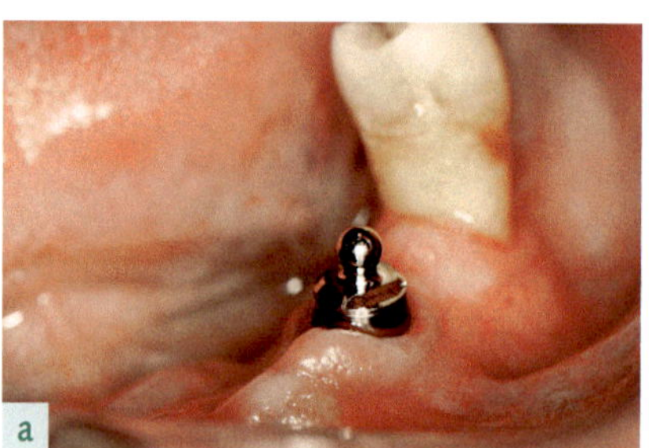

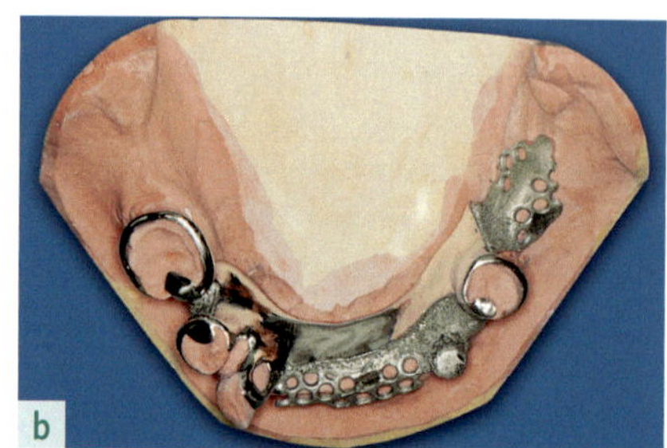

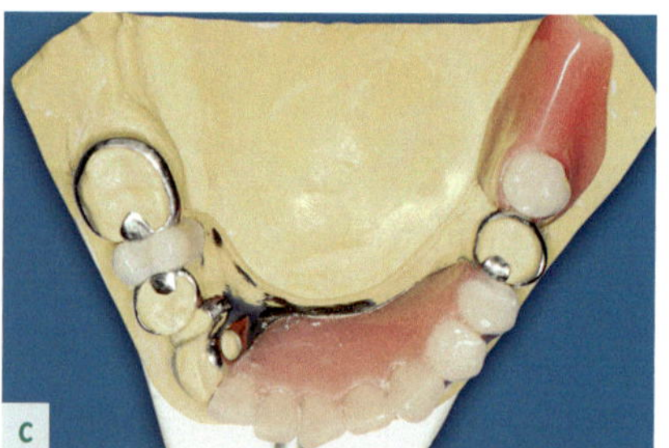

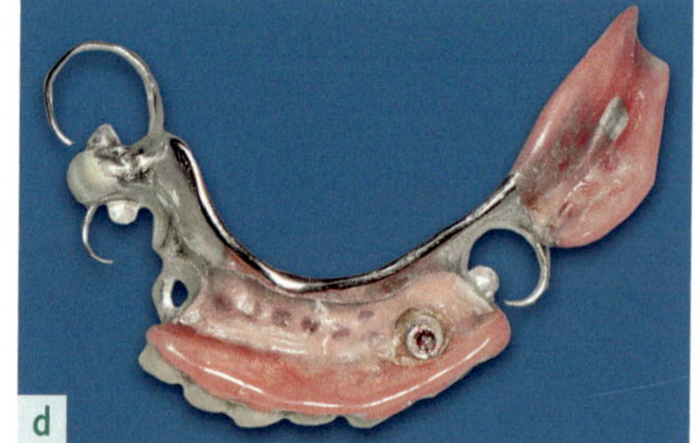

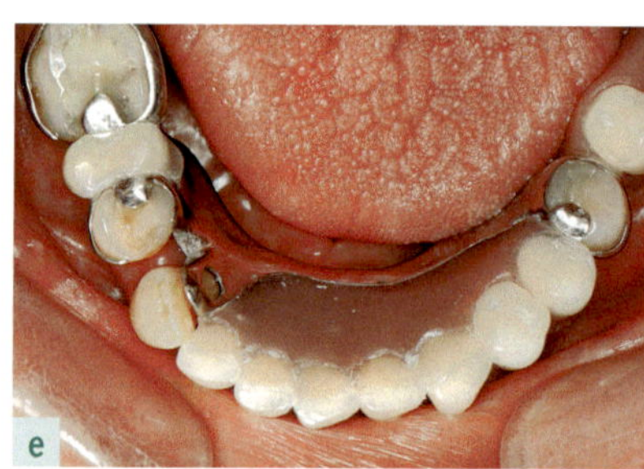

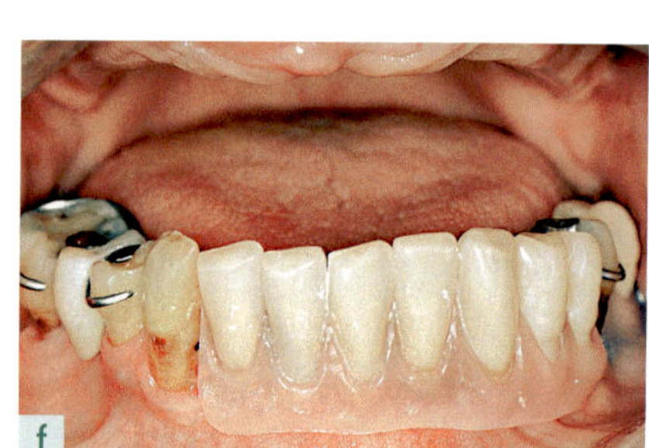

Fig 13-53 With the placement of an implant in the mandibular left canine, the stability and retention is improved for an RPD, guaranteeing a better structural profile. (a) An intraoral view of the implant and a 2.25-mm ball atttachment. (b) The master cast with a metal structure in place showing protection for the attachment. (c) The master cast with the complete RPD. (d) Internal view of the RPD showing the matrix cemented with resin composite. (e) Occlusal view of the completed case. (f) Frontal view. Loss of bone has made an extension of the prosthetic body necessary for lip support.

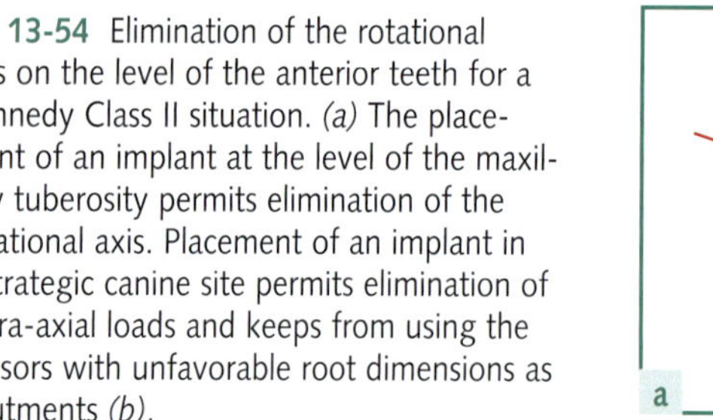

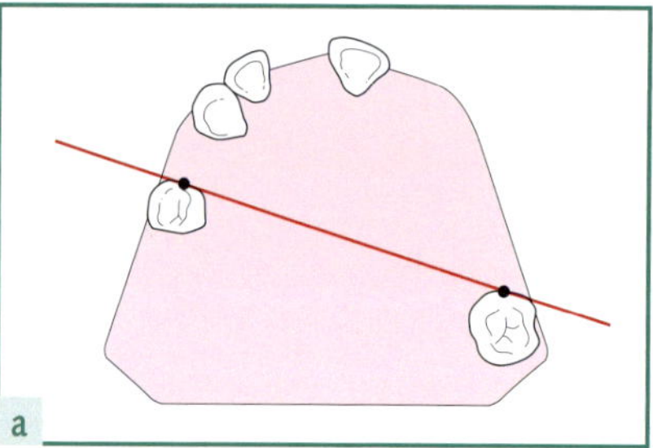

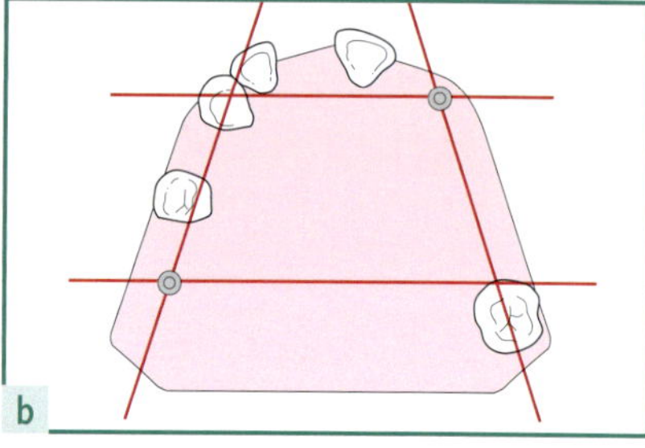

Fig 13-54 Elimination of the rotational axis on the level of the anterior teeth for a Kennedy Class II situation. (a) The placement of an implant at the level of the maxillary tuberosity permits elimination of the rotational axis. Placement of an implant in a strategic canine site permits elimination of extra-axial loads and keeps from using the incisors with unfavorable root dimensions as abutments (b).

Fig 13-55 *(a)* Occlusal view of a maxilla. Placement of implants in the right second molar and left canine sites modifies the edentulism to Class III with polygon support. Two 2.25-mm patrices are attached to the right second molar implant and the root of the right second premolar, and a UCLA pillar (Noble Biocare) with a 2.2-mm over-fused ball attachment (Bredent) is placed on the left canine implant to compensate for the buccal inclination. *(b)* The master cast with similar implant placement and plaster stumps of the natural teeth.

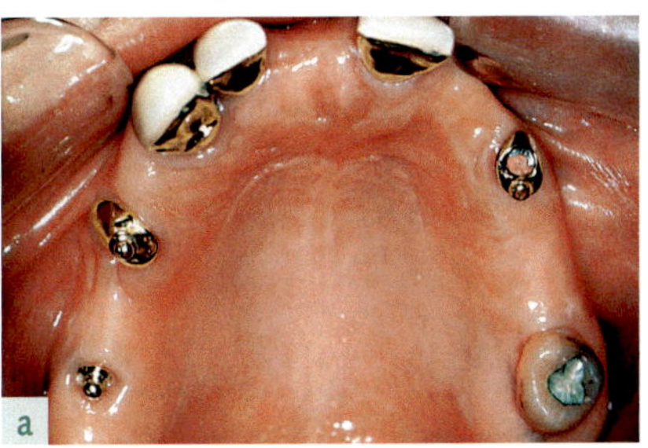
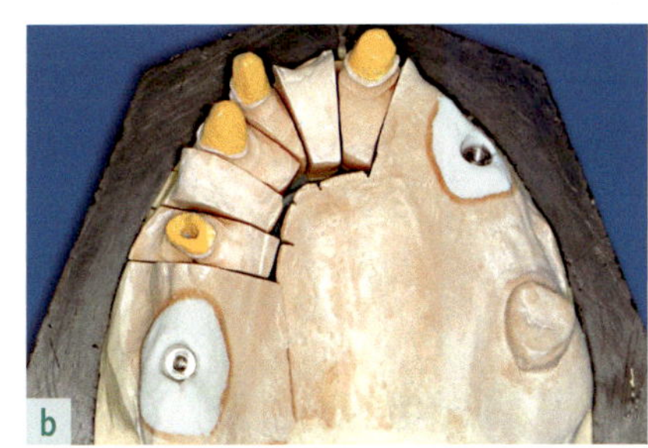

Fig 13-56 *(a)* Occlusal view of a completed RPD with metallic protection of the attachment at the left canine. *(b)* Internal view of the RPD showing the matrix attachment on the right second molar and second premolar and the Bredent attachment on the left canine. The loss of bone at the edentulous gaps requires an overdenture prosthetic body for support of the cheeks and lips. An overdenture that permits accessibility for home hygiene is the best solution for respecting the periodontal tissues. *(c)* Occlusal view of the completed case. *(d)* Frontal view.

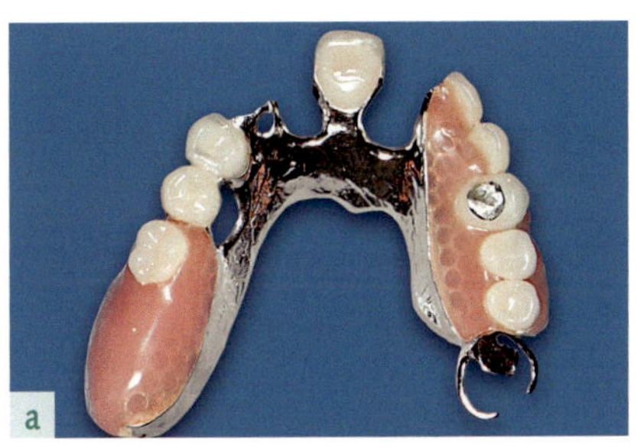
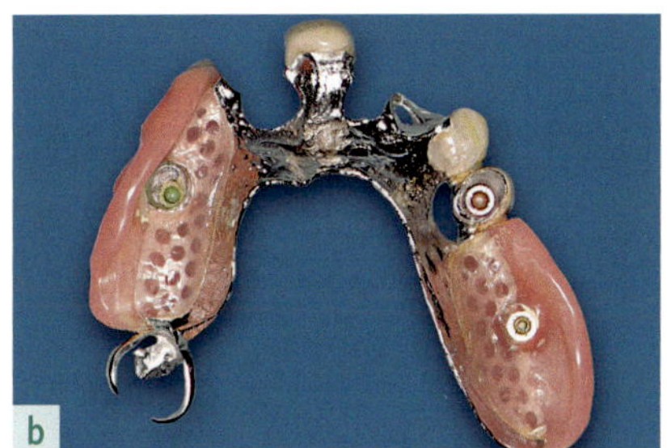

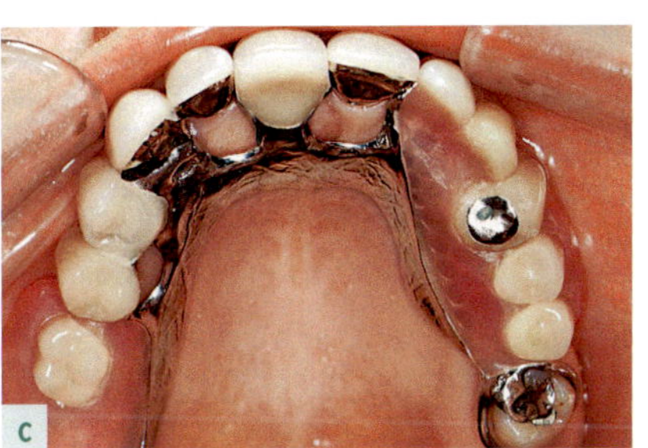
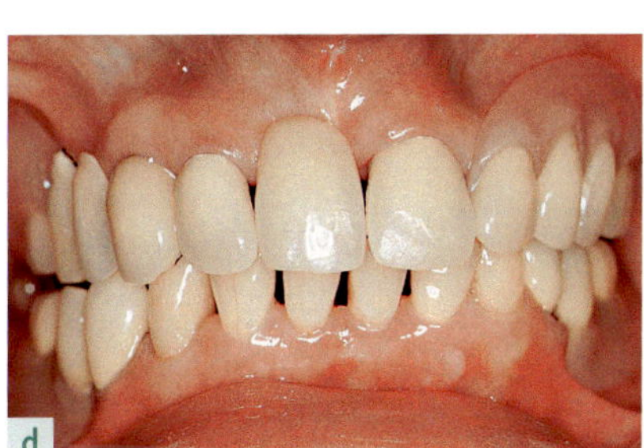

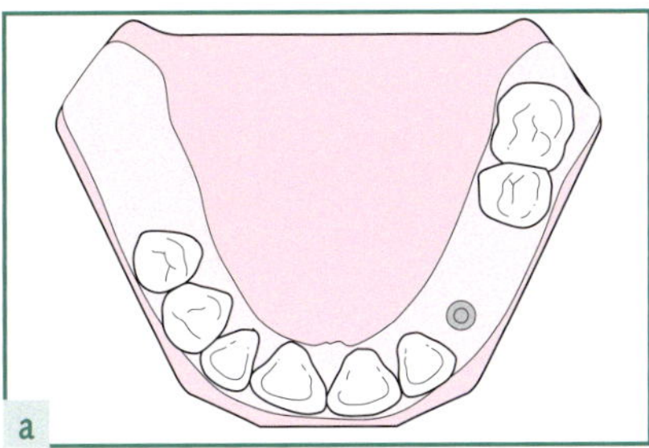
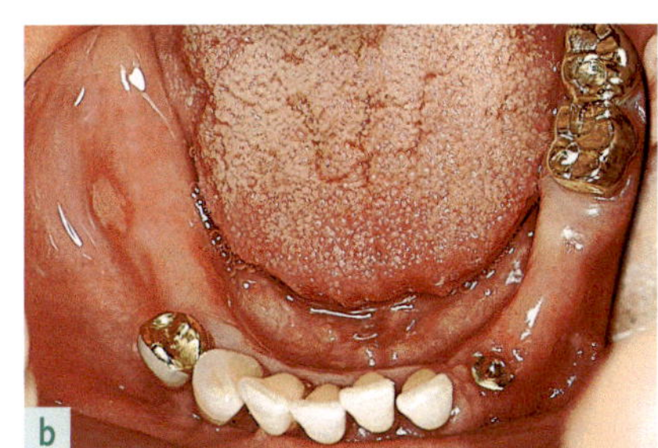

Fig 13-57 Restoration missing a strategic anterior abutment. A missing canine requires the preparation of an RPD without compromising biomechanics or esthetics. *(a)* Diagram of Kennedy Class II situation with a missing mandibular left canine, which leaves a lateral incisor—not ideal for added occlusal loading. *(b)* Restoration with an implant in the canine site avoids anchorage of the RPD with a clasp, which would be esthetically and biomechanically unfavorable for the lateral incisor.

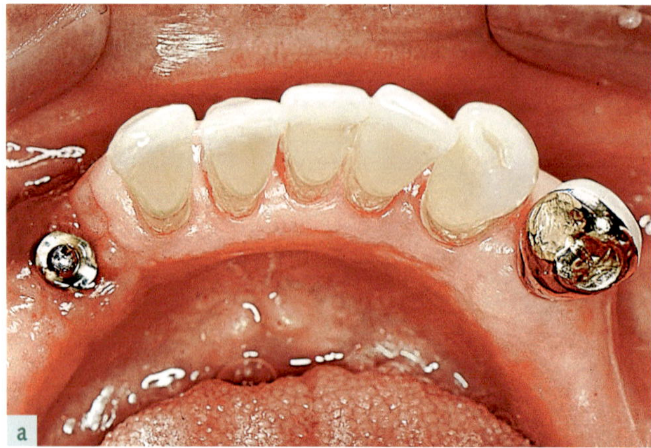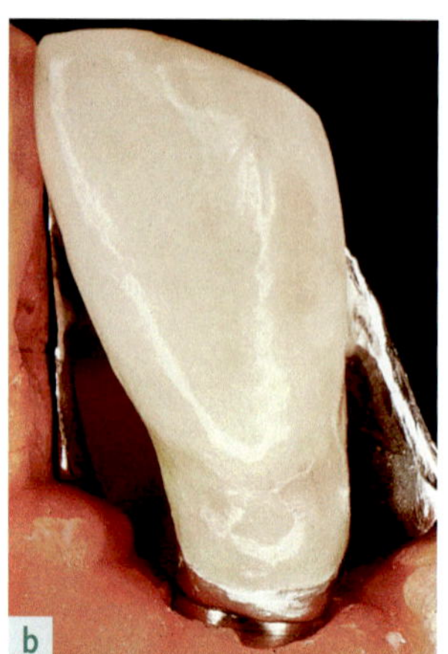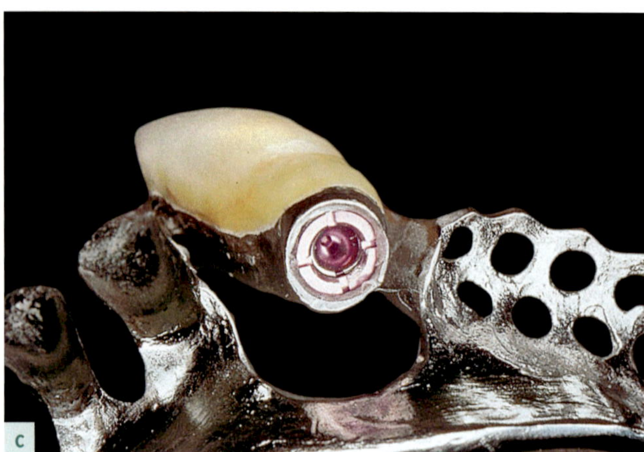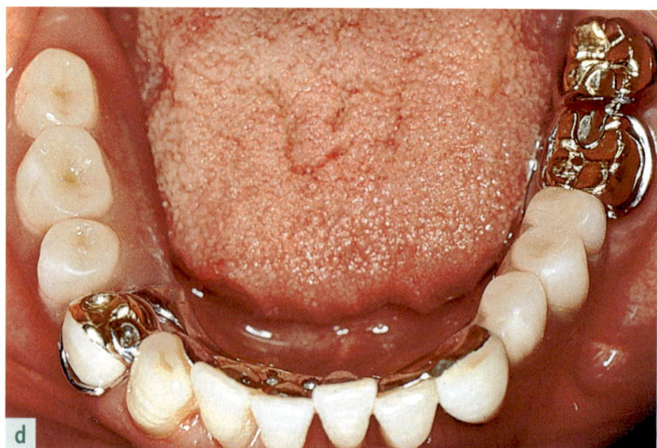

Fig 13-58 (a) Occlusal view of a 2.25-mm ball attachment on the left canine implant. The compromised periodontal tissue of the incisors does not permit clasp anchorage. (b) Lateral view of the master cast of the RPD at the implant level. The perioverdenture respects the marginal tissues and allows enough space for hygiene. (c) Internal view of the matrix attachment cemented with composite resin in the area of the left canine crown. (d) Occlusal view of the completed RPD in situ; the primary connector is a lingual step-back plate, which is useful for diastema or anterior gingival recession that may expose the metal support.

3. Resorting to the cantilever FPD must be evaluated in terms of the characteristics of the anchorage abutment and the conditions of the antagonist.

4. The RPD with clasps is biologically and economically favorable. Its versatility and the possibility of being easily and affordably modified make it the most recommended method for elderly patients.

5. Using precision attachments must be limited to patients with a high degree of esthetic requirements or when teeth need to be restored with crowns.

6. Using adhesive attachments is a simple method that is moderately invasive and is an alternative to clasps without the inconveniences of the traditional attachment.

7. Implant placement is an excellent choice for patients who have enough quality bone (and sufficient economic resources).

8. Sophisticated techniques that increase osseous quantity can be used for implants when indicated, but these measures can only be carried out by specialists. There are no published longitudinal studies supporting these techniques.

9. Placement of a limited number of implants in a strategic position allows modification of the biomechanics of the RPD.

Part II: Edentulous Gaps

Edentulous gaps are the spaces that remain after the loss of permanent teeth. The loss of a tooth does not always bring about a permanent gap; in 20% of dental extractions in adults, the space closes spontaneously.[1,2] Interdental spaces can also be present among a full set of teeth, as, for example, in the case of diastema. Öwall[3] defined an *edentulous gap* as a space at least half as wide as a premolar (3.5 mm).

Edentulous gaps are more frequent in the posterior regions. Gaps following the loss of molars are prevalent in the mandible, whereas those caused by the loss of premolars, canines, and incisors are prevalent in the maxilla. Single-tooth gaps are more frequent than multitooth gaps[1,2] (Fig 13-59). Despite greater care and prevention, reports indicate an increase in the number of edentulous gaps,[4,5] possibly because of the increase in average lifespan.

Need for treatment

Edentulous gaps in the anterior region must always be rehabilitated for esthetic and phonetic reasons. Even the missing incisors can have a negative effect on the subjective perception of health and oral function.[6] Gaps in the posterior region do not always need rehabilitation. The decision to proceed or not with rehabilitation must be made after having evaluated the magnitude of the dental-periodontal damage and its influence on the functionality of the dental complex.

Edentulous gaps can cause migration, inclination, and rotation of teeth on either side and extrusion of opposing teeth without occlusal contact (Figs 13-60 to 13-62). These alterations can give rise to periodontal pathologies, damage from dental decay, variations in the vertical occlusal dimension, and signs and symptoms of craniomandibular disorders. The onset of such pathologies is extremely variable and can be influenced by local factors,[7] such as localization and number of missing teeth, type of maxillomandibular relationship, position of the tongue, and tendency toward parafunctional activity.

In the past it was believed that the loss of one or more teeth could compromise functionality of the dental complex. Based on this belief, for many years the therapeutic approach revolved around the integral restoration of the dental arches.[8] Epidemiologic research in recent years, however, has shown how many factors, such as age, adaptive ability, neuromuscular tolerance, and favorable psychologic conditions can often limit or avoid the negative effects of tooth loss, allowing the dental complex to adapt itself in time to the new situation.[9]

Studies have shown that maintenance of normal functionality of the dental complex can be achieved in a significant percentage of patients with distal extension edentulism.[10,11]

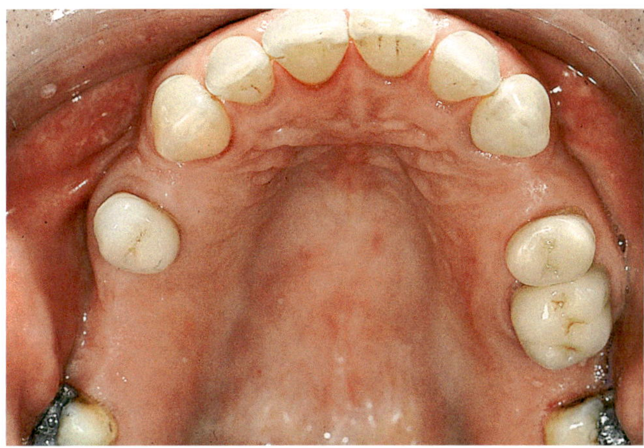

Fig 13-59 Maxillary arch with single- and multiple-tooth gaps.

The functional consequences of the edentulous gaps adjacent to natural teeth in the posterior regions have instead been the subject of more limited investigations, probably because of the difficulty of finding homogenous samples and the greater number of variables (eg, number and position of the missing teeth).

Theoretically, edentulous gaps between or adjacent to natural teeth should not be more functionally compromising than distal extension edentulism. Rather, it should allow greater masticatory effectiveness due to the maintained posterior support of the teeth distal to the gap. Nevertheless, the occlusal situation is made unstable by the presence of such teeth because their position changes over time. These migrations can create interferences, forcing the mandible into nonphysiologic positions and altering the stability of the oposing teeth.[12] The stability of the teeth opposing or adjacent to the gap is considered risky,[13] especially in pediatric patients, in whom it is advisable to restore the arch after full growth has been attained.

In adult and elderly patients, however, the choice of intervention needs to be based on the following considerations:

- Dental migrations usually occur in the first 6 to 12 months after the loss of teeth[14,15] and stop once a new occlusal balance has been reached (Fig 13-63).
- The tongue can mitigate the extrusion of teeth without an antagonist.
- Even if inclinations of the teeth are considerable, they do not generally cause periodontal illness.[16]
- Only gaps that are extended bilaterally in the presence of 20 or fewer permanent teeth can diminish masticatory efficiency.
- In the presence of limited gaps, which can also be bilateral,[17,18] masticatory efficiency can be obtained because of compensating mechanisms, such as increase in the number of contacts

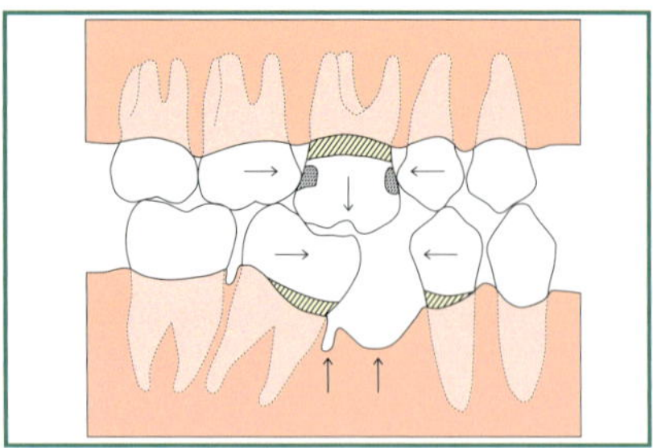

Fig 13-60 Roberts diagram: Possible movement of the adjacent and antagonistic teeth as a result of the noncompensated loss of the mandibular first molar. The outlined area indicates the zone in which there are caries lesions and periodontal pathologies. (Modified from Shillingburg et al.[29])

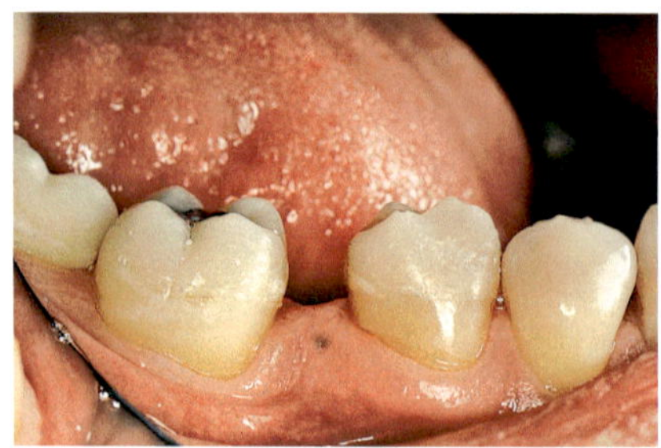

Fig 13-61 Gaps in the mandibular arch at the mandibular right first molar; the migration of adjacent teeth have reduced the width of the gap.

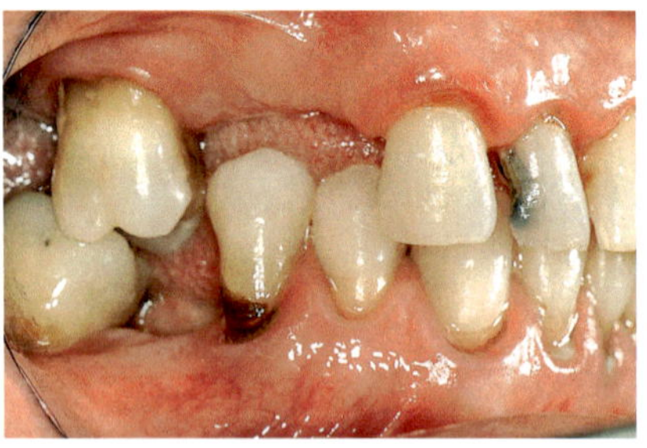

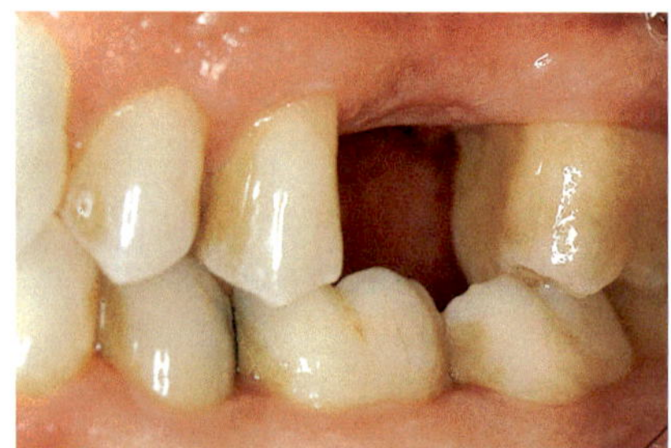

Fig 13-62 Single- and multiple-tooth gaps; the movement of residual teeth has induced caries lesions, periodontal pathologies, and vertical and horizontal reduction of the spaces.

Fig 13-63 Single-tooth gap due to missing maxillary left first molar for more than 5 years. The movement of the residual teeth has been limited by a new occlusal equilibrium.

between residual teeth, increase in the frequency of masticatory cycles, and swallowing of more voluminous boluses.

- The correlation between occlusal interferences in partial edentulism, deriving from the migration of the residual teeth and the onset of signs and symptoms of craniomandibular disorders, has not been well substantiated in the literature.[19–23]
- The survival of teeth adjacent to the gap does not seem to be influenced by prosthetic rehabilitation: Shugars and colleagues[24] examined 569 patients for 8 years postextraction, and Aquilino and colleagues[25] evaluated 317 patients for 10 years. In both studies, the subjects had been subjected to first molar or second premolar extractions and had a maximum of five missing teeth (excluding the third molars or premolars extracted for orthodontic reasons). Both studies showed that there are no significant differences in the survival of the teeth adjacent to gaps among patients who had not been treated with an FPD.

Conclusion

- Treatment for posterior gaps that have been present for at least 1 year is not recommended in the presence of physiologic occlusions[26,27] or if there is satisfactory oral function, occlusal stability, and adaptive capacity.

- Prosthetic rehabilitation is recommended when the loss of teeth is recent, because the capacity to adapt to the new situation is not predictable.
- Rehabilitation is recommended when the gaps have induced a pathologic occlusion in which one or more alterations of the dental complex are present and can be correlated to the loss of teeth.

Types of Rehabilitation

The rehabilitation of an edentulous gap can be achieved through:
- FPD with dental anchorage
- Fixed partial adhesive denture (FPAD) with dental anchorage
- IS-FPD
- RPD

Fixed partial dentures

Indications

FPD closely imitates the natural set of teeth and allows for excellent restoration of the masticatory, phonetic, and esthetic functions. It is easily integrated into the oral cavity, providing the patient with maximum functional and psychologic comfort.

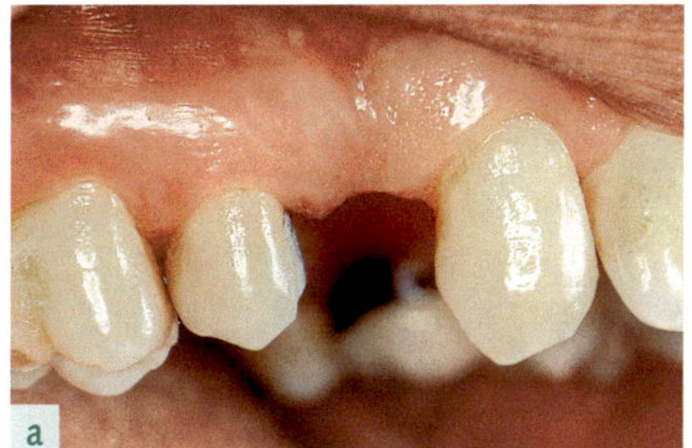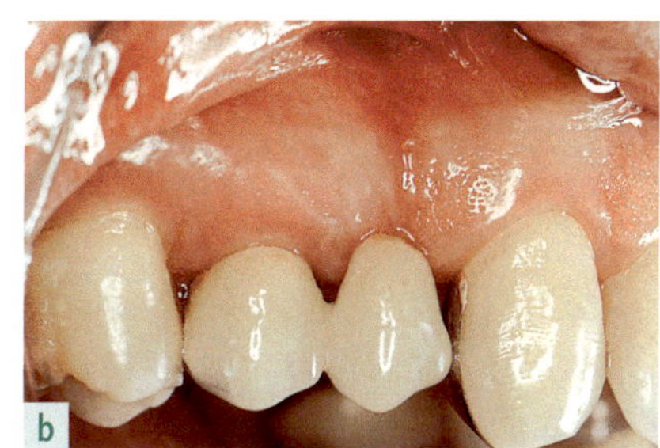

Fig 13-64 *(a)* Edentulous gap corresponding to a missing maxillary right first premolar. *(b)* Restoration with a fixed prosthesis.

For this reason, it is the type of rehabilitation most requested by patients.[28] FPD is the therapeutic means most frequently used in the treatment of edentulous gaps and is especially recommended for the rehabilitation of a single- or double-tooth gap (Fig 13-64).

Despite having clear advantages when compared with other types of prostheses, however, FPD presents some inconveniences. The creation of suitable anchorage requires the extraction of healthy dental tissues of the abutment teeth; thus, it is a biologically disadvantaged restoration. Also, numerous and lengthy sittings are necessary. Some operative phases are complicated and may be traumatic, especially for patients who are elderly and/or anxious. Cost is another concern because of the lengthy laboratory and surgical time and the use of materials such as gold alloys and dental ceramics. Furthermore, elderly patients can present limitations that make an FPD unadvisable, such as difficulty maintaining proper oral hygiene in interdental spaces; minor functional and esthetic requirements; and partial edentulism that needs another type of prosthesis. In this case, the biologic and economic costs of FPD make it unadvisable, given that it does not allow for complete rehabilitation of all types of edentulism. It is advisable, however, to substitute the missing teeth with an RPD.

Indications for using FPD can be summarized as follows:

■ Esthetic and functional requirements on behalf of the patient
■ The possibility of maintaining adequate oral hygiene at home
■ Anatomic and periodontal conditions of the residual teeth, extension of the gaps, and functional characteristics of the dental complex that favor long-term success.

Biomechanical considerations

The functional forces that would usually be absorbed by the missing teeth are transmitted to the abutment teeth through the components of the FPD: intermediate elements, connectors, anchors, and fixing cement.[29] Because the capacity of the prosthetic components to absorb the occlusal loads is different from that of the natural structure to which they are anchored,[30] concentrated forces can compromise the integrity of the prosthesis and support structure. Evaluating the extension of the gap and the number of teeth that can be used for support is fundamental in the planning of the treatment.

The variety of clinical situations for which an FPD is used means that there are no universally applicable parameters. The only guideline still considered valid is the rule as put forward by Ante in 1926, according to which: "the useful radicular surface of the supporting teeth must be equal to or greater than that of the teeth to be substituted."[31,32]

The useful radicular surface, calculated by Jepsen,[33] is the area of roots sustained by the periodontal tissues (Fig 13-65). This is an index of the periodontal state of the tooth. The root-crown ratio (relationship between the clinical crown and the extension of the radicular surface supported by the periodontal tissues) is 2:3, and 1:1 is considered the minimum acceptable ratio to define a reliable supporting tooth (Fig 13-66). The evaluation of abutment teeth must also include radicular morphology and height of the clinical crown. Molars with divergent roots are more favorable from the biomechanical point of view than those with convergent roots (Fig 13-67). Abutment teeth must have crowns at least 3 mm high in the anterior teeth and 4 mm in the posterior teeth.[34] For an FPD of single-tooth gap in the posterior region, Ante's rule must always be respected (see Figs 13-127 to 13-141). The substitution of two teeth is possible in most cases. The involvement of other abutment teeth may be recommended when it is necessary to increase the useful radicular surface. The auxiliary (secondary) abutment must have a useful radicular surface that is not inferior to that of the primary abutment.

The substitution of more than two teeth is generally unadvisable because it is difficult for the abutment teeth to support the mechanical stress, particularly in the mesiodistal direction, consequent to the bending of the pontic. Thicker pontics are therefore needed, but because of the limited vertical space, is not always possible. The problem is more evident in metal-ceramic prostheses where, given the different module of elasticity between the two materials, even minimum bending of the metal can cause infractions or fractures of the more rigid ceram-

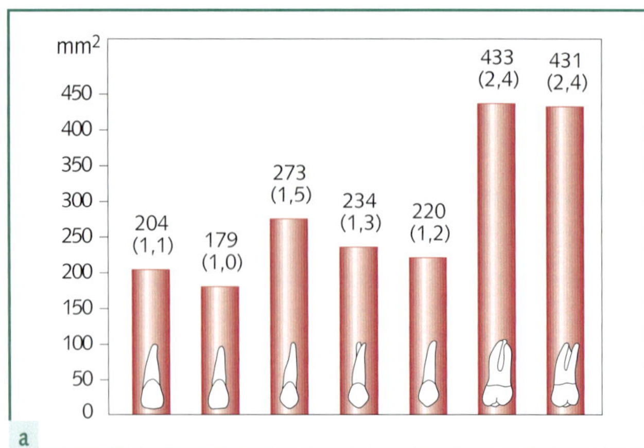

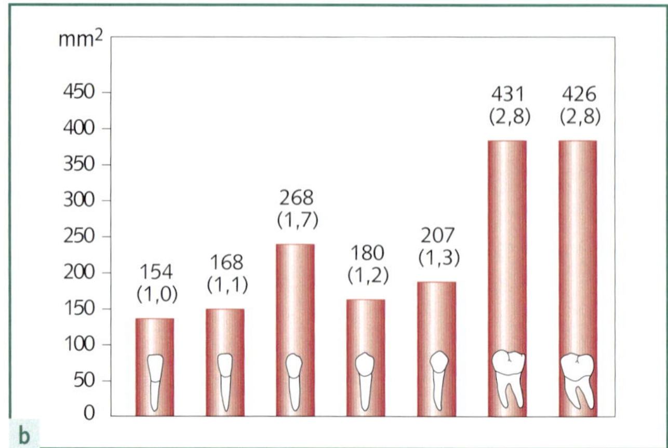

Fig 13-65 *(a)* Relationship between the extension of the maxillary radicular surfaces and that of the lateral incisors, with minimal sufaces (value = 1). *(b)* Relationship between the extension of the mandibular radicular surfaces and the central incisors (value = 1). (From Jepsen[33] modified by Shillingburg et al.[29])

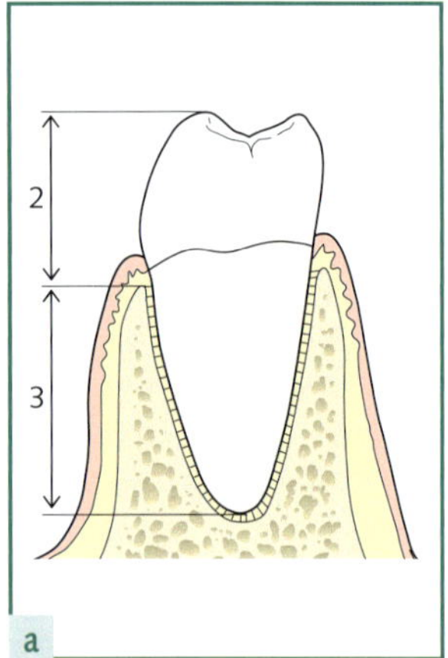

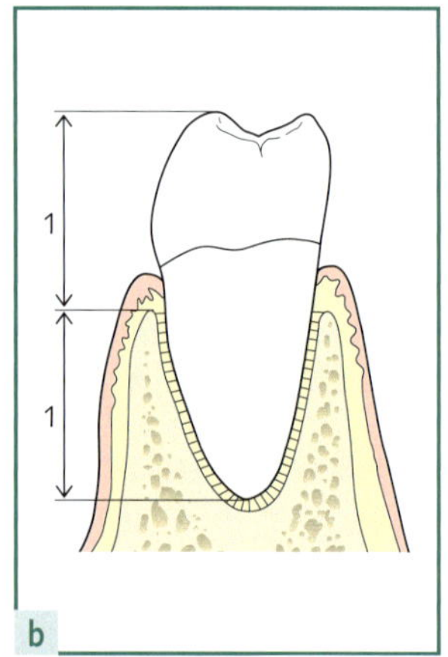

Fig 13-66 Crown-root relationship. *(a)* The optimal relationship is 2:3; *(b)* 1:1 is the minimal acceptable relationship. (Modified from Shillingburg et al.[29])

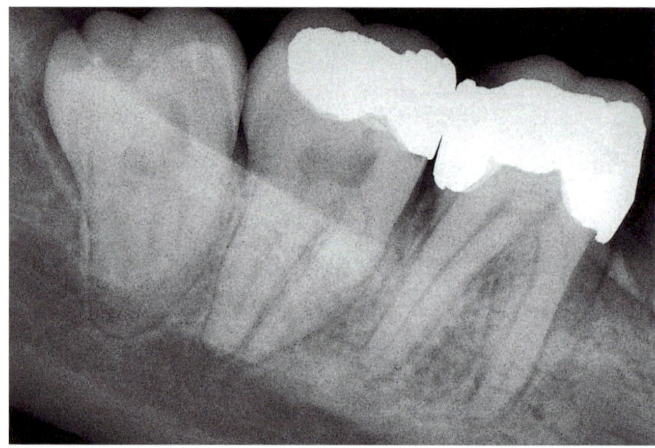

Fig 13-67 Configuration of convergent and divergent roots.

ics. In the rehabilitation of mandibular gaps, the metal pontic is not able to compensate for the movements of the supporting teeth during function. The mandible is subjected to rotations and bending caused by muscular action, both in a mesial and anteroposterior direction. This elastic deformation can modify the position of the supporting teeth even by a few microns. The movements are insignificant for a single- or two-tooth gap but become significant when more teeth are involved. Due to its rigidity, the FPD can become decemented,[35–39] or abutments can become mobilized.

Ante's rule has been clinically corroborated by Leempoel and colleagues.[40] After a 12-year period of monitoring 1,640 FPDs, the authors reported a significantly higher success rate for those observing the rule.

The parameters described above also apply to the posterior regions. In this area, the shape of the ridges is rectilinear, and the functional loads have a predominantly axial direction. The shape of the ridges in the anterior regions, on the other hand, is often curvilinear, and thus, function can result in tangential forces. The intermediate elements, which act as arms of leverage, induce a twisting movement on the supporting teeth, which increases as the curvature of the ridge increases. To oppose this movement, the replacement of the four maxillary incisors often requires the involvement of canines and the first premolars as secondary abutments.

The replacement of the maxillary canines with an FPD is generally problematic for various reasons. The maxillary canines endure the greatest tangential loads in a buccal direc-

190

tion because they are positioned at the point of the greatest curvature. Also, the adjacent teeth (lateral incisors and first premolars) have a reduced radicular surface. Replacement of the incisors and mandibular canines presents minor difficulties because the curvature of the arch offers greater resistence to the lingually directed tangential forces.

Until now, the criteria have been based primarily on the evaluation of the useful radicular surfaces. The teeth with little radicular support are not considered biomechanically able to act as abutments.

Many patients with edentulous gaps adjacent to natural teeth have widespread periodontal disease. The Goteborg School of Periodontology[41–44] showed that it is possible to use few teeth with advanced bone resorption and a high degree of instability as abutments in fixed, even extended, rehabilitation. The prosthetic treatment was aimed at restoring masticatory function and stabilizing the periodontally compromised teeth. This therapeutic approach is based on the premise that the functional threshold of the periodontal mechanical receptors and the alveolar bone in teeth with reduced periodontal support is less than that of teeth with normal support. Such a reduction, acting on the musculature, would constitute a protective mechanism for the residual teeth.[45] The selected patients were able to obtain optimum oral hygiene, with the total removal of bacterial plaque.

The therapeutic approach of the Swedish school contrasts in many ways with that of the more traditional, purely mechanical one. However, because that research has been carried out on selected patients and in highly specialized centers, it must not be considered as a generic alternative but as a therapeutic option for the rehabilitation of previously selected patients with severe periodontal disease. Limits in its applicability are linked to the difficulty in encouraging patients to maintain adequate hygiene.

Functional considerations

The success of an FPD largely depends on the ability of the prosthesis to absorb and distribute the functional loads to the supporting structures. The following factors should therefore be considered:

- Parafunctional activity considerably increases the force and duration of the occlusal loads.[46]
- With aging, the muscular forces generally decrease.[47]
- The type of occlusal relationship can influence the distribution and extent of the occlusal loads; for example, in the presence of a deep bite the horizontal forces exerted on the maxillary teeth are greater.
- When the antagonist is an RPD with mixed support or a complete denture, the extent of the functional loads is less.

Diagnosis and treatment plan

The FPD treatment plan makes use of a diagnostic procedure based on medical history, objective examination, functional evaluation, and instrumental investigation (periodontal survey and evaluation of dental mobility, radiography, and study casts). Intraoral radiographs must be obtained, because a precise evaluation of the periodontal and endodontic conditions and the radicular morphology of every supporting tooth is necessary. In complicated cases, important information can be obtained from a diagnostic waxup[48] (see Fig 13-148), which produces an accurate wax reproduction of the FPD and all of its components. The wax model is built on the supporting teeth, which are prepared in the laboratory using the study cast.

Through the diagnostic waxup the available vertical and horizontal space can be determined; thus, pretreatment with orthodontics and/or corrections of the antagonistic occlusal plane can be avoided, and the material decided in the treatment plan can be used, maintaining an abutment height sufficient to guarantee adequate retention, stability, and esthetic quality. The diagnostic waxup also acts as a construction guide for the provisional FPD. The transformation of the waxup into a provisional prosthesis allows the clinician to evaluate the validity of the treatment from a functional and esthetic point of view before manufacturing the definitive prosthesis.

The treatment plan includes two phases: *(1)* the preparatory phase and *(2)* the prosthetic phase. In the preparatory phase, certain interventions may be required before the FPD can be placed, including extractions, restorative and/or endodontic treatments, orthodontics, and periodontal surgery. For corrective surgery of the mucosa profiles, a provisional FPD is needed during the healing stage. It is important to encourage the patient to maintain optimal oral hygiene during the preparatory phase.

The evaluation results and diagnosis point to the following key components of the treatment plan: the material to be used; the choice of preparation; the number of supporting teeth; and how many abutment teeth will be involved (taking into account the biomechanical considerations described previously).

Choice of material

Gold and metal alloys with an optional ceramic or resin coating are used to construct the FPD.[49–54]

The uncoated gold alloy has certain advantages:

- Modulus of elasticity and hardness that are similar to that of natural enamel[55]
- Malleability, which allows a conservative preparation and respects the healthy residual tissues as much as possible
- Thin and angled preparation margins (eg, bevelled margins) with precision and without distortions
- Biocompatibility

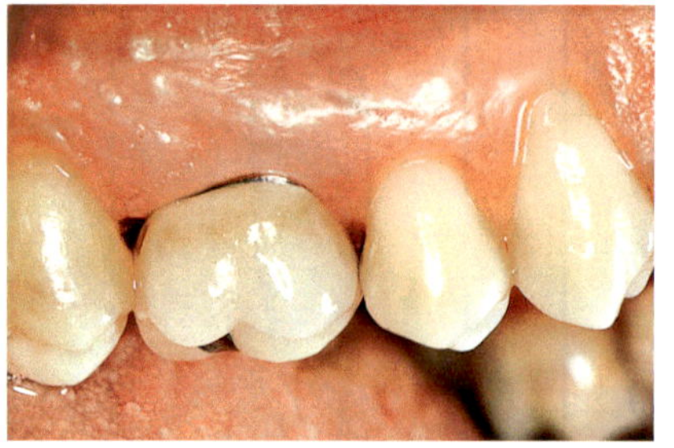

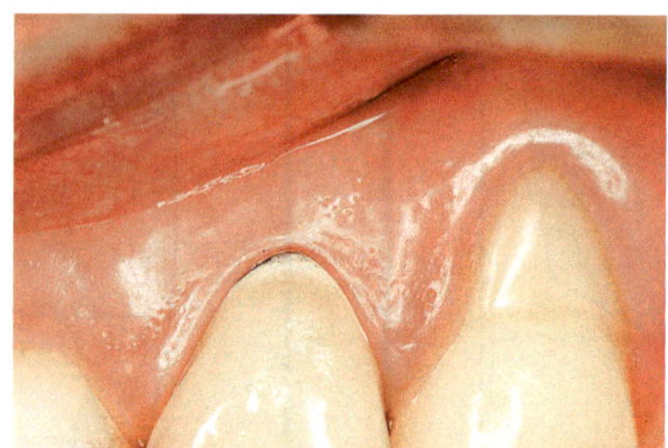

Fig 13-87 Metal-ceraminc crown on the maxillary right first molar. The metal substructure corresponds with the gingival margin.

Fig 13-88 Metal-ceramic crown on a maxillary left canine. The ceramic on a metal margin corresponds to the shoulder design, creating a overcontour that does not resolve the esthetic problem.

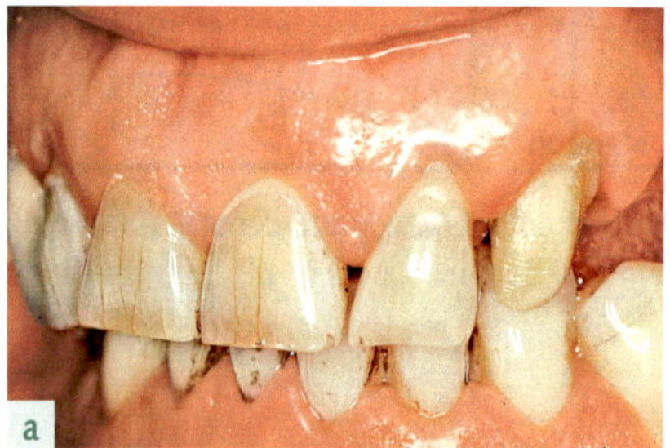

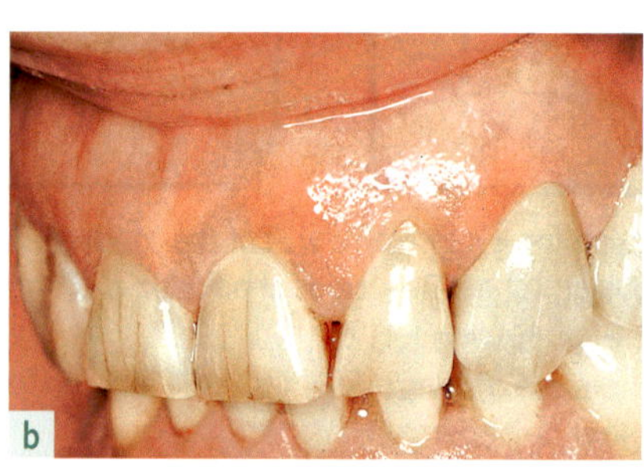

Fig 13-89 (a) Margin preparation with 130 degrees on the maxillary left canine. (b) Definitive prosthesis in situ.

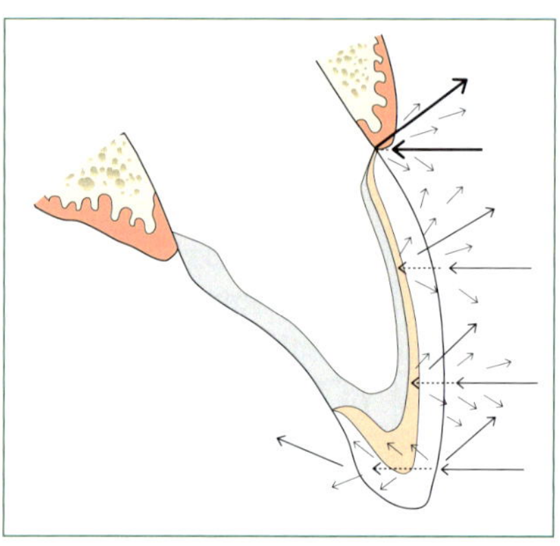

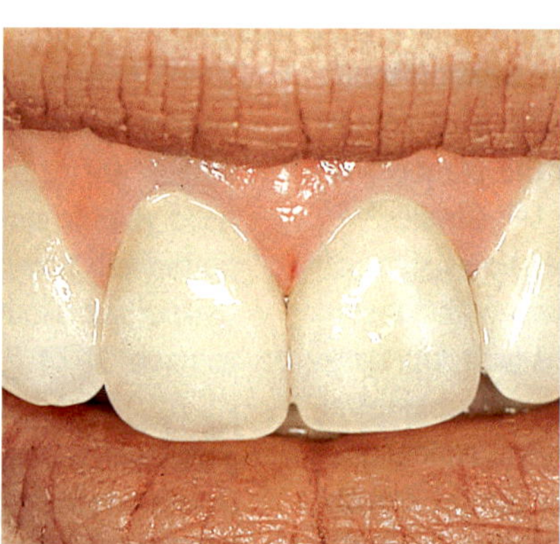

Fig 13-90 Behavior of incidental light. The light is predominantly absorbed in a margin preparation of 130 degrees.

Fig 13-91 Metal-ceramic crown on a maxillary incisor. There is a dark shadow on the gingival margin.

130-degree shoulder

Proposed by Kuwata[95,96] (Fig 13-89) is the preparation most used in both anterior and posterior regions. If the axial wall of the tooth and the marginal surface are connected with a curve rather than an angle, it is called a *deep chamfer*. These margins, compared with the 90-degree bevelled shoulder, have the following advantages:

- They have the same vertical inclination of the bevel and therefore the same marginal precision.
- They have sufficient depth to allow complete coverage of the metal with ceramics without creating overcontours.
- They are technically easier to prepare.
- They require less dental tissue to be removed.

The main limitation of this margin is the possibility of creating overcontours in teeth with linear emergence profiles and thin gingival tissues at the margin of the crown, where metal and ceramics overlap with an acute angle. Furthermore, because of the lack of thickness of the gingiva and ceramic layer, light is absorbed by the underlying metal, limiting refraction and causing the appearance of a dark shadow on the gingival margin (Figs 13-90 and 13-91). To resolve this problem, metal frameworks made of high-gold alloys have been proposed, which are obtained through electrodeposition [97–99] or interstitial deposition[100,101] (Fig 13-92). These metals allow good marginal precision,[102] reduced thickness (0.3 mm), which in turn allows the application of a thicker ceramic coating, and a light-yellow chroma that reflects the light with golden shadows, similar to those of dental tissue. The minor resistance to bending of these metals compared with traditional alloys limits their use to the rehabilitation of single teeth and the use of short-extension FPDs in anterior regions (Fig 13-93).

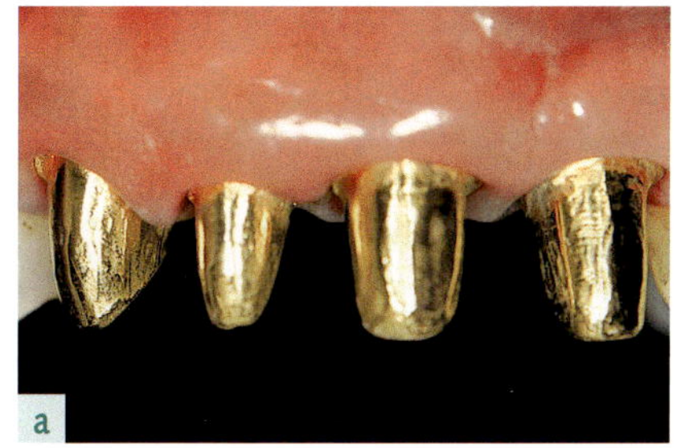
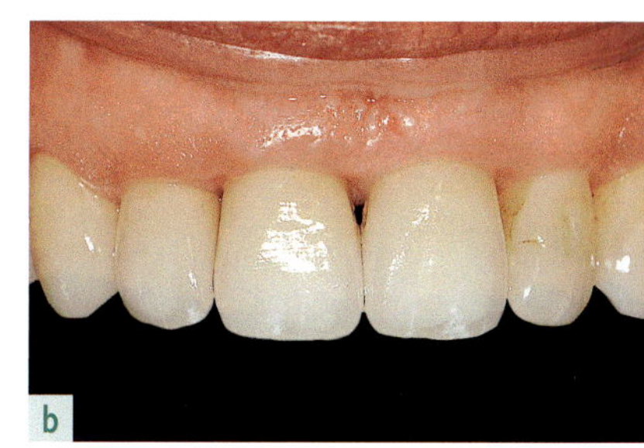

Fig 13-92 *(a)* Electrodeposited metal substructure. *(b)* Definitive crowns.

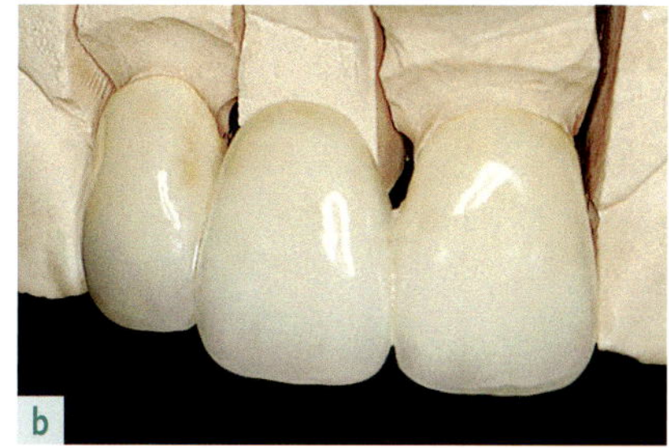

Fig 13-93 *(a)* Restoration to replace a missing maxillary right central incisor with an electrodeposited metal substructure. Corresponding abutments constructed from metal. Soldering was done by laser. *(b)* Definitive prosthesis.

Fig 13-94 In the abscence of a metal substructure, light at the margin is transmitted and not absorbed.

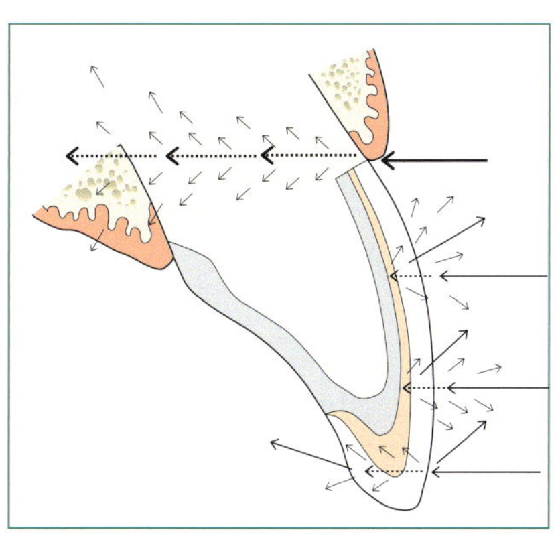
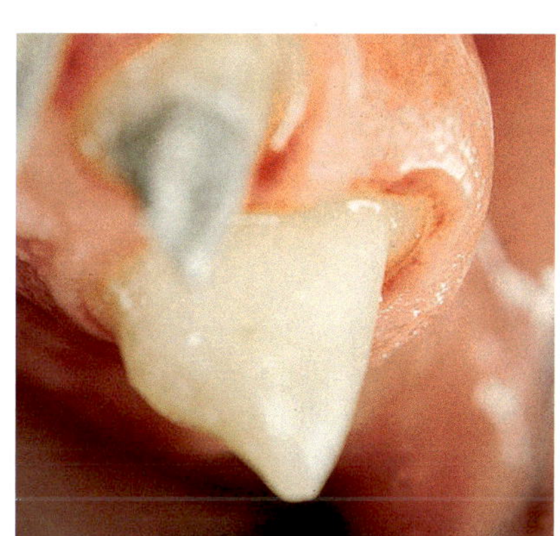

Fig 13-95 A mixed preparation of a maxillary left canine.

Net 90-degree shoulder

This margin gives the best esthetic results because the metal structure ends in the internal portion of the shoulder and therefore allows greater refraction and transmission of light in the marginal ceramics (Fig 13-94). The 90-degree shoulder is less precise compared with other types of margins. For this reason, it is only prepared on labiobuccal aspects, which is the most critical from an esthetic point of view. On the palatolingual aspect of the tooth, the margin can be prepared with a 130-degree shoulder or a 90-degree bevelled shoulder. Preparation with different types of margins is defined as *mixed*[103,104] (Fig 13-95). To remedy the poor precision at the net 90-degree shoulder, marginal ceramics are used, which are subject to less contractions during baking than traditional ceramics and have a melting point about 20°C higher. The use of this type of ceramics allows clinically acceptable marginal seals (< 50 μ).

Chamfer

The chamfer margin is the most recommended for purely metal reconstructions (see Fig 13-85d). Its morphology is similar to that of the deep chamfer but with less depth and is suitable for holding the metal on its own.

In conclusion, the first choice of margin for metal and ceramic restorations is the conservative 130-degree shoulder. For all-metal restorations, the most recommended margin is the chamfer.

FPD pontics

Pontics of the FPD substitute missing teeth. The form of the pontic must respect esthetic and functional requirements and the possibility of maintaining hygiene.[105,106] An incorrectly made pontic can lead to the accumulation of plaque on the restoration surfaces, causing inflammation of the edentulous

199

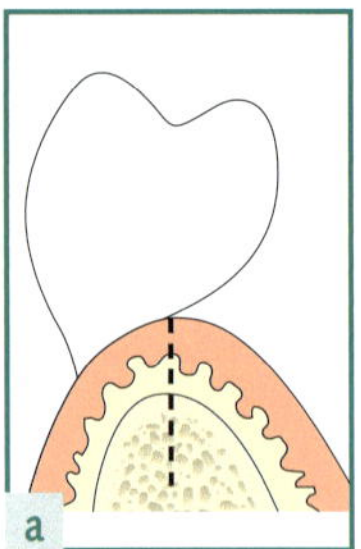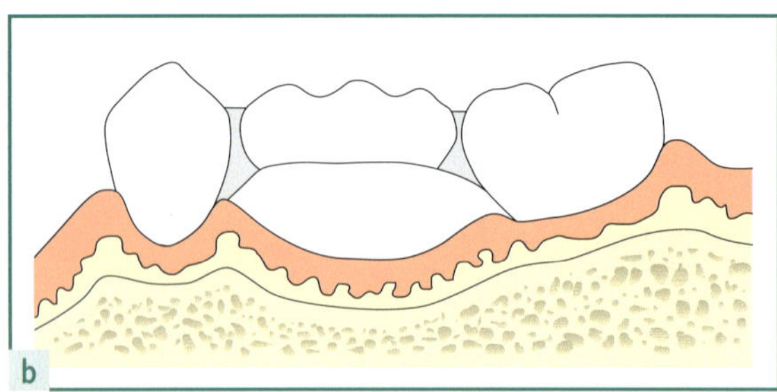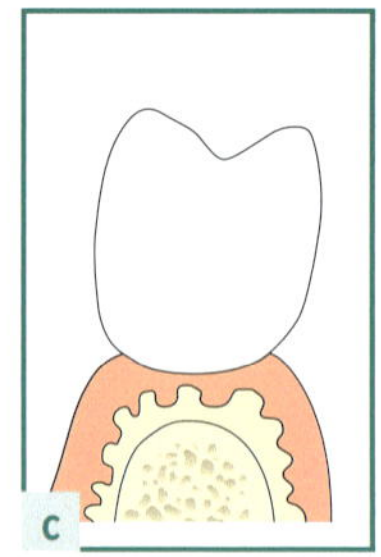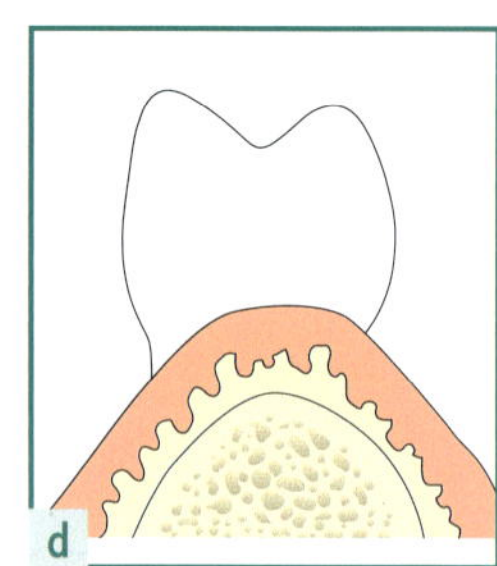

Fig 13-96 Pontic types: *(a)* modified ridge-lap; *(b)* hygienic; *(c)* ovoid; *(d)* saddle.

mucosa. Plaque accumulation can depend on the type of material with which the pontic is made[107–110] or, more frequently, on its morphology.[105,106,111,112]

Pontics are generally constructed with the same materials used for restorations of the supporting teeth. The materials most suitable in terms of direct contact with edentulous mucosa are glazed ceramics and gold.[107–109] Resin, on the other hand, is absolutely not recommended[105,107–109] because of its coarseness, which encourages the accumulation of plaque. Adaptation of the pontic to the soft underlying tissue determines the future health of the tissue; for this reason, the extension and the form of contact are extremely important to ensure success of the rehabilitation[108]:

- The area of contact with the tissue must be minimal[105,111] and slightly wider in a mesiodistal direction.
- The portion of the pontic in contact with the edentulous crest must be convex[112,113] to make hygiene maintenance easier.
- To avoid formation of an ulcer, the cervical margin of the pontic must be placed on the keratinized mucosa without exceeding the mucogingival line.
- The pontic must not exert any pressure on the mucosa.[105,106,111] To prevent the tissues in contact with the pontic from becoming inflamed, scrupulous upkeep of hygiene must be maintained.[105,112,114] To ease access for cleaning, the interproximal spaces at the papilla and the lingual space of the pontic must be sufficiently open to allow the passage of dental floss.[106,112]

Various designs have been suggested for the construction of the pontic, including the modified ridge-lap, the hygienic, the ovate, and the distal extention.

The modified ridge-lap (Fig 13-96a) gives the illusion of a tooth, but all or almost all of its surfaces are convex, which makes cleaning easier and establishes selective contact only on the buccal side of the crest. The lingual surface has a slightly convex outline to minimize the accumulation of plaque. Contact on the edentulous ridge must not extend lingually beyond the peak of the ridge. This design, which has a por-

celain restoration, is the most commonly used in the anterior of both jaws.[108,111] It requires an edentulous ridge that has a regular profile and minimal resorption.

The hygienic pontic does not come into contact with the edentulous ridge. This type of design is used in the posterior for short extension gaps.[108,111,113] The hygienic pontic has a convex lower face both in a vestibulolingual and a mesiodistal sense. The surfaces allow the passage of the dental floss, a task that is extremely difficult with flat surfaces or angles.

The pontic's occlusogingival vertical thickness must not be less than 3 mm if sufficient resistance is to be obtained. The space between the cervical surface and the ridge must be at least 2 mm.[115] For this reason the hygienic pontic can only be used when there is sufficient space on the vertical plane. The FPD should be checked several days after cementing, as the pontic can become an area of food accumulation or tongue insertion.

A hygienic modified pontic design (Fig 13-96b)[116] has been proposed, in which the lower face is concave in the mesiodistal direction and convex in the vestibulolingual direction. This design calls for a greater thickness in the connector area so that the resistance increases and the stress is significantly reduced, while at the center, the pontic is more resistant to bending. Also, hygiene is easier to maintain with this design.

The ovate pontic (Fig 13-96c) is rounded at the ends and is used mainly in the anterior regions where esthetics is of primary importance.[117] The face in contact with the tissue is rounded and is placed in a depression on the ridge crest, obtained artificially by means of a provisional FPD. The provisional FPD is applied immediately after extraction or after the surgical correction of the edentulous mucosa if it is intact.[117] This depression simulates the interdental papillae and the natural emergence of the tooth, and allows adequate cleaning with floss.

Ridge-lap morphology (Fig 13-96d) allows complete coverage of the ridge buccolingually. This type is no longer used because it prevents hygienic intervention below the pontic.

The occlusal surface of the pontic can be reduced in a buccolingual direction to diminish the area subjected to occlusal loads. This tactic reduces stress on the abutment teeth and is

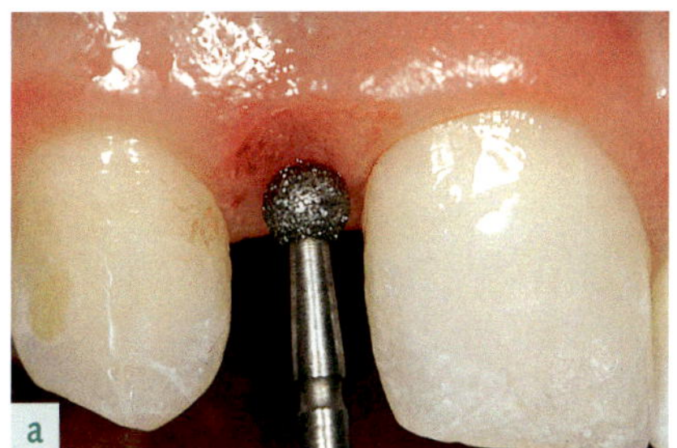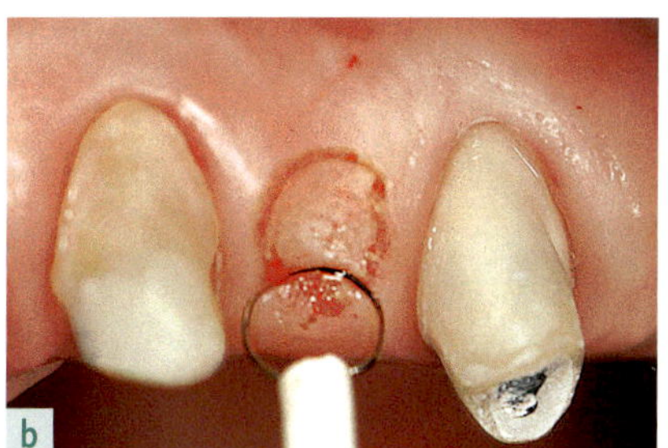

Fig 13-97 *(a)* Gingivoplasty by a diamond bur. *(b)* Use of an electroscalpel.

recommended in the case of extended gap in which the supporting elements have a root-crown ratio that is not optimal, or where, due to diminished prosthetic space, the framework has a reduced thickness.

Following the loss of a tooth, the alveolar process undergoes resorption and remodeling, the interdental papillae disappear, and the edentulous mucosa loses its characteristic aspect of an "orange peel." Strong modifications of the edentulous ridge, by shortcoming or excess, can interfere with lodging of the pontic. Excessive hypertrophy of the mucosa reduces the prosthetic space available, whereas a marked resorption, often following the loss of teeth due to trauma or periodontal illness,[118] excessively increases the vertical dimensions of the element to be rehabilitated. In these cases, it is advisable to surgically intervene before beginning rehabilitation,[119] to make placement of the pontic and its cleaning easier as well as improving the esthetics.

If the ridge is not very resorbed, gingivoplasty is performed as part of the preparation of the site to receive the pontic.[117] A diamond bur or electrosurgery is used to create a concave bed, the sides of which reproduce interdental marginal papillae (Fig 13-97). Gingivoplasty requires the mucosa to be at least 3 mm thick.[120] Healing comes about by applying a surgical dressing or a provisional prosthesis. In some cases there are areas of hypertrophic gingiva adjacent to edentulous gaps. These areas need surgical correction to avoid constructing connectors that are too thin in the vertical dimension and to allow for hygiene maintenance after the pontic is in place.

Surgical techniques that increase the edentulous ridge include:

- Flap inlay graft[121–123]
- Flap graft of deepithelialized connective tissue or the "roll technique"[124]
- Subepithelial tunnel[125]
- Onlay graft[126,127]
- Membrane or metallic mesh[128]

Grafts can consist of full-thickness connective tissue, bone, or synthetic materials (eg, hydroxyapatite). Surgical correction of the edentulous ridge must be done in excess to compensate for contraction during healing, which occurs in the sixth to eighth week following surgery.

The most recommended donor sites for bone grafts are the mental symphysis, the retromolar pads, and the maxillary tuberosity; the palatal mucosa is the first choice area for connective tissue grafts.

If surgery is not possible, the pontic must be modified for use in severely resorbed ridges to avoid the creation of black triangles in the interproximal areas. Besides being esthetically displeasing, black triangles are areas where plaque accumulates, and they reduce the rigidity of the FPD. Prosthetic correction of the pontic can be accomplished by means of *(1)* adding pink porcelain supported by metal or pink acrylic resin on the tissue-bearing surface, which stimulates the interdental papilla; and *(2)* creating a gingival pad with either soft or hard resin, which can be adapted and fixed in the interdental zones.[128] These corrective procedures are often unsatisfactory, because it is difficult to achieve adequate morphologic characteristics.

Preparation techniques

Instruments

To carry out the preparations, rotating burs of various materials, morphologies, and dimensions are used. Diamond or tungsten-carbide burs may be used.[70,129] Diamond burs are more abrasive and therefore more suitable for the enamel; the granules vary in coarseness from 30 to 200 µm (Fig 13-98). The effectiveness of the bur depends on the dimensions of the granules: the larger the grain, the greater the quantity of tissue removed and the coarser the preparation. Fine-grained diamond burs are usually used to polish prepared surfaces.

Cylindrical or conic burs are used for most preparations because of their greater precision. Tapered conic burs allow correct inclination of the axial surfaces to be obtained while keeping the bur parallel to the major axis of the tooth. The tips of both types of burs, which can be flat, round, or at an acute angle, determine the morphology of the preparation margin. In

201

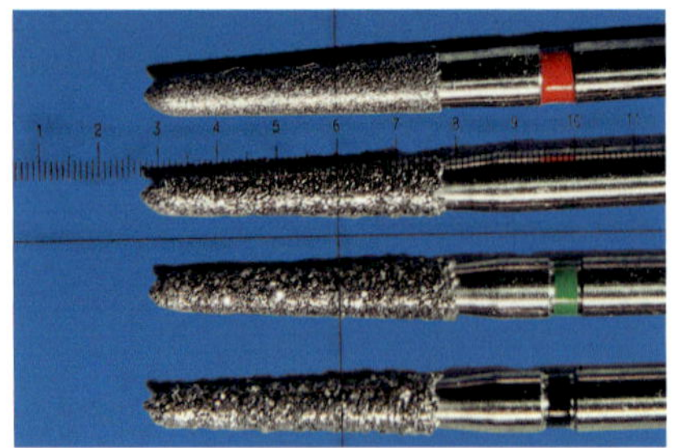
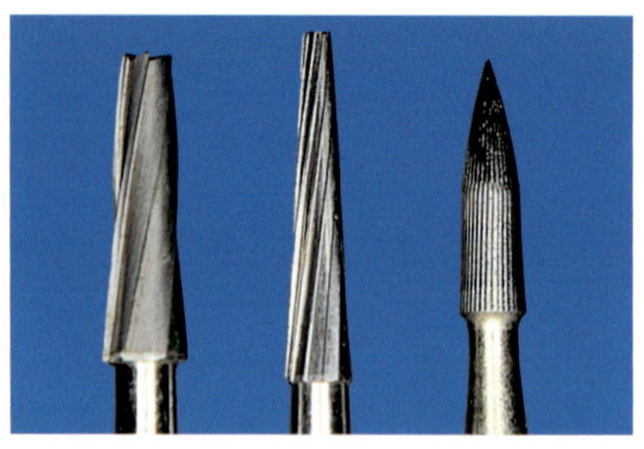

Fig 13-98 Diamond burs with granulation in decreasing coarseness from bottom to top.

Fig 13-99 Tungsten-carbide burs..

some phases of the preparation, it is recommended that football- or flame-shaped burs be used.

The diameter of the diamond burs can be between 0.1 mm to over 2 mm. The size of the diameter of the conic burs refers to the major base. It is also important to know the diameter of the minor base in order to evaluate the exact quantity of tissue removed. The height of the working end of the bur varies between 3 and 12 mm. The choice of bur must take into account the dimensions of the tooth to be prepared.

Tungsten-carbide burs have blades welded to a steel rod. These burs operate with less force and so are suitable for acting on the dentin and for polishing the surfaces. The number of blades varies from 8 to 40; the greater the number of blades, the greater the polishing effect (Fig 13-99). The forms and dimensions are, for the most part, the same as those of the diamond burs. Their use is limited in the preparation of the FPD, because polishing is needed only for the margin preparations.

Phases of preparation

The phases of preparation in sequential order are:

1. Occlusal or incisal reduction
2. Axial buccal reduction
3. Axial lingual reduction
4. Separation and axial proximal reduction
5. Definition and polishing of margins

To achieve occlusal and axial reduction, the most common technique is that of the guide grooves. This technique involves the creation of a series of parallel grooves on the surfaces of the teeth to be prepared, which are then joined together.

Once the caliber of the burs to be used is known, it is easy to set the depth of the preparation and keep it uniform using this technique. For the reduction of occlusal or incisal surfaces, a conic bur with a round tip is recommended. For the reduction of the lingual surfaces of the canines and the incisors, a round bur is recommended to create the guide grooves and a football-shaped bur to join the grooves together.

Buccal and lingual axial reductions require a conic bur whose end corresponds to the marginal preparation desired.

The separation is achieved with a very thin flame-shaped or conic bur. It can be useful to insert a metallic matrix in the interproximal space to protect the adjacent teeth. The interproximal axial reduction consists of correcting the separation with a conic bur with the same working head as that used for the buccal and lingual axial reductions.

Definition and polishing of the margin is carried with the same bur used for the axial reduction along with the matching tungsten-carbide bur.

Anterior region: Incisors and canines
Mixed shoulder preparation

1. Incisal reduction: The initial phase consists of the preparation of the guide grooves with a conic bur with a round tip (314 018). The diameter at the base of the bur is used as a reference for the depth of the grooves, which must deepen on the incisal margin by about 2 mm (Fig 13-100).

2. Buccal reduction: The guide grooves must follow the different directions of the buccal profile. One series must be parallel to the cervical portion of the labial surface and the other to the incisal margin. The grooves must have a minimum depth of 1.2 mm (Fig 13-101). After having joined the guide grooves it is important to correct the passage between the two planes so that an edge does not remain (Fig 13-102).

3. Lingual reduction: Guide pits are created on the incisal margin with a small round diamond bur (314 023), inserting it a little less than half way (Fig 13-103). The pits obtained with the round bur are joined using a football-shaped bur (314 023) (Fig 13-104). On the cervical portion, 0.5-mm-deep guide grooves are created with the round-tip conic bur (314 018) and then joined using the same bur (Fig 13-105).

4. Proximal reduction: Access to the proximal areas and separation from the adjacent tooth is obtained by means of a flame-shaped bur (314 010) (Fig 13-106).

5. Margin definition: To create the buccal 90-degree shoulder, three types of burs have been proposed: flat tip with right angle, round tip, and flat tip with rounded sides. The first is not recommended because it has the tendency to form notches on curved surfaces. If inserted more than halfway, the round-tip bur tends instead to form an unsupported overhang of enamel,

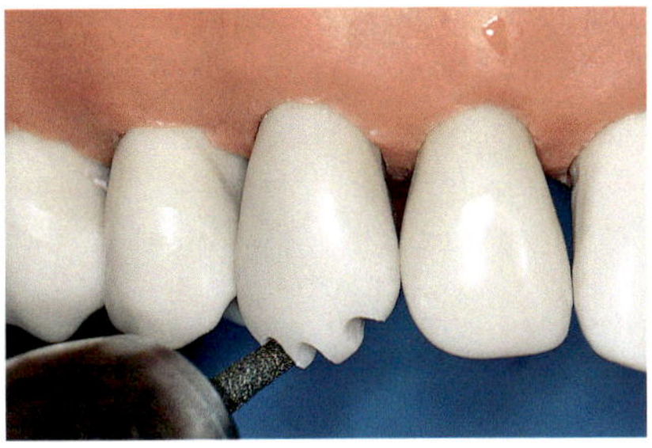

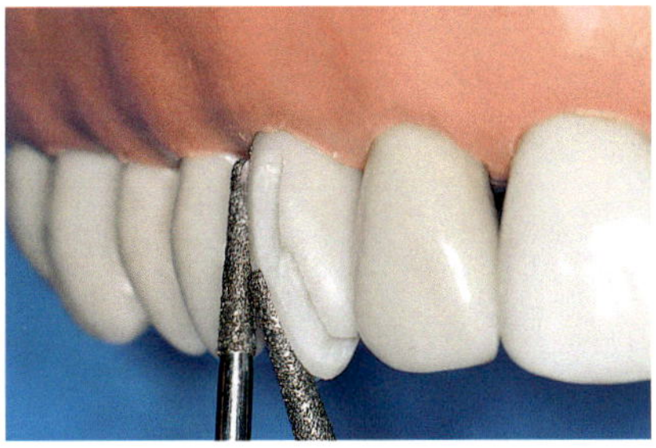

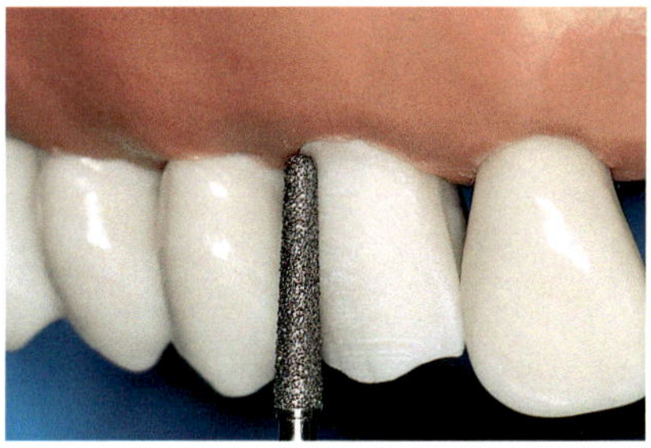

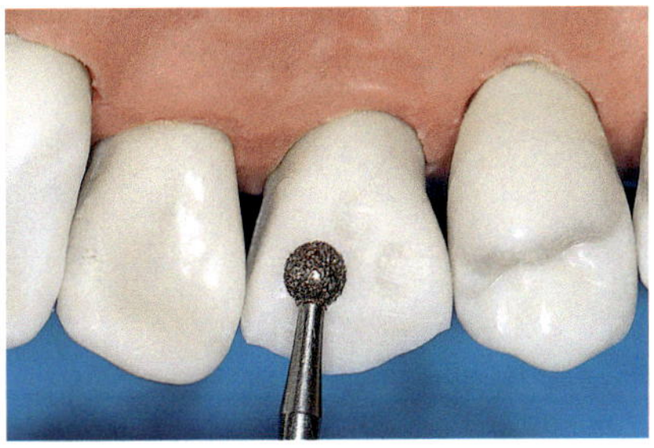

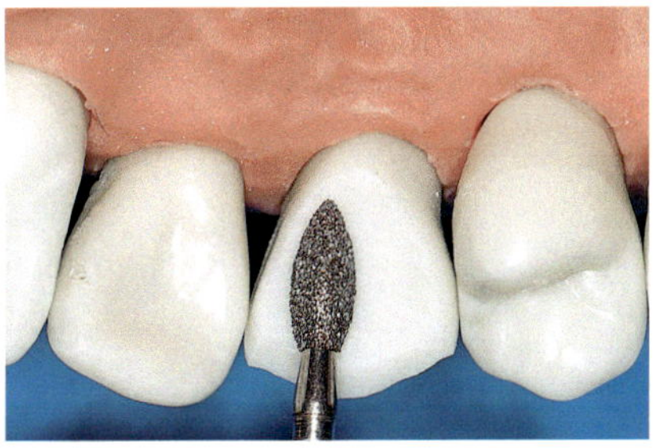

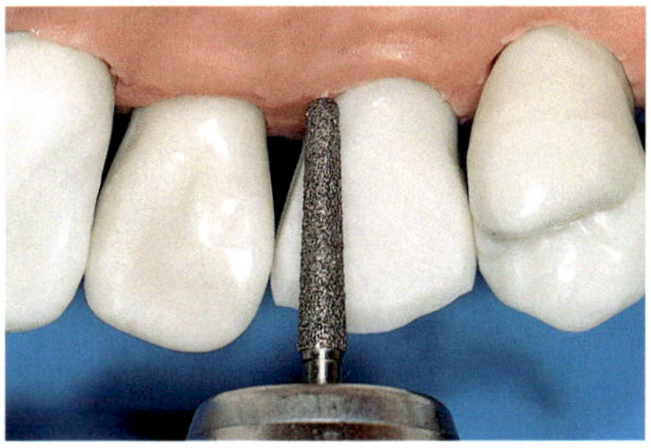

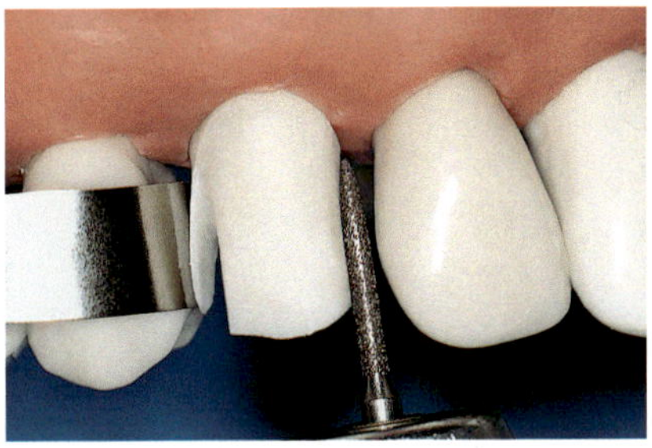

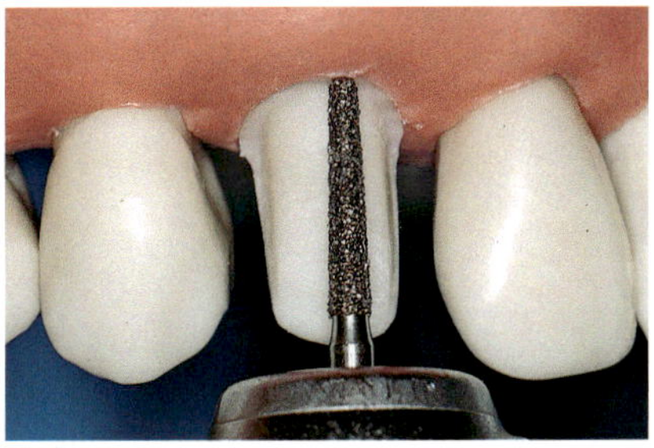

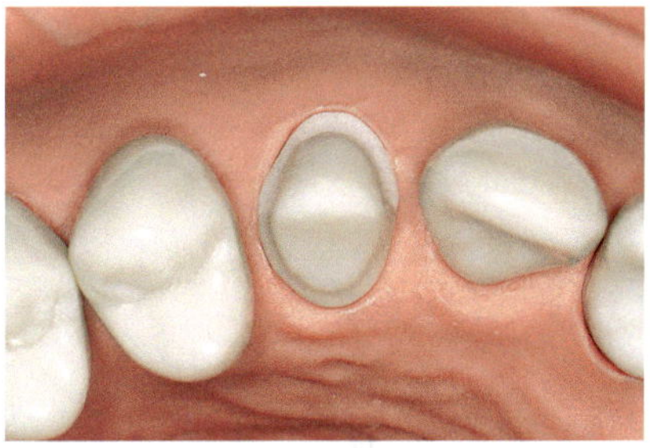

Fig 13-100 to 13-109 Preparation phases.

Fig 13-110 Arkansas stones.

which, if not refined, compromises the precision of the preparation. For the implementation of the shoulder, the most useful is the flat-tip bur with rounded margins, which avoids the formation of notches and overhangs (Fig 13-107). To create a 130-degree shoulder or lingual chamfer, a no. 314 016 bur is used (Figs 13-108 and 13-109).

Polishing: The only part of the preparation that must be polished is the margin. It is recommended that the rest of the abutment be moderately coarse. Polishing is achieved by means of fine-grain diamond or tungsten-carbide burs or with Arkansas stones (Fig 13-110).

Posterior region: Molars

130-degree shoulder

For occlusal reduction:

1. Guide grooves are created with a round-tip conic bur (314 018) on the triangular ridges and on the primary developmental grooves. The reduction for gold-ceramic restorations must have a depth of 1.5 to 2.0 mm on the occlusal cusps (palatal in the maxillary and buccal in the mandible) and 1.0 to 1.5 mm on the guide cusps. For purely metallic crowns, there must be at least 1.5 mm for the occlusal cusps and 1 mm for the guide cusps (Fig 13-111).

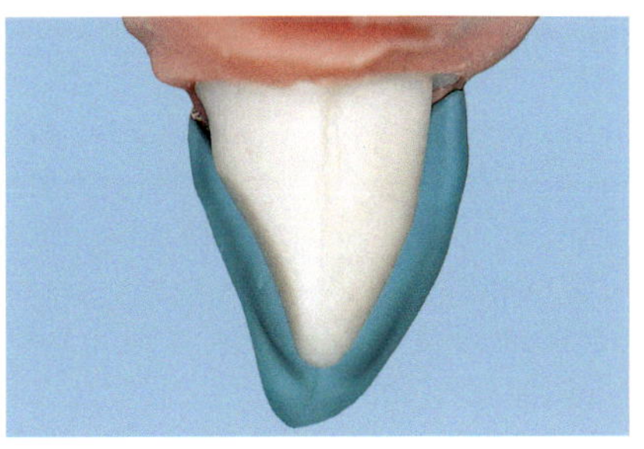

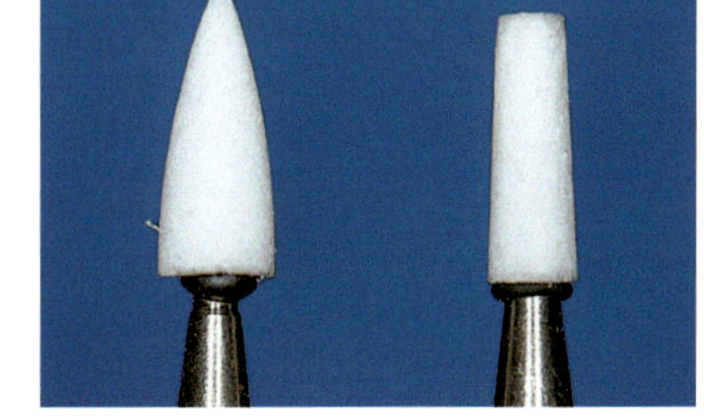

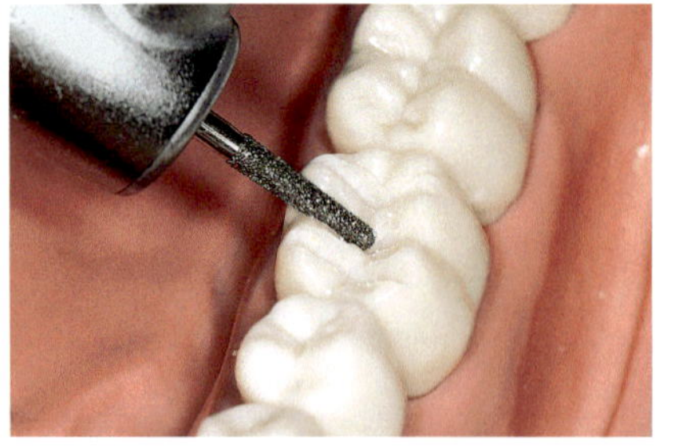 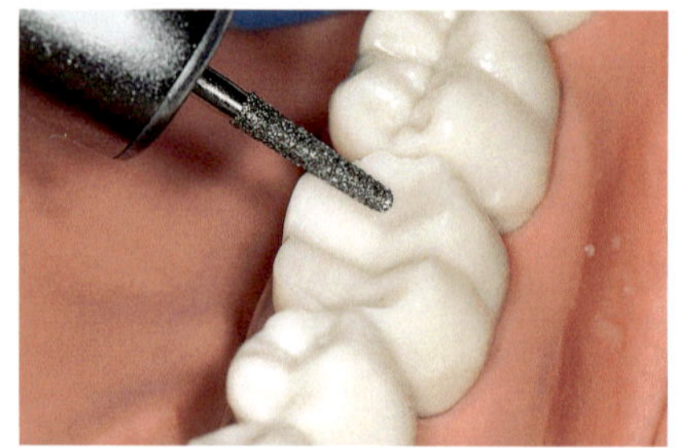 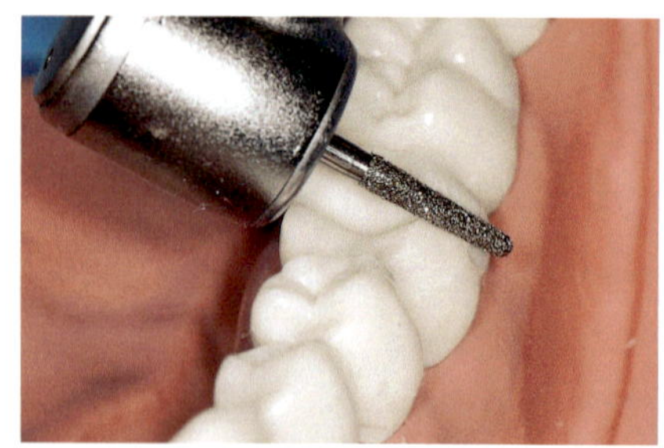

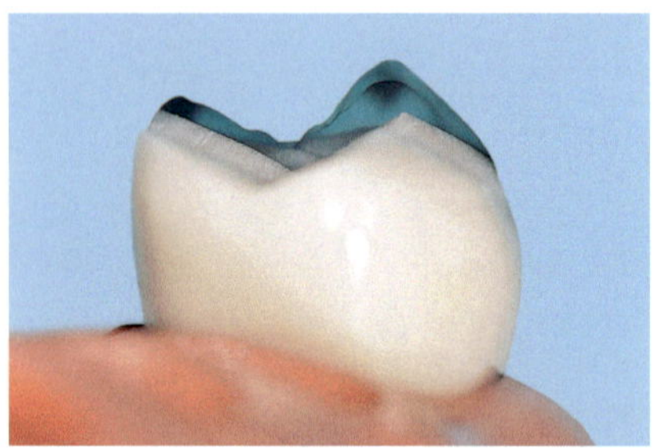 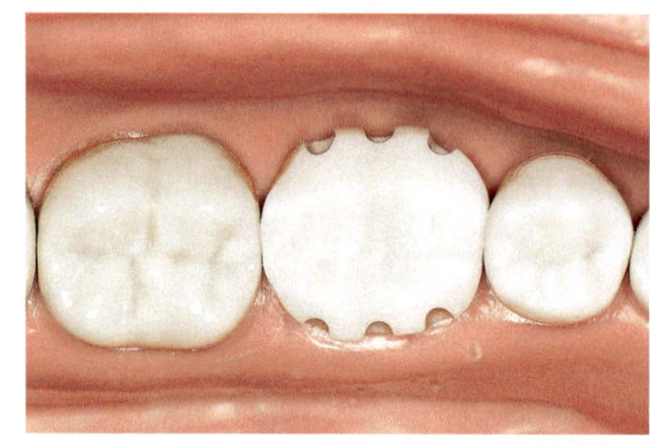 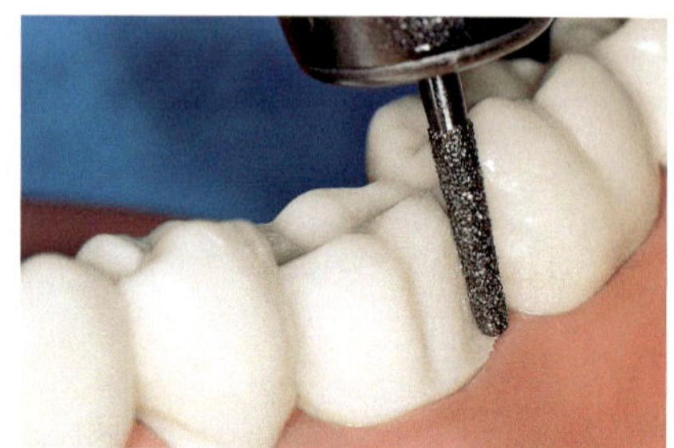

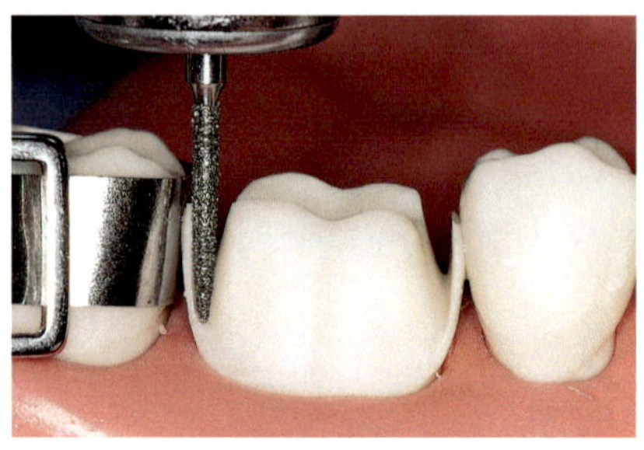 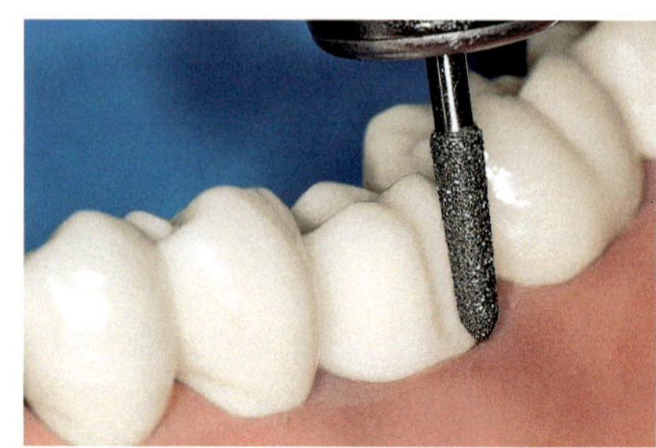

Fig 13-111 to 13-118 Preparation phases continued.

2. **Join** the guide grooves with the same bur used to join the grooves, following the inclination of the cusp of the tooth (Fig 13-112).

3. **The chamfer** is then created, the depth of which varies from between 1.5 and 2.0 mm on the occlusal cusps, depending on whether a metal or metal-ceramic restoration is planned. The inclination of the chamfer follows the occlusal inclination of the guide cusps. Any angles or sharp borders on the preparation must be rounded or they could cause problems with impression taking, restoration fabrication, cementing, and the placement of the completed crown (Figs 13-113 and 13-114).

Axial reduction (buccal and lingual)

1. **Guide grooves:** A conic diamond bur with a round tip (314 018) is used. The reduction must not be less than 1.4 mm for metal-ceramic restorations to avoid an opaque and overcontoured restoration. Because of the lingual inclination of many mandibular molars, the shoulder should be less pronounced (Fig 13-115).

2. **Joining** of the guide grooves: The same round-tip bur is used to join the guide grooves in the buccal and lingual zones. The axial reduction must be extended as much as possible toward the proximal side without damaging the adjacent tooth (Fig 13-116).

Proximal Reduction

1. **Separation:** Use of a flame-shaped bur (862 314 010) with a reduced diameter avoids damaging the adjacent teeth. The handpiece can be guided with an alternate occlusal-cervical movement on the vestibular surface of the interproximal dental structure or with a vestibulolingual movement on the occlusal portion. Once a sufficient space has been obtained, it is advisable to pass the bur a number of times. The bur should not be inclined toward the center of the tooth so as to avoid excessively reducing the preparation (Fig 13-117).

2. **Joining:** The 130-degree shoulder bur (314 016) is used.

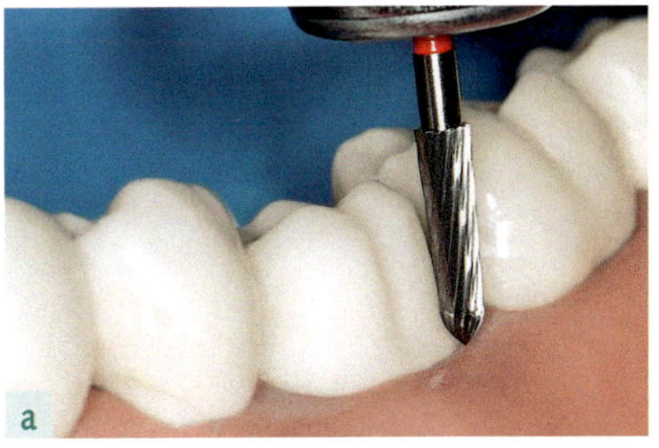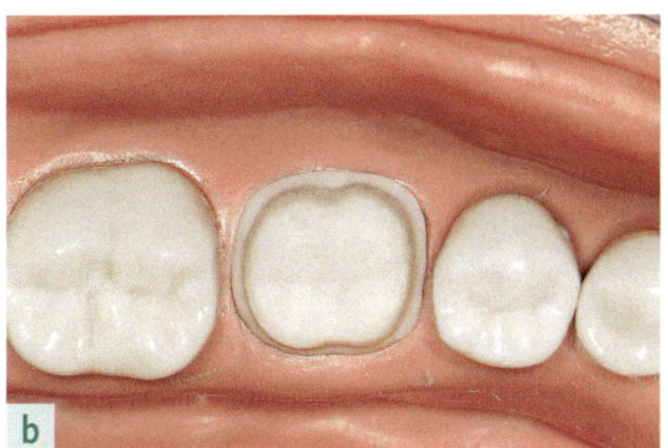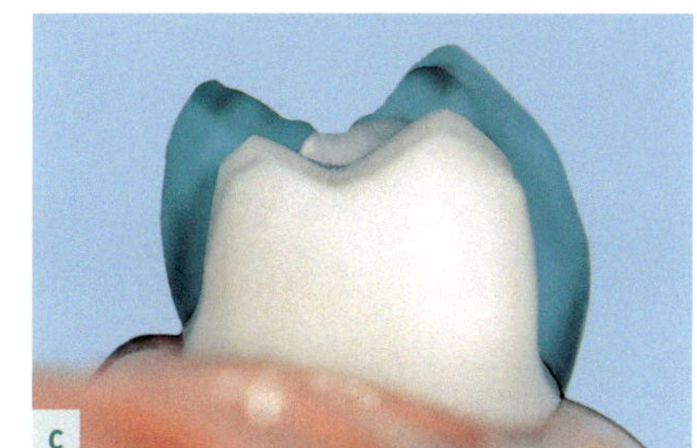

Fig 13-119 *(a)* to *(c)* Preparation phases continued.

Definition of the margins

On the buccal aspect, a 130-degree shoulder or a deep chamfer (no. 314 021) bur is used, with the respective tungsten-carbide burs to coat the margin. The margin should be prepared first supragingivally, and if subgingival positioning is necessary, it can be deepened after finishing the axial reduction. A space is thus obtained in the sulcus so that the diamond bur can be used without damaging the gingiva (Fig 13-118).

Coating

The preparation is completed using a tungsten-carbide bur (no. 314 021) on the axial sides, while the Arkansas burs are used on the occlusal surfaces. The angles of the preparation should be rounded down, and a continuous margin should be obtained (Fig 13-119).

On the buccal aspect, a stabilization groove can be created by completely sinking a bur with a flat tip (847 314 014) at the level where the cusps meet. This groove, which must stop at 0.5 mm from the margin, has three functions: *(1)* It makes the insertion of the crown easier, *(2)* it makes the flow of cement easier, and *(3)* it increases the retention and stability of the preparation.

Provisional crowns and FPD

A provisional prosthesis is used while the definitive prosthesis is being constructed.

The provisional prosthesis protects and stabilizes the prepared abutment teeth and allows functional and esthetic evaluation of the treatment plan.[29,60,96,130]

Types of provisional prostheses

There are various modalities of provisional rehabilitation depending on whether the clinical case is simple or complex. For simple cases, the rehabilitation does not involve changes in occlusal relationships, except those linked to the substitution of the missing teeth. The main functions of a simple provisional prosthesis are that of protection and spatial stabilization of the supporting teeth. It is defined as the "first" provisional prosthesis even if it is often the only one.

Complex rehabilitation involves changes in occlusal relationships, such as vertical and/or horizontal mandibular repositioning; restoration of the majority of the occlusion by means of substitution of numerous missing teeth; and stabilization of the complement of teeth after orthodontic treatment. In complex cases, the first provisional prosthesis is followed by the second or *therapeutic* provisional prosthesis. The latter prosthesis is the means by which the new occlusal relationships are formulated and the degree of adaptation of the stomatognatic system to the new situation is evaluated[96] (Figs 13-120 to 13-124). Generally, this therapeutic phase lasts for a few months; for this reason, the therapeutic provisional prosthesis must be constructed in a way that guarantees its integrity over time.

Materials used

The most common material for the provisional prosthesis is polymethylmethacrylate.[29,60] Other materials with different qualities may be used,[29,130] such as polyisobutylmethacrylate, epoxy resin, and composite resin. The choice of the most suitable material also depends on the construction method applied.

A common limitation for all resin materials is the poor resistance to fracture of the provisional teeth.[131] To remedy this inconvenience, it is possible to reinforce the resin structure with Kevlar fibers, carbon fibers, or metallic thread.[131,132] For the therapeutic provisional prostheses, it is advisable to use cast metal frameworks and metal or composite occlusal surfaces to avoid occlusal wear, which could induce variations in the vertical dimensions.

Construction techniques

The provisional prosthesis has two surfaces: the external surface, which reproduces the crown, and the internal surface, which adapts to the form of the abutment.[130] The two parts are united through different tehniques, such as direct techniques, indirect techniques, and mixed techniques.

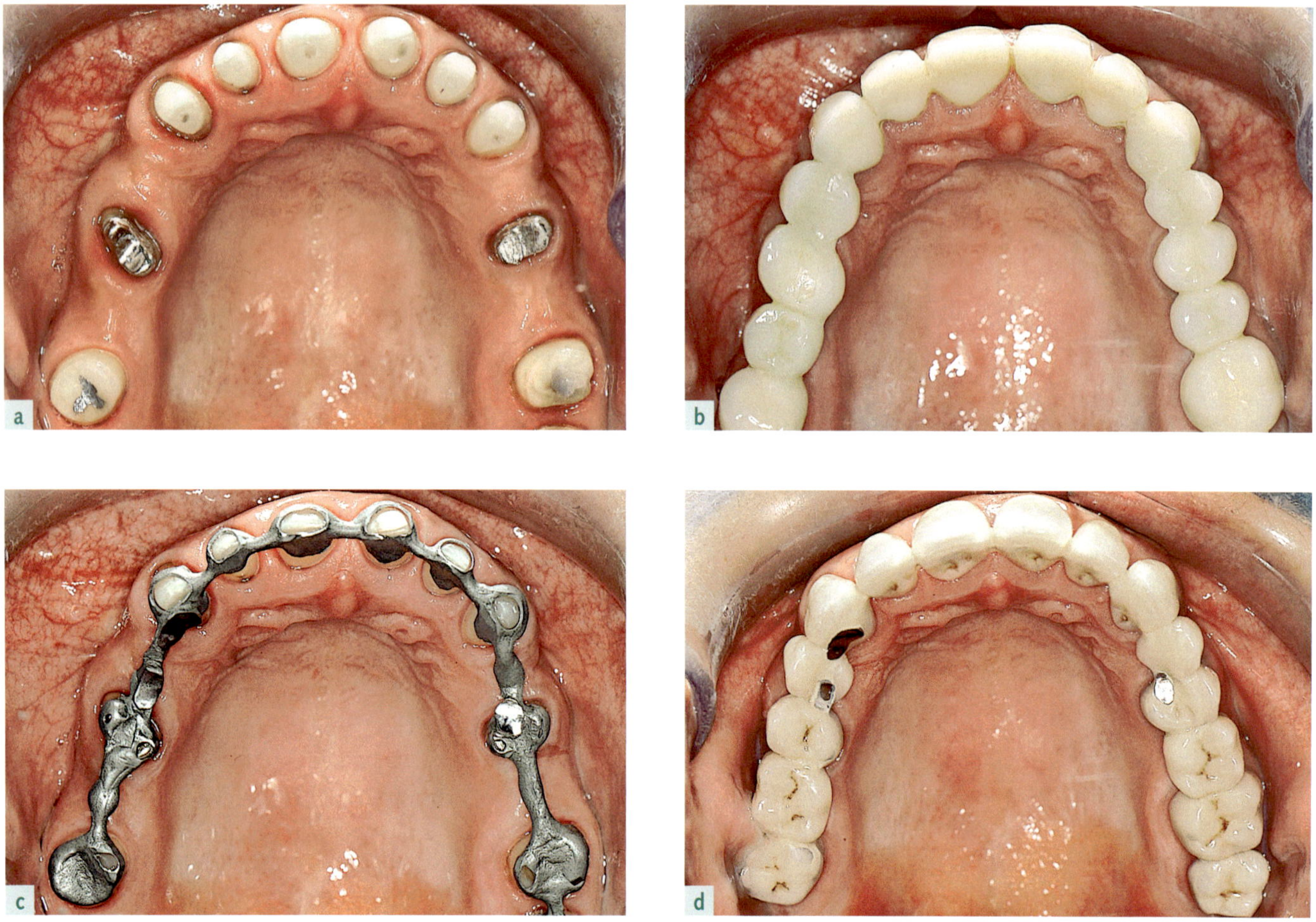

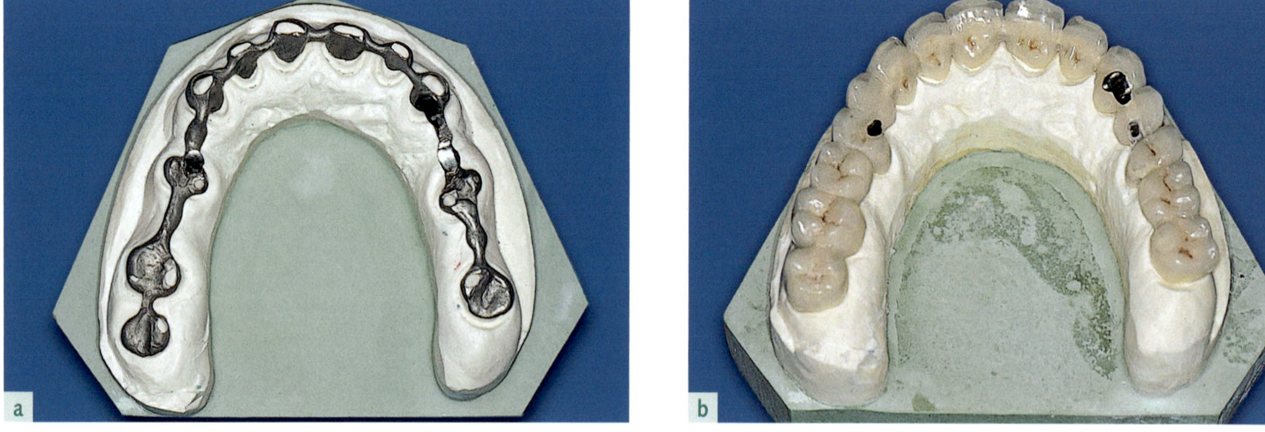

Fig 13-120 Occlusal view of a maxillary arch to be rehabiltated with an FPD. *(a)* Tooth preparation. *(b)* First provisional prosthesis in acrylic-resin. *(c)* Try-in of the metal structure of the therapeutic provisional prosthesis. *(d)* Therapeutic provisional prosthesis in situ.

Fig 13-121 Preparation of a therapeutic provisional prosthesis. *(a)* Metal armature on the plaster cast. *(b)* Completed therapeutic provisional prosthesis.

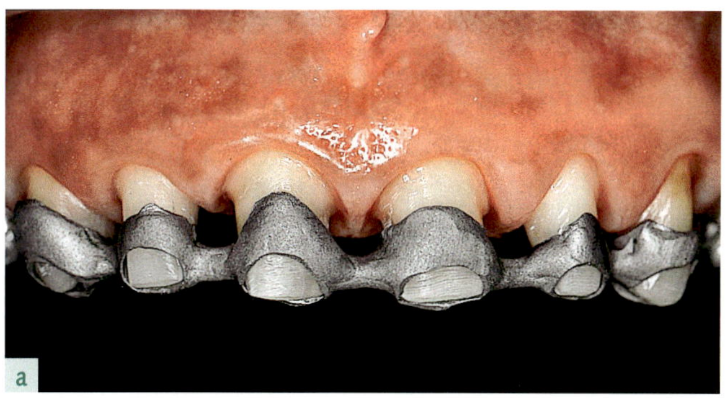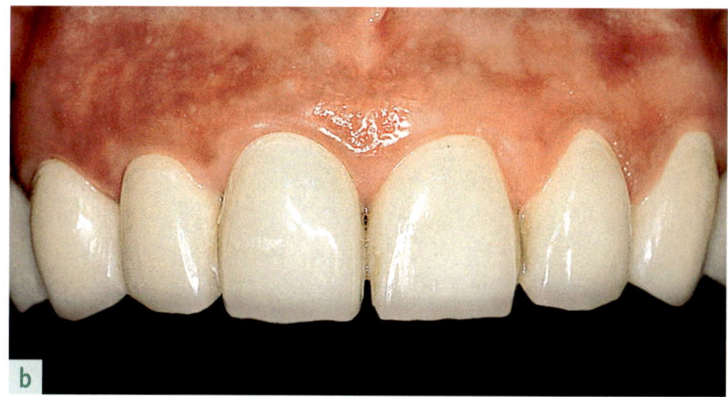

Fig 13-122 Buccal view of the anterior structure. *(a)* Testing the metal structure. *(b)* The therapeutic provisional prosthesis completed.

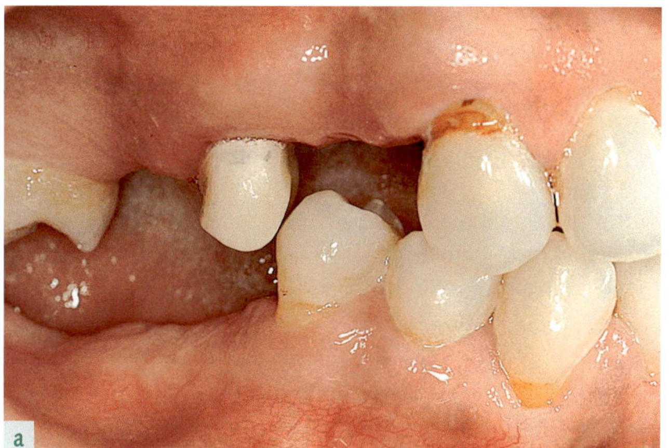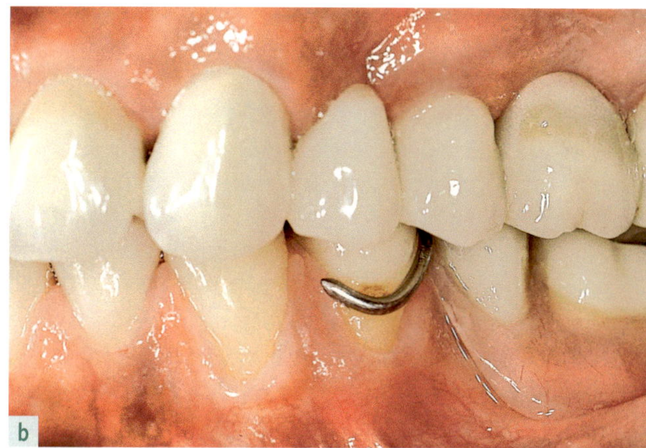

Fig 13-123 *(a)* Right lateral view before the placement of the provisional prosthesis. *(b)* Provisional FPD and RPD with mandibular clasps.

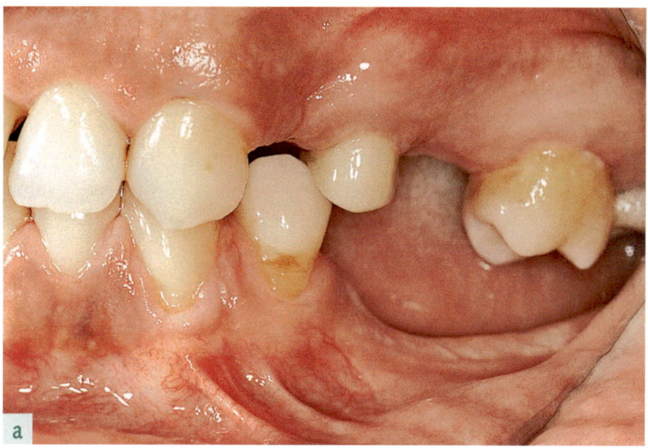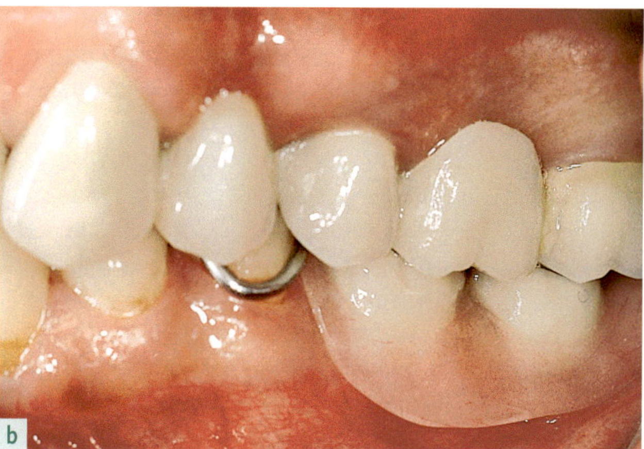

Fig 13-124 *(a)* Left lateral view before the placement of the provisional prosthesis. *(b)* Provisional maxillary FPD and provisional mandibular RPD with clasps.

Direct techniques are carried out entirely in the patient's mouth. They must use an impression as a shell for the external form, created before beginning the dental preparation. For the internal form, they must use the prepared abutments.[133,134] Indirect techniques are carried out entirely outside the mouth, using an impression taken on a cast before the preparation of the abutments. This cast can, if necessary, be corrected with a diagnostic waxup.[135] The silicone index (external form) is applied on the cast of the prepared abutments (internal form).[130,134] Mixed techniques are carried out outside the mouth for the external form and fitted intraorally for the internal form. Examples of mixed techniques are the preshaped crowns or the provisional crowns built before teeth preparation.[136,137] The external form is created in the laboratory, and the internal form is obtained through direct relining on the prepared teeth.

The indirect technique (see Figs 13-120 to 13-124), is often preferable to the direct technique because the patient can avoid the unpleasant sensations (heat and smell) caused by direct relining, and because it offers better adaptation to the abutment.[29,130,138–141]

Direct technique

The direct technique requires an impression of the teeth to be included in the provisional restoration before the prosthetic preparation, possible extractions, or removal of a pre-existent prosthesis.[130,133,134] This impression is not cast and will constitute the mold for the external surface of the provisional prosthesis.

A blade is used to modify the impression, which may involve removing the interdental areas or other elements not involved in the prosthetic preparation.

Then the dentin of the vital teeth is protected with an appropriate varnish, and the abutments are coated with petroleum jelly.

The resin is poured into the area of the impression corresponding to the teeth to be included in the provisional prosthesis, paying attention not to incorporate air. After a few seconds, the resin loses its surface shininess. This process, together with the application of the petroleum jelly, prevents the adhesion of the resin to the abutment. The impression is positioned correctly in the impression tray using the references obtained previously.

As already mentioned, the provisional prosthesis must be removed from the mouth before the resin hardens completely to reduce the thermal stress of the last phase of polymerization. When the impression is removed, the provisional prosthesis may be stuck to the impression tray, in which case, more time is needed to complete the hardening phase. If it remains on the arch, it must be removed before complete hardening without causing distortion. Once polymerization has ended, the excess resin is removed. A pencil can be used to help mark the preparation margin.

The contraction of the resin makes complete rehabilitation with a provisional prosthesis difficult and frequently causes imprecision at the margins. These can be eliminated by relining the prosthesis. If the defect is minimal, resin can be added directly on the margin using a pen dipped alternately in liquid and powder. If the marginal defect is more significant or if the provisional prosthesis does not seat correctly on the prosthetic abutment, it is necessary to slightly reduce the inside of the prosthesis. The adaptation of the provisional prosthesis to the abutment is therefore perfected by relining it. In this phase, the provisional prosthesis must be inserted and removed more than once during polymerization so that excess resin engaged in the undercuts does not block the prosthesis and make its removal difficult. Once the resin has hardened completely, the interproximal surfaces are refined further.

To ensure that oral hygiene can be maintained, resin is removed apically at the interproximal point of contact, without excessively weakening the structure, to allow for the use of the cleaning brush (Fig 13-125). Control of the occlusion and final polishing using simple silicone rubbers complete the process.

Mixed techniques

A provisional prosthesis is based on the plaster cast of the arch to be rehabilitated or produced industrially. In both cases, it must be fitted directly in the oral cavity of the patient.

Once the teeth have been prepared, the provisional prosthesis is seated, verifying that occlusal interferences are not created (the correct maxillomandibular relationship of the opposite side is checked). Then it is relined using a procedure similar to that described for the direct technique (Fig 13-126).

Clinical application of constructive principles

Two case reports illustrate the clinical application of the constructive principles.

Clinical case 1 is shown in Figs 13-127 to 13-141 and clinical case 2 is shown in Figs 13-142 to 13-171.

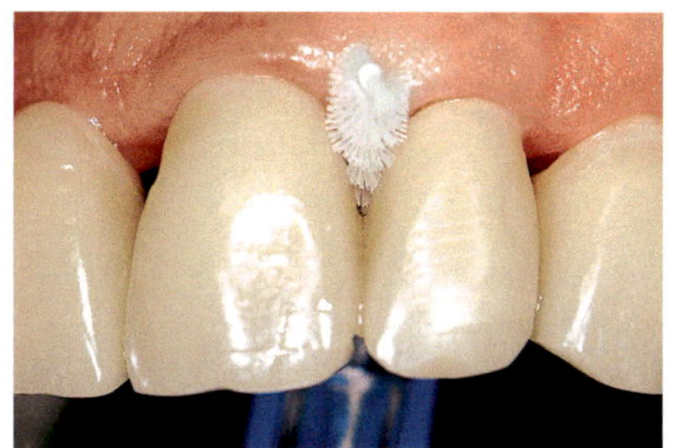

Fig 13-125 Design of the interproximal spaces to allow hygiene.

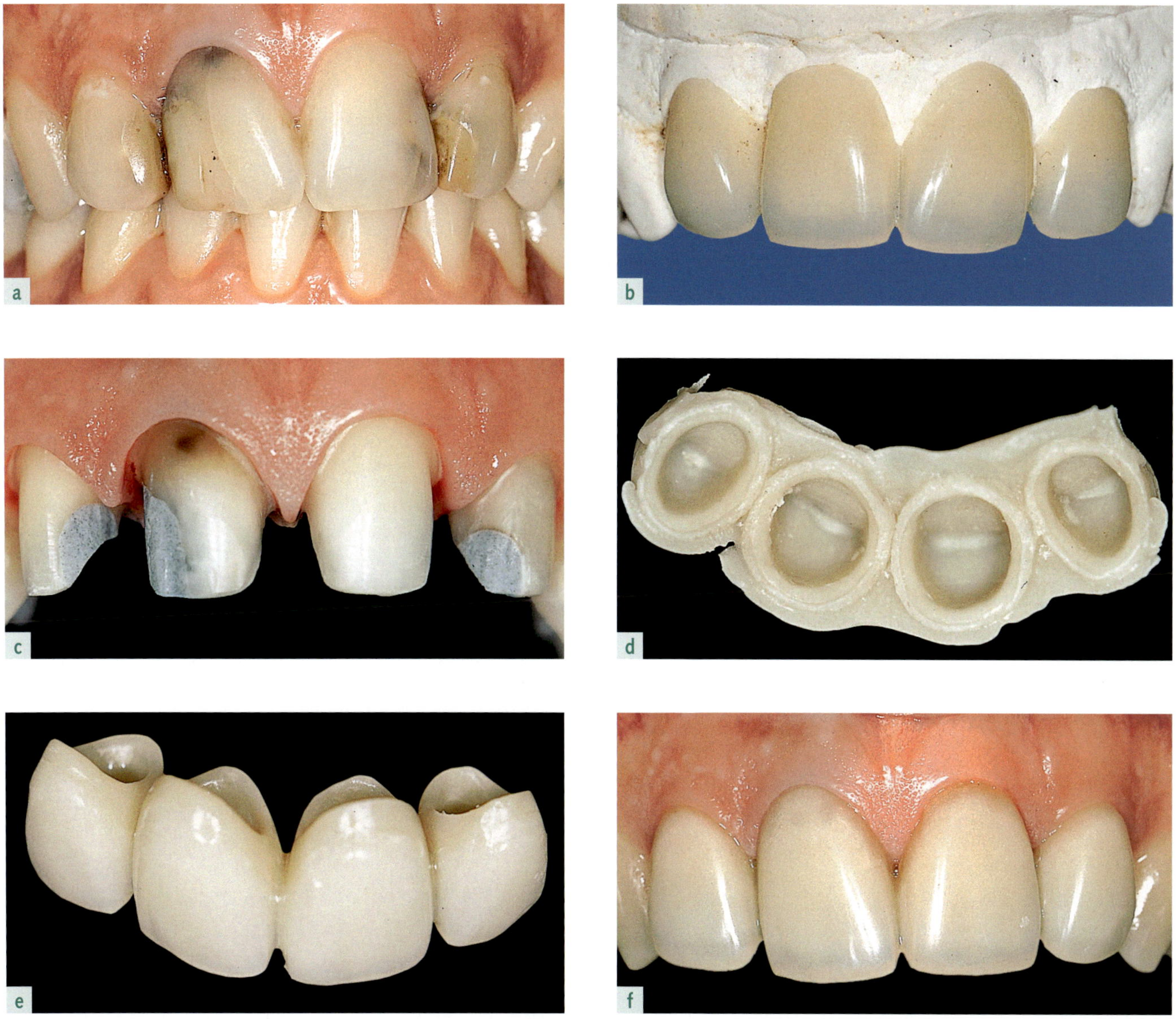

Fig 13-126 Mixed technique. *(a)* Initial clinical situation. *(b)* Provisional prosthesis, before preparation, on the plaster cast. *(c)* Tooth preparation. *(d)* Direct relining with acrylic resin. *(e)* Finishing and polishing the provisional prosthesis. *(f)* Provisional prosthesis in situ.

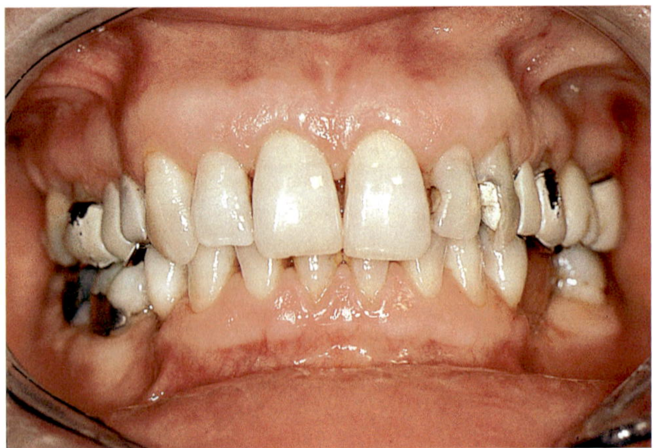

Fig 13-127 A 45-year-old patient in need of a posterior restoration. Frontal view in maximal intercuspidation.

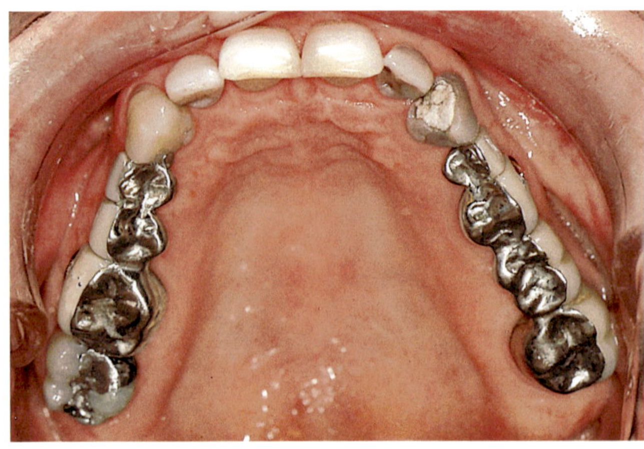

Fig 13-128 Maxillary arch.

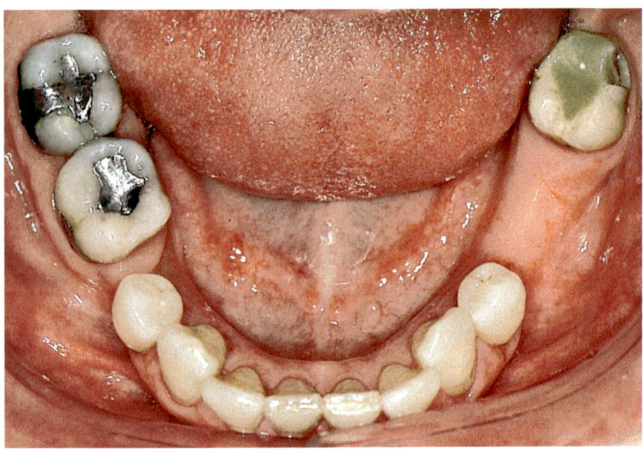

Fig 13-129 Mandibular arch.

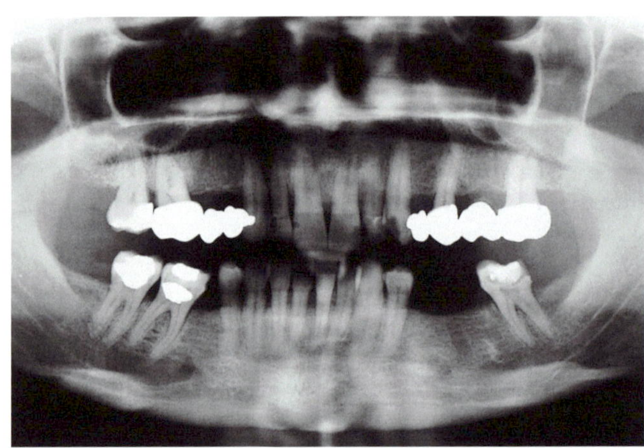

Fig 13-130 Radiographic analysis.

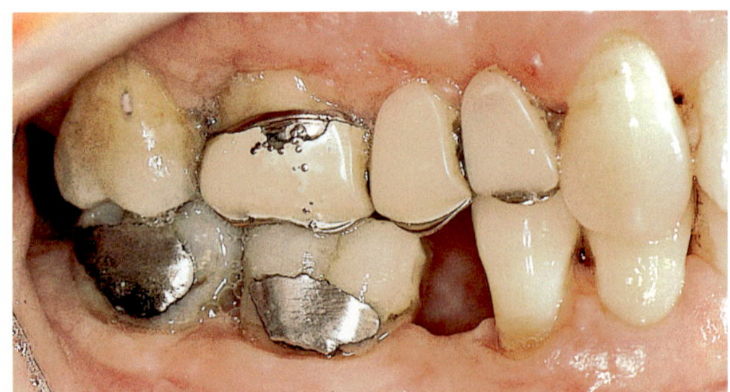

Fig 13-131 Right lateral view in maximum intercuspidation before the rehabilitation.

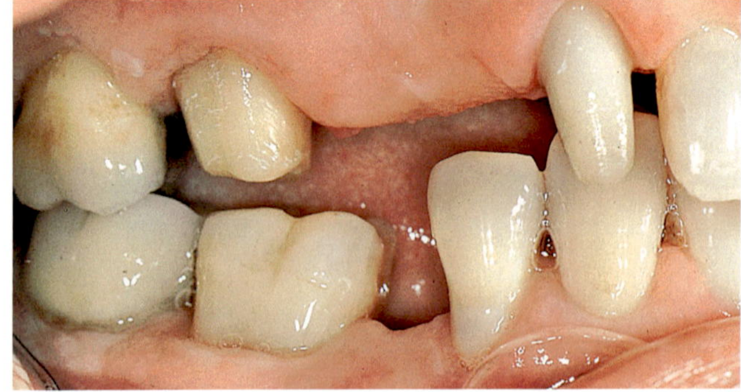

Fig 13-132 Preparation of abutment teeth. The maxillary right canine and first molar are used as abutments in replacing the right first and second premolars. FPD restoration is considered favorable from a biomechanical point of view.

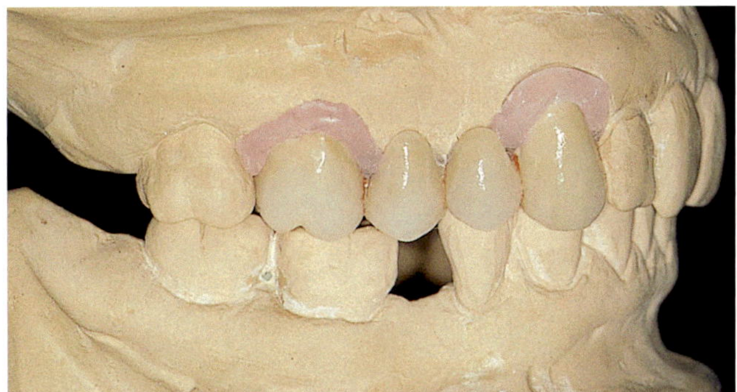

Fig 13-133 Metal-ceramic FPD.

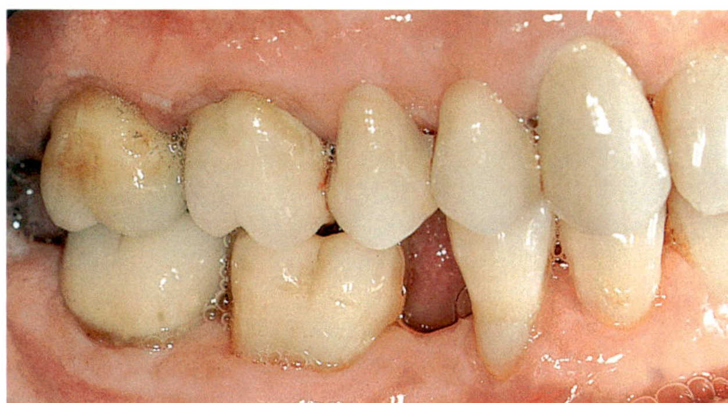

Fig 13-134 Definitive restoration, lateral view. The mandibular right second premolar has not been restored because the gap is reduced, and there are no functional or esthetic indications. The mandibular right first molar has a direct reconstruction in composite material, and the mandibular right second molar has an indirect reconstruction with a reinforced composite crown.

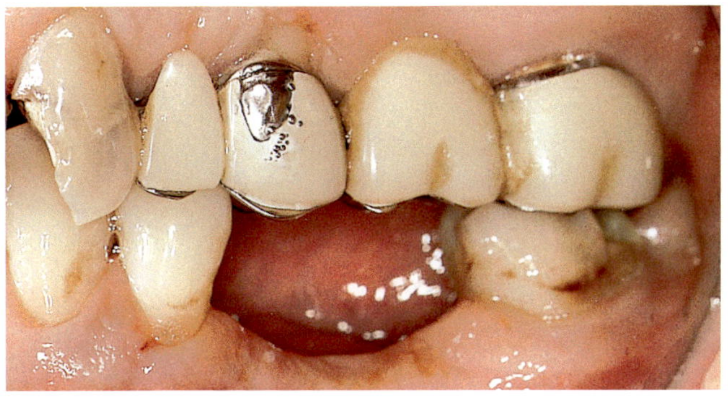

Fig 13-135 Left lateral view in maximal intercuspidation before rehabilitation.

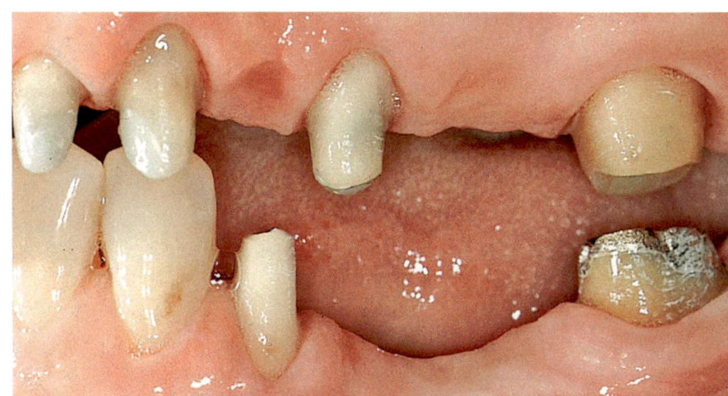

Fig 13-136 Prepared abutment teeth. Also, the maxillary lateral incisor has been restored because of destructive caries lesions. In the mandible, the left first premolar and second molar are used as abutments in replacing the left second premolar and first molar. Such a situation is consdiered to be at the limit of acceptabilty.

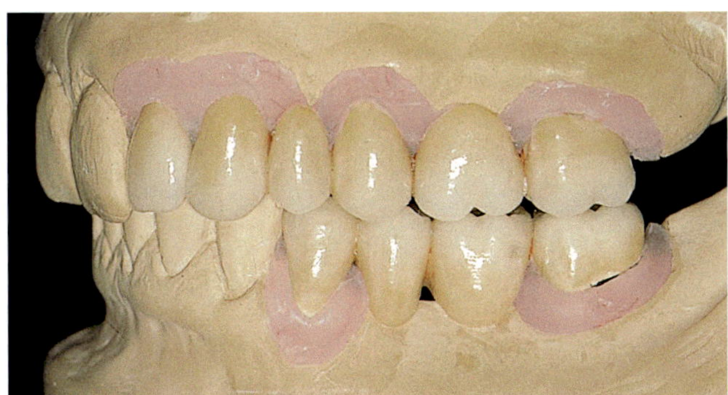

Fig 13-137 Metal-ceramic FPD.

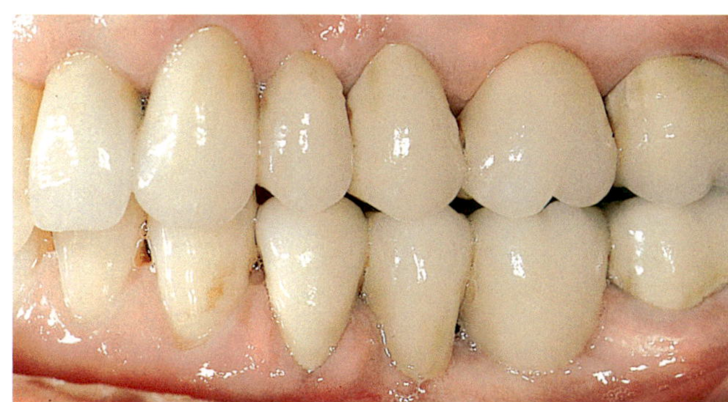

Fig 13-138 Definitive restoration in situ.

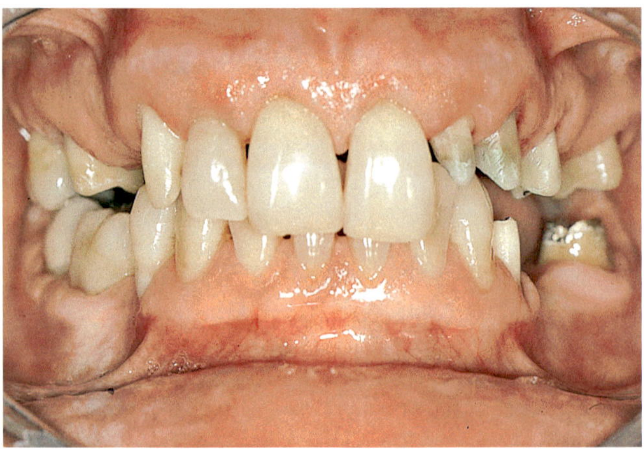

Fig 13-139 Frontal view in maximal intercuspidation before the insertion of the prosthesis.

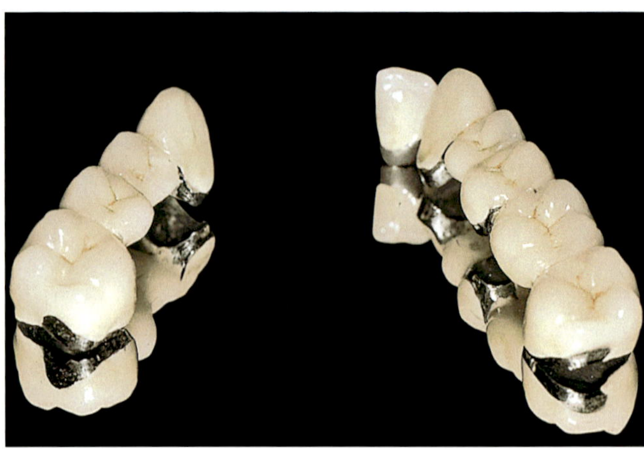

Fig 13-140 Maxillary prostheses before cementing.

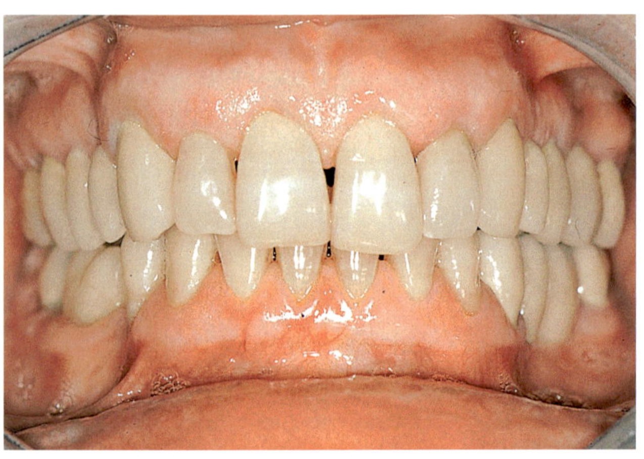

Fig 13-141 Frontal view of the definitive prosthesis.

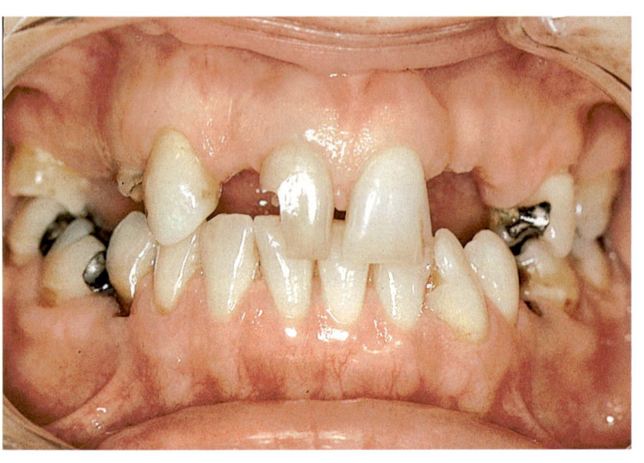

Fig 13-142 Frontal view of the arches in maximum intercuspidation of a 40-year-old female patient. There are several edenutlous gaps interposed that have been present for a long time. There are no signs or symptoms of craniomandibular disorders. The patient indicated functional problems related to diminished mastication, esthetic problems due to the absence of anterior teeth, and the presence of destructive caries lesions on remaining teeth. From the first visit, the patient expressed a desire to have a fixed prosthesis.

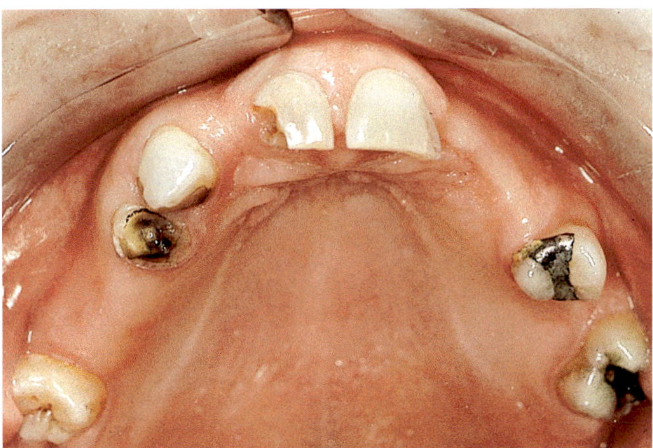

Fig 13-143 Maxillary occlusal view. Note the absence of the right lateral incisor, second premolar, and first and third molars as well as the left lateral incisor, canine, second premolar, and second and third molars. There are extensive caries lesions on the right central incisor, canine, and first premolar as well as the left central incisor, first premolar, and first molar.

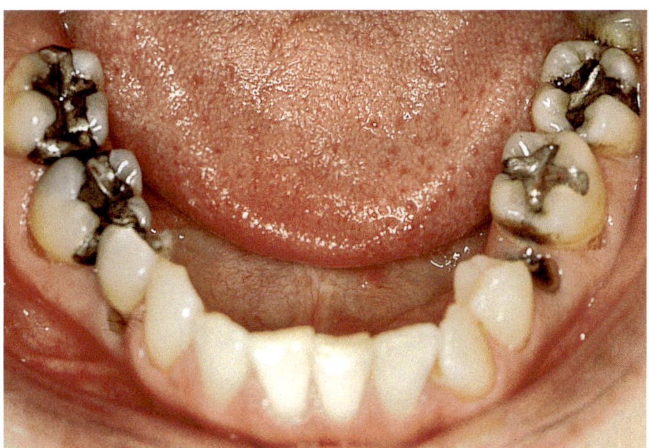

Fig 13-144 Mandibular occlusal view. Note the absence of the left second premolar with the narrowing of the corresponding gap, the absence of the right third molar, the presence of extensive reconstructions in silver amalgam on posterior teeth, and the absence of the crown on the right second premolar.

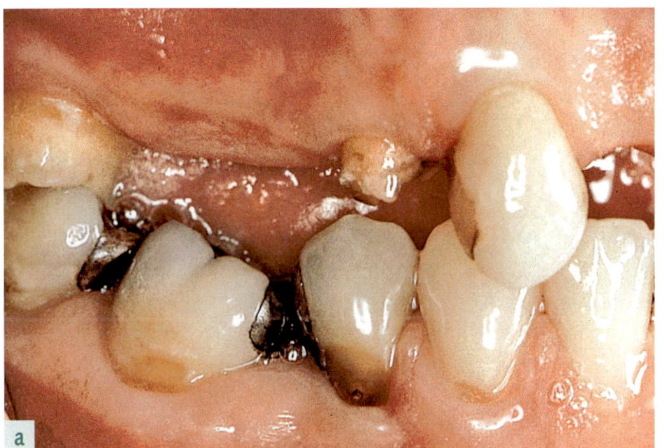

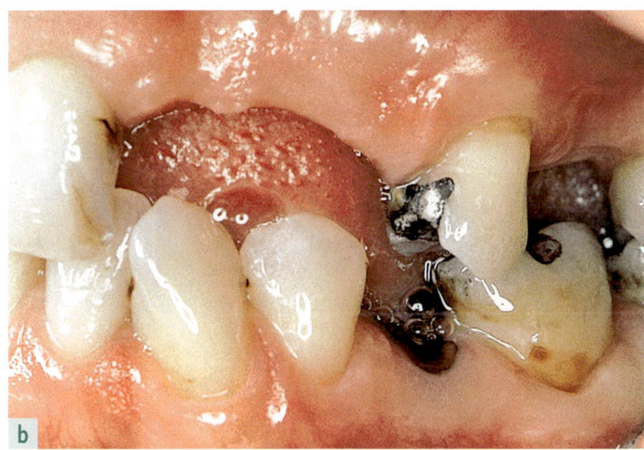

Fig 13-145 *(a)* Right lateral view. *(b)* Left lateral view. Note the movement of residual teeth having caused occlusal disharmony, with alterations of the compensation and reduction of the edentulous spaces on both the vertical and horizontal planes.

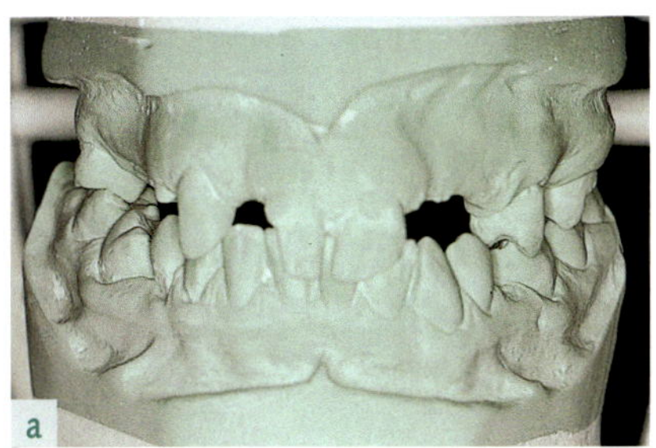

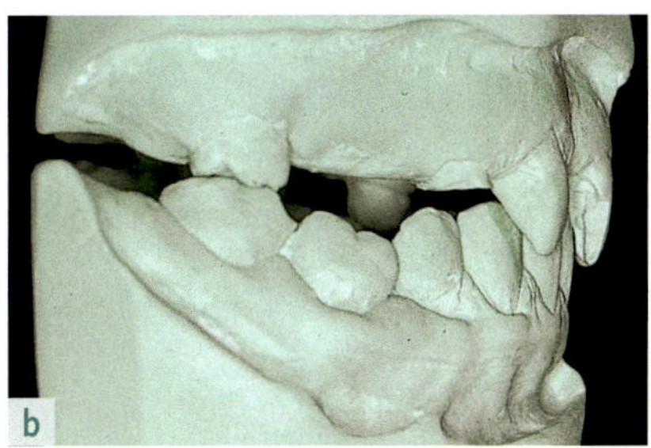

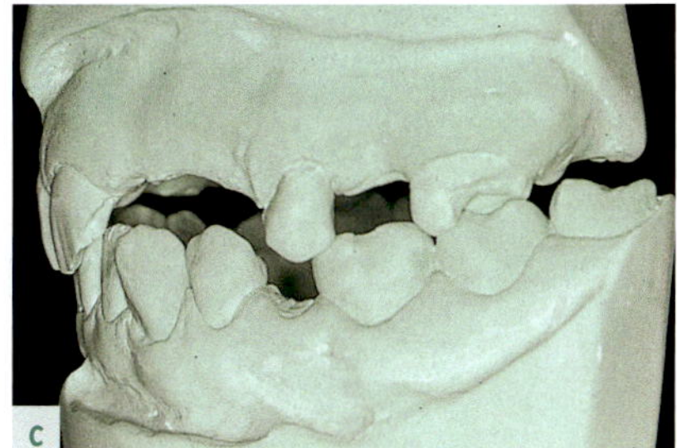

Fig 13-146 Study casts: *(a)* frontal view; *(b)* right lateral view; *(c)* left lateral view.

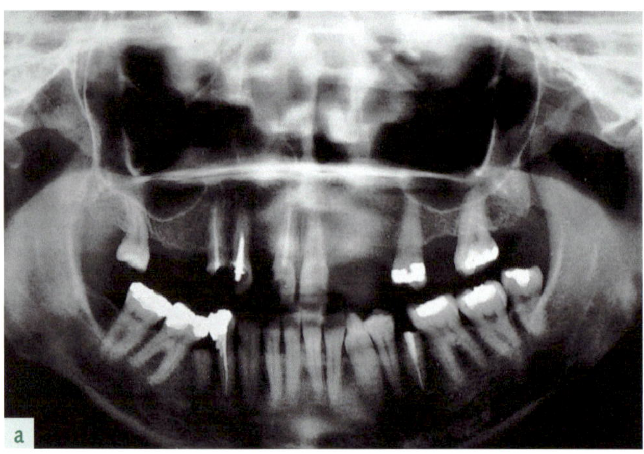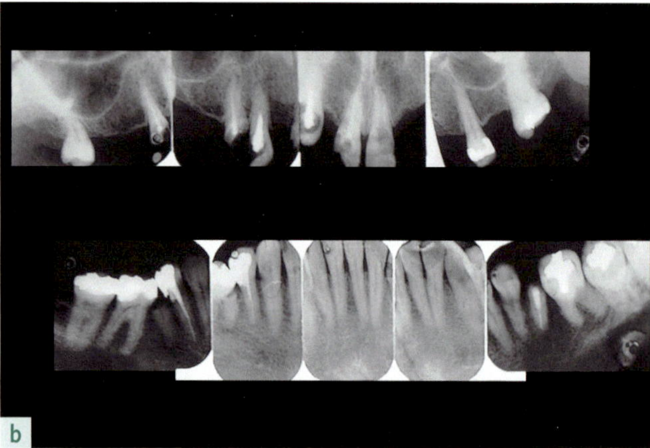

Fig 13-147 *(a)* Panoramic radiograph; *(b)* intraoral radiographs. Note the presence of numerous inadequate endodontic treatments on the maxillary right central incisor, canine, and first premolar; extensive caries lesions on the maxillary central incisors, right canine, and first premolar and on the mandibular right first premolar; and residual root treatment of the mandibular right second premolar.

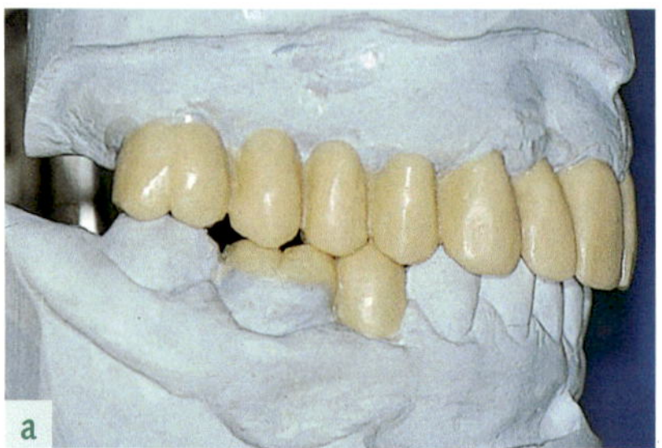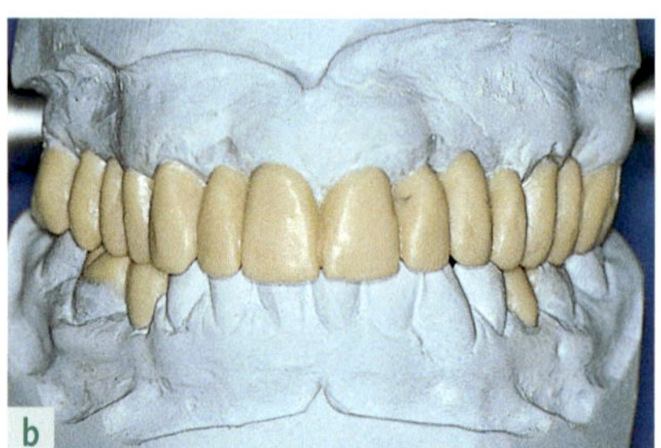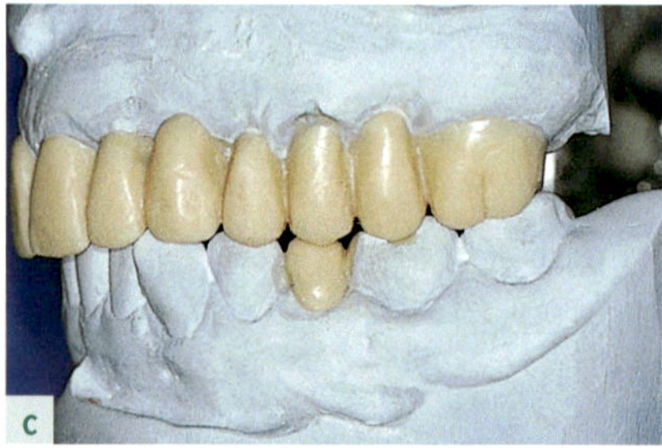

Fig 13-148 Diagnostic waxup to ensure that all residual maxillary teeth and the mandibular left second premolar and second and third molars as well as the right first premolar and first and second molars are included as abutments. The diagnostic waxup shows the desired occlusal plane and substitution of missing teeth except for the mandibular right second premolar. In the maxilla, a fixed prosthesis, even in the absence of the left canine, was planned and designed because the edentulous gap was in a straight line. In the mandible, there was also a plan for the application of full crowns on the left second premolar and the right first premolar and partial crowns for the first and second on both sides. The cast was mounted in an articulator after having registered the intraoral and extraoral relationships of the jaws. *(a)* Right lateral view; *(b)* Frontal view; *(c)* Left lateral view.

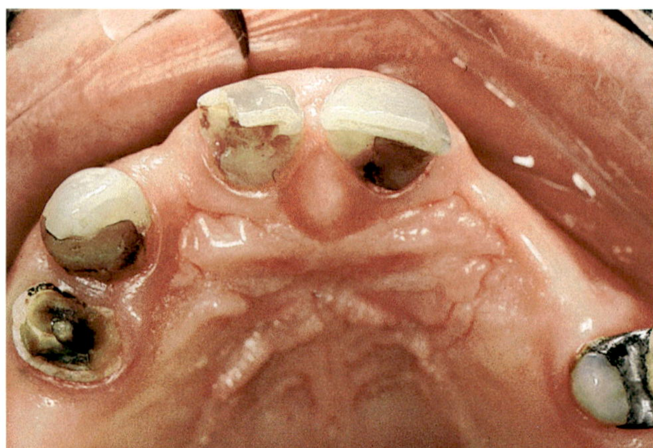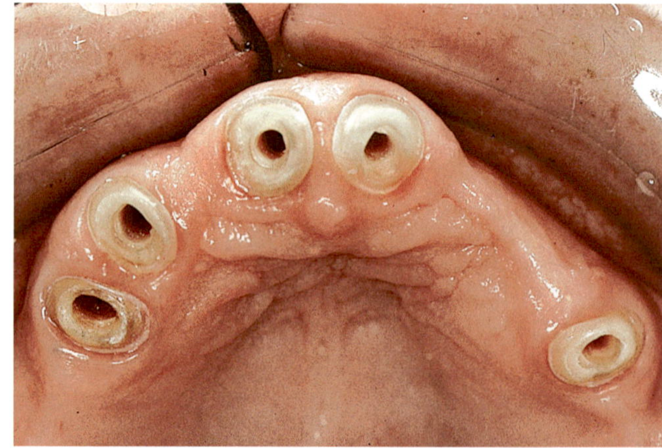

Fig 13-149 Occlusal view of endodontically treated maxillary teeth.

Fig 13-150 Preparation for a reconstruction with post restorations in fused gold alloy.

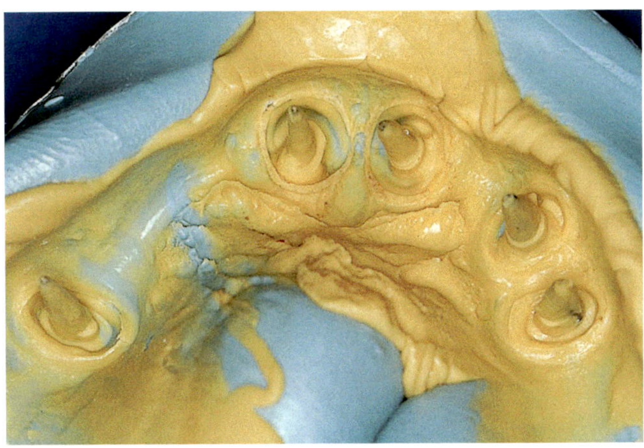

Fig 13-151 Silicone impression for adding the reconstructed fused cement.

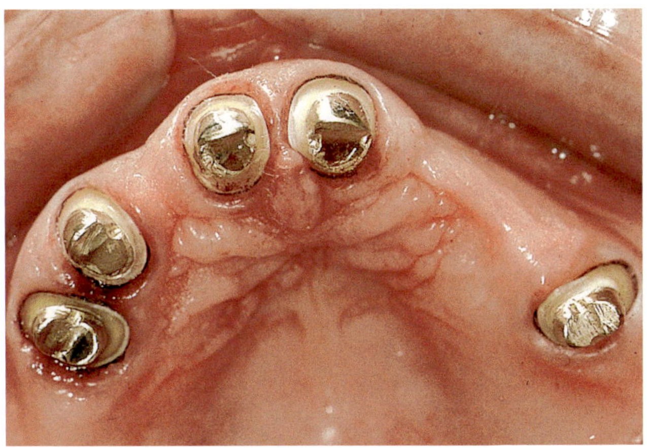

Fig 13-152 Occlusal view of fused and cemented post restoration.

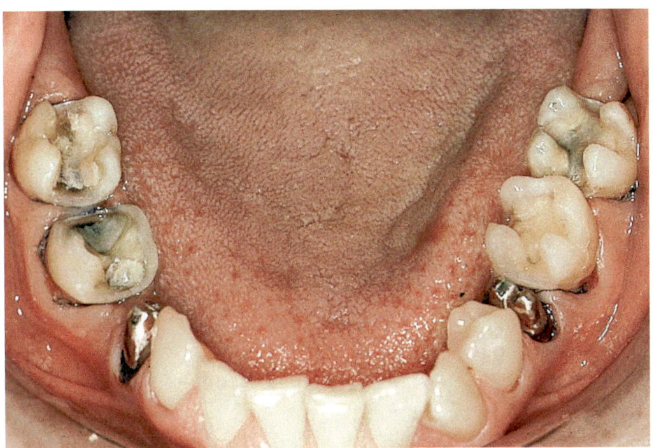

Fig 13-153 Partial preparation of mandibular first and second molars on both sides and reconstruction by post restoration of the left second premolar and right first premolar.

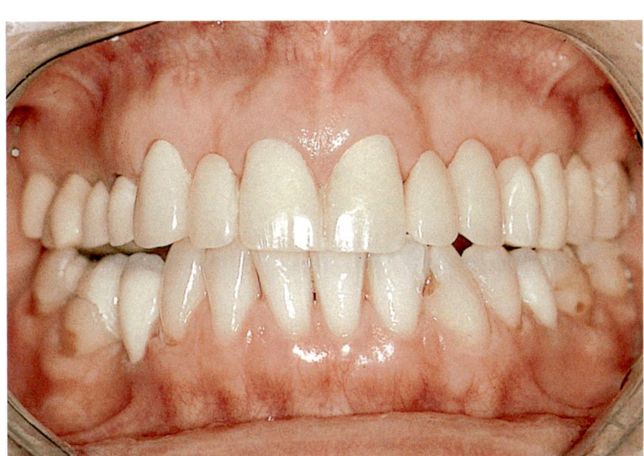

Fig 13-154 Application of indirect provisional restorations on the base of the diagnostic waxup.

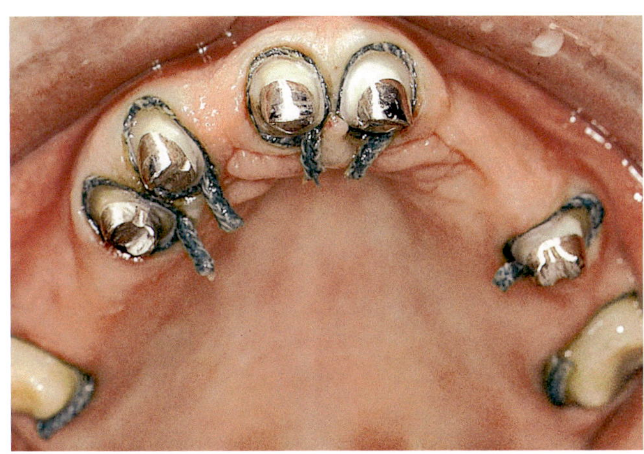

Fig 13-155 Gingiva is retracted during the impression of the maxilla by using double cords in the gingival sulcus.

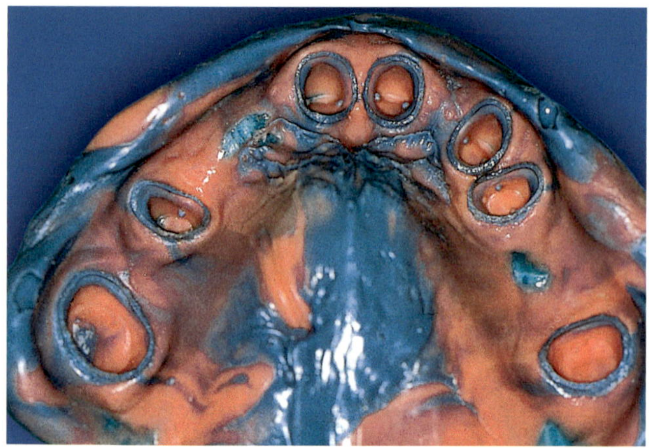

Fig 13-156 Polymer impression for the maxillary master cast.

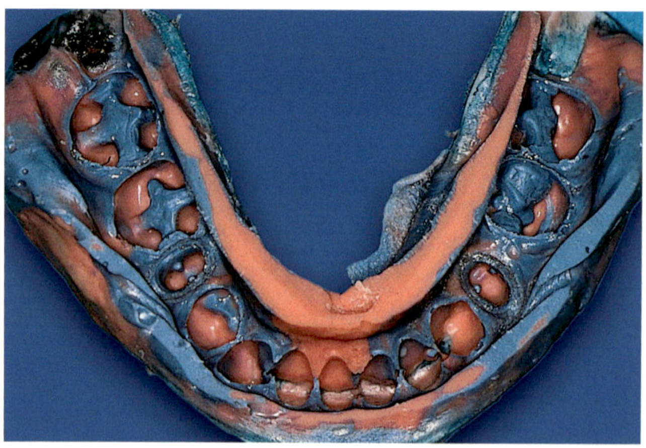

Fig 13-157 Polymer impression for the mandibular master cast.

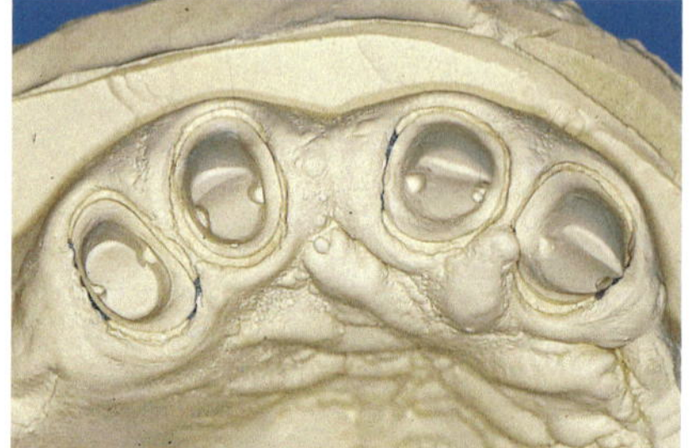

Fig 13-158 Maxillary master cast of the anterior teeth.

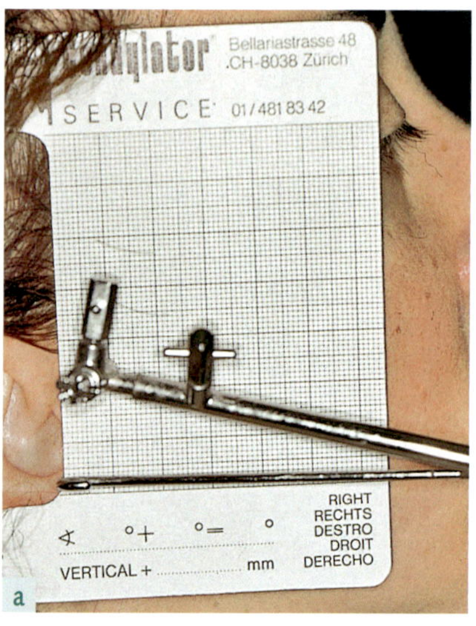

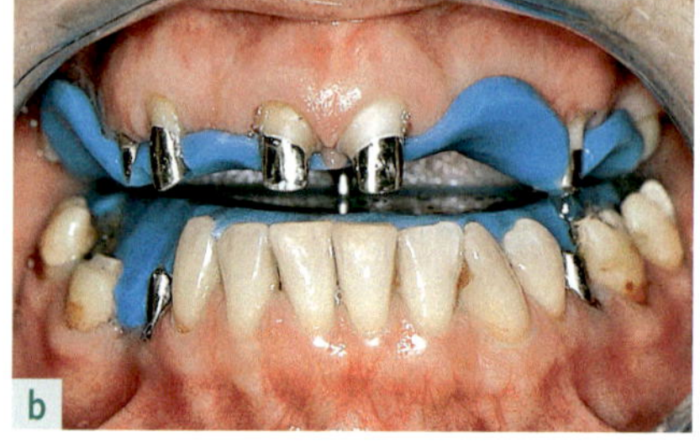

Fig 13-159 Registration of the maxillomandibular relationships: *(a)* extraoral examination *(b)* intraoral examination (gothic arch).

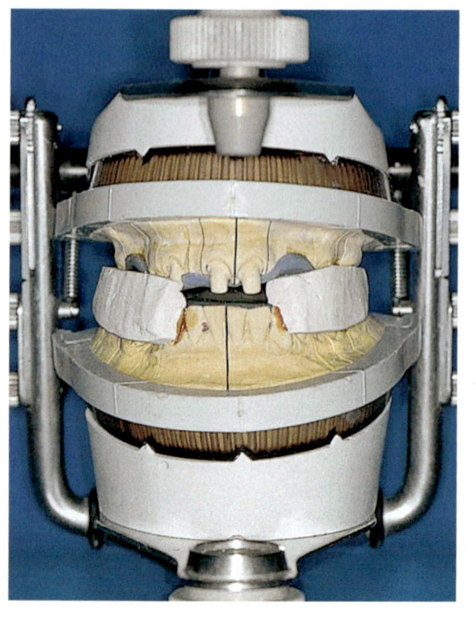

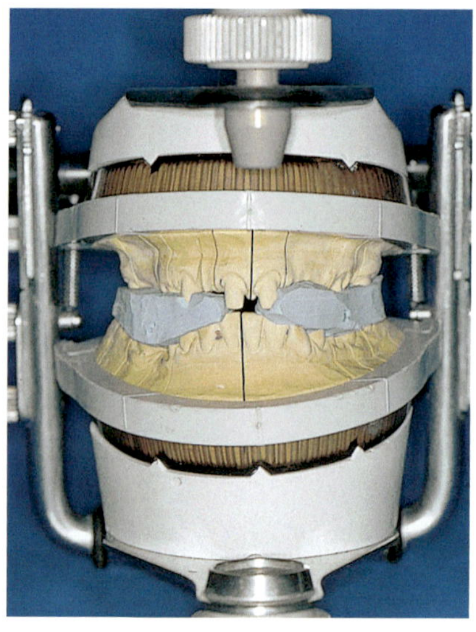

Fig 13-160 Master cast in the articulator with auxiliary keys in plaster.

Fig 13-161 Occlusal keys in silicone constructed in the articulator to check the clinical registration.

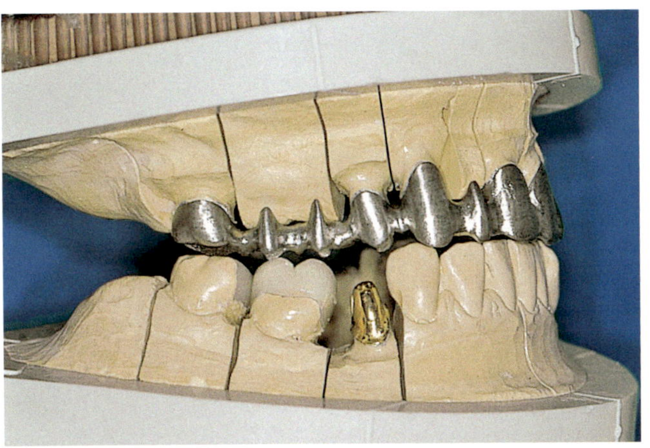

Fig 13-162 Right lateral view of the fused metal framework and partial ceromer crowns in position on the master cast.

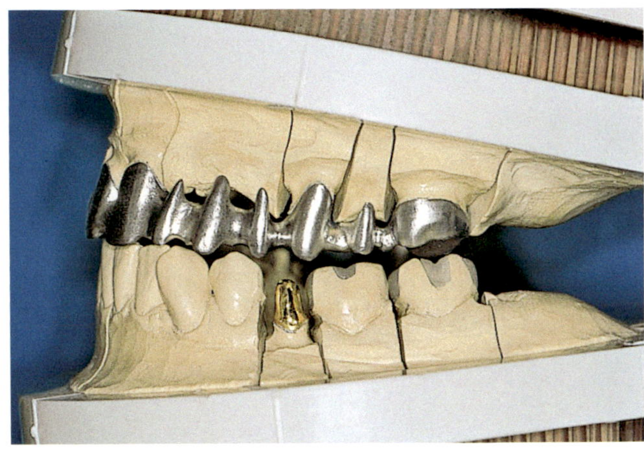

Fig 13-163 Left lateral view of the fused metal framework and partial ceromer crowns in position on the master cast.

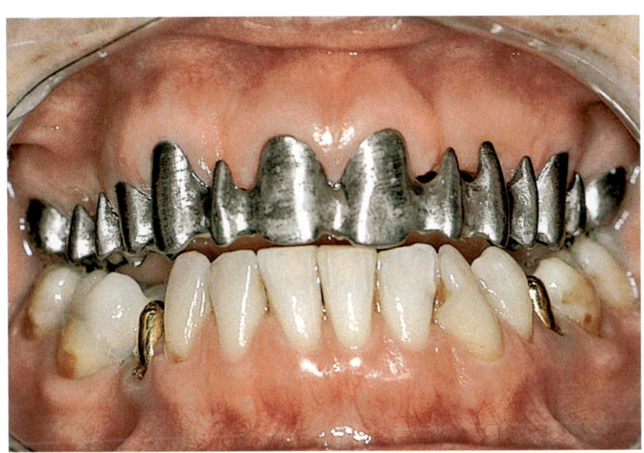

Fig 13-164 Frontal view showing the metal substructures obtained by electrodeposit for the mandibular left second premolar and right first premolar as well as the partial ceromer crowns on the mandibular first and second molars on both sides positioned in the oral cavity.

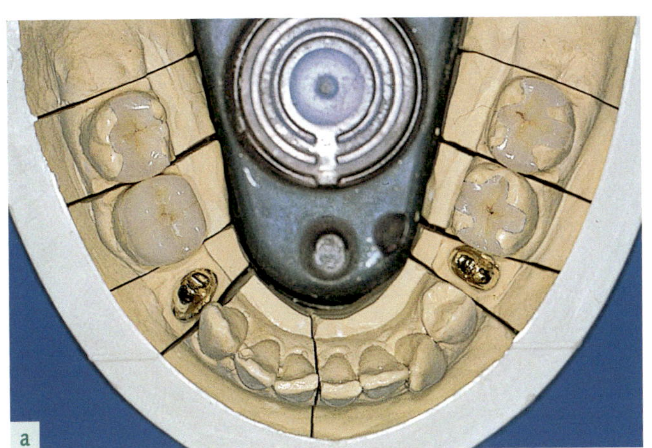

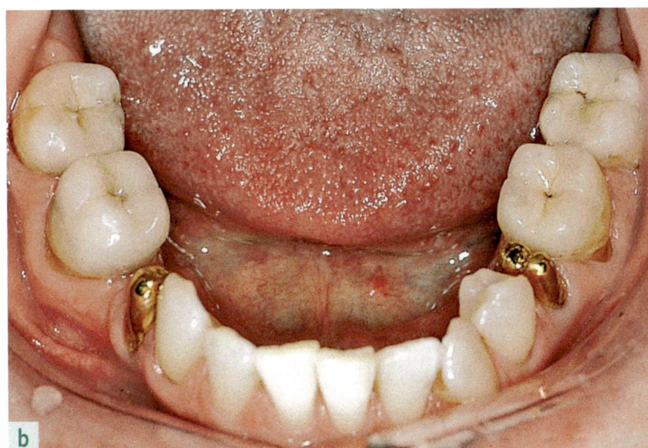

Fig 13-165 Occlusal view of partial crowns on the mandibular first and second molars on both sides, and the metal understructure on the left second premolar and the right first premolar on the master cast (a) and in the oral cavity (b).

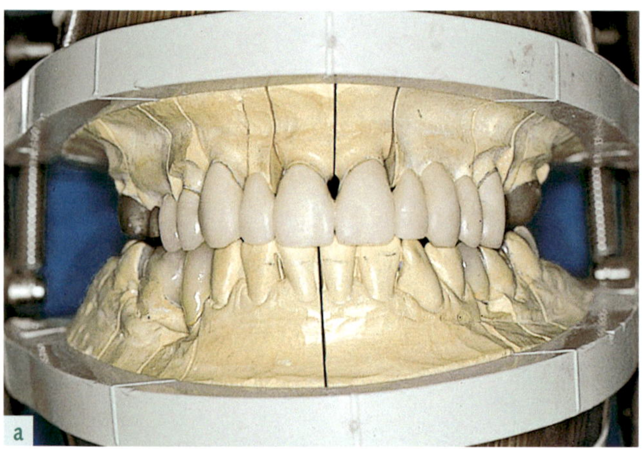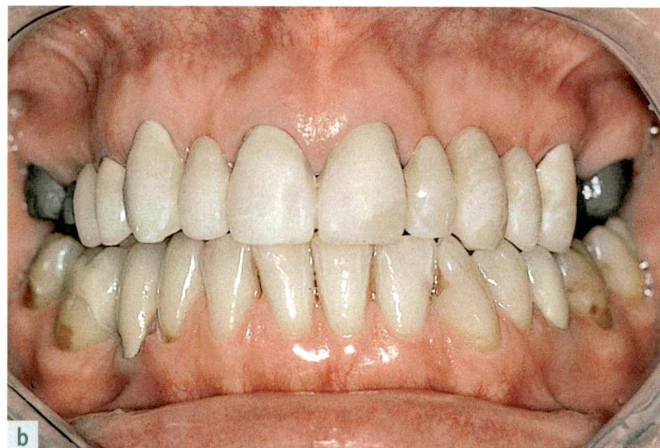

Fig 13-166 Unglazed ceramic prostheses. *(a)* On the master cast. *(b)* Intraoral biscuit test.

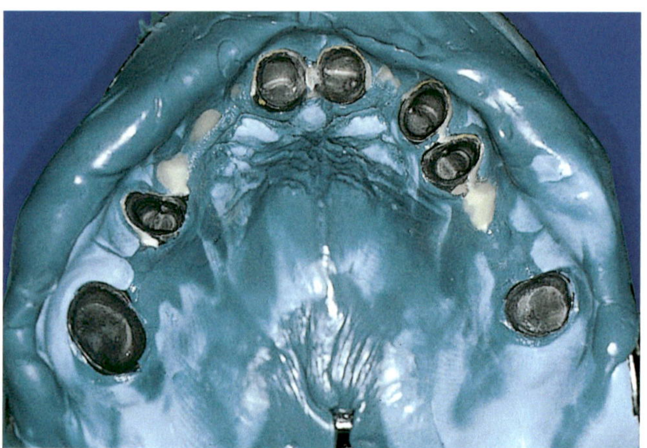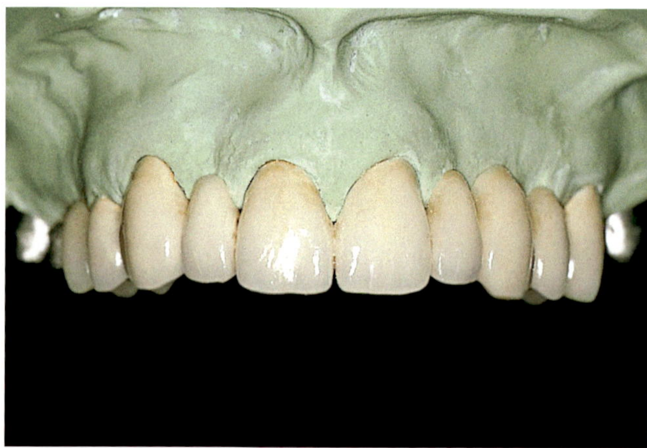

Fig 13-167 Impression in silicone for remounting in the articulator.

Fig 13-168 Definitive FPD in ceramic from the right second premolar to the left second premolar on the remounted impression. A ceromer esthetic material will be used to cover the metal structure.

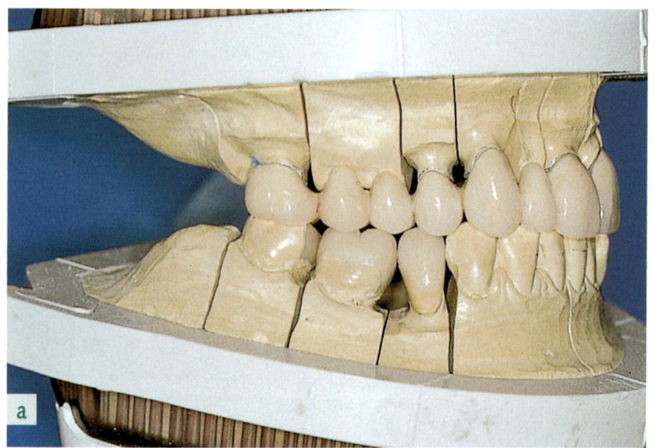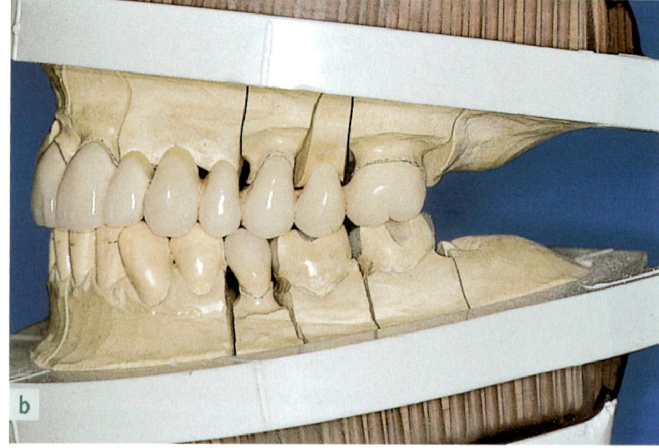

Fig 13-169 FPD positioned on the master cast. *(a)* Right lateral view. *(b)* Left lateral view.

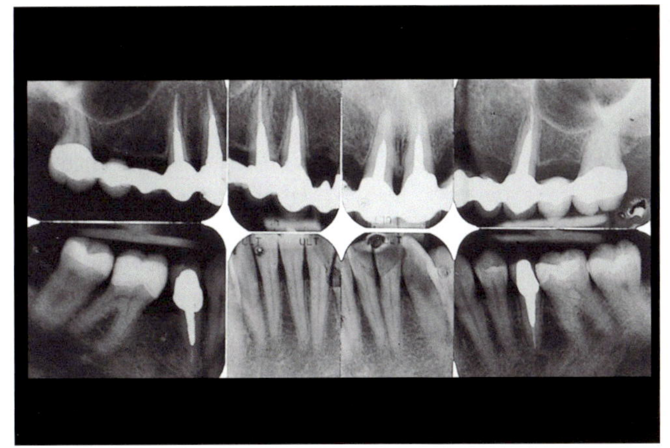

Fig 13-170 A systematic intraoral radiograph at the completion of the prosthetic restoration.

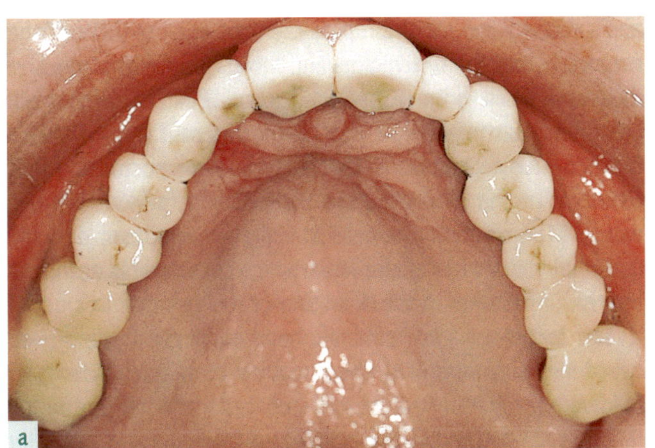

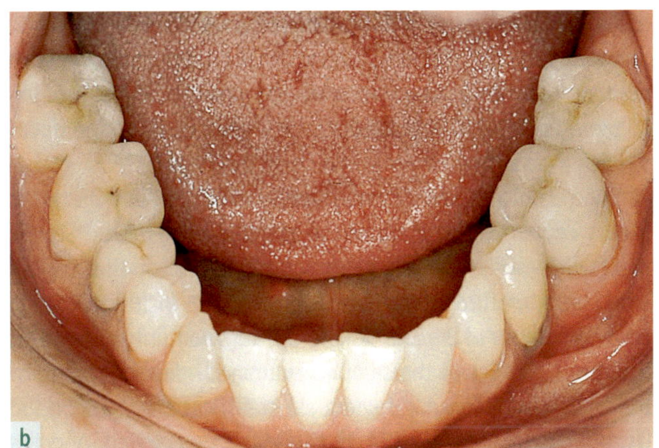

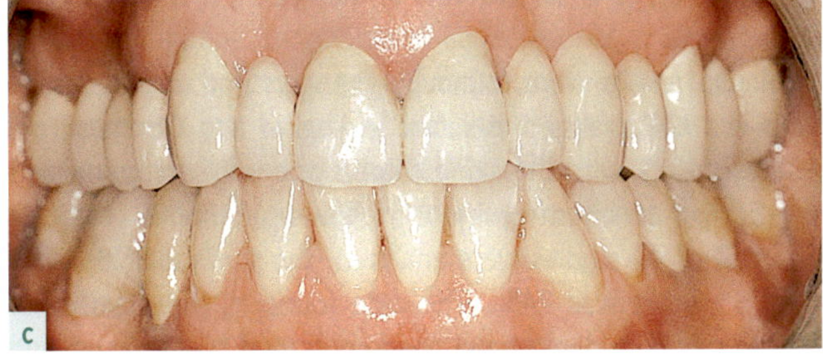

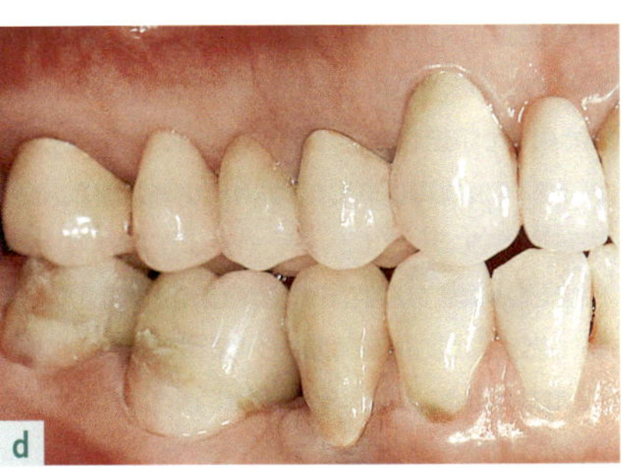

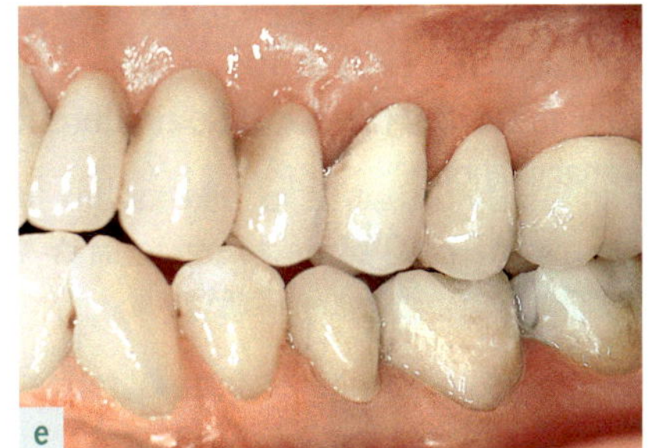

Fig 13-171 Definitive prosthesis in the mouth: *(a)* maxillary occlusal view; *(b)* mandibular occlusal view; *(c)* frontal view in maximum intercuspidation; *(d)* right lateral view; *(e)* left lateral view; direct Class 5a reconstructions in composite corresponding to the mandibular left first and second molar.

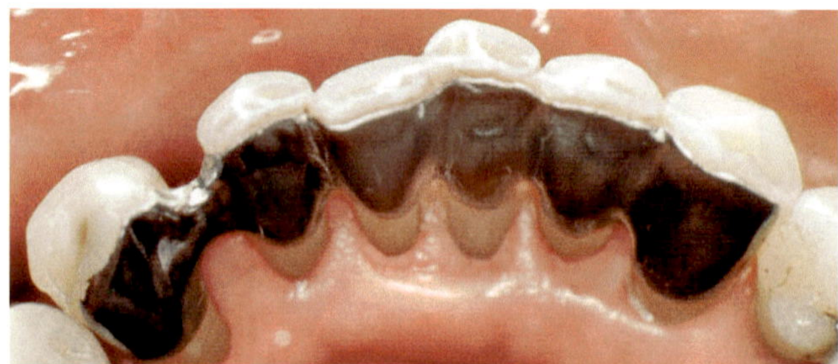

Fig 13-174 An adhesive technique used to stabilize teeth affected by periodontal disease.

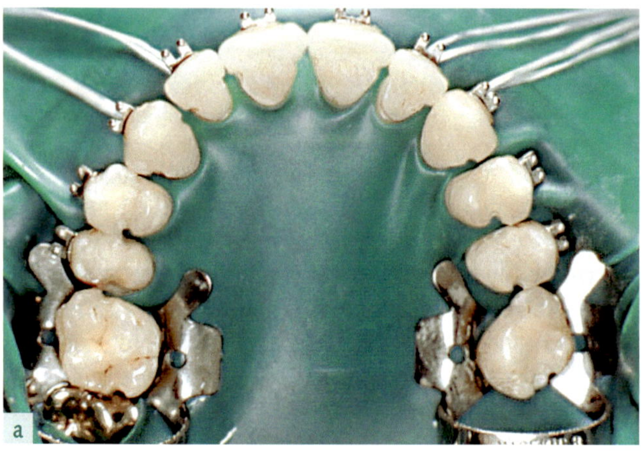

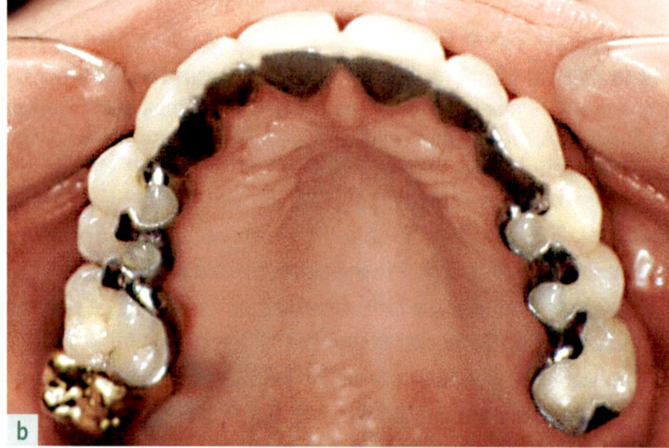

Fig 13-175 Occlusal view of the maxilla after orthodontic treatment and preparations of abutment teeth for an adhesive prosthesis the right first molar to the left first molar. *(a)* The arch has been prepared for cementing. *(b)* Occlusal view of the adhesive prosthesis following cementation.

■ Retention of teeth with reduced (or insufficient) periodontal support (Fig 13-174)

■ Stabilization of the result of an orthodontic treatment (Fig 13-175)

For many years, FPAD has been considered an experimental technique and has often been applied as a sophisticated and costly provisional prosthesis. Most authors considered it appropriate for the replacement of only one tooth in posterior regions or at the most, two teeth in anterior regions. Improvement in preparation and adhesive cementation techniques today has allowed for indications to be extended to include even FPDs with greater extension.

The main contraindications of this technique are:

■ Supporting teeth with extensive fillings. Supporting teeth that have reduced height in which the enamel available—the main element of adhesive resistance—may be insufficient.

■ Supporting teeth with excessively transparent enamel so that the esthetic result may not be satisfactory.

■ Worn supporting teeth in patients with bruxism or with traumatic occlusion. There are no sufficient data on long-term mechanical resistance.

The advantages of this technique are tissue preservation, relative simplicity and speed of execution, respect for the natural esthetics of the patient, and cost, which makes it a widely used prosthetic solution.

Preparation techniques

The preparation must have the maximum extension possible in FPAD. It must also be compatible in terms of esthetics and must preserve the periodontal tissues. The greater the useable surface of enamel for adhesion of the cement, the greater the retention; the inclusion of more than 180 degrees of the circumference of the supporting teeth guarantees good stability.

The ideal condition is when the supporting tooth is undamaged and the preparation is limited to the enamel.[171] If the supporting tooth is damaged, all of the possible preexistent fillings must be replaced with new composite restorations. The preparation margins must always be supragingival to allow for an efficient adhesion and to facilitate oral hygiene.

Proximal grooves and occlusal rests are able to effectively oppose the masticatory load because they distribute the forces vertically on the supporting teeth, increasing retention, stability, and resistance of the prosthesis.[167] For didactic simplicity

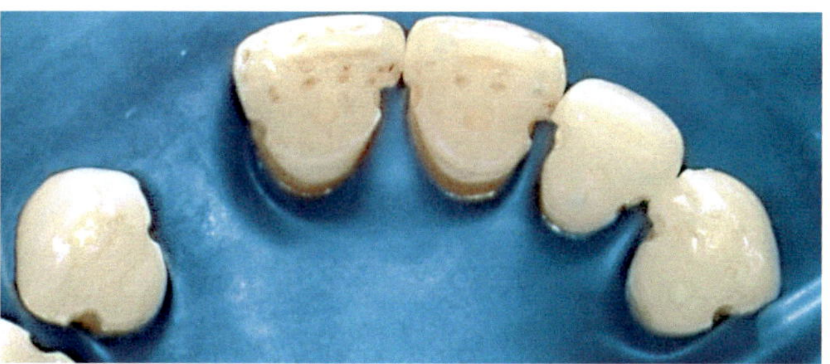

Fig 13-176 Occlusal view of the preparation of FPAD from the maxillary right canine to the central incisor. Treatment with a coloring agent shows the salient points clearly.

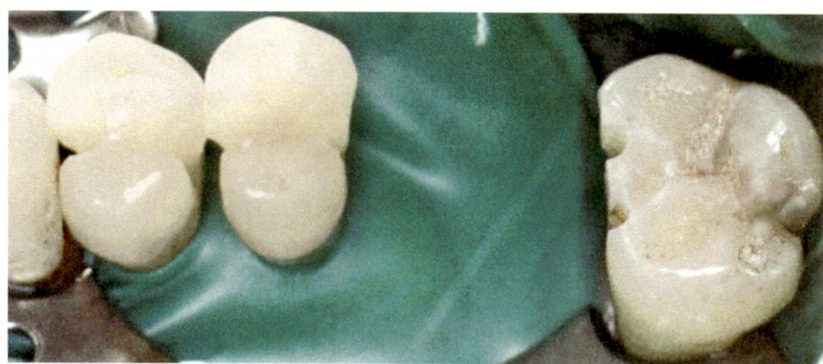

Fig 13-177 Occlusal view of the preparations for an FPAD for maxillary first premolar to second molar. Two parallel grooves on the second molar provide adequate retention.

Fig 13-178 *(a)* Parallelometer: The articulating arms control the movement of the drill to maintain the parallel position of the bur. *(b)* The drill tip is placed on the cast of the impression to ensure parallel planes. *(c)* The support is anchored on the opposing arch while a guide groove is made on the abutment tooth.

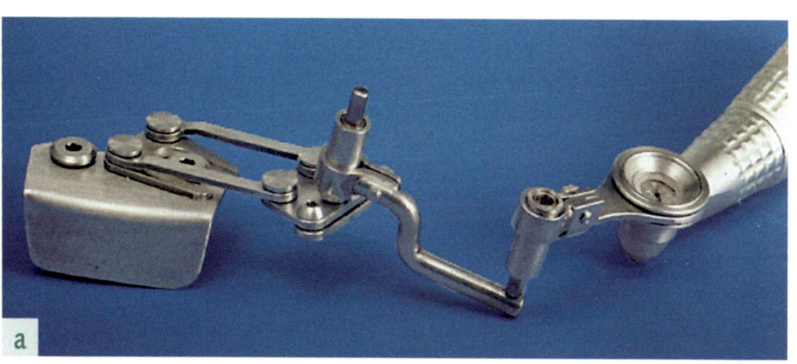

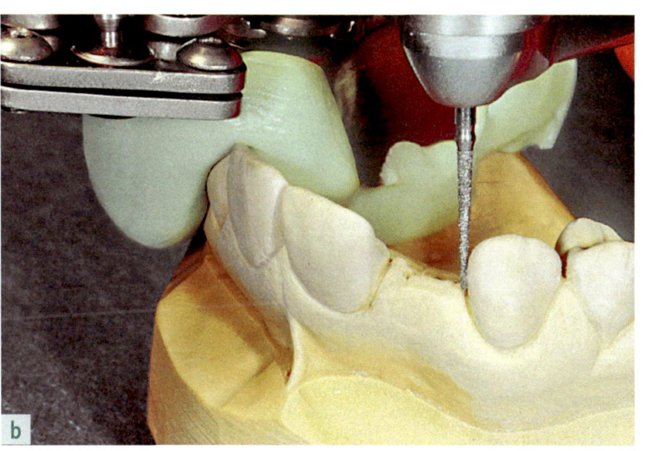

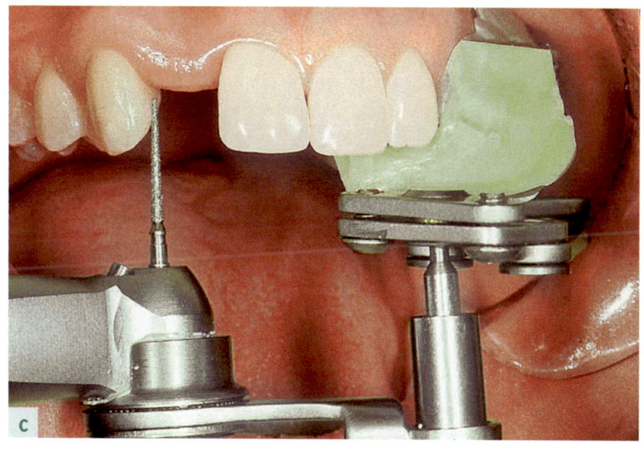

it is useful to subdivide the preparations for FPAD into two types[172,173]: *(1)* preparation for anterior teeth (incisors and canines) (Fig 13-176) and *(2)* preparation of posterior teeth (premolars and molars) (Fig 13-177).

The first phase, which is common to both types of preparation, consists of establishing the insertion axis, which must be kept constant during the process. Preparation must be carried out freehand with the help of an intraoral and extraoral parallelometer. This instrument is indispensable if the teeth to be prepared are both numerous and distributed over all the arch.

The intraoral parallelometer (Parallel-A-Prep, Dentatus) used for the preparation of an FPAD with short extension[174] is made up of an occlusal rest linked to a guide for the handpiece (Fig 13-178). It must first be calibrated on the master cast. This measure allows the creation of parallel grooves in case of little involuntary movements of the patient but is usable only on reduced portions of the arch. The extraoral parallelometer or the oral parallel pantograph (Axidrive, Teknital), introduced more recently in clinical practice,[158] (Fig 13-179a) is made up of a support that is attached to the back of the clinician's chair and a pantograph equipped with a series of adapters for the connection of any commercial handpiece (Fig 13-179b).

The pantograph is attached to the main support, and the handpiece is connected only when the axial walls of the prepa-

223

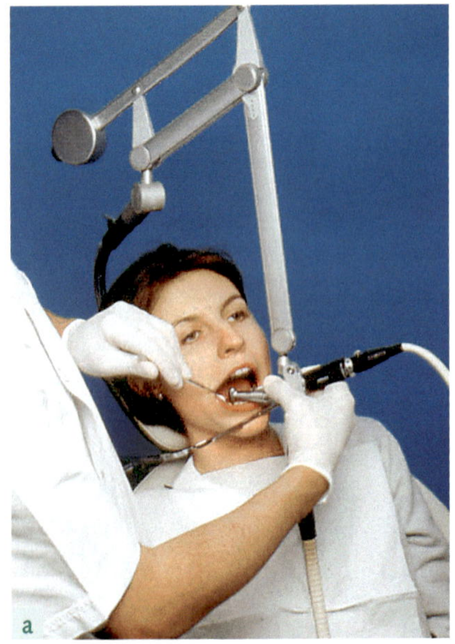

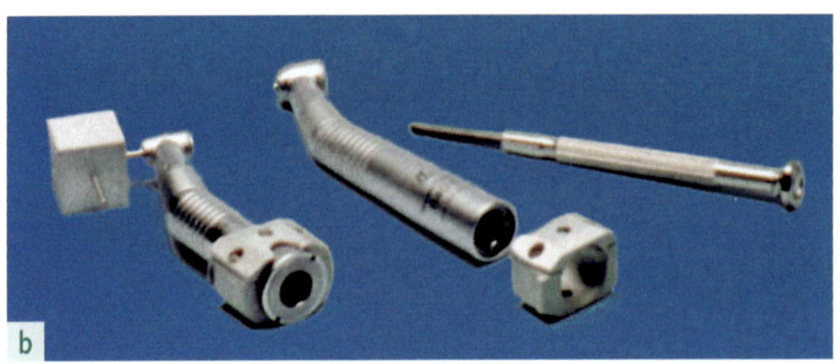

Fig 13-179 *(a)* Oral parallel pantograph ensures parallel planes. The posterior part of the device is anchored to the back of the dental chair. The pantograph allows the movement of the contra-angle tip to be connected in all operative fields, always orienting the axis of the bur as it has been set. The bar supporting the anterior part of the patient's mandible prevents accidental movements. *(b)* An extraoral pantograph for parallelizing the mechanism. A series of connectors allows the use of any drill or handpiece.

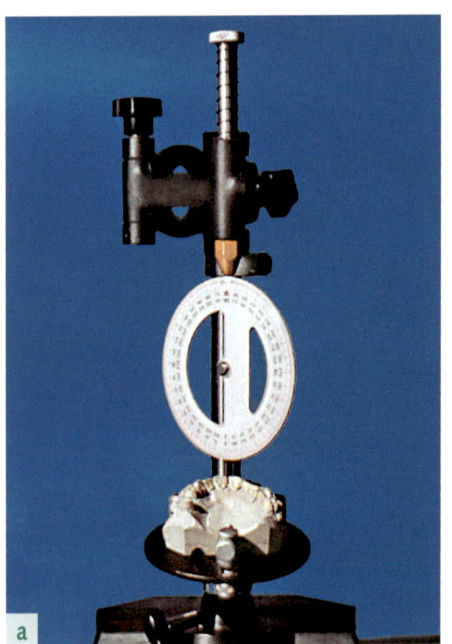

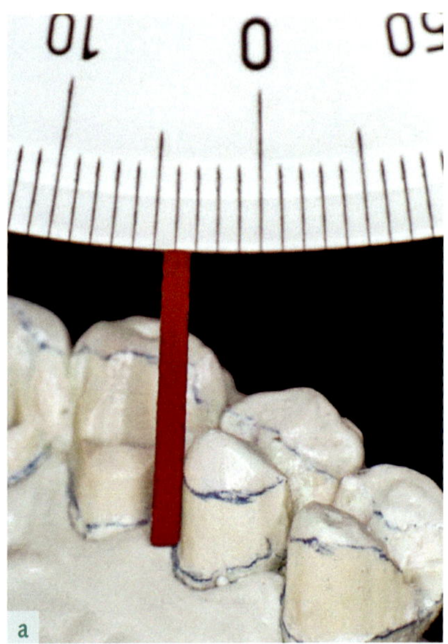

Fig 13-180 *(a)* Goniometer specially modified and mounted on a parallelometer. *(b)* The particularity of the measurements of the inclination of the planes and of the prepared grooves. By ensuring parallel planes, the results will be very close to the optimal tapering values, even in cases with a number of preparations.

ration are prepared. Adjustments are made to align the axis of the bur with the predetermined axis of insertion. Then the patient's head is stabilized by means of a chin bar, and the drilling is completed.

The bur is guided and always kept parallel to the preset axis. By using a bur with standard tapering of ± 3 degrees, uniform tapering is conferred on the preparation, as verified on the master cast through a goniometer attached to the parallelometer (Fig 13-180).

Preparation of incisors and canines

Preparation extends to all palatal or lingual surfaces of the tooth and also slightly on the proximal surfaces (Fig 13-181). The cervical margins are placed at least 1 mm from the gingiva to allow the application of rubber dam during the cementation phase and to avoid the periodontal tissues.

The incisal margins extend to 1 mm from the incisal edge of the tooth. The extension is reduced for very thin teeth to prevent the metal from showing through, or increased up to the incisal margin (distal or canine) in the less visible areas for greater occlusal support.

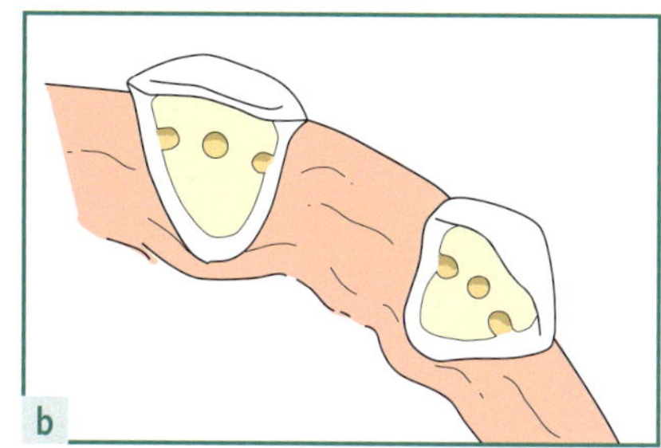

Fig 13-181 *(a)* The palatal design of the preparation for the maxillary incisors and canines. *(b)* The occlusal view of the preparation of the maxillary incisors and canines.

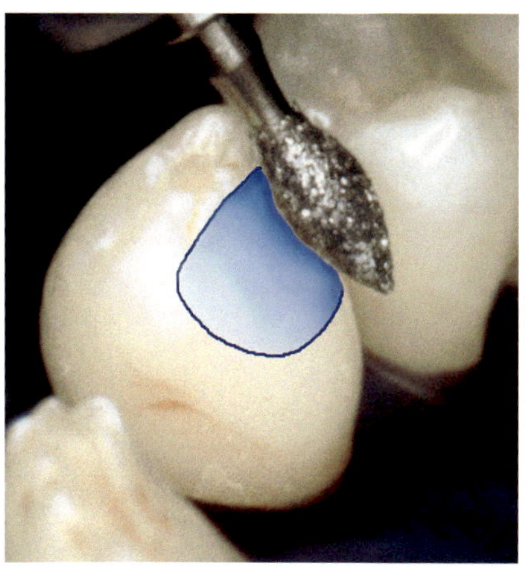

Fig 13-182 Lingual or palatal reduction of a maxillary canine. This reduction must be deep enough to guarantee sufficient space for the thin metal layer on the load surface.

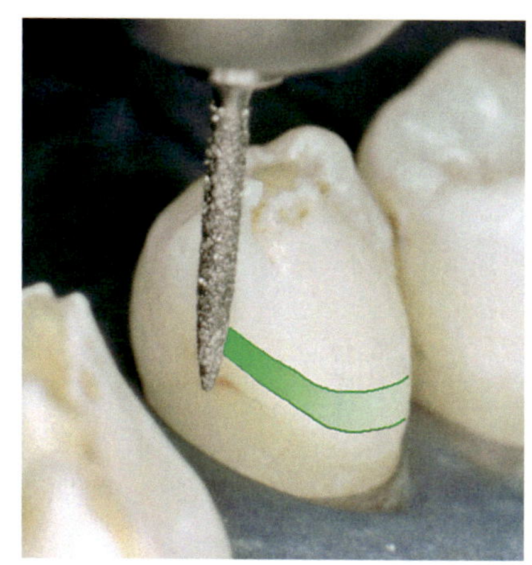

Fig 13-183 Axial reduction of a maxillary canine.

The proximal margins extend up to the contact area with the adjacent tooth, leaving sufficient access for adequate hygiene.

On every proximal surface, a groove is prepared parallel to the insertion axis. The proximal surfaces, opposing one another, are the components of the preparation most responsible for its stability. The stability is at its maximum if the contact is above 180 degrees.

In the case of the incisors, a satisfactory contact must be obtained by "intruding" in a labial sense for esthetic reasons, in an area of little dimension. Sometimes a compromise must be accepted between maximum stability and an acceptable esthetic result.

In the same portion of the lingual or palatal surface, at the cingulum, a support must be prepared that increases stability of the prosthesis and makes the positioning of the framework during cementation easier.

Preparation phases

Lingual or palatal reduction

This phase aims at preparing the incisal portion of the lingual or palatal surface of the tooth. The depth of the preparation, especially for the maxillary teeth, must create a space at least 1 mm in maximum intercuspidation and during lateral and protrusive movements. The following procedure is performed with a football-shaped diamond bur and can be done freehand (Fig 13-182). The wider undercuts on the abutments must be eliminated, as well as those caused by mild rotations or malposition of the teeth, which would excessively constrict in the insertion axis.

Axial preparation

A mildly tapered diamond bur with a round tip is mounted on a handpiece and attached to the extraoral parallelometer (Fig 13-183).

The preparation of all abutments of the same FPD must have the same insertion axis; it is therefore convenient to do the entire preparation in the same sitting. The preparation margins must have a knife edge. The transition from untouched enamel and the prepared enamel must be clear and highly visible in order to be reproduced on the master cast.

Execution of proximal grooves and cingulum rest

A mildly tapered diamond bur with a flat tip is used. Generally, two grooves are prepared, one mesial and one distal, with a diameter of about 1 mm, keeping the bur parallel to the insertion axis. The grooves are made 0.5 mm from the labial margin of the prepared surface, and they should be placed 0.5 to 1.0 mm from the cervical preparation margin (Fig 13-184).

It is important that the angle between the groove and the adjacent axial wall remains clear and well defined to guarantee

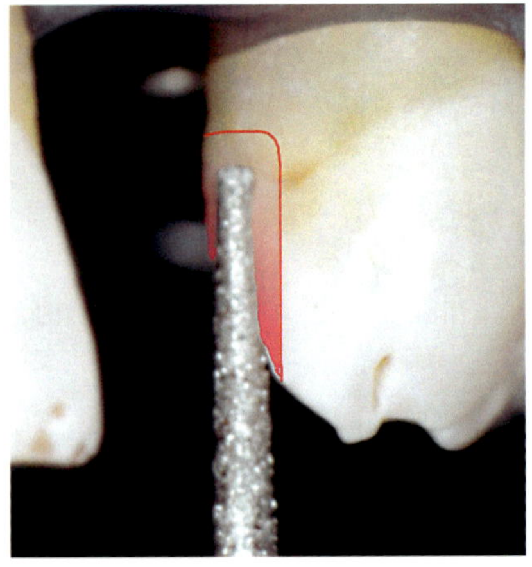

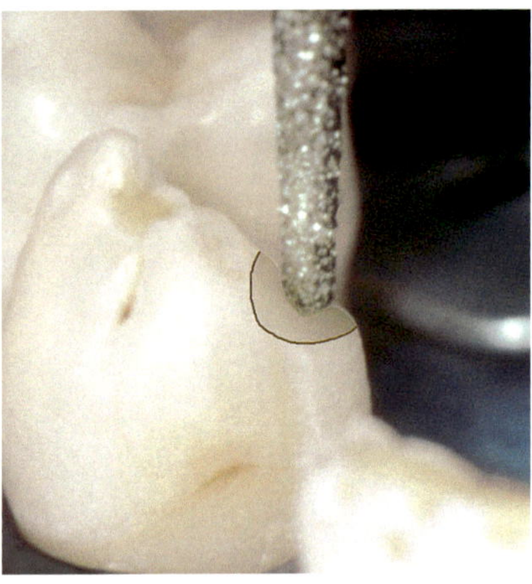

Fig 13-184 Preparation of a groove on a maxillary canine. A different type of bur is used but with the same orientation.

Fig 13-185 Preparation in a maxillary canine of the occlusal support that guarantees stablilization of the occlusal vertical load.

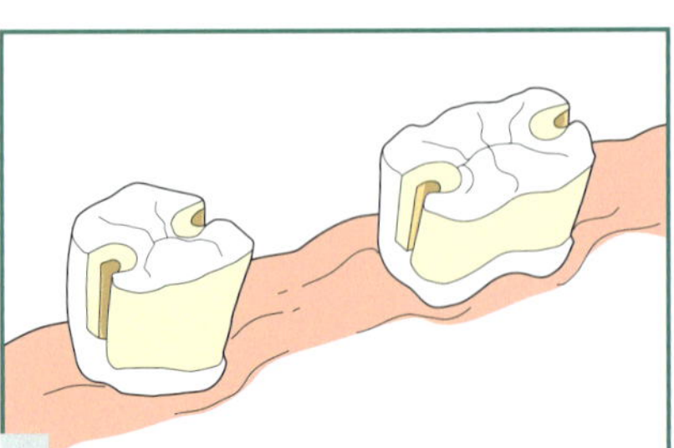

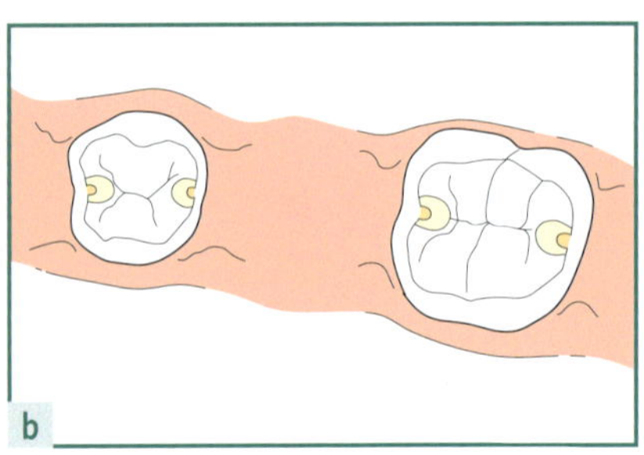

Fig 13-186 (a) Palatal view of the preparation design for mandibular premolars and molars. (b) Occlusal view of the preparation design for mandibular posterior teeth.

maximum stabilization and avoid sideways forces, which can cause displacement of the metal framework.

With a diamond bur of the same shape but with a greater diameter than that used for the grooves, a notch is created, about 1 mm in diameter, 0.5 mm in depth, with an axis parallel to that of insertion (Fig 13-185), and placed in the same portion of the lingual or palatal surface. This procedure serves to improve the distribution of the occlusal load.[175]

Preparation of premolars and molars

The preparation for premolars and molars includes almost the entire palatal or lingual surfaces of the tooth and partially covers the proximal and occlusal surfaces at the rests.

The anatomy of these teeth makes it simpler to obtain a contact greater than 180 degrees, increasing the retention and stability of the prosthesis.[176] The occlusal rests, placed on the marginal crests, are able to effectively oppose the vertical forces exerted on the framework during function (Fig 13-186).

Phases of preparation

Axial preparation

A mildly tapered diamond bur with a round tip is installed on a handpiece and connected to the extraoral parallelometer. If the teeth are not parallel to each other, the insertion axis is determined by following the inclination of the tooth with reduced dimensions.[177]

Axial reduction of the palatal or lingual surface is done, keeping within the thickness of the enamel, with a depth of 1.0 to 1.5 mm measured at the height of contour of the tooth (Fig 13-187).

The edges of the preparation margins must be knife edged and placed about 1 mm from the gingival margin. To increase the resistance of the framework, given the reduced depth of the preparation, an increase in the thickness of the palatal or lingual portion far from the margins is necessary, creating a mild overcontour (Fig 13-188).

Using a very thin flame-shaped diamond bur, the axial preparation is extended to the mesial and distal surfaces of the tooth until the areas of contact with the adjacent tooth are passed, to obtain a contact of more than 180 degrees.

Implementation of the proximal grooves

With a mildly tapered diamond bur with a flat tip (ISO N° 806 314 171524012), two grooves are prepared, one mesial and one distal, with a diameter of about 1 mm, positioned 0.5 to 1.0 mm from the cervical margin of the preparation (Fig 13-189).

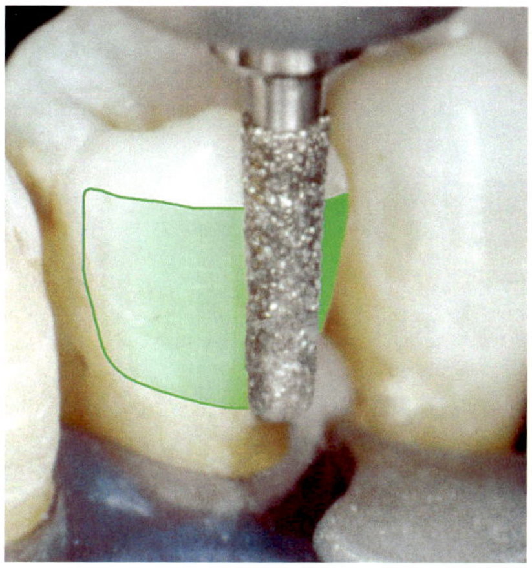

Fig 13-187 Axial reduction of a maxillary premolar that must have the same orientation as the other abutments.

Fig 13-188 Part of the preparation to create space for the metal substructure to increase the thickness with a slight addition in the modeling phase. This procedure confers greater mechanical resistance.

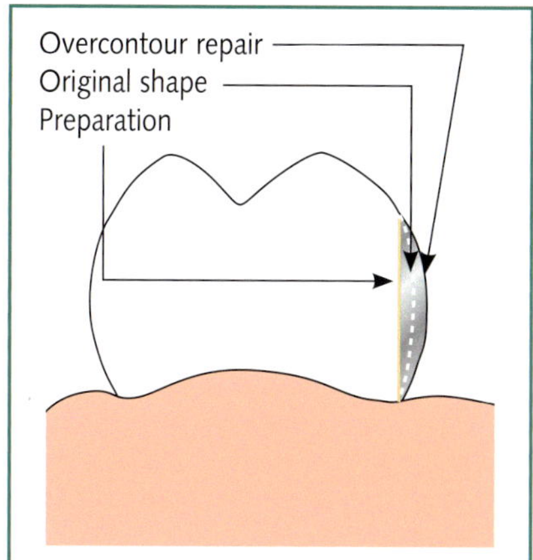

Fig 13-189 Preparation of a groove on a maxillary premolar.

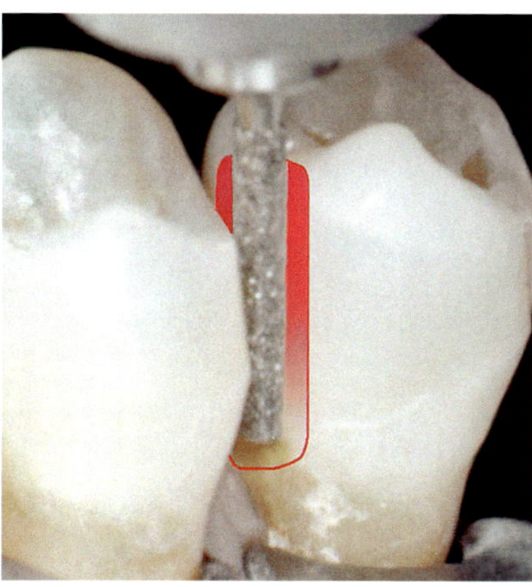

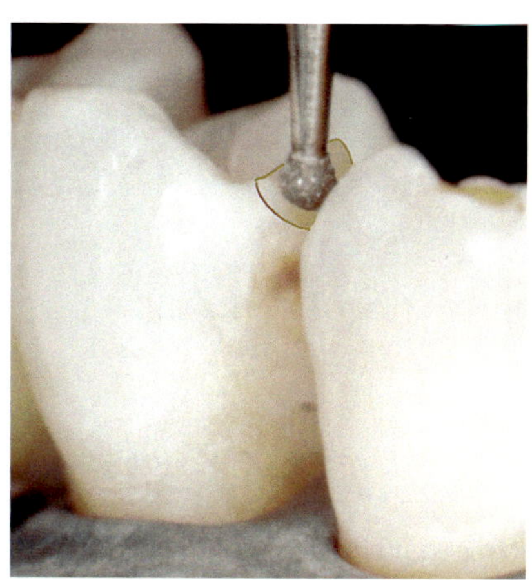

Fig 13-190 Preparation on a maxillary premolar with occlusal morphology that provides optimal support for the occlusal load.

Implementation of the occlusal rests

For the implementation of the occlusal rests, a round diamond bur is used. It is half sunk into the marginal crest at the proximal limit of the preparation (Fig 13-190).

Finishing the preparation

Once the preparation is finished, it is recommended that a check-up be done with the pantograph without activating the handpiece to verify that all grooves are parallel. This checkup is especially important in the case of multiple abutments, and if necessary, corrections should be made. To polish, rotate the bur at low speed while carefully avoiding the grooves (Fig 13-191).

Impression technique

Although the impression technique for adhesive prostheses requires similar materials as conventional fixed prostheses, certain aspects need special consideration. Given that the preparation for this procedure is usually supragingival, retraction techniques are not necessary. The impression tray must be fabricated in acrylic resin, allow for 2 to 3 mm of impression material, have three occlusal rests for correct positioning, and be varnished with a suitable adhesive to avoid detachment of the material.

The impression material must not be subjected to distortion during the removal of the impression itself. If necessary, a sheet of soft wax can be applied to the labial and buccal part of the region concerned (Fig 13-192). The impression tray must not have a buccal flange. The material that flows into the interdental space from the lingual or palatal side should not come in contact with that from the buccal side (Fig 13-193). The removal should be uneventful to ensure optimal interproximal morphology (Fig 13-194).

For an orthodontic apparatus fixed labially, wax prevents the material from incorporating it or else it would be impossible to remove the impression without damaging it. A "safety" impression tray made up of two portions screwed together could be used and then disassembled if difficulties arose during removal.

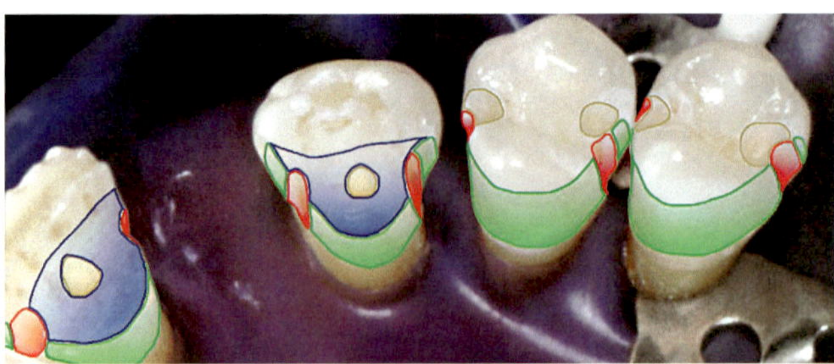

Fig 13-191 Occlusopalatal view of the completed preparations:. occlusal reduction *(blue)*; axial reduction *(green)*; parallel retention grooves *(red)*; and occusal supports *(brown)*.

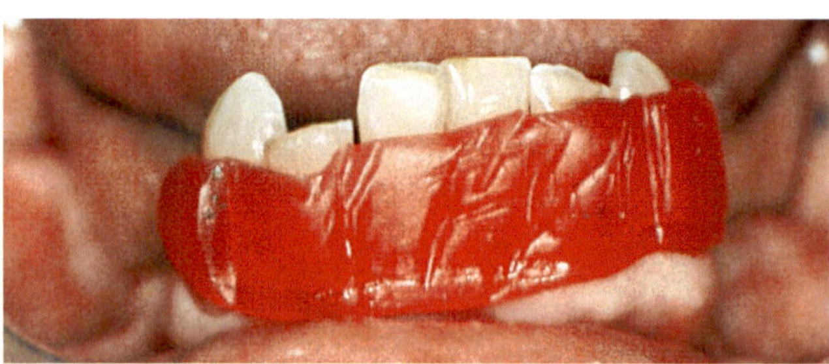

Fig 13-192 Preparation of anterior dentition before impression. A layer of soft wax placed labially maintains the correct interdental space so that the impression material records the lingual and palatal morphologiy without risking stress during removal.

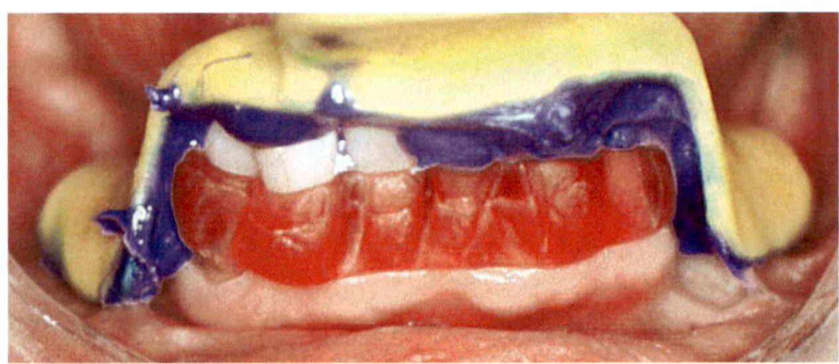

Fig 13-193 Taking the impression. The labial part of the custom tray is shortened to permit the material to flow without impeding the interdental spaces.

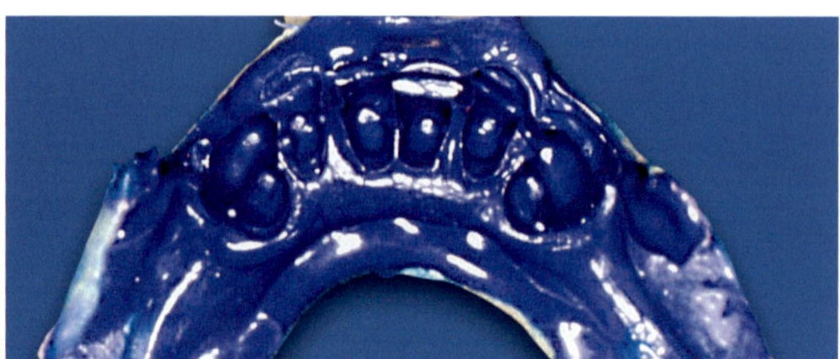

Fig 13-194 A correctly made impression.The material does not reach the labial part but faithfully reproduces the morphology of the prepared surface.

This impression technique is not always able to correctly record the anatomy of the edentulous spaces and buccal surfaces of the abutment teeth. It is therefore advisable to take a follow-up impression after the trial phase of the metal framework.

In the cases involving dental teeth with increased mobility, it is important before preparation and impression to splint them togeher at the interdental points with a drop of composite resin. The integrity of the block is verified beforehand so that stability can be guaranteed.

For a correct recording of the finer details of the preparation, grooves, and rests, an elastomer syringe with a very fine tip is used to avoid the formation of bubbles. The evaluation of the impression includes correct adhesion of the material to the impression tray, integrity of the interdental septi, absence of bubbles, and the correct recording of grooves.

Laboratory procedures

There are two different systems for constructing FPADs in the laboratory. Both use the lost wax casting technique. In the first system, recommended for a prosthesis with reduced extension

(up to three or four teeth), the framework is modeled, attached to the sprue former, removed, and coated. In the second system, recommended for prostheses with greater extension, the framework is cast directly using refractory material obtained through duplication of the master cast. In the first case, the master cast is developed with very hard plaster; on the prepared parts, a thin layer of spacing varnish is applied up to 1 mm from the margin. Thickness can slightly increase at the net angles where excessive attrition could more easily occur.

The wax cast is critical and must be constructed with care. Wax for modeling and auto- and light-curing acrylic resin are used. The two components are united to obtain a precise framework that does not deform or fracture during removal from the cast and during the coating procedure (Fig 13-195).

Preventive modeling of the isolated grooves (Fig 13-196), entailing their removal, repositioning, and the modeling of the rest of the framework, may prevent the wax cast from fracturing at the grooves.

The technique of the refractory cast can only use a wax cast (Fig 13-197). The disadvantage of this procedure is that the refractory cast must be duplicated from the master cast or be cast for a second time from the precision impression. The cast

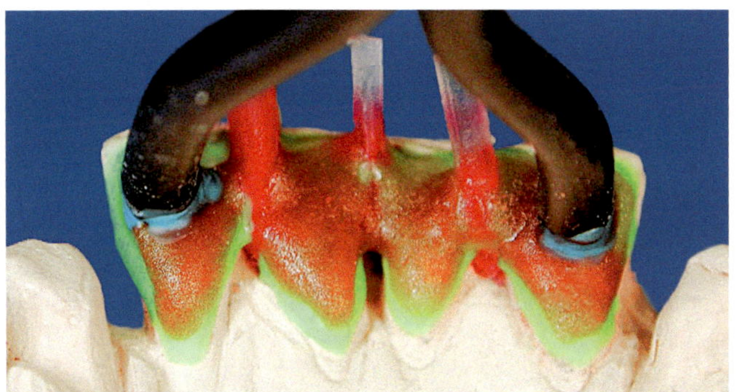

Fig 13-195 Cast of resin-bonded prosthesis with wax and autopolymerizing resin that provides adequate resistance to the structure by means of fused pins.

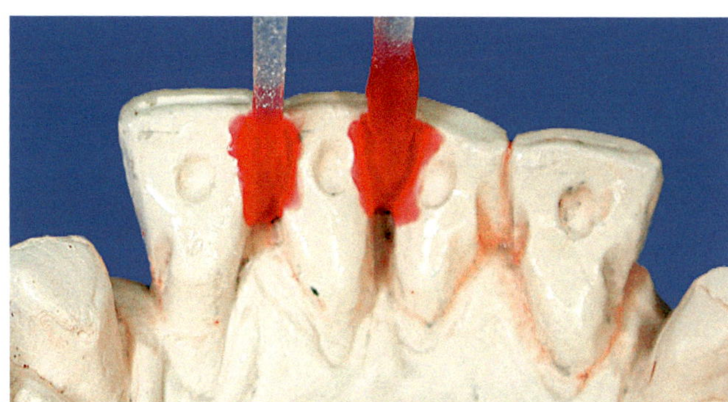

Fig 13-196 For easy removal of the cast without breaking the wax, the grooves are modeled first, removed one by one, repositioned in their seating, and then united with the rest of the model.

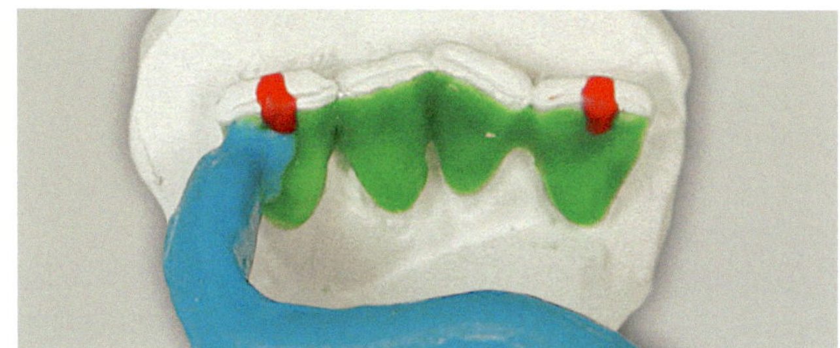

Fig 13-197 The metal framework can also be modeled in wax but only on a duplicate of the master model in refractory material, which can then be covered for the fusion.

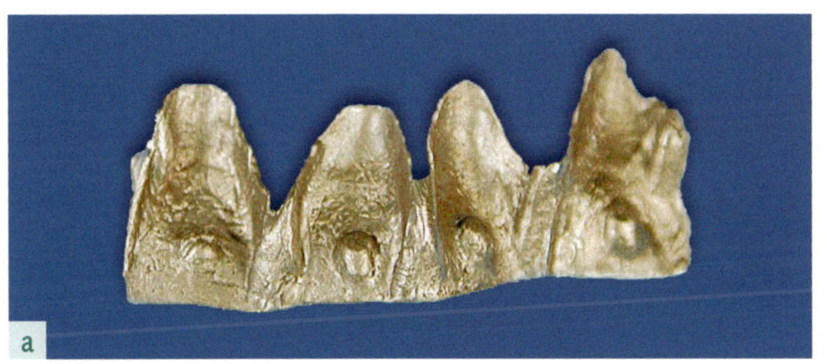

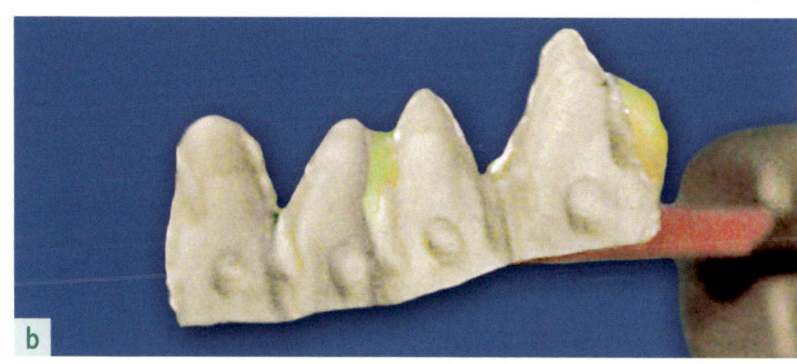

Fig 13-198 (a) The metal framework is cleaned and tried in situ. (b) After electrolytic treatment with a coloring agent, the metal frameworkhas a characteristic opaque look due to the superficial microretention.

metal framework must then be adapted to the master cast, and this indirect process can lead to imprecision. The technique should therefore be limited to extended frameworks, whose wax cast would be difficult to remove from the master cast.

The surface treatment of electrolytic etching[178] yields excellent results in terms of adhesion and allows the prosthodontist to correct the framework before treatment without altering the quality of surface conditioning (Fig 13-198). If it is not possible to effect electrolytic etching or it is considered too complicated,[179] a chemical etching technique can be used instead, with similar results.[162] The perforated framework technique is not recommended because it is less retentive,[180,181] although one study[182] observed the same survival rate of perforated FPDs and etched FPDs when preparation of the grooves was not done.

The sand-bath technique can easily pollute the metal,[183] and using salt crystals in the cast does not allow for modifications, as with the spheric macroretentions technique,[184] which also requires excessive thickness of the framework.

The metals used are predominantly nonnoble alloys such as nickel-chromium-cobalt or cobalt-chromium to reduce the risk of metal sensitivity.[185] These alloys combine the qualities of lightness, rigidity, and precision with the possibility of being etched electrolytically. This type of alloy does not seem to suffer from the thermic treatment necessary for ceramics.[186,187] Recently, however, there has been a tendency to use composite materials so that repairs can easily be made.

The try-in of the framework is an opportunity to check its precision (Fig 13-199). Adaptation, which must be optimal, is

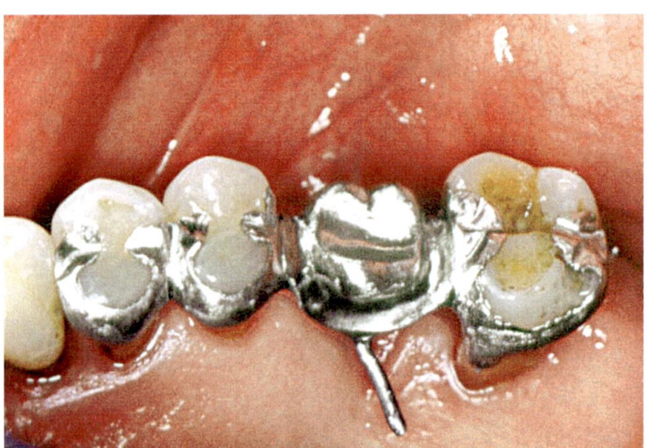

Fig 13-199 Try-in of the metal framework to check the fitting.

Fig 13-200 Definitive prosthesis, polished and treated with a coloring agent.

verified with a silicone pressure indicator. Small modifications of the metal can be made at this point, and each metal groove can be checked for precise lodging of the prepared tooth.

The marginal adaptation of the framework should have no excessive parts, overcontours, occlusal precontacts, or interferences. Electrolytic etching can then be performed, which makes the inner surface retentive (Fig 13-200).

Cementation

There are many cements recommended for definitive fixing of the prosthesis, and their characteristics have been carefully evaluated by numerous authors. Hardness and adhesion to enamel, dentin, composite material, amalgams, and metal pretreated with different modalities have been taken into consideration. The best technique uses rubber dam, etching of enamel and dentin, and electrolytic etching of metal.

Very often, preparation for FPADs intrudes on the dentin because of the retaining grooves. Enamel/dentin adhesives can be used together with composite cements. The latest adhesive systems, whether one- or two-component systems, all involve acid etching of the dentin. The acid removes the smear layer and opens the dentinal tubules, which become partially occupied by the fluid resin and form the hybrid layer. This dentin and resin layer has superior mechanical characteristics compared with those of the single materials that make it up, giving the bond a resistance comparable to that obtained with resin and etched enamel. The two-component enamel/dentin adhesive system (All-Bond 2, Bisco Dental Products) is broadly applicable and has been used together with a two-component self-curing resin cement (C and B cement, Bisco Dental Products).

A fixed orthodontic apparatus can make the application of rubber dam difficult. In this case it is necessary to remove the

metal wire beforehand. If there is an increase in mobility of the abutments, it is necessary to reconstruct the arch temporarily without excessively tightening the ligature so as to avoid creating incongruities with respect to the previous position.

In the cementation seating, the FPD must only be handled with metal instruments to avoid contamination of the etched framework.

After applying rubber dam and scrupulously cleaning the prepared surfaces of the teeth, the cementing process begins, progressing through the following phases:

1. Etching of the enamel
2. Rinsing and drying
3. Applying the enamel/dentin adhesive
4. Applying the resinous cement on the pretreated surface of the metal framework
5. Inserting the FPD in the oral cavity
6. Keeping the FPD in position
7. Polymerization

There are numerous adhesive systems and resinous cements available. If the best results are to be obtained, the instructions for each one must be followed meticulously.

The cement must be opaque to mask the metal of the framework, which could otherwise show through the enamel of the supporting teeth. Another way of rectifying this inconvenience could be with golding,[188] which does not seem to significantly compromise the retention of the etched metal surfaces.

Immediately after the FPD has been positioned in the oral cavity, keeping it firmly in position, the excess cement is removed with a little brush. A layer of glycerine gel is then applied to all the margins to isolate the cement from contact with oxygen, which would partially inhibit polymerization. Once the hardening is completed, sharp cutting instruments are

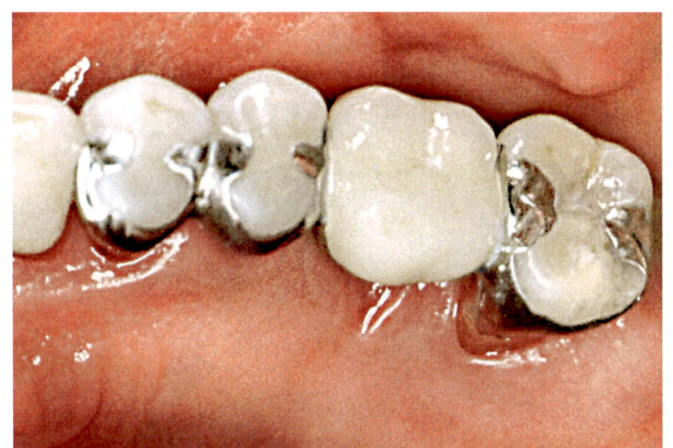

Fig 13-201 Definitive FPD in place from the maxillary left first premolar to the second molar, with a restoration of the left first molar.

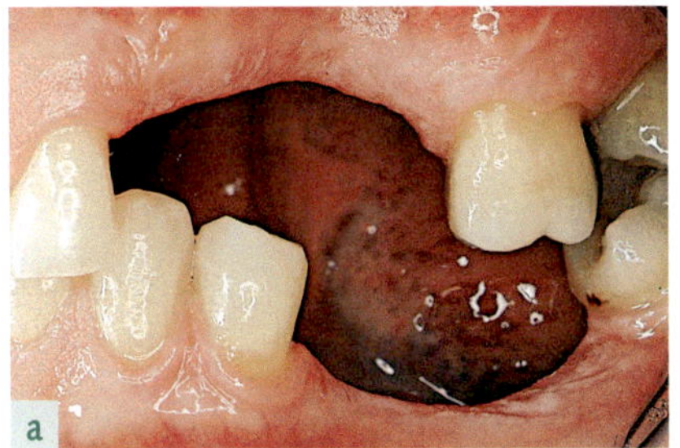
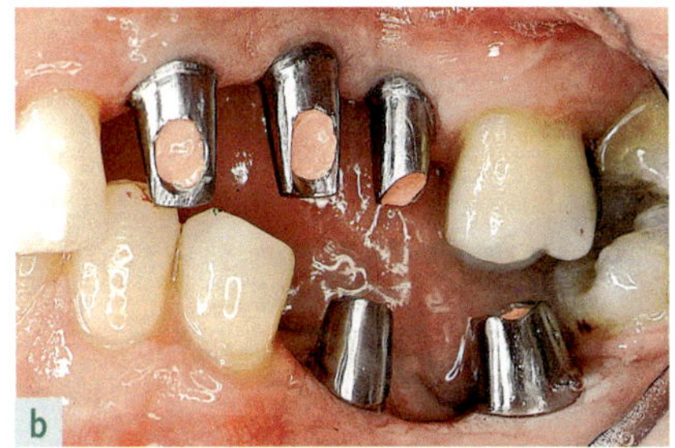
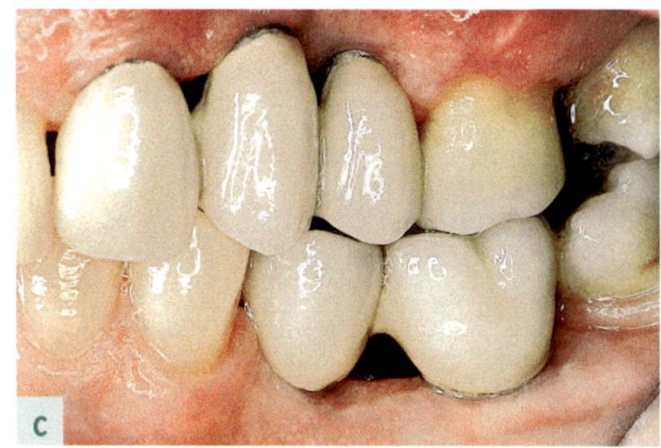

Fig 13-202 *(a)* Interposed edentulous gaps. *(b)* Placement of osseointegrated implants. *(c)* Definitive FPD.

used to remove residues and excess cement. Rubber dam can then be removed (Fig 13-201).

Recementation, if necessary, must be preceded by the complete removal of the FPD, taking care to not deform it,[189] and careful removal of all cement residue on the supporting teeth.

The framework is tried in the mouth again to verify that there have not been any deformations or loss of retention and, only if these conditions are satisfied, can reconditioning and recementation of the old FPD be done. Otherwise, a new FPD must be prepared.[190] Failure of a restoration with an FPD allows an almost complete preservation of preexistent tissues and does not usually compromise the possibility of switching to a conventional prosthesis at a later point.

Implant-Supported FPDs

Osseointegration offers a rehabilitation strategy for edentulous spaces adjacent to natural teeth, especially wide gaps for which RPDs or FPDs of uncertain prognosis were used. IS-FPD is a permanent solution to edentulism (Fig 13-202).

As reported in cases of distal extension edentulism, the success rate of IS-FPD is encouraging. Retrospective and prospective clinical studies report that the success rate of the implants is between 92% and 99% for the mandible and between 87% and 96% for the maxilla. The success rate for the prosthesis is between 94% and 100% for the mandible and between 92% and 99% for the maxilla.[191–200]

The surgical and prosthetic considerations that guide rehabilitation of the extended edentulous gap adjacent to natural teeth are the same as for distal extension edentulism. Of course, esthetic considerations are mainly applied to anterior rehabilitation (Fig 13-203).

In the case of a single missing tooth, and in the presence of sound adjacent teeth, IS-FPD is the number one choice of treatment because it preserves the natural, healthy dentition (Fig 13-204). Clinical studies corroborate the effectiveness of this solution.[201–203] Henry and colleagues[203] reported a cumulative success rate of 96.6% in the maxilla and 100% in the mandible in a 5-year multicenter prospective study on 107 implants. A systematic revision of the meta-analysis, carried out by Lindh and colleagues,[204] who evaluated retrospective and prospective

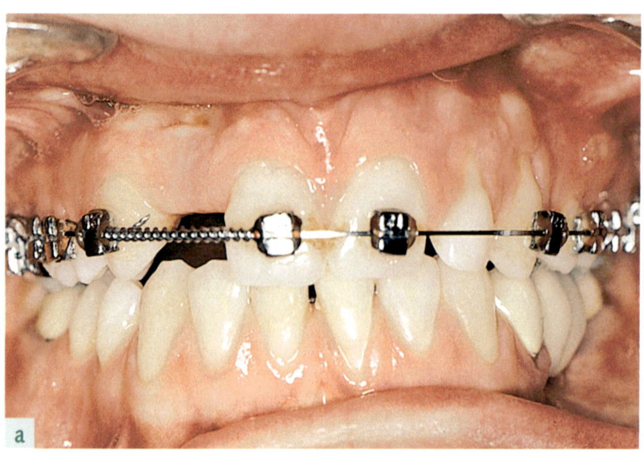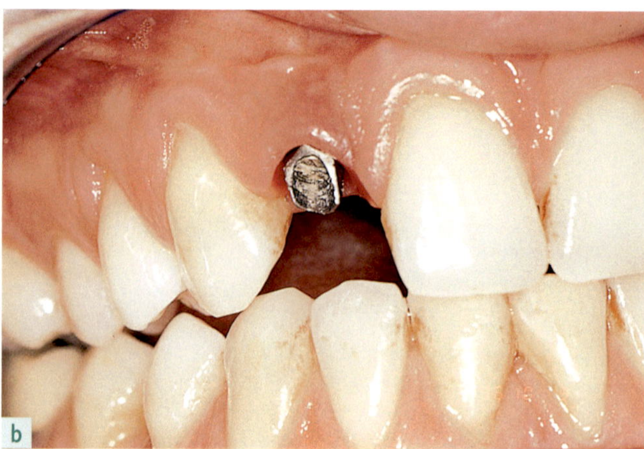

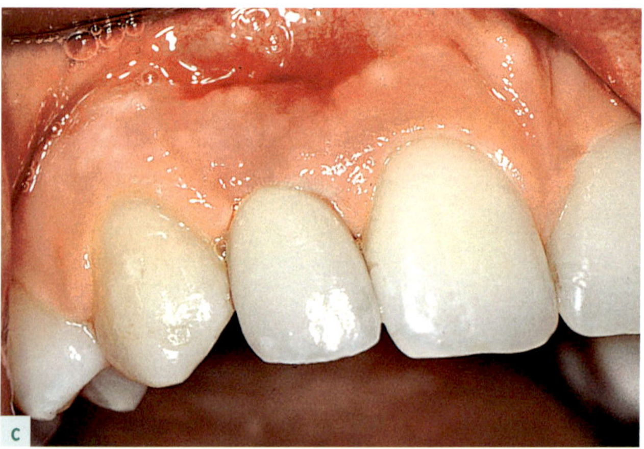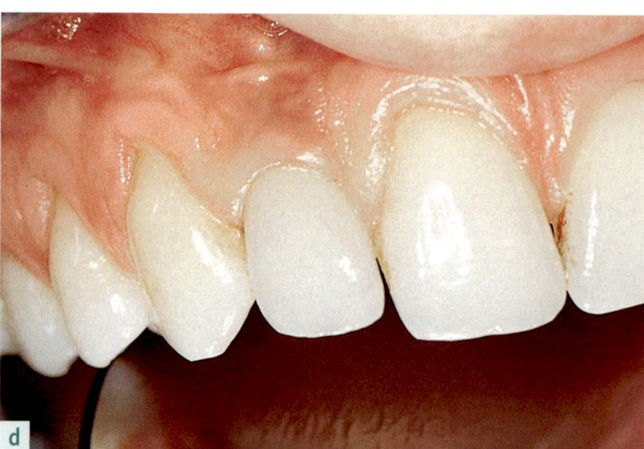

Fig 13-203 Rehabilitation of an anterior edentulous gap requiring a multidisciplinary approach to satisfy the esthetic demands. *(a)* This case of agenesis of a maxillary lateral incisor has been resolved with orthodontic treatment. *(b)* Placement of an osseointegrated implant and *(c)* a metal-ceramic crown. *(d)* Follow-up after 3 years.

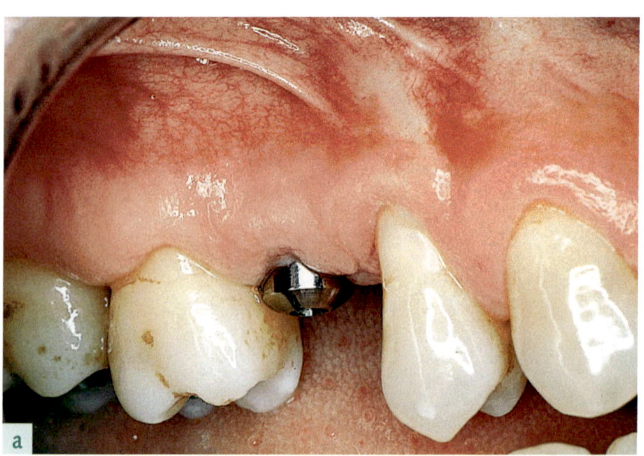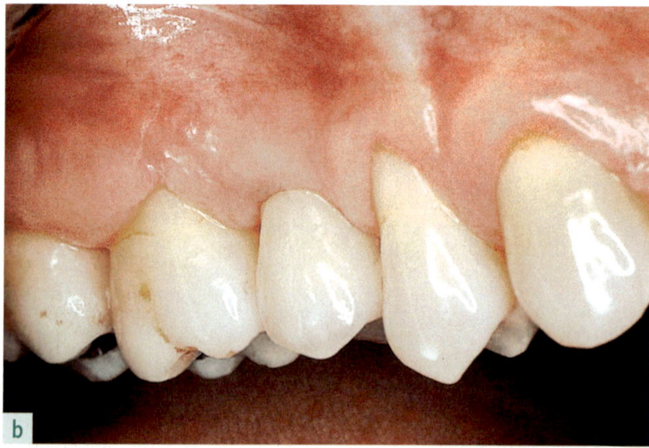

Fig 13-204 Restoration of a maxillary second premolar with a metal-ceramic crown on a single implant. Such a solution permits preserving adjacent teeth.

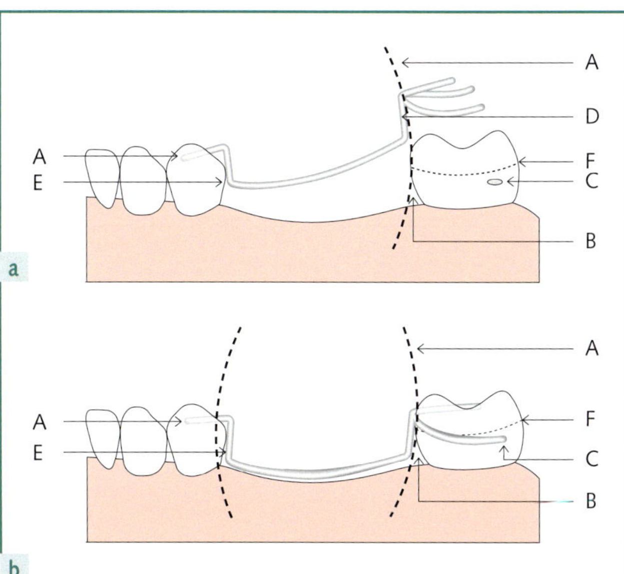

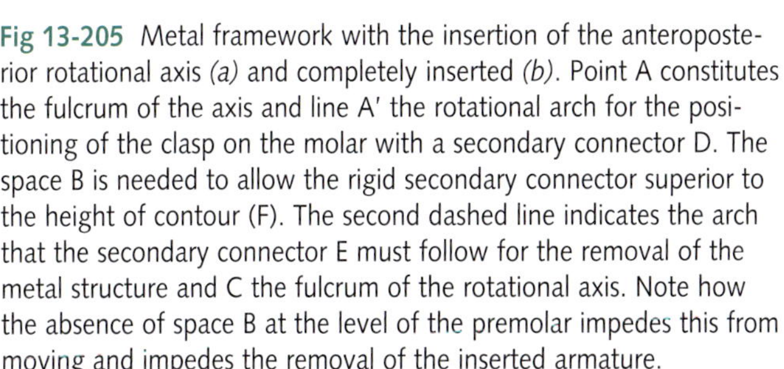

Fig 13-205 Metal framework with the insertion of the anteroposterior rotational axis *(a)* and completely inserted *(b)*. Point A constitutes the fulcrum of the axis and line A′ the rotational arch for the positioning of the clasp on the molar with a secondary connector D. The space B is needed to allow the rigid secondary connector superior to the height of contour (F). The second dashed line indicates the arch that the secondary connector E must follow for the removal of the metal structure and C the fulcrum of the rotational axis. Note how the absence of space B at the level of the premolar impedes this from moving and impedes the removal of the inserted armature.

studies lasting from 1 to 8 years, confirmed a success rate of 97.5% for single crowns supported by implants.

In more complicated cases, clinical experience proves important for obtaining the same results as those reported in the literature.[205] In the case of a single tooth, however, the success rate between inexperienced clinicians and experts is similar.[206]

Removable Partial Denture

Indications

The RPD is recommended in all the situations in which it is not possible to use the FPD or FPAD, including:

- Posterior endentulous gaps adjacent to natural teeth that involve more than two teeth.
- Anterior endentulous gaps that involve more than four incisors, or curved regions of the arch (canine and one or two adjacent teeth).
- Insufficient height of the clinical crown of the supporting teeth.
- Excessive loss of bone at the edentulous zone caused by trauma, or serious periodontal maladaptation to the loss of teeth. In these cases the intermediate teeth of the fixed prosthesis are not sufficient to sustain the lips and cheeks.

When planning the RPD, consideration should be given to the following:

- The biomechanical behavior of the tooth-supported RPD during mastication is analogous to that of the FPD. The distribution of the axial loads is the same; for the transverse loads, however, it is transmitted to the supporting teeth through cross-arch stabilization.
- Hygiene can be easily maintained with RPD if the patient receives adequate instruction and motivation. It has been shown that the incidence of decay or periodontal damage in the residual teeth is no higher for patients with RPDs than for patients with FPDs.[207] The only contraindication for RPDs is the patient's nonacceptance of the restoration for psychologic reasons.
- RPDs are a reversible therapy that does not compromise the residual structures nor impede later rehabilitations with other types of prostheses.
- RPD is adaptable, with simple modifications, if later changes have to be made (for example, adding a tooth that has to be extracted later on) without remaking the entire prosthesis.
- Planning and creating the RPD for edentulous gaps that are adjacent to natural teeth follows the same basic principles as for distal extension situation.

RPDs and rotational path of insertion

In anterior edentulous gaps, RPD with a rotational path of insertion may be used for esthetic reasons. Even though this RPD does not use clasps in the anterior region, it is still stable and retentive (Fig 13-205).

The technique of the rotational path of insertion has been described by many authors over the years,[209–215] but its clinical

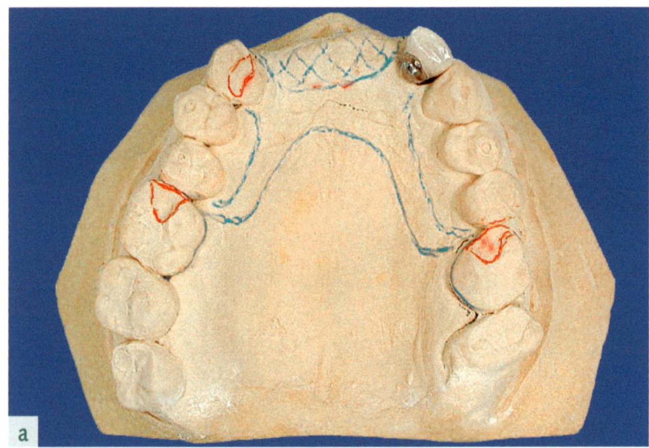

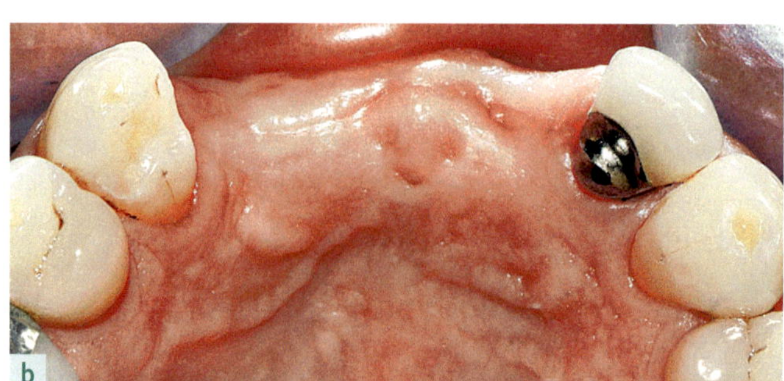

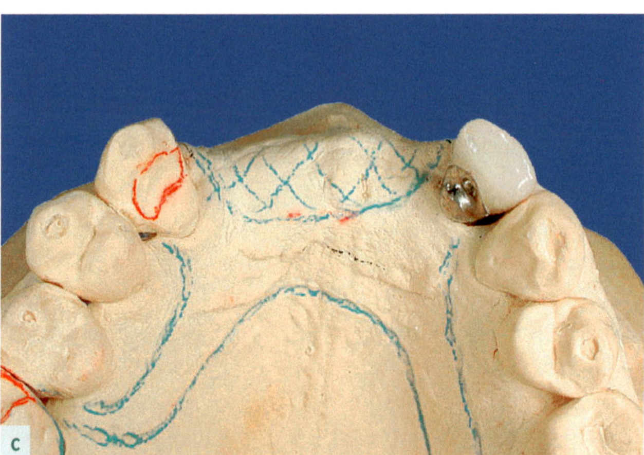

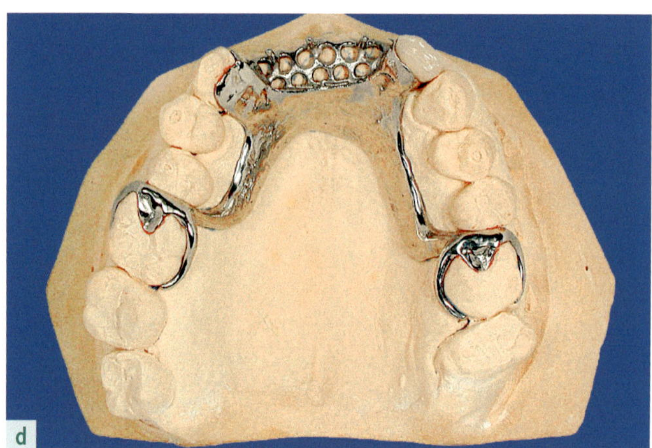

Fig 13-206 *(a)* Preparation of the metal-ceramic crown on the maxillary left lateral incisor and metal framework *(blue)* for an RPD on the master cast. The axis of the rotational insertion permits a rigid metal component (proximal plate) to be positioned in the undercut of the mesiolingual surface of the right canine and left lateral incisor. *(b)* Clinical view. *(c)* Detail of planned framework of the cast. *(d)* Completed framework on the master cast. *(e)* Try-in of the metal framework. *(f)* Clinical situation without RPD. *(g)* Definitive RPD in situ.

application has not been widely diffused.[216] The transfer of the constructive principles of this technique to its clinical practice requires the dentist and the prosthodontist to have specific knowledge, and calls for numerous trials on the cast and in the mouth. With the use of the axis of rotational insertion it is possible to eliminate the retention arm of some clasps with considerable advantages in terms of esthetics and stability (Fig 13-206). This method can be used with the best results in Kennedy Classes III and IV; it cannot be used it in Kennedy Class I, however.[217] The application of the rotational axis in free-extension RPD is described in Kennedy Class II mesial-occlusal-distal situations by Asher,[215] who shows its difficult clinical applicability. This method, in the presence of distal extension situations, does not offer advantages or esthetic improvement.

Conclusion

Anterior edentulous gaps adjacent to natural teeth must always be rehabilitated. Edentulous gaps in the posterior regions must be rehabilitated when they are recent (less than 1 year) or when they have induced a pathologic occlusion.

FPDs are recommended in the following situations:

- Strong esthetic and functional needs (in most young adult patients)
- Single- or two-tooth gap
- Favorable anatomic and functional conditions of the oral cavity from a biomechanical point of view

The materials that are most easily adapted to the construction of FPDs are gold alloy and ceramics.

Partial crown preparations for FPDs are only recommended for single-tooth gaps in the posterior regions, in subjects who

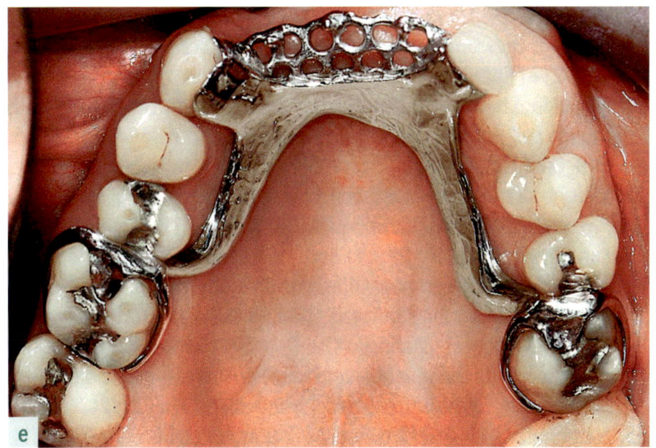

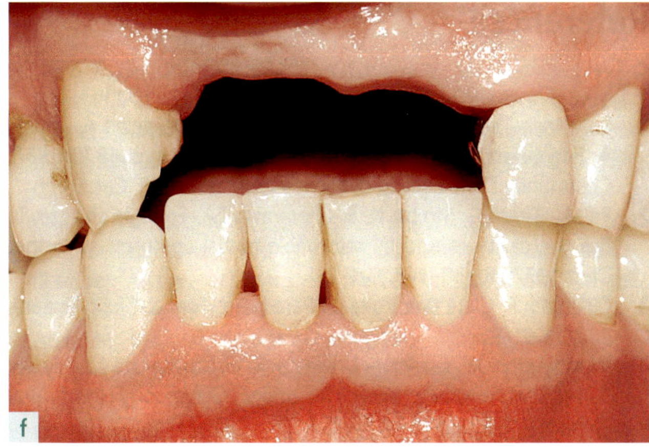

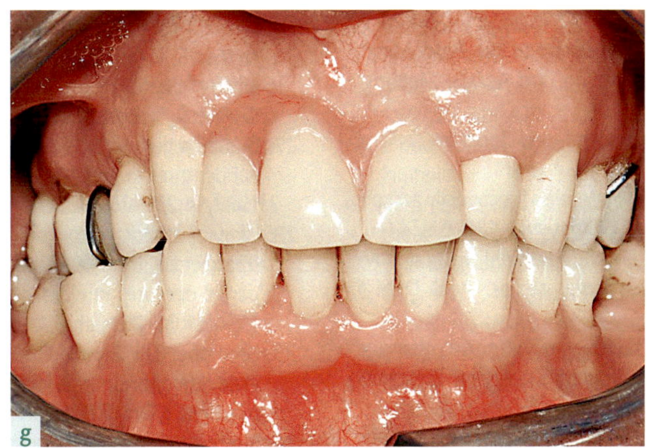

are not carioreceptive, and who do not have particular esthetic needs. In all other situations, complete crown preparations are recommended.

The preparation technique that uses the guide grooves is easy to carry out and is recommended for all types of FPD.

The 130-degree shoulder or the mixed preparation (net 90-degree shoulder buccally and 130-degree shoulder or 90-degree bevelled shoulder in the other regions), are the most adaptive margins for metal-ceramic FPDs.
Indications for the FPAD are:

■ Replacement of a reduced number of missing teeth
■ Anchorage to RPDs through precision attachments
■ Retention of teeth with diminished (or insufficient) periodontal support
■ Stabilization of the result of an orthodontic treatment

The ideal condition is for the supporting tooth to be undamaged and for the preparation to be limited in the enamel area.

The use of an intraoral or extraoral parallelometer eases preparation and execution.

Cementation must be carried out with an adhesive technique using enamel/dentin adhesive systems together with autocuring composite cements.

If there is sufficient bone quantity and quality, it is possible to rehabilitate extended edentulous gaps using an IS-FPD. The presence of undamaged natural teeth adjacent to the gap is an indication for IS-FPD.

RPDs are recommended in all situations in which it is not possible to use FPD or FPAD and when the patient has not specifically requested IS-FPD.

73. Kratochvil FJ. Principles of Removable Partial Denture. Philadelphia: Saunders, 1988. Cat. 7

74. Stewart KL, Rudd KD, Kuebker WA. Clinical Removable Prosthodontics, ed 2. St Louis: Mosby, 1988. Cat. 7

75. Preti G, Pera P. Prótesis parcial removibile. Padova: Piccin Nuova Libraria, 2000. Cat. 7

76. Lindhe J, Ericsson I. The influence of trauma from occlusion on reduced but healthy periodontal tissues in dogs. J Clin Periodontol 1976;3:110–122. Cat. 5

77. Ericsson I, Lindhe J. Lack of effect of trauma from occlusion on the recurrence of experimental periodontitis. J Clin Periodontol 1977;4:115–127. Cat. 5

78. Nyman S, Ericsson I. The capacity of reduced periodontal tissues to support fixed bridgework. J Clin Periodontol 1982;9:409–414. Cat. 4

79. Giargia M, Lindhe J. Tooth mobility and periodontal disease. J Clin Periodontol 1997;24:785–795. Cat. 7

80. Mullally BH, Linden GJ. Periodontal status of regular dental attenders with and without removable partial dentures. Eur J Prosthodont Restor Dent 1994;2:161–163. Cat. 4

81. Yusof Z, Isa Z. Periodontal status of teeth in contact with denture in removable partial denture wearers. J Oral Rehabil 1994;21:77–86. Cat. 4

82. Kapur KK, Deupree R, Dent RJ, Hasse AL. A randomized clinical trial of two basic removable partial denture designs. Part I: Comparisons of five-year success rates and periodontal health. J Prosthet Dent 1994;72:268–282. Cat. 1

83. Kapur KK, Garrett NR, Dent RJ, Hasse AL. A randomized clinical trial of two basic removable partial denture designs. Part II: Comparisons of masticatory scores. J Prosthet Dent 1997;78:15–21. Cat. 1

84. Burgersdijk R, Truin G, Kalsbeek H, van't Hof M, Mulder J. Objective and subjective need for cosmetic dentistry in the Dutch adult population. Community Dent Oral Epidemiol 1991;19:61–63. Cat. 4

85. Taylor CM, Fiske J, Cooper D, Gelbier S. Dental needs of preretirement and retired people in an inner-city area. Public Health 1994;108:413–417. Cat. 4

86. Spang H. Sistemi di attacco nelle protesi parziali. Milano: Scienze e Tecniche Dentistiche Edizioni Internazionali, 1985. Cat. 7

87. Öwall B, Jönsson L. Precision attachment-retained removable partial dentures. Part 3. General practitioner results up to 2 years. Int J Prosthodont 1998;11:574–579. Cat. 4

88. Leupold RJ, Faraone KL. Etched castings as an adjunct to mouth preparation for removable partial dentures. J Prosthet Dent 1985;53:655–658. Cat. 4

89. Taleghani M, Leinfelder KF, Taleghani AM. An alternative to cast etched retainers. J Prosthet Dent 1987;58:424–428. Cat. 4

90. Marinello CP, Scharer P, Meyenberg K. Resin-bonded etched castings with extracoronal attachments for removable partial dentures. J Prosthet Dent 1991;66:52–55. Cat. 4

91. Van Meerbeek B, Dhem A, Goret-Nicaise M, Braem M, Lambrechts P, Vanherle G. Comparative SEM and TEM examination of the ultrastructure of the resin-dentin interdiffusion zone. J Dent Res 1993;72:495–501. Cat. 6

92. Keltjens HM, Käyser AF, Hertel R, Battistuzzi PG. Distal extension removable partial dentures supported by implants and residual teeth: considerations and case reports. Int J Oral Maxillofac Implants 1993;8:208–213. Cat. 8

Part II

1. Björn AL, Öwall B. Partial edentulism and its prosthetic treatment. Swed Dent J 1979;3:15–25. Cat. 4

2. Widström E. Loss of teeth and the frequency and condition of removable and fixed dentures in Finnish immigrants in Sweden. Swed Dent J 1982;6:61–69. Cat. 4

3. Öwall B. Prosthetic epidemiology. Int Dent J 1986;36:230–234. Cat. 7

4. Campion EW. The oldest old. N Engl J Med 1994;330:1819–1820. Cat. 9

5. Steele JG, Treasure E, Pitts NB, Morris J, Bradnock G. Total tooth loss in the United Kingdom in 1998 and implication for the future. Br Dent J 2000;189:598–603. Cat. 7

6. Elias AC, Sheiham A. The relationship between satisfaction with mouth and number and position of teeth. J Oral Rehabil 1998;25:649–661. Cat. 7

7. Öwall B, Käyser AF, Carlsson GE. Prosthodontics: Principles and Management Strategies. Baltimore: Mosby-Wolfe, 1996:40–41. Cat. 7

8. Levin B. The 28th syndrome—Or should all teeth be replaced? Dent Surv 1974;50:47. Cat. 9

9. Öwall B, Käyser AF, Carlsson GE. Prosthodontics: Principles and Management Strategies. Baltimore: Mosby-Wolfe, 1996:45–46. Cat. 7

10. Käyser AF. Shortened dental arches and oral function. J Oral Rehabil 1981;8:457–462. Cat. 4

11. Witter DJ, Creugers NHJ, Kreulen CM, de Haan AF. Occlusal stability in shortened dental arches. J Dent Res 2001;80:432–436. Cat. 4

12. Shugars DA, Bader JD, White A, Scurria MS, Hayden WJ Jr, Garcia RI. Survival rates of teeth adjacent to treated and untreated posterior bounded edentulous spaces. J Am Dent Assoc 1998;129:1089–1095. Cat. 4

13. Lyka I, Carlsson GE, Wedel A, Kiliaridis S. Dentists' perception of risks for molars without antagonists. A questionnaire study of dentists in Sweden. Swed Dent J 2001;25:67–73. Cat. 4

14. Love WD, Adams RL. Tooth movement into edentulous areas. J Prosthet Dent 1971;25:271–278. Cat. 4

15. Gragg KL, Shugars DA, Bader JD, Elter JR, White BA. Movement of teeth adjacent to posterior bounded edentulous spaces. J Dent Res 2001;80:2021–2024. Cat. 3

16. Lundgren D, Kurol J, Thorstensson B, Hugoson A. Periodontal conditions around tipped and upright molars in adults. An intra-individual retrospective study. Eur J Orthod 1992;14:449–55. Cat. 4

17. Agerberg G, Carlsson GE. Chewing ability in relation to dental and general health. Acta Odontol Scand 1981;39:147–53. Cat. 4

18. Käyser AF In: Öwall B, Käyser AF, Carlsson GE. Prosthodontics. Principles and Management Strategies. Baltimore: Mosby-Wolfe, 1996:41. Cat. 7

19. Kirveskari P, Alanen P, Jämsä T. Association between craniomandibular disorders and occlusal interferences. J Prosthet Dent 1989;62:66–69. Cat. 1

20. Seligman DA, Pullinger AG. The role of functional occlusal relationship in temporomandibular disorders: A review. J Craniomandib Disord 1991;5:265–279. Cat. 7

21. Kirveskari P, Alanen P. Scientific evidence of occlusion and craniomandibular disorders. J Orofac Pain 1993;7:235–240. Cat. 7

22. Pullinger AG, Seligman DA, Gornbein JA. A multiple regression analysis of the risk and relative odds of temporomandibular disorders as a function of common occlusal features. J Dent Res 1993;72:968–979.Cat. 2

23. De Boever JA, Carlsson GE, Klineberg IJ. Need for occlusal therapy and prosthodontic treatment in the management of temporomandibular disorders. Part I. Occlusal interferences and occlusal adjustment. J Oral Rehabil 2000;27:367–379. Cat. 7

24. Shugars DA, Bader JD, White BA, Scurria MS, Hayden WJ Jr, Garcia RI. Survival rates of teeth adjacent to treated and untreated posterior bounded edentulous spaces. J Am Dent Assoc 1998;129:1089–1095. Cat. 4

25. Aquilino SA, Shugars DA, Bader JD, White BA. Ten-year survival rates of teeth adjacent to treated and untreated posterior bounded edentulous spaces. J Prosthet Dent 2001;85:455–460. Cat. 4

26. Carlsson GE, Haraldson T, Mohl ND (eds). A Textbook of Occlusion. Chicago: Quintessence, 1988:181–182. Cat. 7

27. Ash MM, Ramfjord SP. Occlusion, ed 4. Philadelphia: Saunders, 1995. Cat. 7

28. Cronin RJ, Cagna DR. An update on fixed prosthodontics. J Am Dent Assoc 1997;128:425–436. Cat. 7

29. Shillingburg HT, Hobo S, Witsett LD, Jacobi R, Brackett SE. Basi fondamentali di Protesi Fissa. ed 3. Milano: Scienza e Tecnica Dentistica e Internazionali, 1998. Cat. 7

30. Lindhe I. Parodontologia ed Implantologia. ed 3. Bologna: Martina, 1997. Cat. 7

31. Ante IH. The fundamental principles of abutments. Mich State Dent Soc Bull 1926;8:14–23. Cat. 7

32. Caputo AA, Standlee JP. Biomechanics in Clinical Dentistry. Chicago: Quintessence, 1987. Cat. 7

33. Jepsen A. Root surface measurement and a method for x-ray determination of root surface area. Acta Odontol Scand 1963; 21:35–46. Cat. 6

34. Goodacre CJ, Campagni WV, Aquilino SA. Tooth preparations for complete crowns: An art form based on scientific principles. J Prosthet Dent 2001;85:363–376. Cat. 7

35. Mc Dowell JA, Regli CP. A quantitative analysis of the decrease in width of the mandibular arch during forced movements of the mandible. J Dent Res 1961;49:1183–1185. Cat. 4

36. Burch JG, Borchers G. Method for study of mandibular arch width change. J Dent Res 1970;49:463–464. Cat. 8

37. Goodkind RG, Heringlake CB. Mandibular flexure in opening and closing movements. J Prosthet Dent 1973;30:134–138. Cat. 4

38. De Marco TJ, Paine S. Mandibular dimensional change. J Prosthet Dent 1974;31:482–485. Cat. 4

39. Abdel Latif HH, Hobkirk JA, Kelleway JP. Functional mandibular deformation in edentulous subjects treated with dental implants. Int J Prosthodont 2000;13:513–519. Cat. 4

40. Leempoel PJ, Käyser AF, Van Rossum GM, De Haan AF. The survival rate of bridges. A study of 1,674 bridges in 40 Dutch general practices. J Oral Rehabil 1995;22:327–330. Cat. 4

41. Nyman S, Ericsson I. The capacity of reduced periodontal tissues to support fixed bridgeworks. J Clin Periodontol 1982;9:409–414. Cat. 4

42. Nyman S, Lindhe J, Lundgren D. The role of occlusion for the stability of fixed bridges in patients with reduced periodontal support. J Clin Periodontol 1975;2:53–66. Cat. 2

43. Nyman S, Lindhe J. A longitudinal study of combined periodontal and prosthetic treatment of patients with advanced periodontal disease. J Periodontol 1979;50:163–169. Cat. 2

44. Randow K, Glantz PO, Zoger B. Technical failures and some related clinical complications in extensive fixed prosthodontics. An epidemiological study of long-term clinical quality. Acta Odontol Scand 1986;44:241–255. Cat. 2

45. Hannam AG. Periodontal mechanoreceptors. In: Anderson DJ, Matthews B (eds). Mastication. Bristol: Wright & Sons, 1976. Cat. 7

46. Gibbs CH, Mahan PE, Mauderli A, Lundeen HC, Walsh EK. Limits of human bite strength. J Prosthet Dent 1986;56:226–229. Cat. 8

47. Resnick NM. Geriatric medicine. In: Harrison's Principles of Internal Medicine: Self-Assessment and Board Review. New York: McGraw-Hill, 2001. Cat. 7

48. van Zyl J, Geissberger M. Simulated shape design. Helping patients decide their esthetic ideal. J Am Dent Assoc 2001;132:1105–1109. Cat. 8

49. Craig RG. Restorative dental materials, ed 10. Chicago: Mosby, 1997. Cat. 7

50. O'Brien WJ. Dental Materials and Their Selection, ed 4. Chicago: Quintessence, 2008. Cat. 7

51. Summitt JB, Robbins JW, Hilton TJ, Schwartz RS. Fundamentals of Operative Dentistry: A Contemporary Approach, ed 3. Chicago: Quintessence, 2006. Cat. 7

52. Preston JD. Perspectives in Dental Ceramics. Proceedings of the Fourth International Symposium on Ceramics. Chicago: Quintessence, 1988. Cat. 7

53. Yamamoto M. Metal-Ceramics: Principles and Methods of Makoto Yamamoto. Chicago: Quintessence, 1985. Cat. 7

54. Crispin BJ. Contemporary Esthetic Dentistry: Practice Fundamentals. Chicago: Quintessence, 1994. Cat. 7

55. Ekfeldt A. Incisal and occlusal tooth wear and wear of some prosthodontic material. An epidemiological and clinical study. Swed Dent J Suppl 1989; 65:1-62. Cat. 2

56. Tjan AH, Miller GD, The JG. Some esthetic factors in a smile. J Prosthet Dent 1984;51:24–28. Cat. 4

57. Witter DJ, Van Elteren P, Käyser AF, Van Rossum GM. Oral comfort in shortened dental arches. J Oral Rehabil 1990;17:137–143. Cat. 2

58. Carossa S, Pera P. Preparazioni Parziali in Oro e Ceramica. Milano: Masson, 1997. Cat. 7

59. Nevalainen M, Ruokolainen T, Rantanen T, Mäkilä M, Könönen M. Comparison of partial and full crowns as retainers in the same bridge. J Oral Rehabil 1995;22:673–677. Cat: 4

60. Rosenstiel SF, Land MF, Fujimoto J. Contemporary Fixed Prosthodontics, ed 2. St Louis: Mosby, 1995. Cat. 7

61. Kaufman EG, Cohelo DH, Colin DH. Factors influencing the retention of cemented gold castings. J Prosthet Dent 1961;11:487–502. Cat. 6

62. Jørgensen KD. The relationship beween retention and convergence angle in cemented veneers crowns. Acta Odontol Scand 1955;12:40–53. Cat. 6

63. Potts RG, Shillingburg HT, Duncanson MG. Retention and resistance of preparations for cast restorations. J Prosthet Dent 1980;43:303–308. Cat. 8

64. Lorey RE, Myers GE. The retentive qualities of bridge retainers. J Am Dent Assoc 1988;76:568–592. Cat. 6

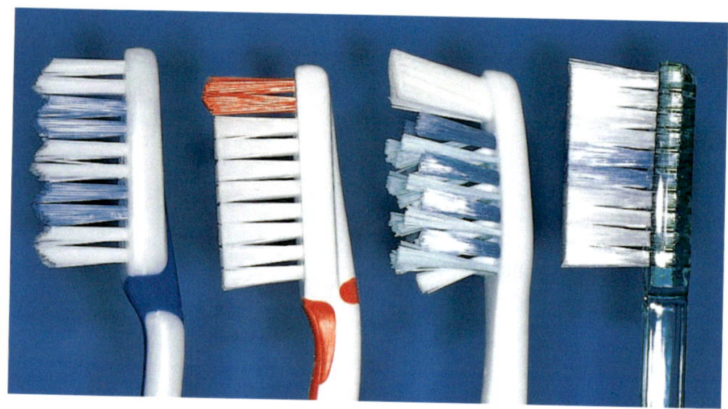

Fig 14-16 Manual brushes with varied profiles and bristle inclinations.

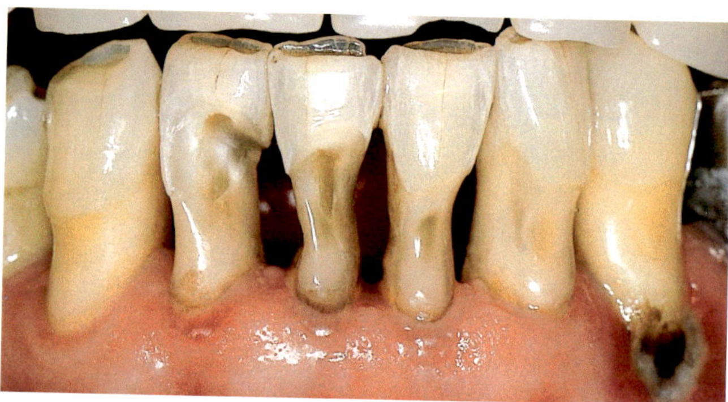

Fig 14-17 Serious dental abrasion caused by use of a toothbrush with very hard bristles and an excessive brushing technique.

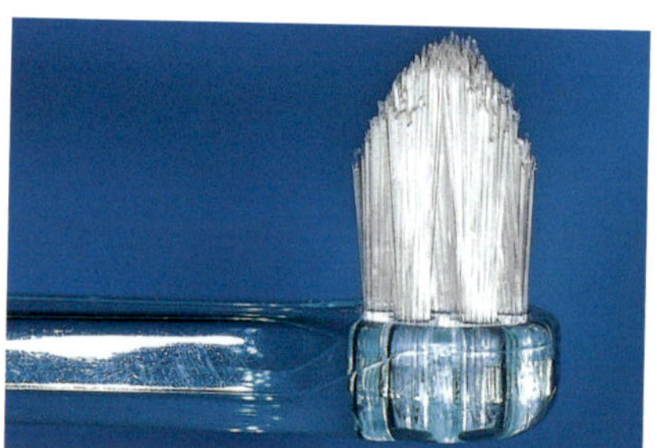

Fig 14-18 Monotuft toothbrush.

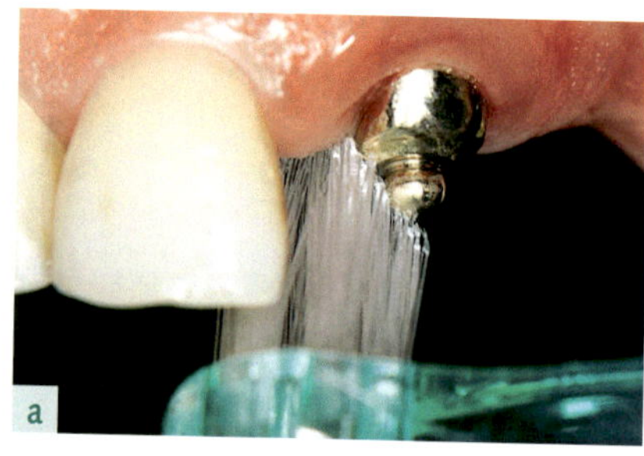

Fig 14-19 Using a monotuft toothbrush. *(a)* Cleaning a ball attachment for an maxillary overdenture. *(b)* Cleaning an attachment for a mandibular overdenture.

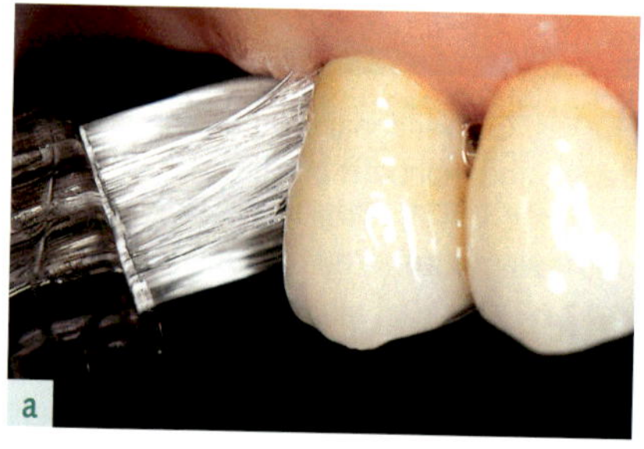

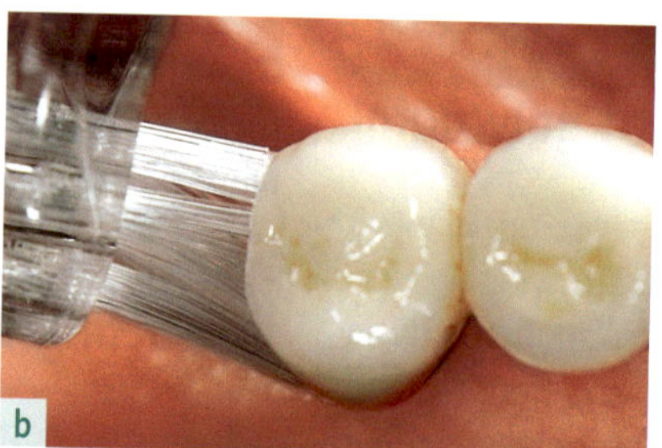

Fig 14-20 Monotuft brush used to clean the distalmost tooth bordering a posterior edentulous gap. *(a)* Buccal view of metal-ceramic crowns on the maxillary right first and second premolars. *(b)* Occlusal view.

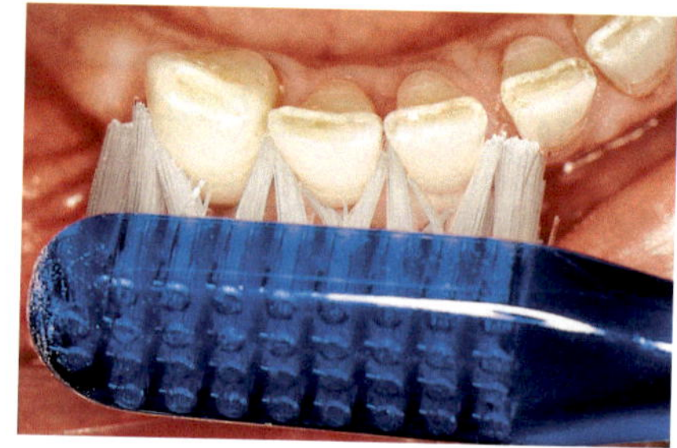

Fig 14-21 Traditional toothbrush, which cannot clean the interdental space completely.

by the brushing technique used. Although it is important to remove bacterial plaque thoroughly, the integrity of the tissues must be respected. Brushing too aggressively or brushing with a hard-bristled toothbrush abrades the oral tissues (Fig 14-17). A soft or medium-soft toothbrush is preferable because it is just as effective but causes less damage.[50,51]

A prosthesis requires a toothbrush with soft synthetic bristles with round tips and a small head that can be maneuvered easily in posterior regions and areas that are hard to access. For this reason, the monotuft toothbrush is often recommended (Figs 14-18 to 14-20). The traditional toothbrush is effective on the buccal, lingual, and occlusal surfaces, but it has little effect in the interproximal areas, which are harder to reach (Fig 14-21). Patients who have a removable prosthesis should use specifically designed toothbrushes. A cone-shaped toothbrush with rigid bristles is used to clean around the parts of removable partial prostheses (Figs 14-22 and 14-23).

A larger toothbrush that has two groups of bristles on the same handle is advised for the resin prosthetic bodies of removable prostheses (Figs 14-24 and 14-25). The harder bristles are used to clean external surfaces, and the softer bristles serve to remove remains from the internal surfaces of the prosthetic body.

Careful maintenance of the removable prosthesis is essential. If residue is not removed, it becomes food for bacteria on the

Fig 14-22 Conic brush with rigid bristles for an RPD.

Fig 14-23 Using a conic brush to clean the metal surfaces of an RPD.

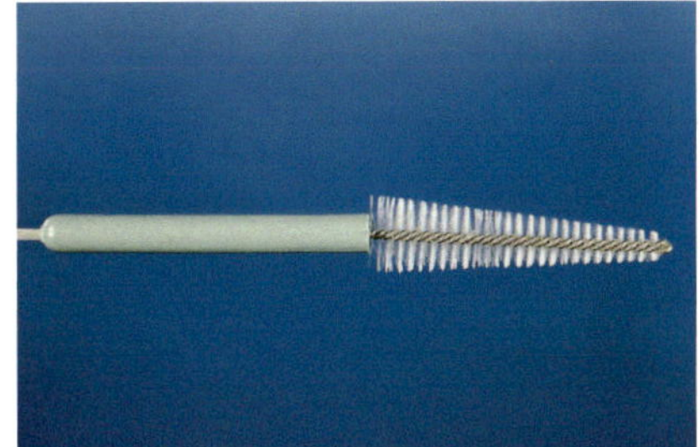

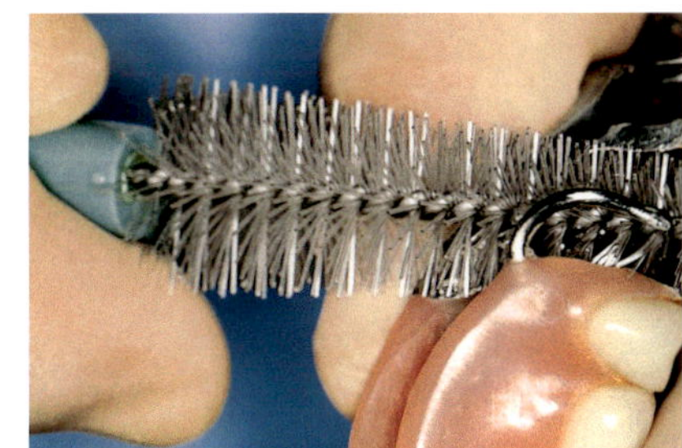

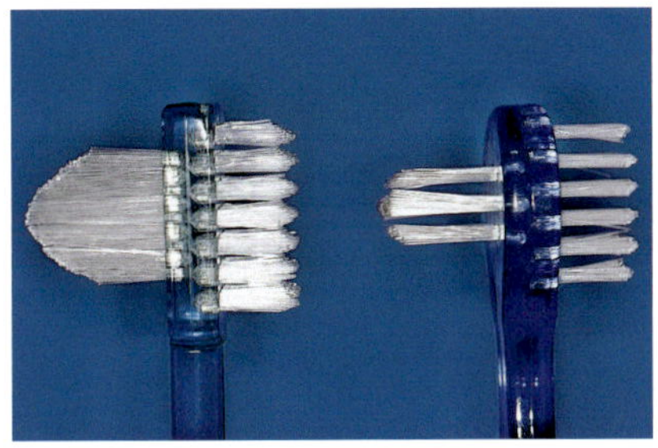

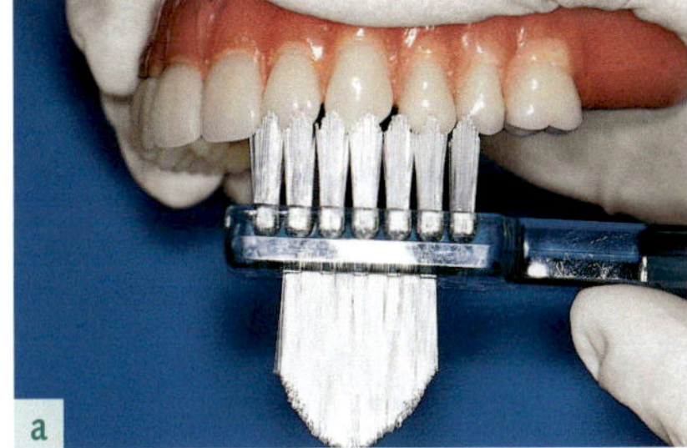

Fig 14-24 Brushes with two groups of bristles for cleaning an RPD.

Fig 14-25 (a) Hard bristles are used to clean the external surfaces of the prosthesis. (b) Softer bristles are used to clean the internal surfaces of the prosthetic body.

Fig 14-26 Head of an electric toothbrush.

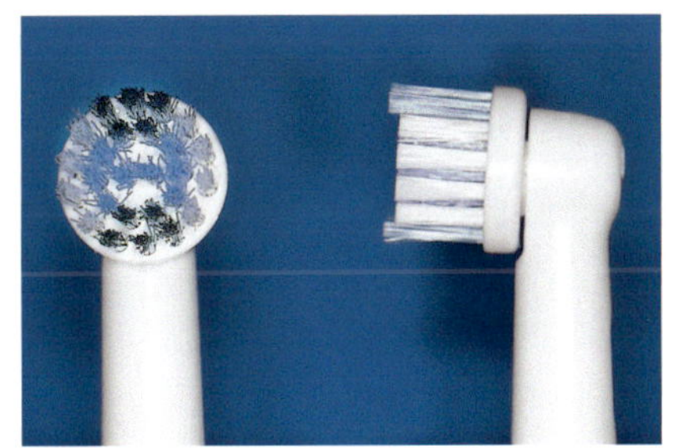

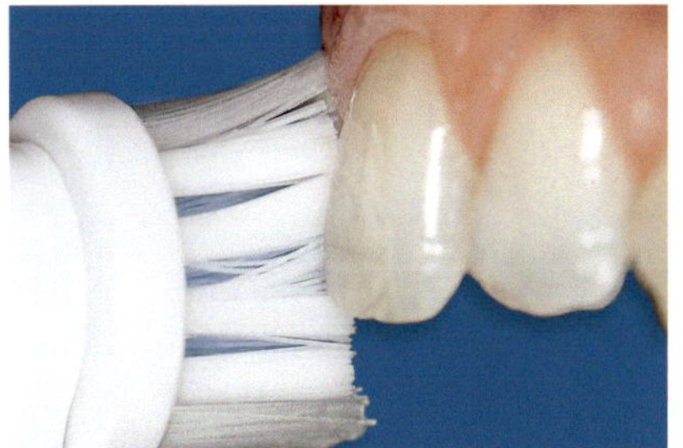

Fig 14-27 Clinical use of an electric toothbrush.

supporting mucosa, which is already stressed by functional and parafunctional loads.

Electric toothbrushes

Short-term studies have demonstrated that electric toothbrushes are as effective as conventional ones, and if they are used correctly they can be even more effective. They can be particularly advantageous for patients who lack manual dexterity, who have orthodontic appliances or a complex prosthetic restoration, and who have plaque retention.[52-56] Electric brushing can be used with any technique, but it is advisable to use a slow movement with light pressure that will not bend the bristles.

There are various types of electric toothbrushes with rotary, oscillating, or pulsating movements, and with tufts of bristles pointing in different directions (Figs 14-26 and 14-27). Modern electric brushing cannot be matched by manual brushing. The filaments of the rotary or oscillating head vibrate and oscillate thousands of times a minute. This action transfers enough energy to break down the electrostatic and electrochemical bonds responsible for the adhesion of plaque to the dental-periodontal surfaces. Despite the increased frequency of movement and increased energy transmitted to the tissues, electric toothbrushes create less damage than incongruous manual brushing.[57,58]

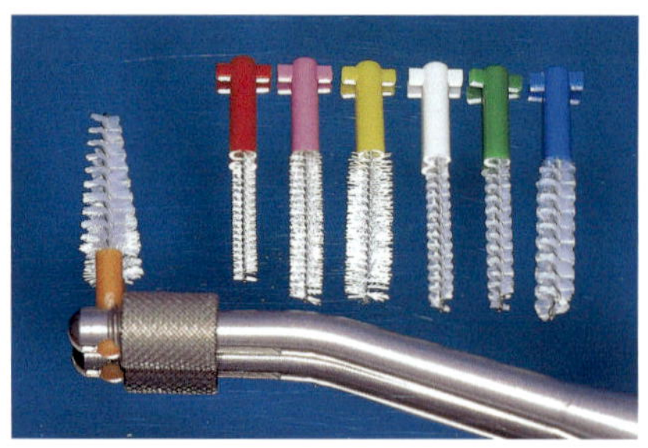

Fig 14-28 Interdental brushes of different forms and dimensions.

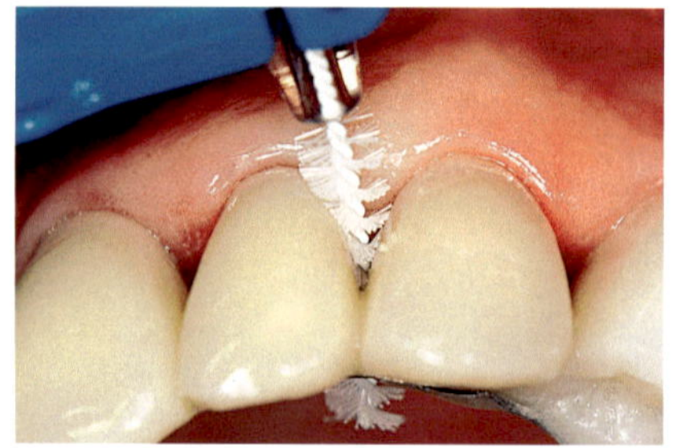

Fig 14-29 Clinical use of an interdental brush between teeth of a provisional fixed partial denture in resin.

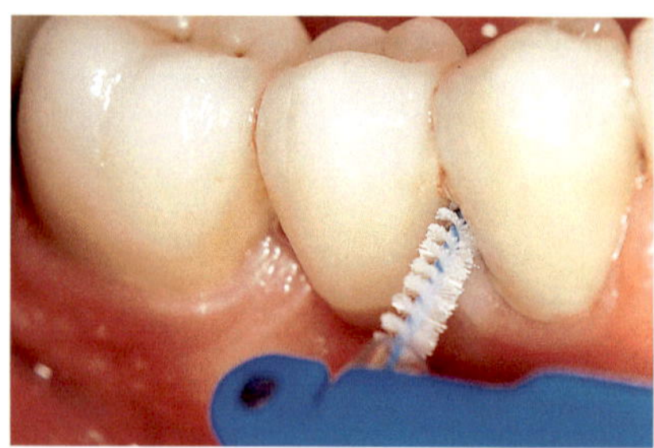

Fig 14-30 Clinical use of an interdental brush to clean between teeth in a definitive metal-ceramic fixed partial denture.

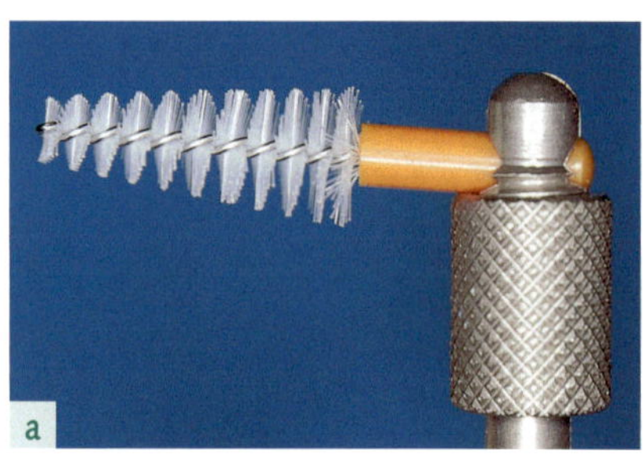

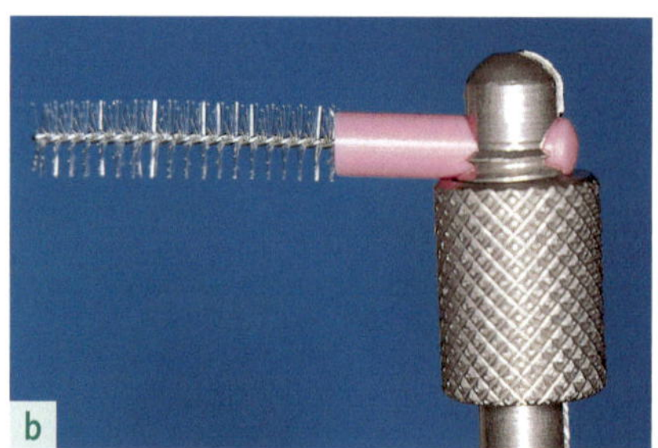

Fig 14-31 Interdental brushes with uncoated metal cores. *(a)* Conic brush with bristles set in a spiral. *(b)* Cylindrical brush with bristles set in radiating rows.

Fig 14-32 Interdental brushes with plastic-coated cores.

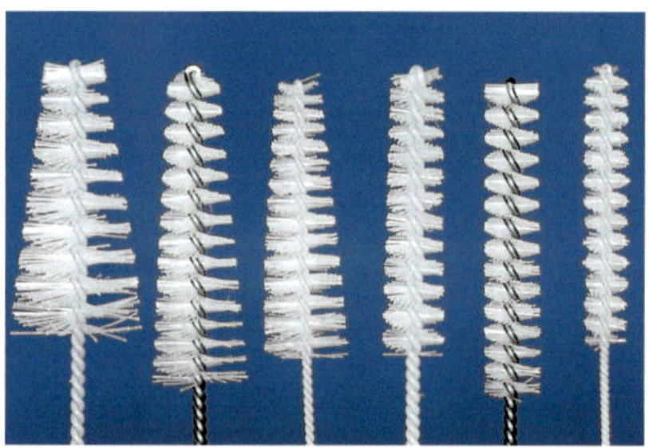

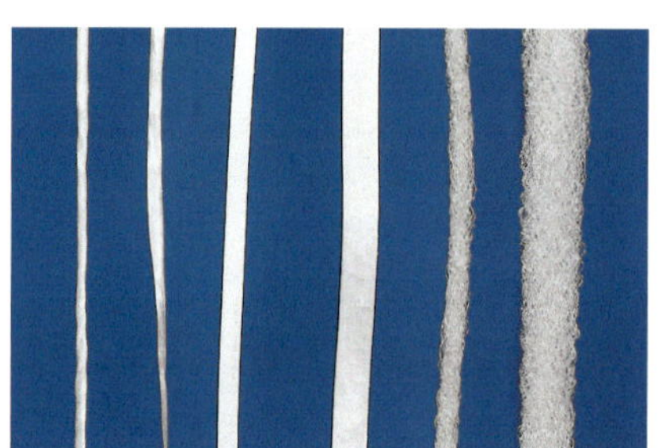

Fig 14-33 Types of dental floss *(left to right)*: Waxed, unwaxed, normal tape, and spongy tape.

Interdental brushes

The interdental brush can effectively substitute floss on natural and prosthetic teeth. It removes bacterial plaque from spaces between the teeth or from the areas around fixed and removable prostheses. The choice of shape (eg, conic or cylindrical) and size must be selected according to the width of spaces to be cleaned[59] (Figs 14-28 to 14-30).

The interdental brush has a central core of entwined metal wire in which bristles are arranged in a spiral or in rows radiating out from the core (Fig 14-31). The metal core may be coated in plastic to avoid damaging tissues or scratching the titanium surface of implants. If the layer of surface oxides of the titanium is altered, it becomes more vulnerable to corrosion. The interproximal toothbrush with soft nylon bristles does not significantly alter the titanium surfaces (Fig 14-32).

Dental floss

Floss is an effective instrument for the removal of bacterial plaque between teeth and the papillae spaces.[59] It is only efficient on the convex surfaces, and it is often insufficient in the posterior regions, given the presence of interproximal concavity.[60]

There are various types of floss, mostly made of interlaced nylon or silk filaments in the form of a thread or tape and that may be coated with wax (Fig 14-33). Research has shown that there is no difference in the effectiveness of waxed versus unwaxed floss[61-63] (Figs 14-34 and 14-35).

Spongy interdental floss with hard tips is especially recommended for patients who have a fixed prosthesis on natural teeth and on implants, but it can also be useful for cleaning the abutments of overdentures and perio-overdentures.

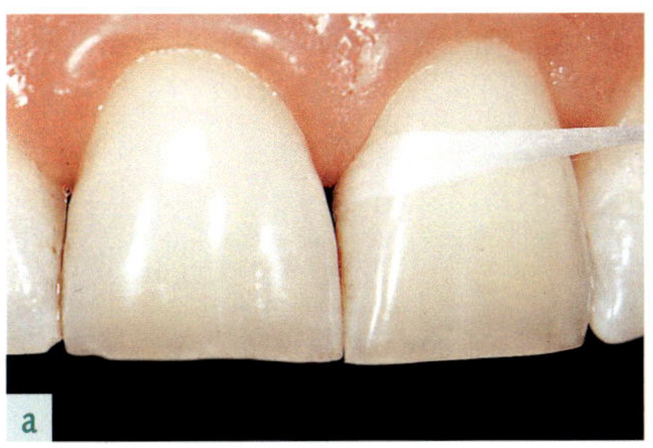 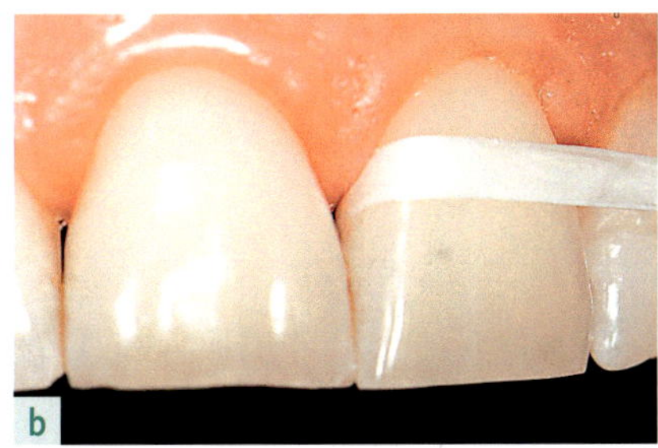 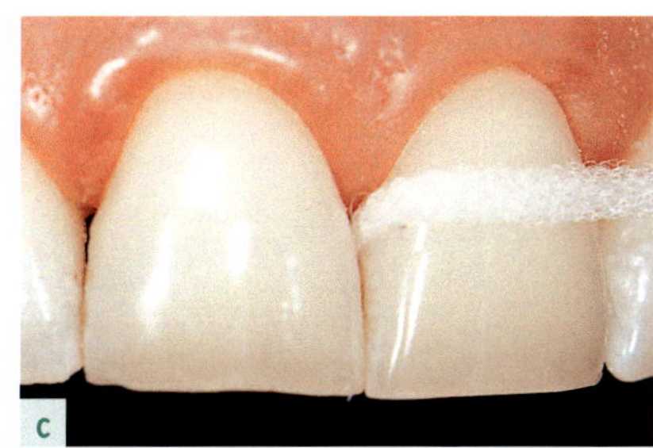

Fig 14-34 Using dental floss between natural teeth. *(a)* Unwaxed tape floss. *(b)* Large tape floss. *(c)* Spongy floss .

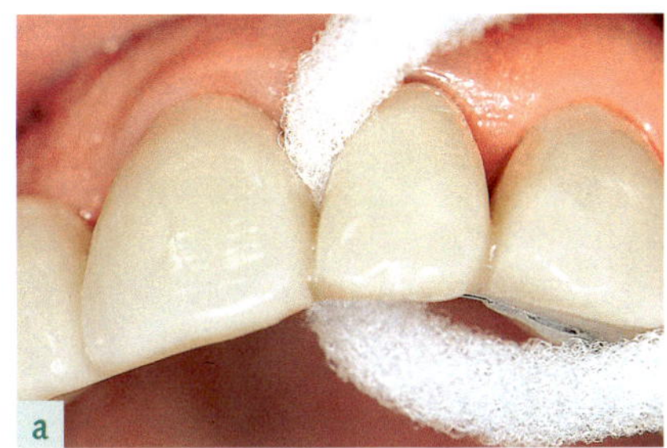 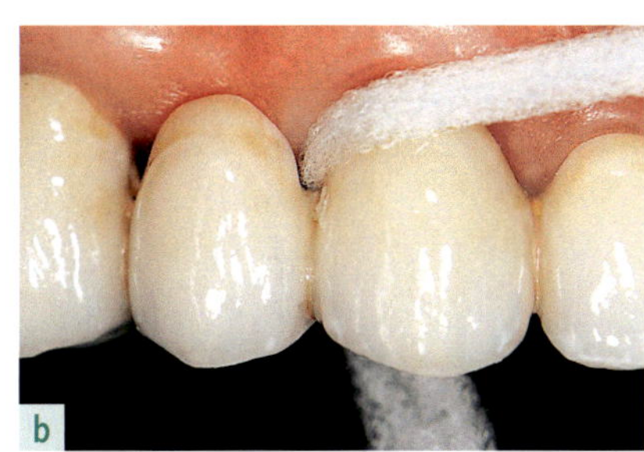

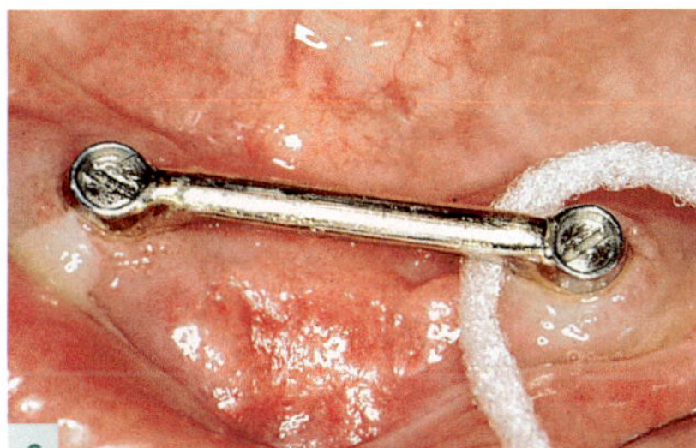 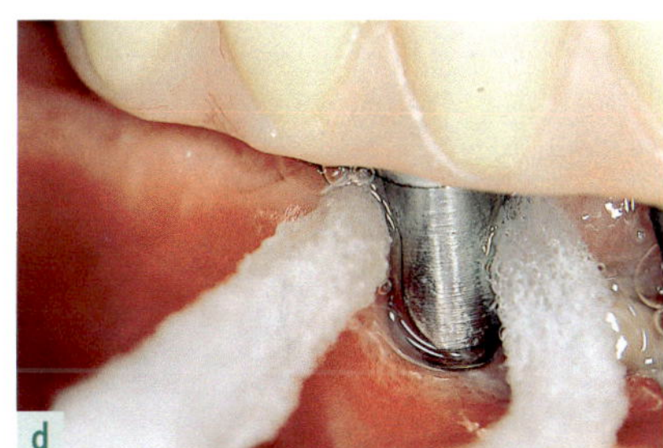

Fig 14-35 Using spongy floss with rigid ends for a provisional fixed partial denture in resin *(a)*, definitive metal-ceramic fixed partial denture *(b)*, a Dolder bar for retention of an overdenture *(c)*, and an implant abutment *(d)*.

Fig 14-36 Cleaning and massaging an edentulous gap with gauze soaked in hypertonic sodium chloride solution.

Fig 14-37 Cleaning the distal area of an abutment with gauze soaked in antiseptic solution.

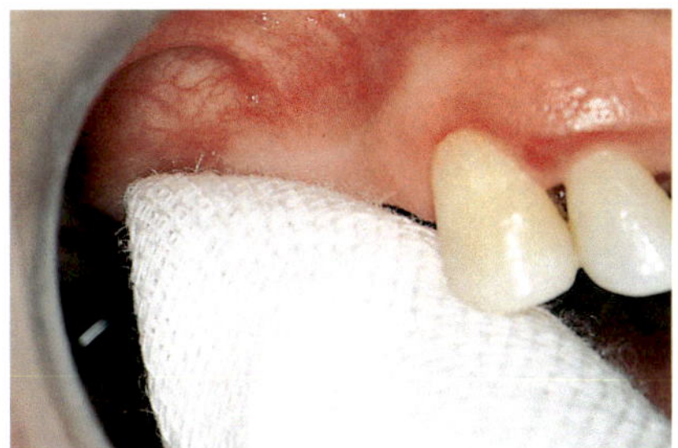 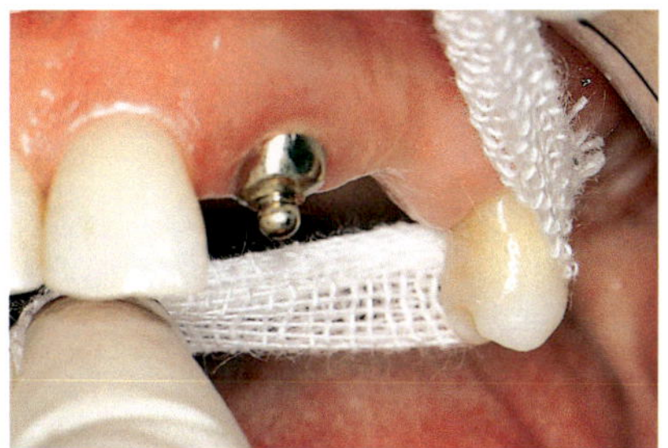

Gauze

Gauze is recommended for cleaning and massaging the edentulous mucosa. It may be used to apply a hypertonic sodium chloride solution, which has an antiedematous effect (Fig 14-36). Patients who complain of periodic inflammation or a massive accumulation of plaque between the lingual papilla can benefit from the daily use of sterilized gauze soaked in a disinfectant solution of chlorhexidene and fluoride.

The distal aspects of the posterior teeth, especially when acting as abutments for the removable prosthesis, can be best cleaned using tape-covered gauze soaked in a disinfectant solu-

253

tion. This method removes the plaque more delicately than can be achieved with a toothbrush (Fig 14-37).

Brushing techniques

There is no one technique that can be applied by every patient. The ideal brushing technique can be defined as that which enables the quickest and most complete removal of buccal, lingual, and occlusal bacterial plaque, applying enough pressure to be effective but without damaging the tissues.

Each patient must establish how often brushing takes place, but teeth should be brushed at least twice per day to control bacterial plaque and prevent halitosis. Effective plaque removal largely depends on how long brushing lasts. In general, 5 minutes are necessary with a manual toothbrush and 2 minutes with a high-quality electric toothbrush.[64] Brushing pressure can vary from person to person.

The choice of brushing technique depends on the amount of keratinization of the attached gingiva. Use of the roll technique and apical positioning of the bristles is recommended for thin gingival biotypes, whereas a modified Bass technique is recommended for thick biotypes. In the presence of extragingival prosthetic margins and open interproximal spaces, the Charters method works well.

Brushing techniques can be classified in terms of movement and position of the toothbrush. The most common methods are:

- Horizontal
- Vertical (Leonard)
- Roll
- Circular (Fones)
- Stillman
- Charters
- Bass
- Occlusal
- Tongue brushing

Brushing techniques to avoid
Horizontal technique
This technique is still in use, but should be avoided because it only cleans part of the crown and completely neglects the cervical areas where most plaque accumulates. Horizontal brushing is potentially damaging in that it can abrade the enamel and gingiva (Fig 14-38).

Vertical technique
Comparable to horizontal brushing, vertical brushing is still often used even though it should be avoided. It is not only ineffective in removing plaque in the cervical areas, but it also carries the risk of pushing microorganisms into the cervical areas. Also, using too much pressure can cause gingival recession (Fig 14-39).

Brushing techniques to use
Roll technique
This technique is effective in removing plaque without traumatizing the tissue. The toothbrush is positioned apically on the gingiva at a 45-degrees angle to the long axis of the tooth and then brushed with a rotating movement in the coronal direction with moderate pressure. This movement removes soft deposits. The roll method is recommended when the gums are healthy as well as in cases of gingival recession, for sensitive teeth, around implants surrounded by alveolar mucosa, after surgical periodontal intervention, and for very thin and vulnerable gums (Fig 14-40).

Fones technique
This is a circular roll technique in which the buccal and labial surfaces are approached with the jaws closed, and brushing is applied with light pressure, moving in wide circles from the gums of the maxilla to those of the mandible. It is easy to carry out and is therefore generally recommended for children, especially those in their first years, elderly people, people with poor manual skills, and disabled people. The technique can be modified by brushing with the jaws open rather than closed. Open jaws are essential for reaching the lingual and palatal areas. The technique, however, could damage the dental structure and the soft tissues if applied too vigorously and may not be effective in reaching the proximal areas.

Stillman technique
The simple Stillman technique was invented to massage, stimulate, and clean the cervical areas. The bristles must be set on the gingival margin, and modest pressure must be applied with vibrating circular movements. The bristles bend but do not move from their original position. The Stillman technique can also use the roll brushing method, with rotation of the bristles in a coronal direction. This method is recommended for removing plaque from the cervical areas and interproximal surfaces (Fig 14-41).

Charters technique
The original purpose of this technique was to stimulate the gingival margin around each tooth, especially in the interdental spaces, presupposing that there are no interdental papillae. The toothbrush is positioned on the gingiva and on the tooth, but it differs from the Stillman technique in that the bristles are positioned in the opposite direction, toward the crown of the

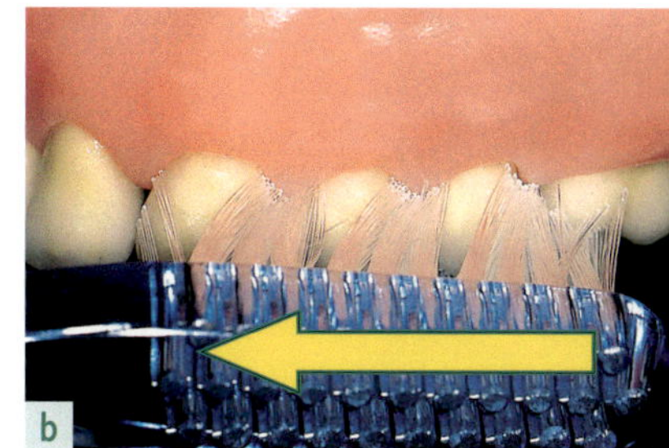

Fig 14-38 *(a and b)* Horizontal brushing technique.

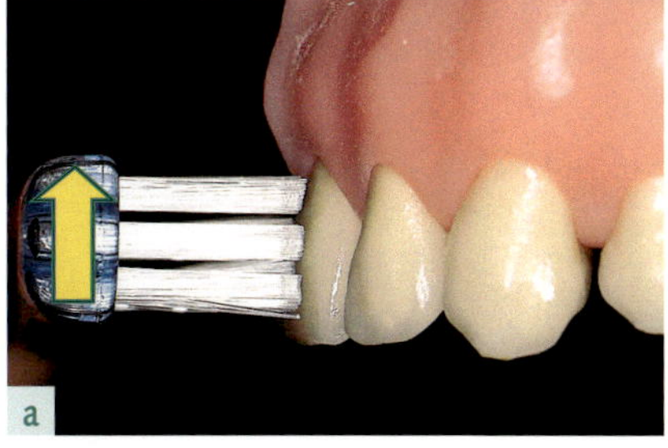
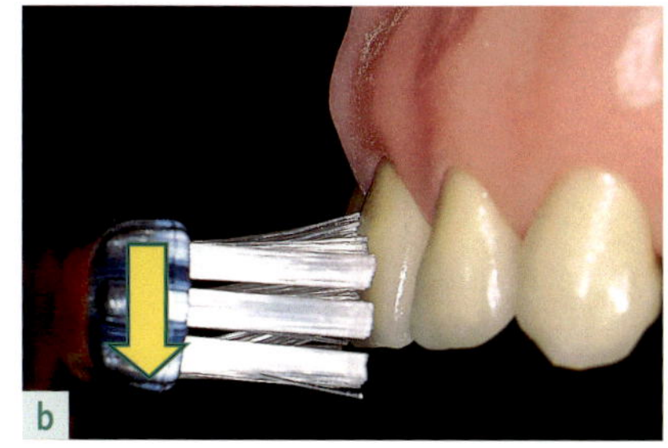

Fig 14-39 *(a and b)* Vertical brushing technique.

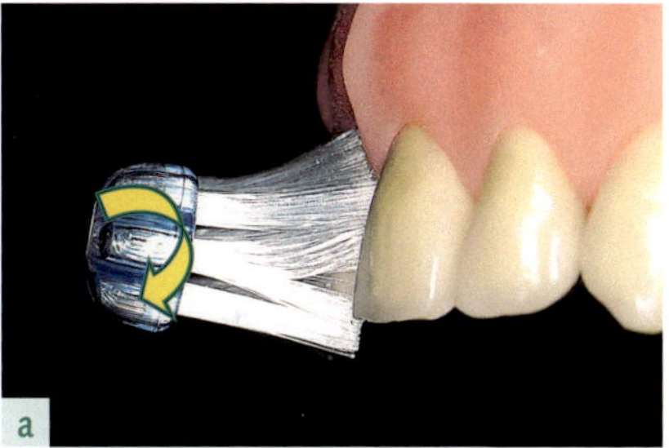
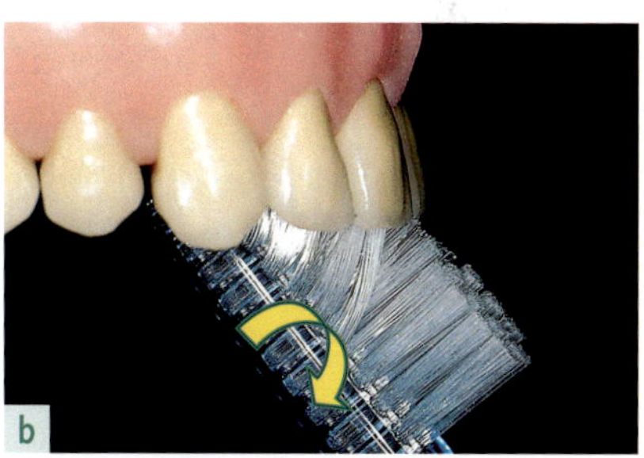

Fig 14-40 *(a and b)* Roll brushing technique.

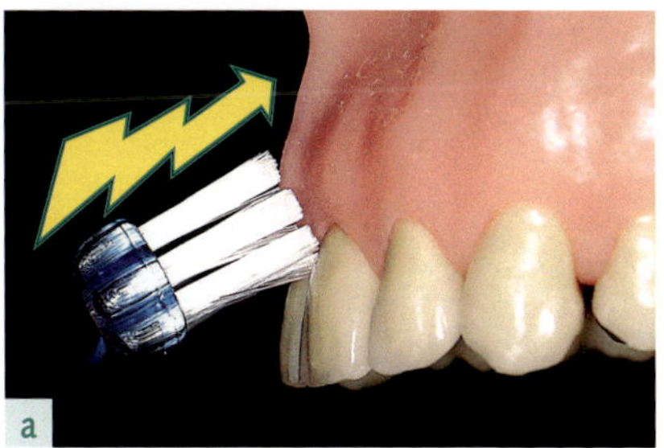
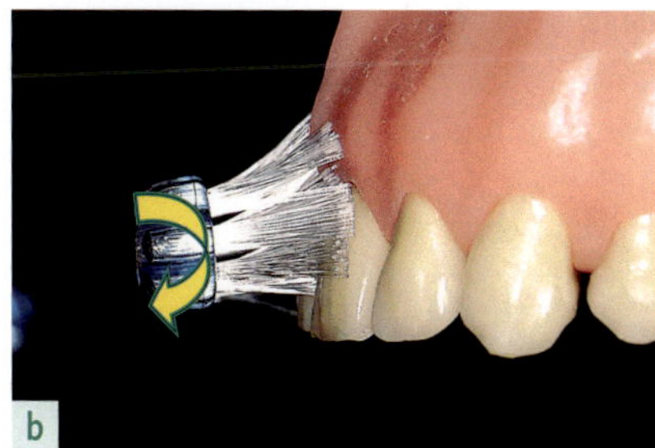

Fig 14-41 *(a and b)* Modified Stillman brushing technique.

tooth. Light pressure is applied to bend the bristles and force their tips between the teeth, while the sides of the bristles are pushed against the gums. Light but fast vibrations are needed, and the tips of the bristles must be kept in contact with the prosthesis (Fig 14-42).

This method is recommended to remove plaque in the interproximal areas when there is scarce interdental papillae, around the abutment of the implants, in the presence of orthodontic attachments under the prosthesis, and especially in the posterior areas. In the case of a fixed prosthesis it is useful to clean the abutment teeth and the gingival areas of a conventional partial denture. With this technique, however, the plaque cannot be removed from the crevice.

Bass technique

This method is the best known and most widely used. This technique allows cleaning of the sulci by introducing the bristles inside the gingival crevice at 45 degrees to the arch. Light pressure and vibrations are applied to remove the bacterial plaque hidden in the inside of the crevice itself.

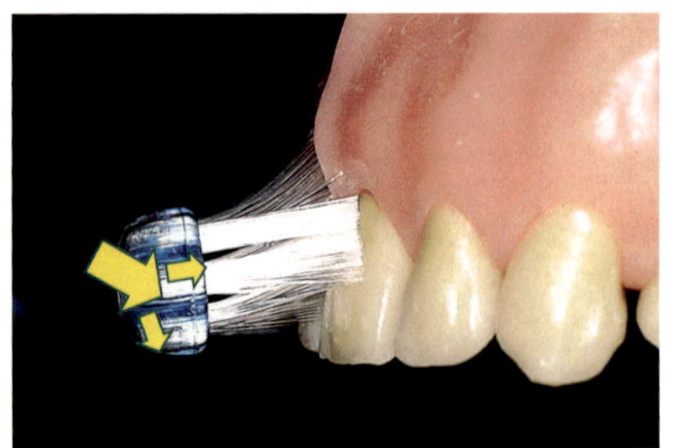

Fig 14-42 Charters brushing technique.

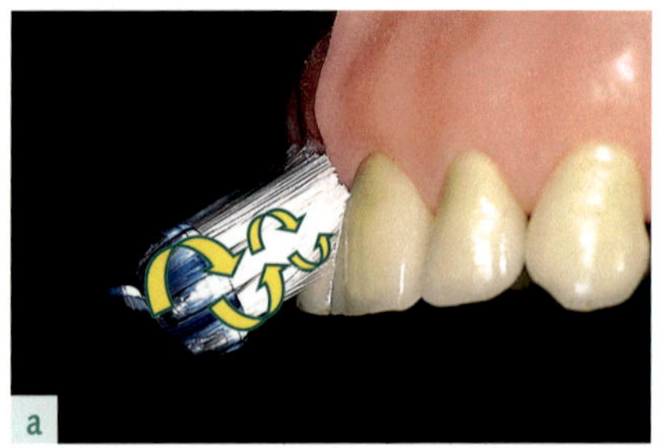

Fig 14-43 *(a and b)* Modified Bass brushing technique.

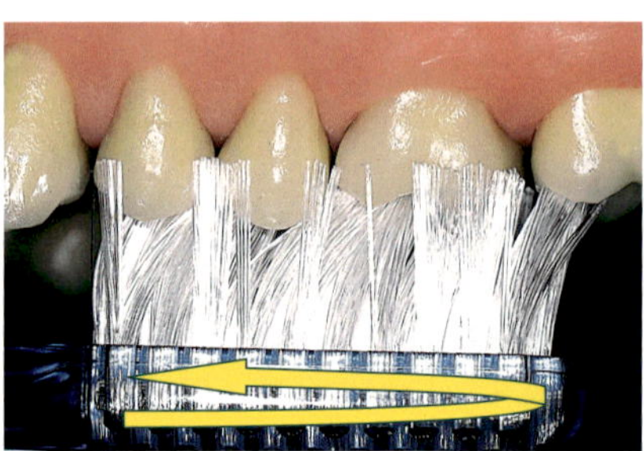

Fig 14-44 Brushing occlusal surfaces.

This technique can be modified by rotating the toothbrush in a coronal direction, similar to the roll method, so that the plaque that has already been broken up by the pressure and vibrations inside the crevice can be efficiently removed. The Bass technique is usually taught with this modification (Fig 14-43).

This technique is recommended for healthy tissue or when periodontal problems subsist, in particular in the presence of deep pockets. The periodontal tissue must be robust and the gums thick and fibrous, however—otherwise the pressure of the toothbrush might provoke gingival recession. For thin gingiva the roll method is recommended.

Occlusal technique

To clean the masticatory surfaces, the horizontal brushing technique would be appropriate, but because the patient may then carelessly apply this movement to other areas of the mouth, a rotary movement is preferred (Fig 14-44).

Tongue brushing technique

Microorganisms in the saliva come mainly from the tongue and influence the bacterial flora of the entire oral cavity.[65] Cleaning the tongue slows down the formation of bacterial plaque, diminishes the total accumulation of plaque, reduces the number of microorganisms, and reduces halitosis. Therefore, the hygienist should remind the patient that cleaning the tongue is part of the regular oral hygiene routine.

Brushing of the tongue is achieved by holding the handle of the toothbrush at a right angle to the midline of the tongue and the bristles facing toward the throat. Applying light pressure, the bristles are rotated forward, until they arrive at the tip of the tongue.

Chemicals, detergents, and disinfectants

Plaque disclosing agents

These products are very useful in the initial patient-motivation phase, in which it is helpful to show the areas that need cleaning. Plaque indicators are also useful for checking the efficiency of the home hygiene plan and evaluating the effectiveness of brushing.

They are available in liquid, tablet, and pill form and contain coloring agents, which, once dissolved in the saliva, are retained by the bacterial plaque deposits. Various coloring agents are used, such as iodine, erythrosin, fluorescein, and merbromin.

Toothpastes

Using toothpaste together with a toothbrush makes the removal of bacterial plaque easier and can distribute substances such as fluoride, antiseptics, desensitizers, and whiteners[66-71] (Fig 14-45).

The particles contained in the toothpaste should have an abrasive caliber of between 25 and 75 relative dentin abrasion (RDA) to safeguard the enamel, the neck of the tooth, and the roots. The abrasiveness depends on the dimensions of the granules in the mixture. With materials that are excessively abrasive, patients who are particularly aggressive in their brushing can cause deterioration of the resin surfaces of the prosthesis.[50,51,57]

It must be made clear to the patient that toothpaste works as a hygiene accessory and that the main work is accomplished through the brushing.

To brush the resin of the prosthetic base, nonalkaline soaps such as Marseille soap are recommended. These soaps, however, leave a nasty after-taste, which patients find difficult to tolerate. Alternatively, toothpastes with a very low level of abrasiveness can be used.

Mouthrinses

Chemical control of bacterial plaque cannot substitute mechanical removal; it can be considered an aid rather than a therapy for periodontal illness.[2,72] Chemical agents with an antimicrobial effect, for example, chlorhexidine, reduce gingivitis associated with the presence of bacterial plaque. These substances control and inhibit the bacterial flora above and below the gingival margins.[17,22,73-75] Chlorhexidine in mouthrinses, gels, toothpaste, sprays, or chewing gum, is the most efficient antiplaque and disinfecting agent. Hydrogen peroxide agents also aid mechanical cleaning of the prosthesis.[22,67,68,76,77]

Chlorhexidine cannot be used over a long period in all patients because of the adverse effects. With continued use of chlorhexidine, areas of dark pigmentation can form on the surfaces of the artificial teeth and the prosthetic body and on the upper surface of the tongue. It may also reduce the perception of taste, and in some subjects it may cause desquamation of the epithelial coating. The red-brown coloring of the upper surface of the tongue is harmless and disappears once the treatment has finished. The alterations in taste and burning sensations of the tongue usually decrease with continued use of the mouthwash. In these cases, the treatment should be interrupted for a period. The eventual pigmentation of the prosthetic resin is more problematic, although it is only superficial and can be removed mechanically with rotating tips or by the hygienist or dental technician.[22,23]

Sodium hypochlorite (5%) solution is an excellent sterilizing solution in terms of the rugosity or porosity of the prostheses. Twice per week the already-cleaned prosthesis should be immersed in the solution overnight. The prostheses must be carefully rinsed under cold running water before being put back into the mouth. High concentrations of sodium hypochlorite can decolorize the resin of the base or the artificial acrylic teeth if used frequently.

Effervescent cleansing tablets are advertised as an adjuvant to home hygiene for patients who are unable to undertake proper mechanical hygiene. These products must not substitute mechanical cleaning of the prostheses. When put in water, these tablets release oxygen, which has a mild mechanical and

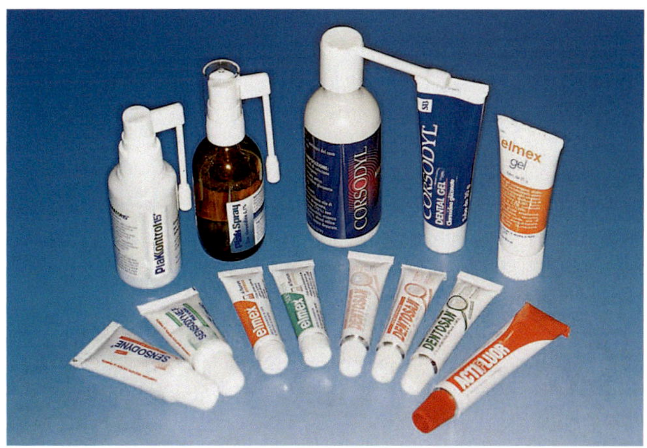

Fig 14-45 Chemical cleaners and disinfectants.

chemical action but not enough to remove all of the residue and bacterial plaque stuck to the prosthesis.

Antimicrobial agents must also be considered as supplements and not substitutes for mechanical cleaning to control subgingival plaque. They are inefficient in treating periodontal illness, which needs professional intervention.[4,16,23,78]

Fluoride

Fluoride is the most effective method for preventing and controlling decay. Furthermore, fluoride has indirect therapeutic and preventive effects on periodontal health, because of its ability to act on microorganisms.[69,79-81]

In the presence of ceramic or resin prostheses, highly concentrated fluoridated agents must be avoided. A pH that is too acidic causes etching on the surface of the prosthesis, which alters its smoothness and makes it easier for plaque to adhere. Accidental or prolonged contact with highly concentrated fluoridated solutions (containing 20 ppm of fluoride ions) could also damage the surface characteristics of titanium by destroying the oxide layer, which makes it more susceptible to corrosion.

Professional Oral Hygiene

Supplementary professional hygiene eliminates the predisposing and aggravating factors in periodontal illness by restoring and maintaining periodontal health through the elimination of gingival bacterial plaque, and the reduction of gingival bleeding, deep pockets, and tooth mobility.[7] The first phases of periodontal rehabilitation are scaling and root planing, which can be done manually or surgically depending on the probing depth of the most serious osseous defects. A third phase, polishing, is carried out on the radicular and dental surfaces to diminish roughness and, consequently, adhesive bacteria.[4,82]

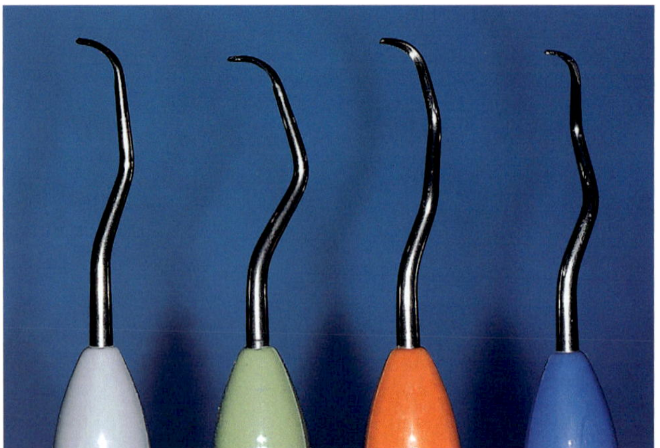

Fig 14-46 Gracey curettes.

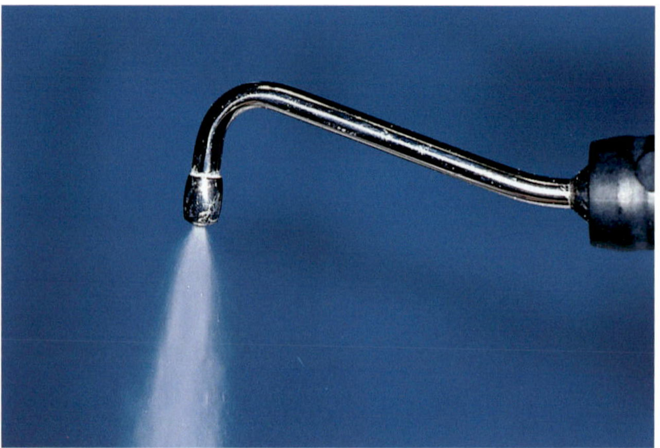

Fig 14-47 Spray of water and bicarbonate powder.

Instruments used in these phases include curettes and scalers, hyposonic, ultrasonic, and rotating instruments, instruments that spray abrasive powder and water, and medicated irrigating solutions and accessories, such as cups, brushes, and polishing pastes.

The frequency with which professional hygiene is needed depends on numerous factors to be determined individually. The literature shows that scaling and radicular smoothing are the most important elements of periodontal rehabilitation. Not all authors agree, however, on which technique is most effective in removing plaque and tartar both above and below the gingiva, which produces the smoothest radicular surfaces, or which causes the least damage to the dental tissues.

Manual instruments

Almost all authors consider the curette to achieve the greatest root smoothing and remove the most cementum.[83] In other research, hand instruments have been shown to be more effective in removing plaque and tartar, even when the elimination of local periodontal irritation factors is excluded.[84] Hand instruments scratch the metal of the prosthetic crown but generally leave the ceramic surfaces intact. The metallic margin may be damaged but less so than with ultrasonic instruments, and the ceramic cervical margin may fracture.[85] Scaling and root-planing (radicular smoothing) are done with the Gracey curette, which must be well sharpened (Fig 14-46). A curette is used to scale near the crowns, moving parallel to the movement of the closure while avoiding crossing the prosthetic margin so as not to damage the restoration margins.[86] Universal currettes or specific curved curettes are preferred because they can go beyond the prosthesis more easily.

Ultrasonic instruments

Ultrasonic instruments (2,300 to 6,300 cycles per second) with plastic-coated tips are efficient in the removal of plaque and tartar around implants without altering the titanium surfaces and the prosthetic structure.

Abrasive spray instruments

These instruments have been shown to be efficient in the removal of plaque and pigments on the surface of the teeth, especially in areas where it is difficult for manual and ultrasonic instruments to reach, such as troughs, crevices, and clefts (Fig 14-47). Studies confirm the increased abrasive effect of these instruments on the cementum and radicular dentin and show the rough surfaces with crater formations. As far as prosthetic restorations are concerned, the literature reports a slight increase in surface roughness of amalgam and gold alloys, for which the effect of the bicarbonate and water spray can be considered clinically minimal.[87] Serious surface damage may be caused even by brief exposure of the acrylic resin and resin composite to the abrasive spray, including considerable increase in roughness, considerable removal of the organic matrices, and evident abrasions.[87]

The action of abrasivespray on ceramic has not always been interpreted the same way in the literature. According to some authors, surface damage is minimal or nonexistent, whereas in more recent research, scratching, indentation, depressions, and broken fragments have been reported, which would make the use of these instruments on ceramic restorations inadvisable.[88]

If abrasive sprays are used correctly and are kept in motion, they do not seem to significantly damage either metal or ceramic restorations. If, however, the spray is used for a longer period of time, surface depression and roughness can appear.

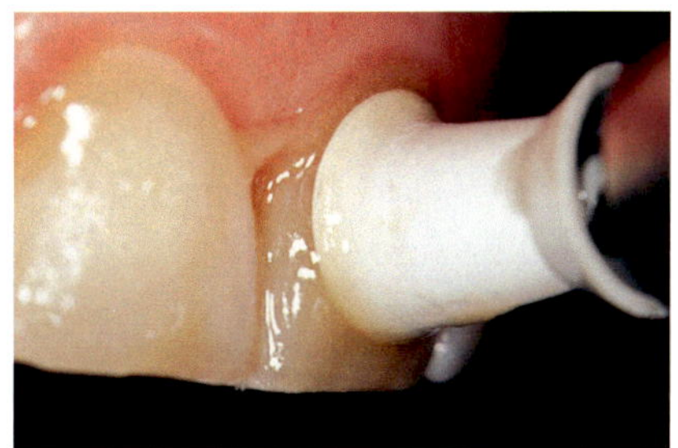

Fig 14-48 Polishing with a rubber cup and low-abrasive prophylaxis paste.

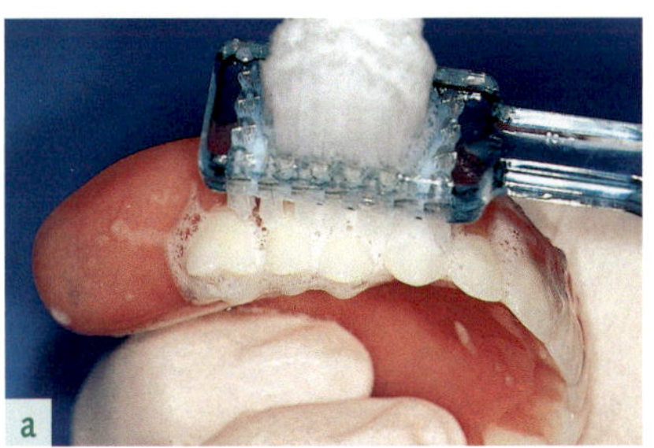
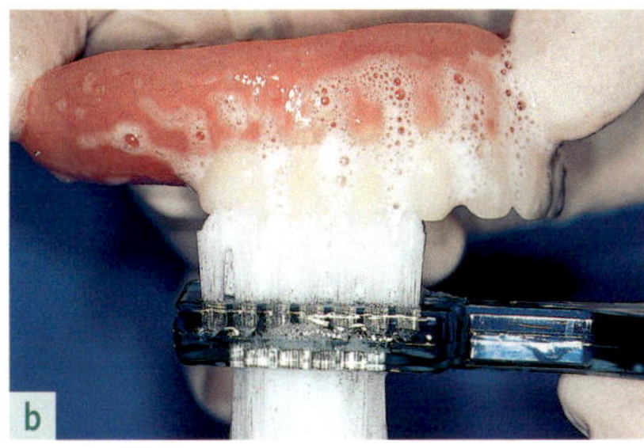
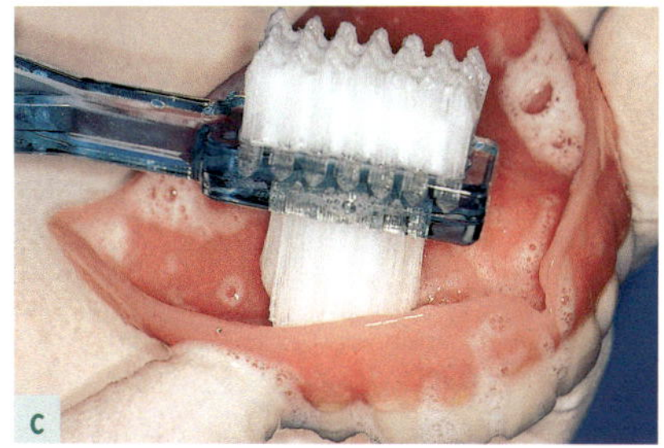

Fig 14-49 Brushing and cleaning a complete maxillary prosthesis with Marseille soap. *(a)* Hard bristles on the external surface. *(b)* Hard bristles on the occlusal surfaces. *(c)* Soft bristles on the internal surface of the prosthetic body.

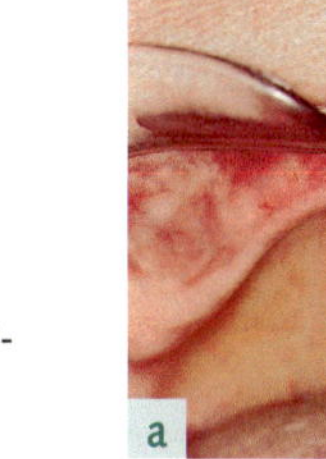
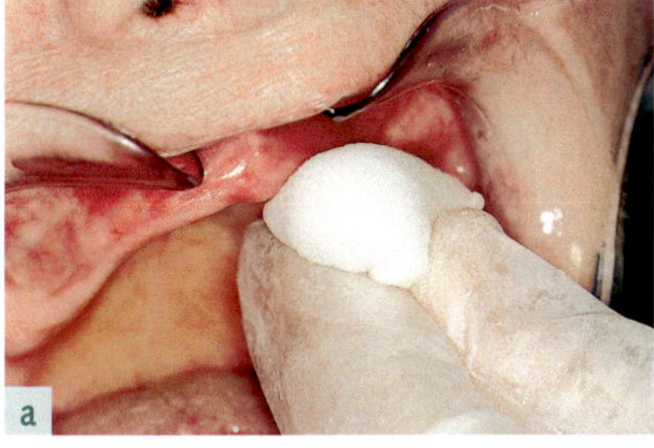
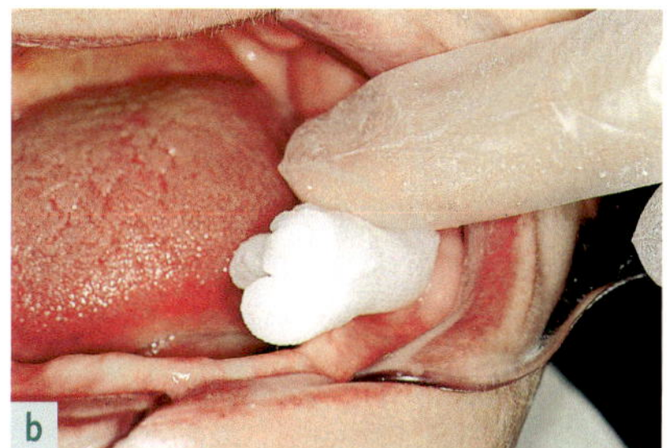

Fig 14-50 Massage and cleaning of edentulous mucosa using gauze soaked in hypertonic sodium chloride solution. The maxilla *(a)* and mandible *(b)* are delicately wiped.

Polishing

Polishing of prosthetic surfaces is recommended to eliminate discoloration and achieve perfectly smoothed surfaces. This step is necessary to limit the accumulation of plaque and tartar in the proximity of the gingival margins. Soft rubber cups are used as well as prophylactic pastes, which are different for each type of material. The degree of abrasiveness can be higher (120 RDA) on ceramic surfaces than on acrylic resin or composite resin surfaces (Fig 14-48).

Subgingival plaque is also removed from the buccal and lingual surfaces with soft rubber cups and from the interproximal surfaces with interproximal toothbrushes, both with a contra-angle.

Patient with a Prosthesis
Complete prosthesis

The formation of plaque on the surfaces of the complete prosthesis that comes into contact with the oral mucosa is the main cause of prosthetic stomatitis.[17,89] There are three ways of controlling plaque on this surface: *(1)* mechanical control, *(2)* chemical control, and *(3)* correct wearing of the prosthesis.[90,91] Patients must be instructed as to how to remove the prosthesis after every meal and how to carefully brush with Marseille soap or nonabrasive toothpaste before reinserting it in the oral cavity (Fig 14-49).

The use of gauze with hypertonic sodium chloride solution, with its antiedematous properties, is recommended for cleaning and massaging the edentulous mucosa on which the prosthesis rests (Fig 14-50).

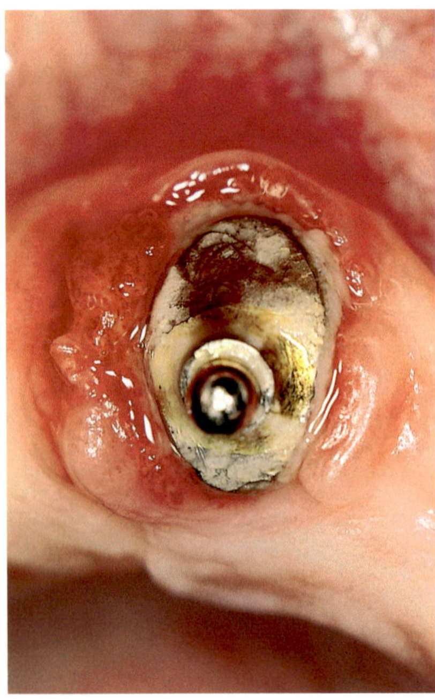
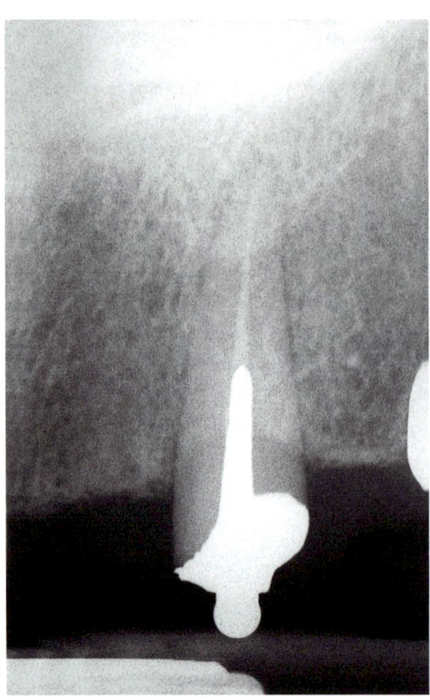

Fig 14-51 Ball attachment for an overdenture that is seriously compromised due to lack of hygiene. *(a)* Clinical view. *(b)* Radiograph.

Because of the frequent negligence of elderly people who have a complete prosthesis, a large number of chemical cleaning substances have been introduced, such as alkaline peroxide, alkaline hypochloride, acids, disinfectants, and enzymes, each of which has adverse effects.[90] To eliminate the disadvantages of the chemical substances listed above, surface reactants and antibacterial agents such as chlorhexidine, benzoic acid, alcohol, eucalyptus, menthol, metasalicylic, thymol, amino alcohol, and glutaraldehyde can be used. These treatments should be combined with mechanical removal of plaque.[91,92]

Continual wear of a complete prosthesis provokes stomatitis and traumatizes the oral mucosa. Mechanical irritation can increase the turnover of the epithelial cells, making the epithelial surface less keratinized and more permeable to toxins and microbic antigens. In prosthetic stomatitis linked to *Candida albicans*, the most important therapeutic measure is a rigorous oral and prosthetic hygiene regimen. Stomatitis is often associated with fungal colonies in the plaque both on the oral mucosa and prosthetic surfaces in contact with the mucosa. Intraoral treatment with antibiotics and antimycotic topical therapy (eg, nystatin, miconazole, amphotericin B, and ketoconazole) and extraoral disinfection of the removable prosthesis with antimicrobial agents (eg, 0.2% chlorhexidine solution or 1% hypochlorite solution) should be used[90,92,93] (see chapter 5).

Overdentures

The abutment teeth of those who have an overdenture or perio-overdenture also run a high risk of decay and periodontal disease because of the greater proliferation of bacteria, such as *Streptococcus* and *Actinomycetales* in the areas of contact between the residual teeth and the prosthesis, where it is also difficult to maintain good plaque control[11,94,95] (Fig 14-51). The bacterial flora of the prosthetic surfaces contain high percentages of *Lactobacillus*, *S mutans*, and *Candida*, which explains the unpredictability of the decay process on teeth in close contact with the prosthetic surfaces.[96]

Longitudinal studies have shown that it is possible to obtain reasonable levels of oral and prosthetic hygiene in elderly people who have overdentures[11,20] (Figs 14-52 to 14-54).

Plaque control can also be effective if chemical agents are used, both on the prosthetic abutments and on the prosthesis itself.[9,79] If the prosthesis is not worn at night, the risk of decay of the natural teeth is reduced because the plaque accumulates less quickly and because the antibodies and antibacterial mechanisms of the saliva protect the abutment teeth.[11,77,97] Motivating patient hygiene before starting this treatment is fundamental, and follow-ups every 3 to 6 months must be planned to evaluate the prosthesis.[9,94-99]

After having constructed the prosthesis, preventive measures in patients who have overdentures are aimed at controlling bacterial plaque on the exposed dentin and radicular surfaces of the abutment teeth.[100]

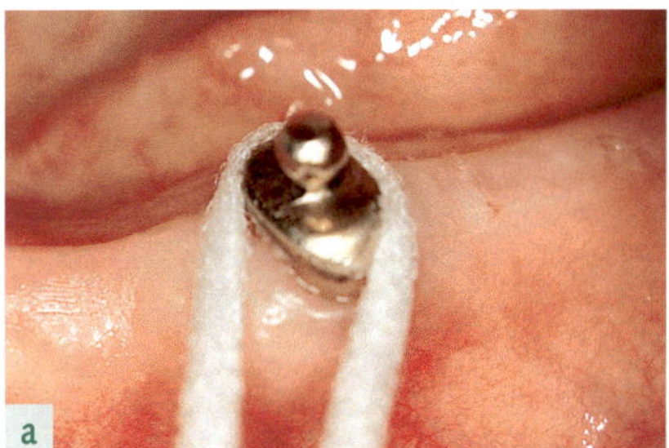 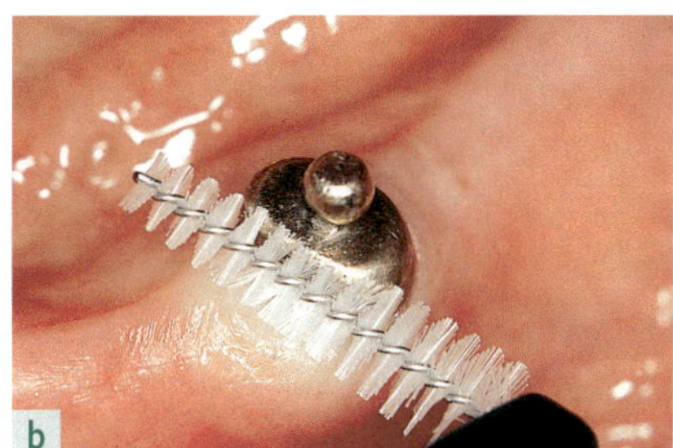 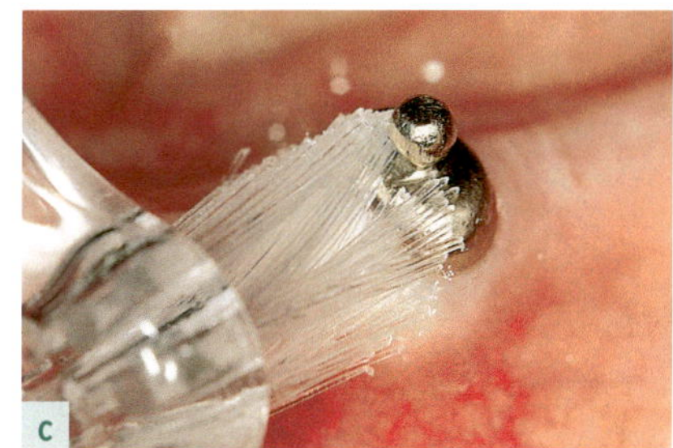

Fig 14-52 Oral hygiene methods to clean the ball attachment for an overdenture. *(a)* Spongy interdental floss. *(b)* Conic interdental brush. *(c)* Monotuft toothbrush.

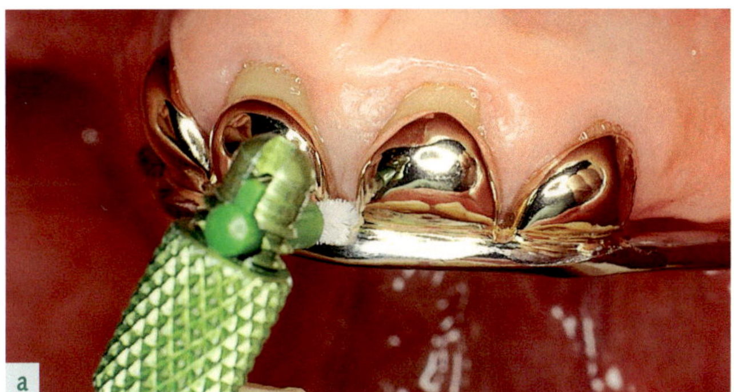 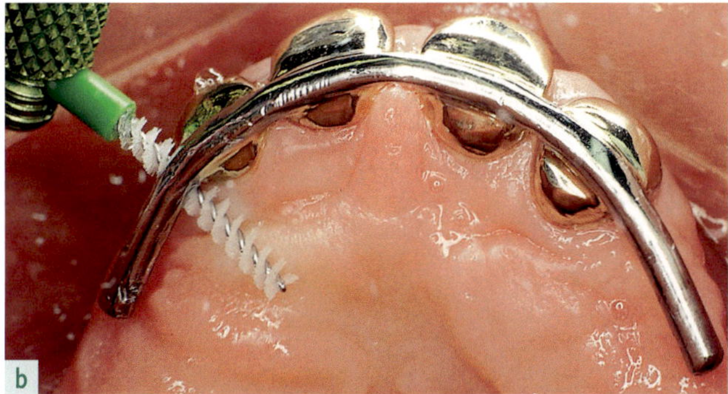

Fig 14-53 Using an interdental brush to clean an overdenture retainer bar. *(a)* Labial view. *(b)* Occlusal view.

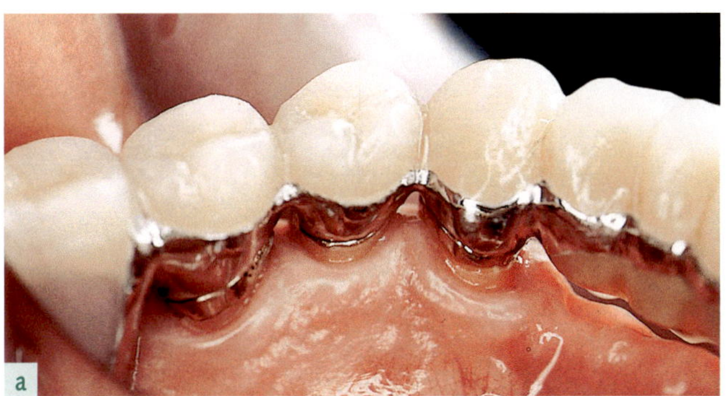 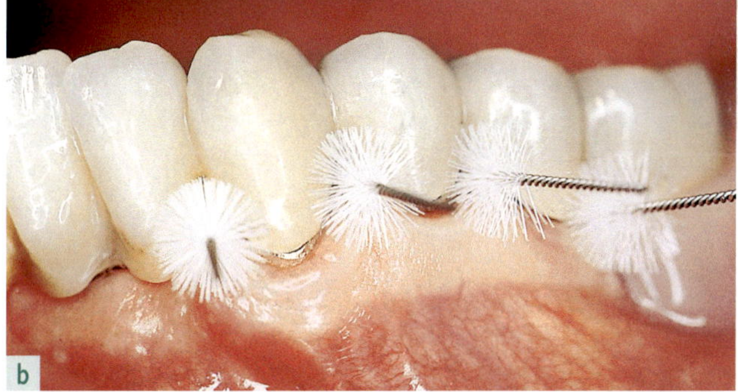

Fig 14-54 Using an interdental brush on a perioverdenture. *(a)* Lingual view. *(b)* Buccal view with interdental brush in the interproximal spaces.

Removable partial denture

It is important to monitor hygiene in areas of the RPD that come into contact with the residual structures and the abutment teeth, especially at the points of gingival recession where radicular surfaces may be exposed.[101]

Periodontal damage and decay of the abutment teeth may result if the RPD has not been well designed or is not sufficiently cleaned intraorally and extraorally[10,33,102-104] (Figs 14-55 and 14-56). As a prophylaxis, the patient should be instructed to use fluoride gel for the clasps, supports, and guides that come into contact with the abutment teeth[80,81] (Fig 14-57).

During the design stage, it is necessary to respect the free gingival margin and ensure that the functional loads are transmitted as vertically as possible to the abutment teeth and edentulous crests.[15,34,105] The RPD on its own does not cause deterioration of the periodontium through the increase of the pressure loads, but together with inflammation causes serious damage to the residual structures of the oral cavity.[10,13,101,103,105]

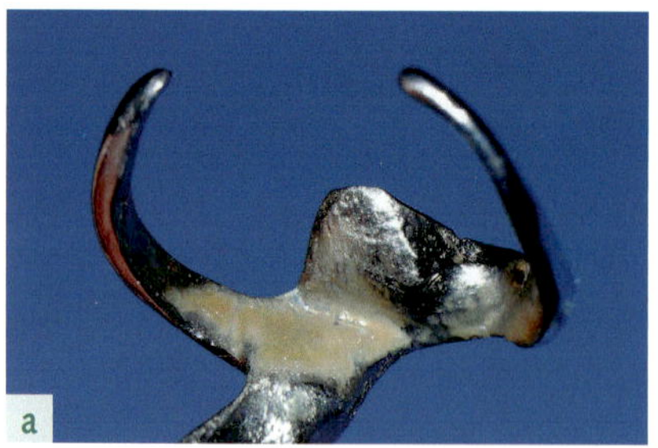

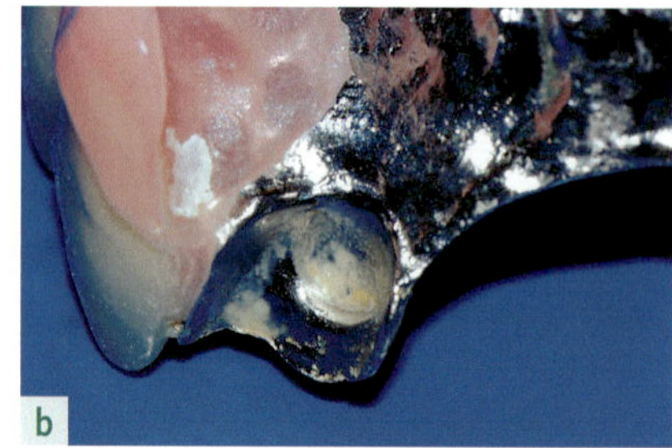

Fig 14-55 Tartar deposit on the metal structure of an RPD. *(a)* Clasp. *(b)* Support and guide plane.

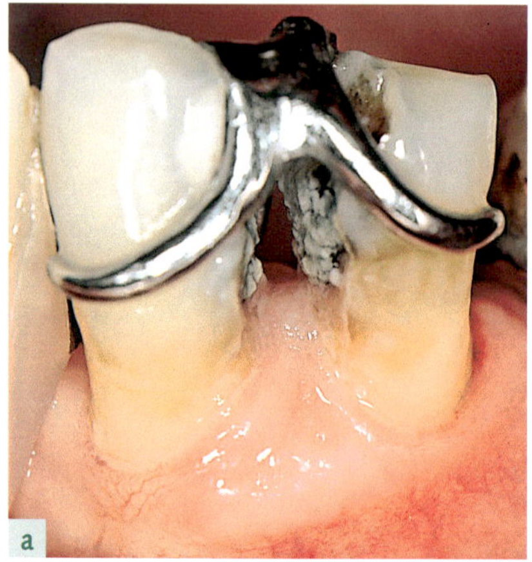

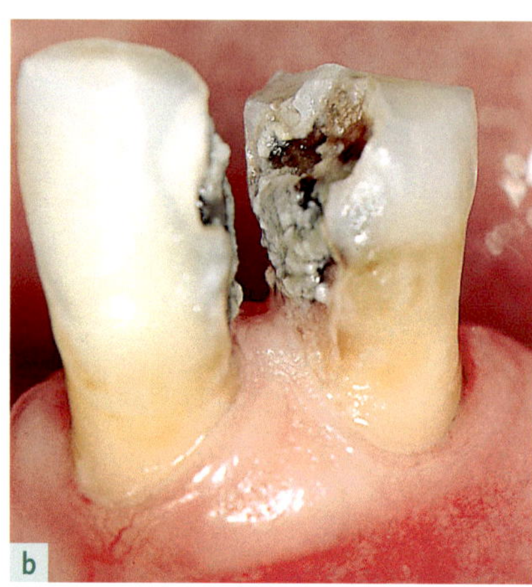

Fig 14-56 Caries lesions caused by an RPD that has not bee properly cleaned. *(a)* Mandibular left canine and first premolar were restored with Bonwill double clasps. *(b)* Caries lesions destroying the teeth.

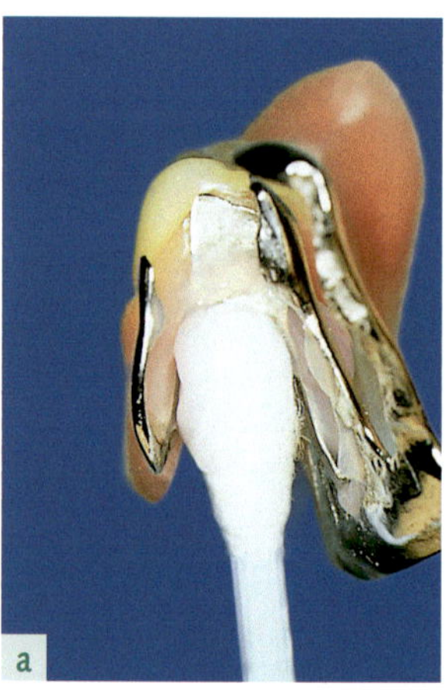

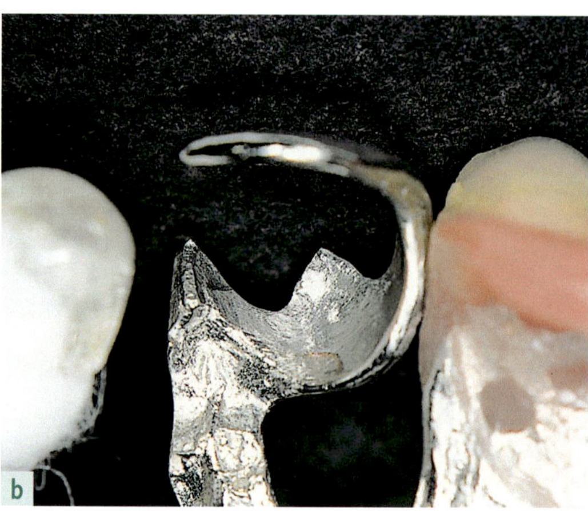

Fig 14-57 Topical application of fluoride gel on the metal parts of an RPD that come in contact with the dental tissues. *(a)* Guide plane and precision attachment. *(b)* Clasps and support.

Fixed partial denture

The fixed partial denture (FPD) must be designed to be functional, esthetic, and easy to maintain. An incorrect emergence profile and the subgingival margins, for example, encourage the retention and accumulation of bacterial plaque, which can cause marginal gingivitis and consequently, loss of periodontal attachment and bone destruction.[21,36,38,41,42,74,106]

Instruction on the use of chlorhexidine, interproximal toothbrushes, monotuft brushes, and spongy interproximal floss should be given, taking into consideration the design of the denture, the anatomy of the interproximal spaces, and the positioning of the coronal margins[63,73,74,76] (Figs 14-58 to 14-62).

Close contact between the denture base and edentulous crest should be established in elderly patients who have poor manual skills and consequently find it difficult to use floss. Likewise, interproximal spaces that are very tight and limit the use of more comfortable interproximal toothbrushes should be rehabilitated.[36,40]

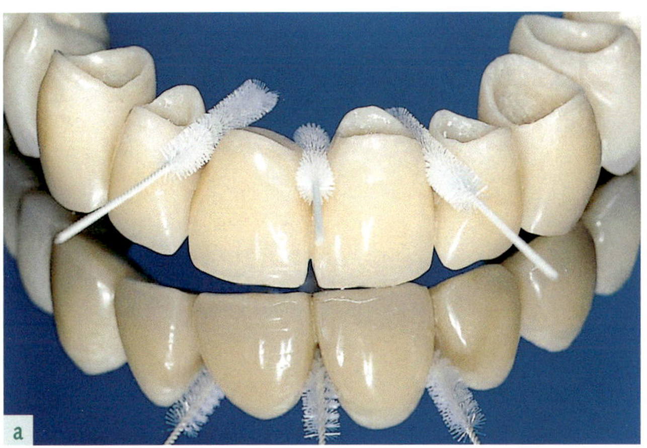
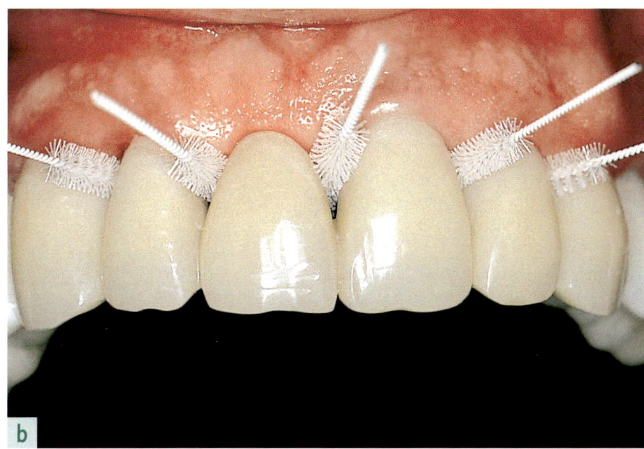

Fig 14-58 Provisional prosthesis in resin must allow easy precise cleaning. Interproximal spaces must permit the passage of the interdental brush. *(a)* Checking the interdental spaces in the laboratory. *(b)* Checking the interdental spaces of the prosthesis in the mouth.

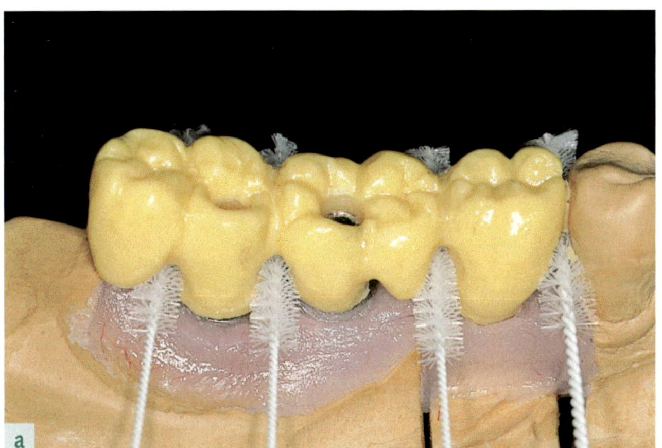
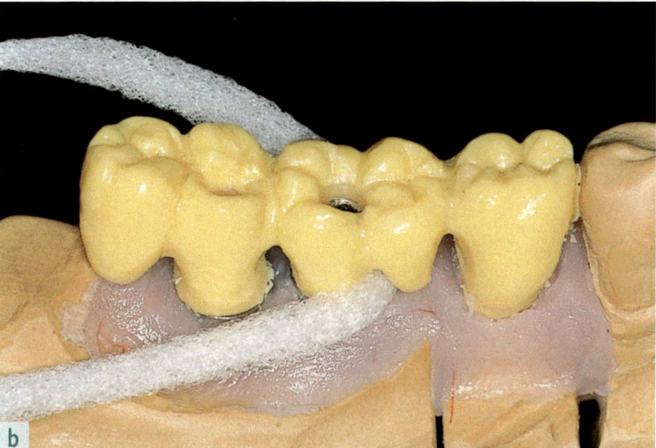

Fig 14-59 Waxing of the metal structure for a fixed partial denture must take into account the interproximal spaces and the correct distance from the edentulous ridge to ensure proper construction. *(a)* Testing with interdental brushes. *(b)* Testing with spongy dental floss.

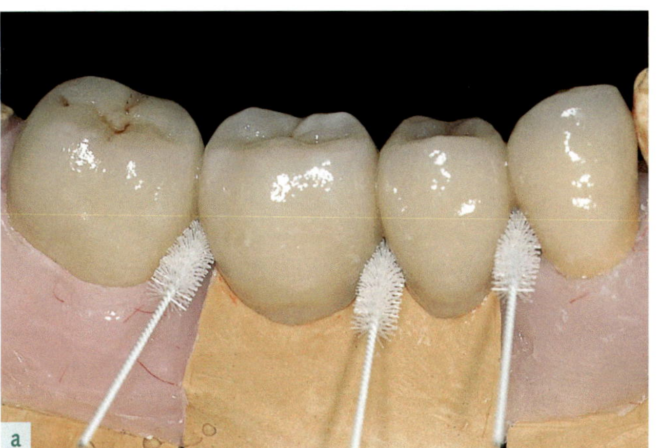
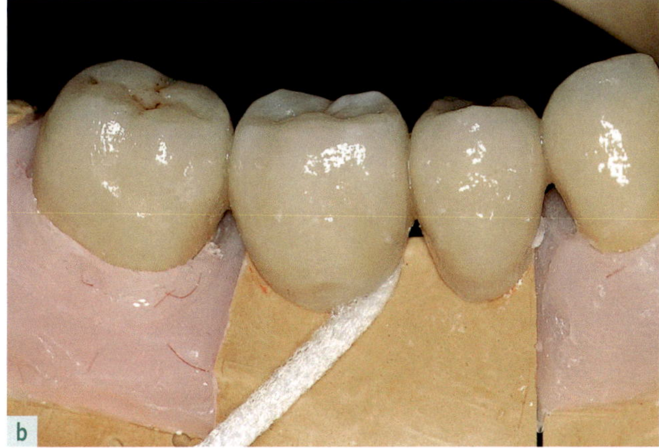

Fig 14-60 The ceramic fixed partial denture must provide the correct interproximal spaces and adaptation of the teeth on the distal extension of the RPD. *(a)* Testing interdental brushes. *(b)* Testing spongy dental floss.

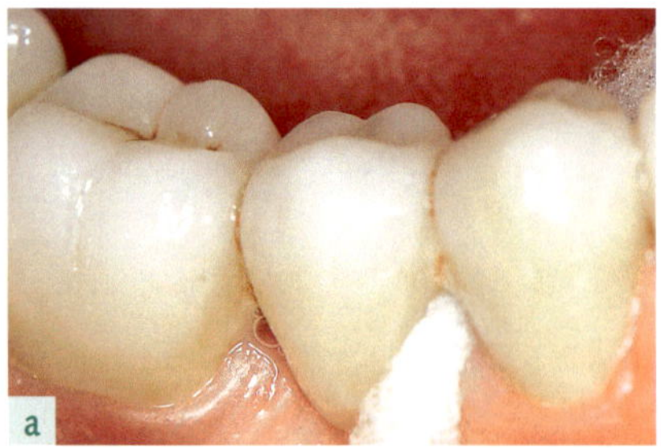

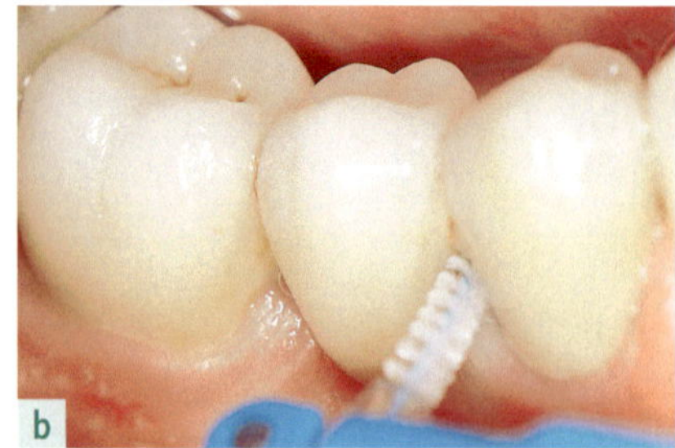

Fig 14-61 Cleaning interproximal spaces of a metal-ceramic fixed partial denture. *(a)* Use of spongy floss with rigid tips. *(b)* Use of an interdental brush.

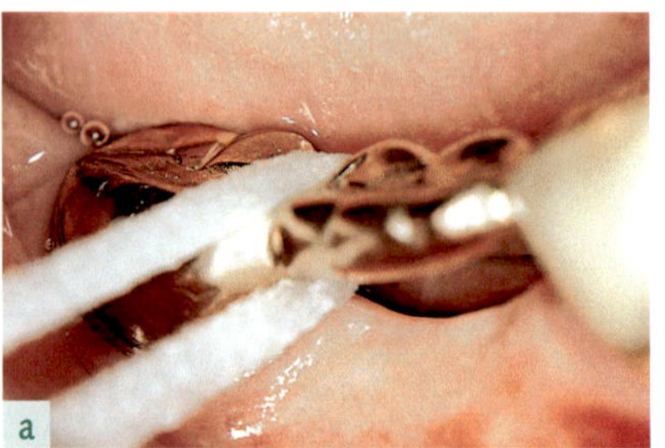

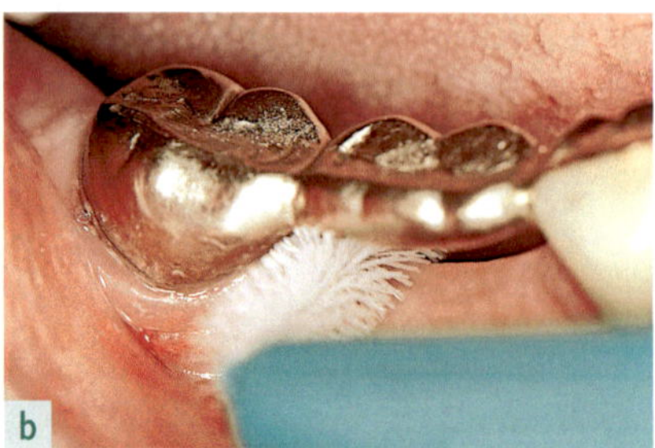

Fig 14-62 Cleaning the interproximal spaces of a fixed partial denture in gold alloy. *(a)* Spongy floss with rigid tips. *(b)* An interdental brush.

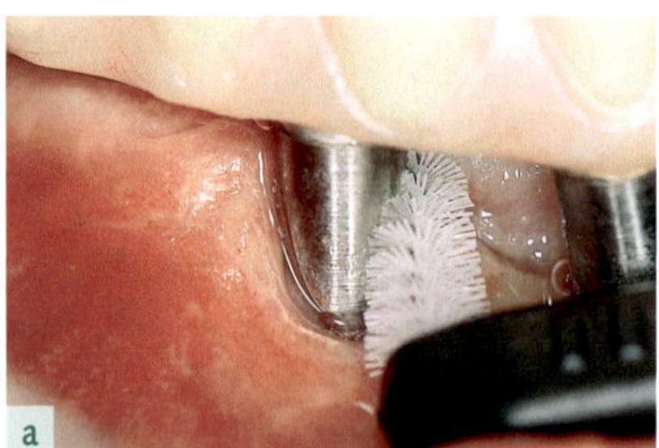

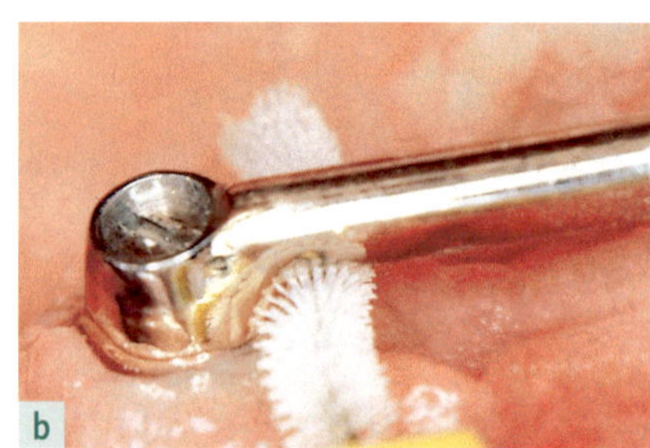

Fig 14-63 Interdental brush with plastic-coated metal core for cleaning titanium-abutment *(a)* and Dolder bar *(b)*.

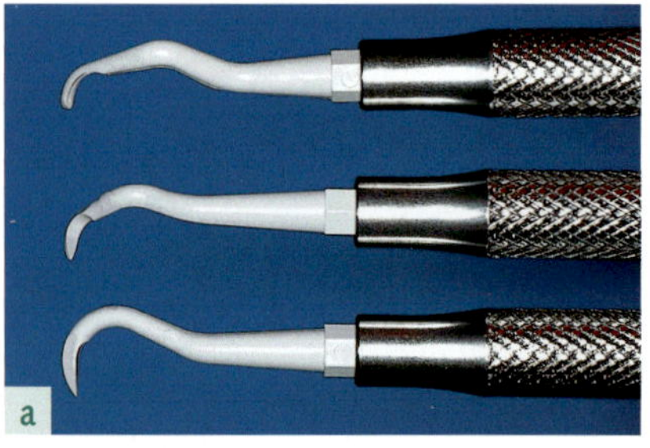

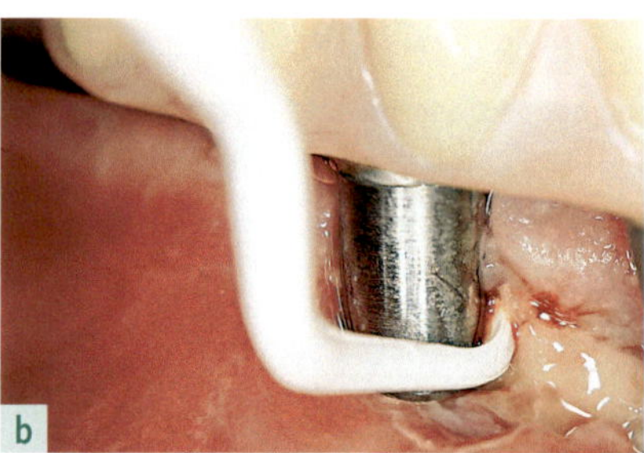

Fig 14-64 Plastic curettes for professional cleaning of implants. *(a)* Available curette designs. *(b)* Clinical use on an abutment.

Implant-supported prostheses

Oral hygiene for these patients is the same as for patients with a fixed partial denture (FPD) or an RPD[8,107-111] (Fig 14-63). Particular attention should be given to the effects of smoking and tobacco on the peri-implant tissues: Patients who smoke have a higher index of bleeding, deeper probing depths, and greater degrees of osseous resorption, with greater risks of developing peri-implantitis, especially in the maxilla.[110]

During professional hygiene sessions it is necessary to pay special attention to the removal of tartar, using instruments made of polymerized materials so as not to scratch or contami-

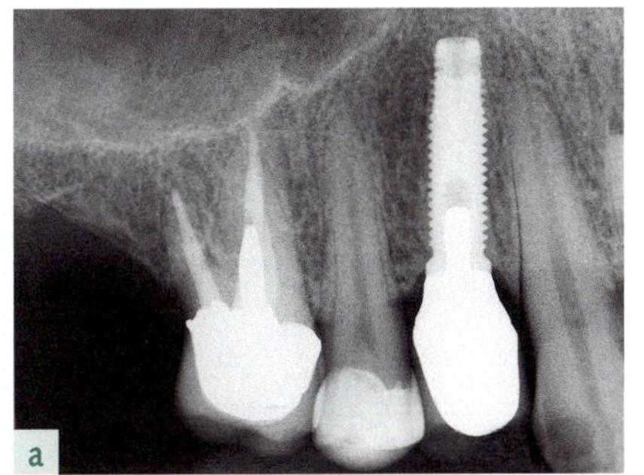
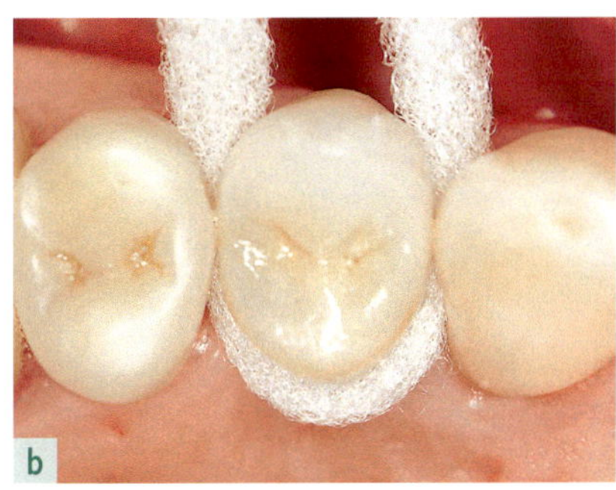

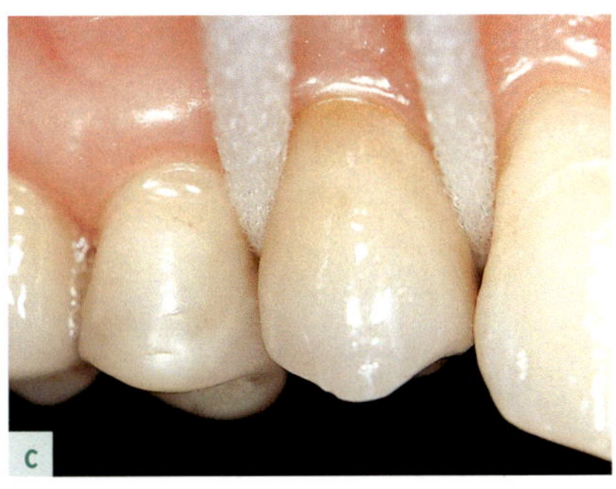
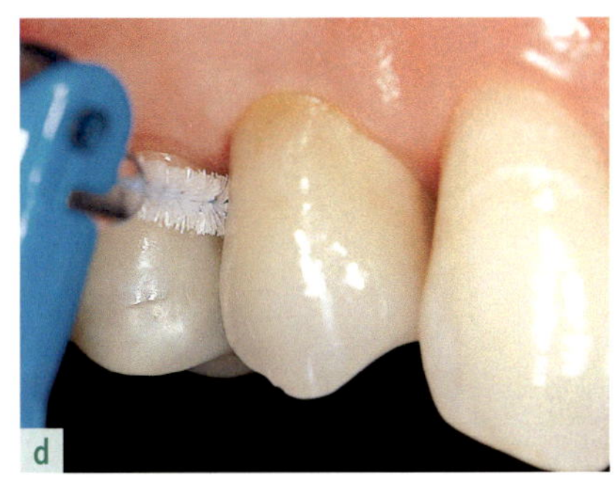

Fig 14-65 Clinical case involving maxillary restorations with an implant in the right first premolar site, a ceramic onlay on the right second premolar, and a metal-ceramic crown on the right first molar. *(a)* Radiographic examination. *(b)* Occlusal view of use of spongy floss. *(c)* Buccal view of spongy floss. *(d)* Interdental brush with a plastic-coated metal core .

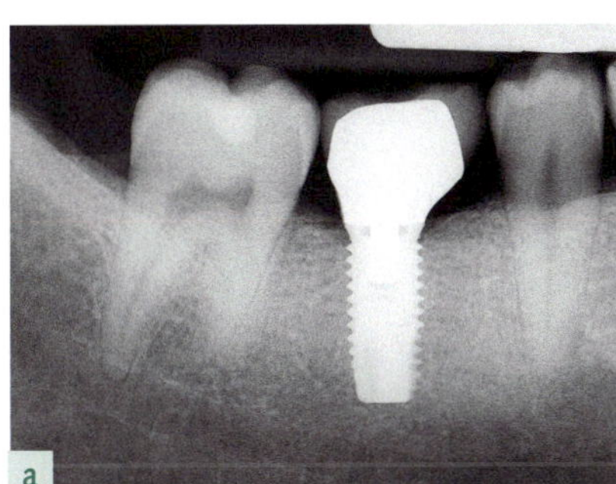
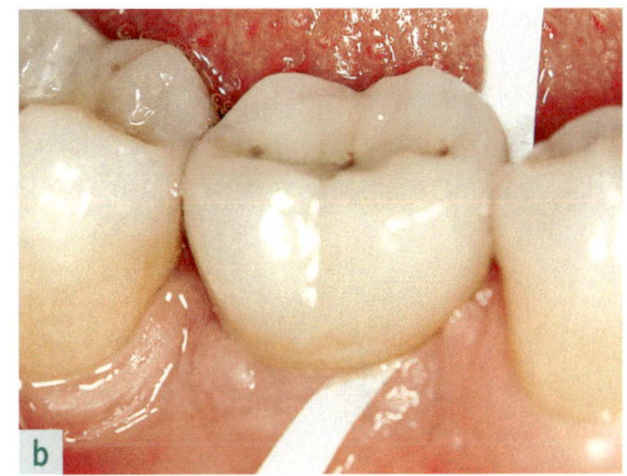

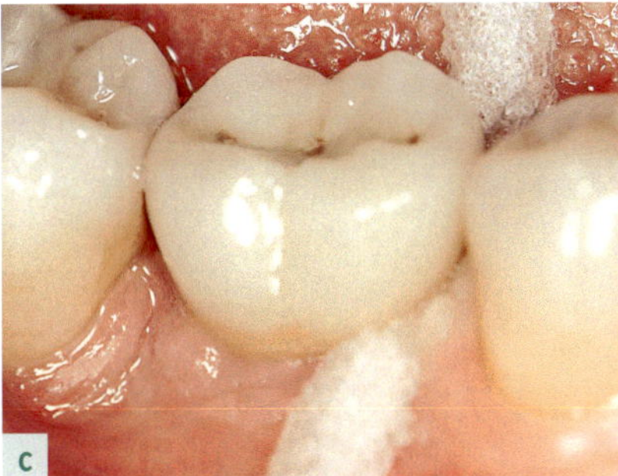
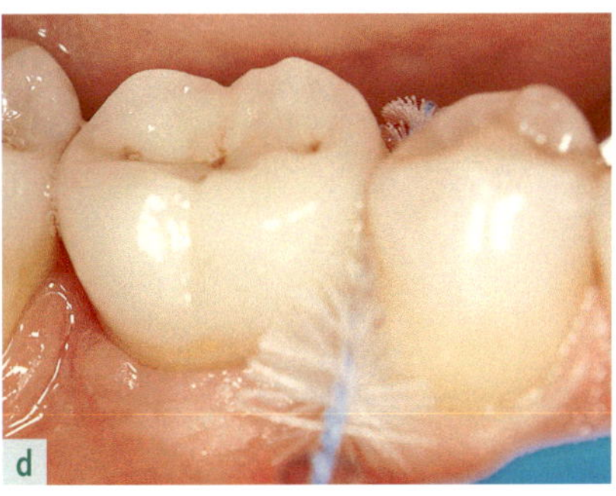

Fig 14-66 Clinical case involving an implant in the mandibular right first molar site. *(a)* Radiographic examination. *(b)* Tape floss for cleaning the deepest part of the transmucosal pathway. *(c)* Spongy floss for cleaning the ceramic surface, not joined to the abutment. *(d)* Interdental brush with plastic-coated metal core.

nate the relatively soft and spongy titanium surface with other metals.[111,112] There are various types of curettes to choose from. Teflon curettes, compared with those in plastic, have excellent rigidity, which enables them to easily remove calcified residue from the implant surfaces. The tips of these curettes are sometimes too big, which makes it difficult to use them subgingivally (Fig 14-64). Hyposonic ablators with plastic tips may also be used effectively. Microscopic analysis of the surfaces treated with these instruments has shown that the surface alterations were minimal and disappeared after polishing with rubber cups and prophylactic pastes.[112,113]

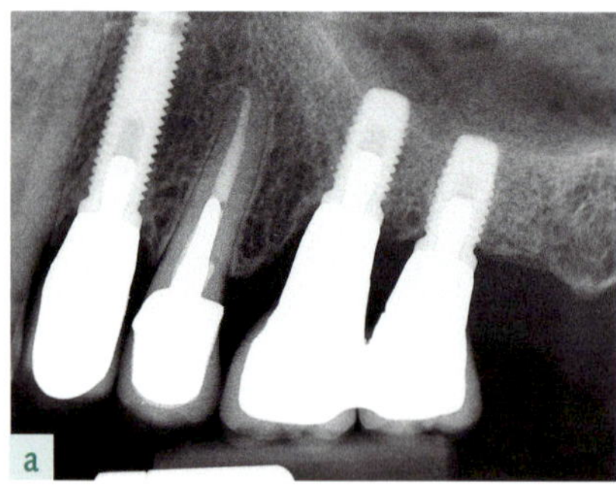

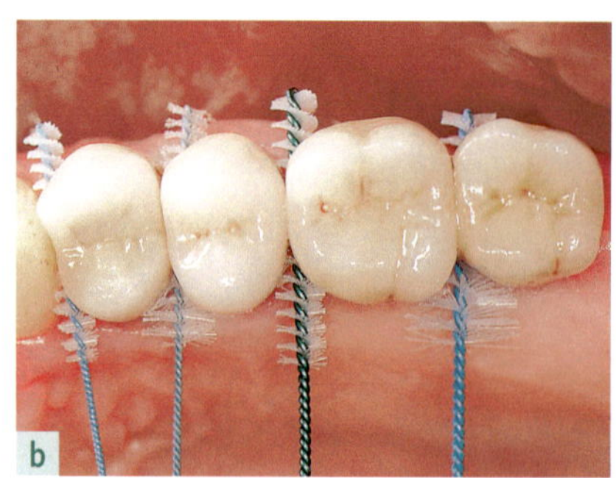

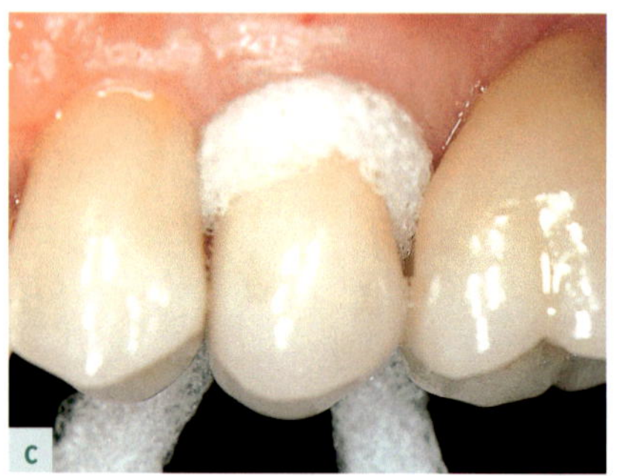

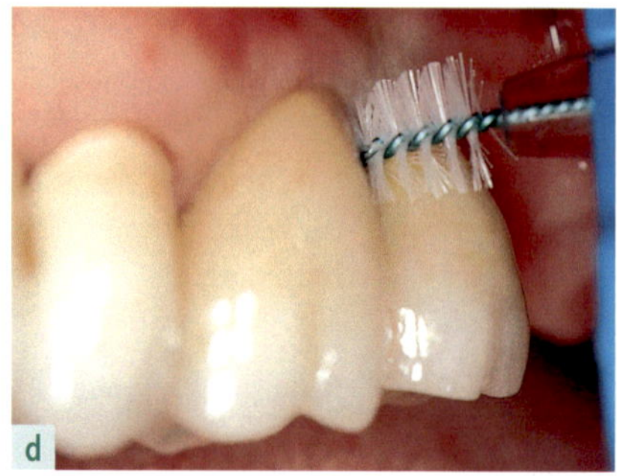

Fig 14-67 Clinical case involving maxillary restorations with. implants in the left first premolar and first and second molar sites and a metal-ceramic crown on the left second premolar. *(a)* Radiograph examination. *(b)* Occlusal view of interdental brushes with a plastic-coated metal core. *(c)* Buccal view of spongy floss. *(d)* Buccal view of interdental brush with plastic-coated metal core.

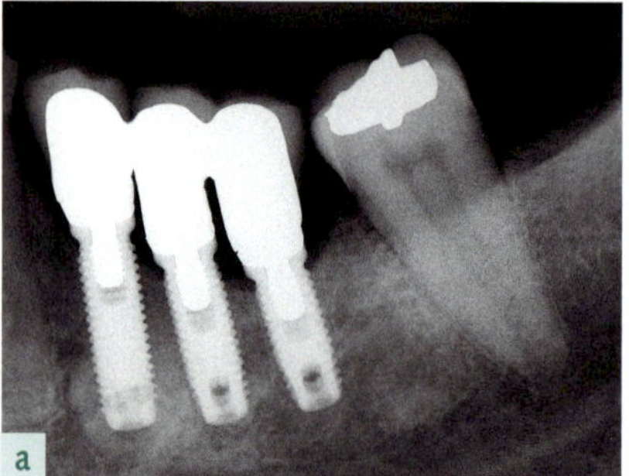

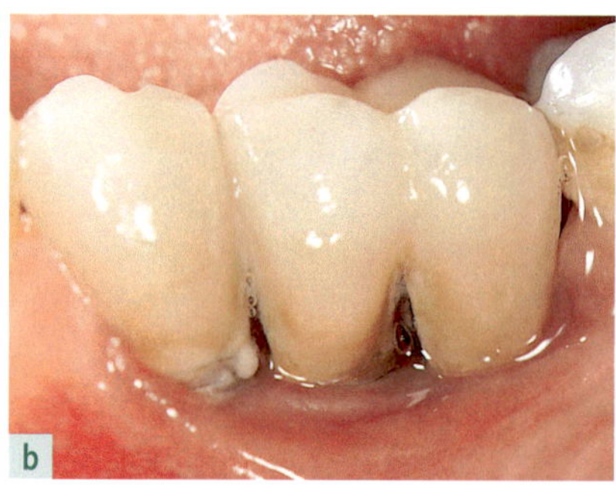

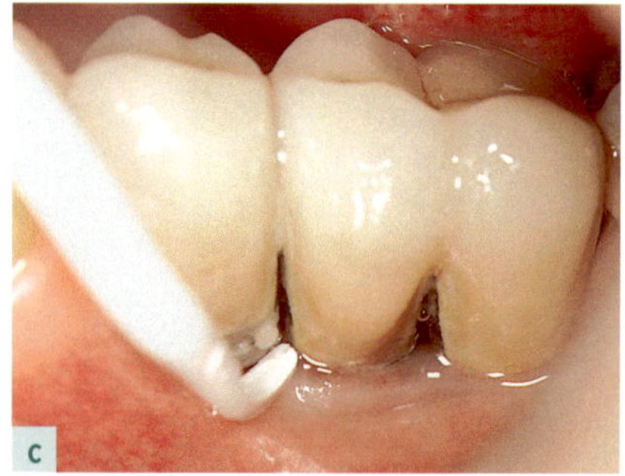

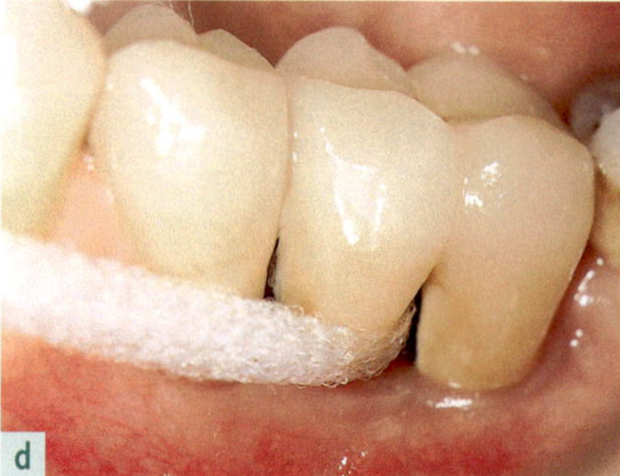

Fig 14-68 Clinical case involving implants in the mandibular left first and second premolar and first molar sites. *(a)* Radiographic examination. *(b)* Deposits of plaque and tartar due to teeth being too close together and thus preventing the passage of the interdental brush between the first and second premolar. *(c)* Professional hygiene with a plastic curette. *(d)* Home care instruction using spongy floss.

Periodic irrigation with 0.12% to 0.2% chlorhexidine solutions can also be carried out in the sulcus around the implant if combined with mechanical therapy to obtain chemical control of the peri-implant bacterial flora. Subgingival irrigation is an effective means of upkeep of the implant surfaces in the presence of rough areas.

Clinical cases

Figures 14-65 to 14-68 show four cases in which oral hygiene techniques were used for the maintenance of fixed prostheses supported by osseointegrated implants.

266

References

1. Renner R. Post-treatment maintenance care. In: Wall B, Kiser A, Carlsson GE (eds). Prosthodontics: Principles and Management Strategies. Baltimore: Mosby, 1996:161. Cat. 7
2. Socransky SS. Relationship of bacteria to the etiology of periodontal disease. J Dent Res 1970;49:203–222. Cat. 7
3. Lang NP, Cumming BR, Löe H. Toothbrushing frequency as it relates to plaque development and gingival health. J Periodontol 1973;44:396–405. Cat. 3
4. Adriaens PE, De Boever JA, Loesche WJ. Bacterial invasion in root cementum and radicular dentin of periodontally diseased teeth in humans. A reservoir of periodontopathic bacteria. J Periodontol 1988;59:222–230. Cat. 2
5. Gibbons RJ. Bacterial adhesion to oral tissues: A model for infectious diseases. J Dent Res 1989;68:750–760. Cat. 6
6. Ramberg P, Lindhe J, Dahlën G, Volpe AR. The influence of gingival inflammation on de novo plaque formation. J Clin Periodontol 1994;21:51–56. Cat. 3
7. Erpenstein H. The role of the prosthodontist in the treatment of periodontal disease. Int Dent J 1986;36:18–29. Cat. 7
8. Palmer R, Palmer P, Howe L. Complications and maintenance. Br Dent J 1999;187:653–658. Cat. 4
9. Ettinger RL, Taylor TD, Scandrett FR. Treatment needs of overdenture patients in a longitudinal study: Five-year results. J Prosthet Dent 1984;52:532–537. Cat. 3
10. Bergman B, Hugoson A, Olsson CO. A 25 year longitudinal study of patients treated with removable partial dentures. J Oral Rehabil 1995;22:595–599. Cat. 3
11. Budtz-Jørgensen E. Prognosis of overdenture abutments in elderly patients with controlled oral hygiene. A 5 year study. J Oral Rehabil 1995;22:3–8. Cat. 3
12. Yi SW, Ericsson I., Carlsson G, Wennström JL. Long-term follow-up of cross-arch fixed partial dentures in patients with advanced periodontal destruction. Acta Odontol Scand 1995;53:242–248. Cat. 4
13. Carlsson GE, Hedegärd B, Koivumaa KK. Studies in partial dental prosthesis. IV: Final results of a 4-year longitudinal investigation of dentogingivally supported partial dentures. Acta Odontol Scand 1965;23:443–472. Cat. 3
14. Grasso JE, Nalbandian J, Sanford C, Bailit H. Effect of restoration quality on periodontal health. J Prosthet Dent 1985;53:14–19. Cat. 4
15. Roberts BW. The recall system. A necessary part of a partial denture service. Br Dent J 1980;149:46–48. Cat. 7
16. Reiker J, van der Velden U, Barendregt DS, Loos BG. A cross-sectional study into the prevalence of root caries in periodontal maintenance patients. J Clin Periodontol 1999;26:26–32. Cat. 4
17. Pietrokovski J, Azuelos J, Tau S, Mostavoy R. Oral findings in elderly nursing home resident in selected countries: Oral hygiene conditions and plaque accumulation on denture surfaces. J Prosthet Dent 1995;73:136–141. Cat. 4
18. Haas R, Haimböck W, Mailath G, Watzek G. The relationship of smoking on peri-implant tissue: A retrospective study. J Prosthet Dent 1996; 76: 592–596. Cat. 4
19. Knabe C, Kram P. Dental care for institutionalized geriatric patients in Germany. J Oral Rehabil 1997; 24: 909–912. Cat. 4
20. Bergman B, Hugoson A, Olsson CO. Caries, periodontal and prosthetic findings in patients with removable partial dentures: A ten-year longitudinal study. J Prosthet Dent 1982;48:506–514. Cat. 3
21. Valderhaug J, Ellingsen JE, Jokstad A. Oral hygiene, periodontal conditions and carious lesions in patients treated with dental bridges. J Clin Periodontol 1993;20:482–489. Cat. 3
22. Van Rijkom HM, Truin GJ, van't Hof MA. A meta-analysis of clinical studies on the caries-inhibiting effect of chlorhexidine treatment. J Dent Res 1996;75:790–795. Cat. M1
23. Christie P, Claffey N, Renvert S. The use of 0.2% chlorhexidine in the absence of a structured mechanical regimen of oral hygiene following the non-surgical treatment of periodontitis. J Clin Periodontol 1998;25:15–23. Cat. 2
24. Löe H, Theilade E, Jensen SB. Experimental gingivitis in man. J Periodontol 1965; 36: 177–187. Cat. 3
25. Socransky SS, Haffajee AD. The bacterial etiology of destructive periodontal disease: Current concepts. J Periodontol 1992;63: 322–331. Cat. 7
26. Morrison LS, Cobb CM, Kazakos GM, Killoy WJ. Root surface characteristics associated with subgingival placement of monolithic tetracycline-impregnated fibers. J Periodontol 1992;63:137–143. Cat. 2
27. Ramberg P, Furuichi Y, Volpe AR, Gaffar A, Lindhe J. The effect of antimicrobial mouthrinses on de novo plaque formation at sites with healthy and inflamed gingivae. J Clin Periodontol 1996;23:7–11. Cat. 2
28. Somayaji BV, Jariwala U, Jayachandran P, Vidyalakshmi K, Dudhani RV. Evaluation of antimicrobial efficacy and release pattern of tetracycline and metronidazole using a local delivery system. J Periodontol 1998;69:409–413. Cat. 2
29. Ghamrawy EE. Quantitative changes in dental plaque formation related to removable partial dentures. J Oral Rehabil 1976;3: 115–120. Cat. 3
30. Brill N, Tryde G, Stoltze K, El Ghamrawy EA. Ecologic changes in the oral cavity caused by removable partial dentures. J Prosthet Dent 1977;38:138–148. Cat. 3
31. Ghamrawy EE. Qualitative changes in dental plaque formation related to removable partial dentures. J Oral Rehabil 1979;6:183–188. Cat. 3
32. Marsh PD, Percival RS, Challacombe SJ. The influence of denture-wearing and age on the oral microflora. J Dent Res 1992;71: 1374–1381. Cat. 2
33. Mojon P, Rentsch A, Budtz-Jørgensen E. Relationship between prosthodontic status, caries, and periodontal disease in a geriatric population. Int J Prosthodont 1995;8:564–571. Cat. 4
34. Atwood DA. Reduction of residual ridges: A major oral disease entity. J Prosthet Dent 1971;26:266–279. Cat. 9
35. Pissiotis AL, Michalakis KX. An esthetic and hygienic approach to the use of intracoronal attachments as interlocks in fixed prosthodontics. J Prosthet Dent 1998;79:347–349. Cat. 9
36. Gade E. Hygienic problems of fixed restorations. Int Dent J 1963;13:318–330. Cat. 7
37. Hirshberg SM. The relationship of oral hygiene to embrasure and pontic design. A preliminary study. J Prosthet Dent 1972;27: 26–38. Cat. 2
38. Becker CM, Kaldahl WB. Current theories of crown contour, margin placement, and pontic design. J Prosthet Dent 1981;45:268–277. Cat. 7

Follow-up Care of Prostheses

Considerations

The clinician and the patient are jointly responsible for maintaining the health of the remaining teeth and the long life of the prosthesis.[1] The success of the prosthesis depends on the capability of the clinician to instruct and motivate the patient to follow an agreed-upon program of maintenance.[2,3]

Lang[4] stressed the importance of a sequential plan of treatment, including a preliminary period of hygiene intervention and maintenance followed by the treatment and then periodic follow-up. Schärer[5] also advised a three-phase plan comprising an urgent phase, a preprosthetic phase, and a maintenance phase.

An individualized maintenance program must include:

1. Continual motivation to follow hygiene guidelines
2. Instruction on the use of the prosthesis
3. Checking the adaptation of the functional aspects of the prosthesis
4. Correction of function as requested by the patient
5. Professional hygiene appointments
6. Follow-up on the health of remaining teeth
7. Correction of any problems resulting from systemic pathology
8. Treatment for any emergency
9. Adaptation to any structural changes resulting from function or parafunction
10. Treatment of any new pathology

The follow-up program is fundamental for the maintenance of the health of the oral structures and, consequently, the entire stomatognathic apparatus.[6,7]

Biologic Aspects of Maintenance

The frequency of follow-up is influenced by several factors:

- Type, extension, and complexity of the prosthesis
- Capacity of the patient to mainatin adequate control of bacterial plaque
- Biologic changes that modify the patient's general health
- Patient's capacity and psychologic attitude

Aging of the residual tissues must also be considered in the maintenance program.[8]

Physiology of aging

Aging brings with it gradual reduction in sensory and motor functions as well as changes in tissue structure and function. In elderly patients, loading has a significant impact on hard tissues, with an increase in fragility and the development of radicular caries. A reduction in the pulp chamber may result in extensive cervical caries lesions that are asymptomatic. The oral mucosa may become more susceptible to chronic trauma, owing to reduced vascularity and saliva, especially in patients with a removable prosthesis that rests on the mucosa. Frequent ulceration or hypertrophy of the supporting mucosa indicate the necessity for clinical modification and reduction in loading periods.[9,10]

Nutrition

Dietary guidelines should be given to the patient, stressing the importance of limiting the amount of sugar and greasy food. An increase in professional cleanings and a more rigorous home maintenance regimen should be advised as well. Malnutrition can interfere with oral health and the prosthesis. Gastric reflux, frequent vomiting by anorexic or bulimic patients, or excessive consumption of acidic drinks can result in serious damage to the residual teeth and to the mucosa.[11,12] The direct and adverse effects of medications must also be considered. Regular use of or chlorhexidene in mouthrinse, and repair can be made with a sealant after treatment with a coloring agent on the ceramic surface. Detachment of the facets or a small part of the covering can be reconstructed in composite or repaired by replacing the covering after removal of the prosthesis. Reconstruction in composite gives satisfactory esthetic results over a long but variable time. Replacement of the entire ceramic overlay is more complex because of the possible clinical complications due to recementation procedures. The use of ultrasonic devices for dissolving the cement and the instruments used for prosthetic removal must reduce the percentage of accidental fractures of the abutments.

Occlusal evaluation

Evaluation of the occlusal relationships is essential, in particular in subjects who have parafunctional habits. The contacts must be evaluated in a centric position to control the interdental relationships responsible for occusal stability and to verify the integrity of guide grooves.

The position of the occlusal surfaces must be checked as well for possible parafunctional habits, which may affect the occlusal contacts. The occlusal evaluation should also include balancing any occlusal protection plates prepared at the end of treatment.

Emergencies

The most frequent emergencies are fractures of the ceramic covering and loss of adhesion. In such cases the prosthetic body must be removed. Recementing can be done if the clinical condition of the abutment is good and the cause of the detachment is eliminated.

Sometimes the patient will arrive complaining of pain. The source, type, severity, and frequency must be determined. The most common cause of pain is pulpal pathology.

Follow-up of the Implanted-Supported Prosthesis

The follow-up and maintenance of patients wearing a fixed or removable prosthesis must continue in 4- to 6-month periods, depending on the type of implant support and prosthesis.[40]

The preventive measures for health and oral hygiene are the same as for patients with a traditional fixed denture or a removable partial denture.[41-43]

Evaluation of plaque control

Plaque and tartar should be removed without scratching or contaminating the titanium surfaces with metal curettes during professional cleaning. Polymer or Teflon instruments should be used so as not to scratch the implant structure.[44-47]

Particular attention must be paid to the effects of smoking on the peri-implant tissues. Patients who smoke tobacco have more elevated indices of bleeding, depth of probing, and rate of osseous resorption, with major risks of developing peri-implantitis, especially in the maxilla.[48]

Clinical evaluation, radiographs, and emergencies

The follow-up of these patients requires attentive clinical and radiographic evaluation every 3 months and then annually to evaluate the bone morphology, peri-implant spaces, pain, or failure of osseointegration. The evaluation principally concerns mechanical yielding and possible loosened screws.[40]

Emergencies usually involve the peri-implant tissues and the implant components. Purely prosthetic problems are rare. Emergencies of the components relate to fracture of parts of the implant, such as screws or fixed components.

Recording Oral Hygiene and Periodic Controls

See tables 15-1 and 15-2.

Table 15-1 Record of personalized oral hygiene checkup for patients wearing a complete denture or an overdenture

		Controls										
		1st visit	delivery	1 day	3 days	7 days	15 days	45 days	3 months	6 months	...	...
Mucosa												
Inflammation	Absent											
	Localized											
	Diffused											
Atrophic												
Ulceration												
Overdenture implants												
Abutments	Plaque < 20%											
	Plaque > 20%											
	Supragingival tartar											
	Subgingival tartar											
Gingival Inflammation	Absent											
	Hypertrophic											
	Periodontitis											
Total points												
Hygiene												
Brushed	yes											
	no											
Interdental brushes/ Dental floss	yes											
	no											
Prosthetic detergent	yes											
	no											
Mouthrinse	yes											
	no											
Brushes the body of the prosthesis	yes											
	no											
Professional cleaning	yes											
	no											
Total points												
Clinical evaluation												
Stabilized	Date											
Retention	Date											
Occlusal contacts	Date											
Radiologic evaluation												
Technique	Observations											
Technique	Observations											
Technique	Observations											
Technique	Observations											

Table 15-2 Record of personalized checkup for patients wearing a removable partial denture, a fixed denture, or an implant-supported denture

		Controls										
		1st visit	delivery	1 day	3 days	7 days	15 days	45 days	3 months	6 months	...	...
Bacterial plaque	Absent											
	Present < 20%											
	Present > 20%											
Tartar	Plaque > 20%											
	Tartar above gingiva											
	Tartar below gingiva											
Gingival inflammation	Absent											
	Gingiva hypertrophic											
	Periodontitis											
Mucosa	Normal											
	Inflamed											
	Hypertrophic/ulcerated											
Total points												
Hygiene												
Brushing	yes											
	no											
Dental floss	yes											
	no											
Interdental brush	yes											
	no											
Mouthrinse	yes											
	no											
Brushing body of prosthesis	yes											
	no											
Professional cleaning	yes											
	no											
Total points												
Clinical evaluation												
Residual teeth	Date											
Prosthesis	Date											
Occlusal contacts	Date											
Radiologic evaluation												
Technique	Observations											
Technique	Observations											
Technique	Observations											
Technique	Observations											

References

1. Roberts BW. The recall system: A necessary part of a partial denture service. Br Dent J 1980;149:46–48. Cat. 9

2. Ettinger RL, Beck JD, Jakobsen J. Removable prosthodontic treatment needs: A survey. J Prosthet Dent 1984;51:419–427. Cat. 4

3. Weintraub AT. Dental needs and dental service use patterns of an elderly edentulous population. J Prosthet Dent 1985;54:226–232. Cat. 4

4. Lang NP, et al. Corone e ponti: Programmazione sinottica. Milano: Masson, 1995. Cat. 7

5. Schärer P, Strub J, Belser U. Elementi fondamentali della moderna riabilitazione protesica con corone e ponti. Milano: Scienza e Tecnica Dentistica Edizioni Internazionali, 1988. Cat. 7

6. Ghamrawy E. Quantitative changes in dental plaque formation related to removable partial dentures. J Oral Rehabil 1976;3: 115–120. Cat. 4

7. Ghamrawy E. Qualitative changes in dental plaque formation related to removable partial dentures. J Oral Rehabil 1979;6: 183–88. Cat. 4

8. Renner R. Post-treatment maintenence care. In: Öwall B, Käyser A, Carlsson GE (eds). Prosthodontics. Principles and Management Strategies. London; Baltimore: Mosby-Wolfe, 1996:161–177. Cat. 7

9. Iacopino AM, Wathen WB. Geriatric prosthodontics: an overview. Part I. Pretreatment considerations. Quintessence Int 1993;24: 259–266. Cat. 7

10. Iacopino AM, Wathen WB. Geriatric prosthodontics: an overview. Part II. Treatment considerations. Quintessence Int 1993b;24: 353–361. Cat. 7

11. Eccles JD, Jenkins WG. Dental erosion and diet. J Dent 1974;2:153–159. Cat. 7

12. Hellstrom I. Oral complications in anorexia nervosa. Scand J Dent Res 1977;85:71–86. Cat. 7

13. Bergman B, Hugoson A, Olsson CO, Caries and periodontal status in patients fitted with removable partial dentures. J Clin Periodontol 1977;4:134–146. Cat. 4

14. Yusof Z, Isa Z, Periodontal status of the teeth in contact with denture in removable partial denture wearers. J Oral Rehabil 1994;21:77–86. Cat. 4

15. Yeung ALP, Lo ECM, Chow TW, Clark RK. Oral status of patients 5-6 years after placement of cobalt–chromium removable partial dentures. J Oral Rehabil 2000;27:183–189. Cat. 3

16. Bergman B. Periodontal reaction related to removable partial dentures: A literature rewiew. J Prosthet Dent 1987;58:454–458. Cat. 7

17. Jacobson TE. Rotational path partial denture design: A 10-years clinical follow-up. Part I. J Prosthet Dent 1994;71:271–277. Cat. 4

18. Jacobson TE. Rotational path partial denture design: A 10 years clinical follow-up. Part II. J Prosthet Dent 1994;71:278–282. Cat. 4

19. Budtz-Jorgensen E, Bochet G. Alternate framework designs for removable partial dentures. J Prosthet Dent 1998;80:58–66. Cat. 8

20. Brill M, Tryde G, Stoltze K, El Ghramraway EA. Ecologic changes in the oral cavity caused by removable partial dentures. J Prosthet Dent 1977;38:138–148. Cat. 4

21. Addy M, Bates JF. The effect of partial dentures and clorhexidine gluconate gel on plaque accumulation in the absence of oral hygiene. J Clin Periodontol 1977;4:41–47. Cat. 4

22. Stipho HDK, Murphy WM, Adams D. Effect of oral prostheses on plaque accumulation. Br Dent J 1978;145:47–50. Cat. 4

23. Bergman B, Hugoson A, Olsson CO. A 25 year longitudinal study of patient treated with removable partial dentures. J Oral Rehabil 1995;22:595–599. Cat. 4

24. Mojon P, Rentsch A, Budtz-Jørgensen E. Relationship between prosthodontic status, caries, and periodontal disease in a geriatric population. Int J Prosthodont 1995;8:564–571. Cat. 4

25. Wright PS, Helleyer PH. Gingival recession to removable partial denture in older patients. J Prosthet Dent 1995;74:602–607. Cat. 4

26. Bergman B, Ericson G. Cross-sectional study of the periodontal status of removable partial denture patients. J Prosthet Dent 1989;61: 208–211. Cat. 4

27. Karlsson S. A clinical evaluation of fixed bridges, 10 years following insertion. J Oral Rehabil 1986;13:423–432. Cat. 4

28. Odman P, Karlsson S. Follow-up study of patients with bridge constructions performed by private dental surgeons and at university clinic, 8 years following insertion. J Oral Rehabil 1988;15:55–63. Cat. 4

29. Palmqvist S, Swartz B. Artificial crowns and fixed partial dentures 18 to 23 years after placement. Int J Prosthodont 1993;6:279–285. Cat. 4

30. Leempoel PJB, Kayser AF, van Rossum GM, de Haan AFJ. The survival rate of bridges. A study of 1,674 bridges in 40 Dutch general practices. J Oral Rehabil 1995;22:327–330. Cat. 4

31. Creugers N, Kayser A, van't Hof M. A meta-analysis of durability data on conventional fixed bridges. Community Dent Oral Epidemiol 1994;22:448–452. Cat. M4

32. Valderhaug J. A 15-year clinical evaluation of fixed prosthodontics. Acta Odontol Scand 1991;49:35–40. Cat. 4

33. Glantz PO, Nilner K, Jendresen MD, Sundberg H. Quality of fixed prosthodontics after 15 years. Acta Odontol Scand 1993;51: 247–252. Cat. 4

34. Axelsson P, Lindhe J. Effect of controlled oral hygiene procedures on caries and periodontal disease in adults. Results after 6 years. J Clin Periodontol 1981;8:239–248. Cat. 4

35. Walton JN, Gardner FM, Agar JR. A survey of crowns and fixed partial denture failures: Length of service and reasons for replacement. J Prosthet Dent 1986;56:416–421. Cat. 4

36. Valderhaug J, Jokstad A, Ambjorsen E, Norheim PW. Assessment of the periapical and clinical status of crowned teeth over 25 years. J Dent 1997;27:97–105. Cat. 4

37. Randow K, Glantz PO, Zoger B. Technical failures and some clinical complications in extensive fixed prosthodontics. An epidemiological study of long term clinical quality. Acta Odontol Scand 1986;44:241–255. Cat. 4

38. Karlsson S. Failures and length of service in fixed prosthodontics after long-term function. A longitudinal clinical study. Swed Dent J 1989;13:185–192. Cat. 4

39. Foster LV. Failed conventional bridge work from general dental practice: Clinical aspects and treatment needs of 142 cases. Br Dent J 1990;168:199–201. Cat. 4

40. Palmer R, Palmer P, Howe L. Complications and maintenance. Br Dent J 1999;187:653–658. Cat. 9

41. Lindhe J, Berglundh T, Ericsson I, Liljenberg B, Marinello CP. Experimental breakdown of peri-implant and periodontal tissues. A study in the beagle dog. Clin Oral Implants Res 1992;3:9–16. Cat. 4

W

Waxup
　for perio-overdenture, 139, 140f, 158, 158f
　for provisional prosthesis, 90, 91f, 214f

X

Xerostomia, 118

Z

Zinc oxide–eugenol paste, 62f
Zygomatic implants, 142, 146